The
MEDICAL and HEALTH
ENCYCLOPEDIA

The MEDICAL and HEALTH ENCYCLOPEDIA

Volume One

EDITED BY

RICHARD J. WAGMAN, M.D., F.A.C.P.

Associate Clinical Professor of Medicine
Downstate Medical Center
New York, New York

THE SOUTHWESTERN COMPANY • NASHVILLE, TENNESSEE

Portions of *The Medical and Health Encyclopedia* have been
previously published under the titles of *The Complete
Illustrated Book of Better Health, The Illustrated Encyclopedia
of Better Health,* and *The New Complete Medical and Health
Encyclopedia,* all edited by Richard J. Wagman, M.D.

Editor

Richard J. Wagman, M.D.,
F.A.C.P.
Associate Clinical Professor of
Medicine
Downstate Medical Center
New York, New York

Consultant in Gynecology

Douglas S. Thompson, M.D.
Clinical Professor of Obstetrics and
Gynecology and Clinical Associate
Professor of Community Medicine
University of Pittsburgh School of
Medicine
Pittsburgh, Pennsylvania

Consultant in Pediatrics

Charles H. Bauer, M.D.
Clinical Associate Professor of
Pediatrics and Chief of Pediatric
Gastroenterology
The New York Hospital-Cornell
Medical Center
New York, New York

Consultants in Psychiatry

Julian J. Clark, M.D.
Assistant Professor of Psychiatry

and

Rita W. Clark, M.D.
Clinical Assistant Professor of
Psychiatry
Downstate Medical Center
New York, New York

Contents

INTRODUCTION

The MEDICAL AND HEALTH ENCYCLOPEDIA is designed to give you clear, accurate answers to your questions about health care. Thorough discussions of major diseases such as cancer and heart problems are included, along with facts about many other less serious diseases and physical problems and how they are treated.

Many people today want to take an active part in their own treatment. This usually takes the form of asking your physician to present the treatment options available to you, then making a decision about which course to follow. Let's assume that your physician is in tune with this approach and willing to relinquish some of the authority doctors traditionally have assumed to tell patients what to do. You will need information to ask intelligent questions and to understand the alternatives being discussed. This encyclopedia. will give you that information.

Fortunately, research in medicine is continually advancing. The MEDICAL AND HEALTH ENCYCLOPEDIA has been revised in this edition to include material on recent advances in medicine and health care.

Becoming ill and being treated are only part of the picture in health care today. More and more, professionals and lay people are putting the emphasis on preventive medicine, doing everything possible to stay well and healthy. To help you and your family stay in the best possible condition, the editors have included detailed information on food and nutrition, dieting, care of skin and hair, and dental health.

Families often have questions about children's health. Parents, stepparents, and grandparents want to know what is normal and expected from a child at various ages in terms of physical, mental, and emotional development. Therefore, the editors have included two chapters, one on younger children, and the other on teenagers, that discuss everything from the common cold to stuttering, from creativity to sexual maturation.

Older people, too, have special health concerns. Senior citizens or their families will want to read the information on diet, daily habits, mental health, activities to pursue during retirement, nursing homes, and retirement homes for the aging.

Generic drugs have been in the spotlight increasingly in recent years. For your convenience in sorting out which drug is equivalent to which, the editors have included a chapter on 100 commonly prescribed generic drugs. The chapter includes information on brand names and the action that each drug has in the body.

These are just a few of the subjects covered in this encyclopedia. How can you make the best possible use of this encyclopedia? First and foremost, do not use this information to treat yourself or anyone else except temporarily in an emergency. (Please note the chapter on Medical Emergencies.) If any symptom of disease is present, no one can take the place of a trained professional.

Use the MEDICAL AND HEALTH ENCYCLOPEDIA for background information on a host of topics, as a handy guide to first aid, and as a reference on where to get further information.

1

Your Body

The Skeleton

Say "skeleton" to children and you probably conjure up in their minds a rickety structure of rigid sticks, or, to the more fanciful child, a clickety-clacketing collection of rattling bones cavorting under a Halloween moon. A look at almost any anatomical drawing of the human skeletal system bears out the child's image: dry sticks of bones, stripped of skin and flesh, muscle and tendon—a grotesque caricature of a living human being.

Our living bones are something quite different. They are rigid, yes, but not entirely so: they also may bend a little and grow and repair themselves; and they are shaped and fitted so that—rather than the herky-jerky motions of a wooden puppet—they permit the smooth grace and coordination power displayed by an accomplished athlete or a prima ballerina.

Our bones do not do just one thing but many things. Some bones, like the collarbone or *clavicle,* mainly give support to other body structures. Others, like the skull and ribs, encase and protect vulnerable organs. Still others, like the *metacarpus* and *phalanges* that make up our hands and fingers, give us mechanical advan-

tages—leverage and movement. There are even bones, the tiny *ossicles* in the middle ear, whose vibrations enable us to hear.

Finally, to think of bone simply as a structural member, like a solid steel girder in a skyscraper, ignores the fact that bone is living tissue. It is one of the busiest tissues in our bodies, a chemical factory that is continually receiving, processing and shipping a wide variety of mineral salts, blood components, and a host of other vital materials.

How the Bones of the Skeletal System Fit and Work Together

Medical textbooks name a total of 206 bones making up the skeletal system of the normal, adult human being. The words "normal" and "adult" are significant. A newborn baby normally has 33 vertebrae making up its backbone (also called *spinal column* or simply *spine*); but by the time a person reaches adulthood, the number of individual vertebrae has shrunk to 26. The explanation: during the growth process, the nine bottom vertebrae

fuse naturally into just two. In like fashion, we "lose" some 60 bones as we grow up. Some otherwise perfectly normal adults have "extra" bones or "missing" bones. For example, although the normal number of ribs is 12 pairs, some adults may have 11; others may have 13 pairs.

Even a practicing physician might be hard-pressed to identify each of our 200-plus bones and describe its function. An easier way to gain a general understanding of the various functions, capabilities—and weaknesses, too—of our bones is to visualize the skeletal system as a standing coatrack, say, about six feet high.

Call the central pole the backbone. About ten inches down from its top (the top of your skull) is a horizontal crossbar (your shoulders—collarbones and shoulder blades), approximately a foot-and-a-half across. Sixteen or so inches below the bottom of the top crossbar is another, shorter crossbar, broader and thicker—the *pelvic girdle.* The coatrack with its two crossbars is now a crude model of the bones of the head and trunk, collectively called the *axial skeleton.* Its basic unit is the backbone, to which are attached the skull at the top, then the bones of the shoulder girdle, the ribs, and at the bottom, the bones of the pelvic girdle.

By hanging down (or appending) members from the two ends of the top crossbar, and doing the same at the lower crossbar, we would simulate what is called the *appendicular skeleton*—arms and hands, legs and feet.

Now, make the coatrack stand on its new legs, cut off the central pole just below the lower bar (if you wish, calling it man's lost tail), and you have the two main components of the skeletal system, joined together before you. Let us look at each more closely.

The Axial Skeleton

Within the framework of the axial skeleton lie all the most vital organs of the body. People have gone on living with the loss of a hand or a leg—indeed, with the loss of any or all of their limbs. But nobody can live without a brain, a heart, a liver, lungs, or kidneys—all of which are carried within the framework of the axial skeleton.

The Skull

The bones of the skull have as their most important function the protection of the brain and sense organs.

There are also, of course, the jawbones that support the teeth and gums and which enable us to bite and chew our food.

Most of the skull appears to consist of a single bone—a hard, unbroken dome. Actually, the brain cage or *cranium* consists of eight individual platelike bones which have fused together in the process of growth. At birth, these bones are separated, causing the soft spots or *fontanelles* we can readily feel on a baby's head. As the baby's brain enlarges, the bones grow along their edges to fill in the fontanelles, finally knitting together in what are called *suture lines,* somewhat resembling inexpertly mended clothes seams. Along the suture lines, the skull bones continue to grow until the individual's mature skull size is reached.

Teeth

The hardest substance in the human body is the *enamel* that covers the exposed surface of a tooth. Below the gum, the tooth's outside surface is composed of somewhat softer *cementum.* Beneath enamel and cementum is a bonelike substance, called *dentin,* which covers the soft interior of the tooth, called *pulp.* Pulp is serviced by blood vessels and nerves through the root or roots of the tooth. The passageway of nerves and blood vessels that lead up through the tooth from the gum sockets is called a *root canal.* Tooth and gum are stuck to each other by a tough, adhesive tissue called *periodontal* (or peridental— "surrounding the tooth") *membrane.* See Ch. 22, *The Teeth and Gums,* for further information on teeth.

The Backbone

At the base of the skull, the backbone begins. The skull is supported by the

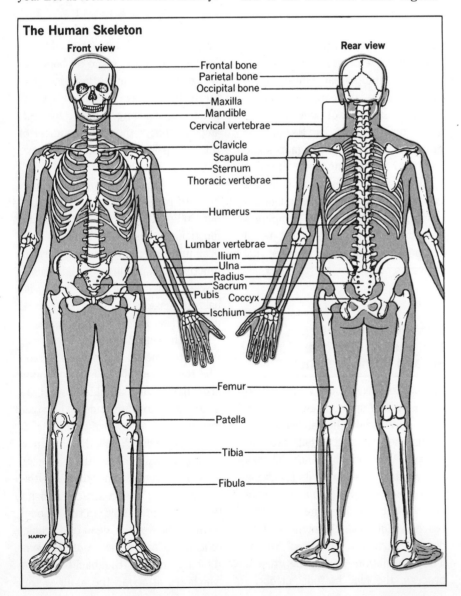

The Human Skeleton

Front view   Rear view

Frontal bone
Parietal bone
Occipital bone
Maxilla
Mandible
Cervical vertebrae
Clavicle
Scapula
Sternum
Thoracic vertebrae
Humerus
Lumbar vertebrae
Ilium
Ulna
Radius
Sacrum
Pubis   Coccyx
Ischium
Femur
Patella
Tibia
Fibula

HARDY

topmost *cervical* (neck) vertebra. The curious thing about a backbone is that the word has come to suggest something solid, straight, and unbending. The backbone, however, just isn't like that: it consists of 26 knobby, hollowed-out bones—*vertebrae,* rather improbably held together by muscles, ligaments, and tendons. It is not straight when we stand, but has definite backward and forward curvatures; and even some of its most important structures (the disks between the vertebrae) aren't made of bone, but of cartilage.

All in all, however, the backbone is a fairly well designed structure in terms of the several different functions it serves—but with some built-in weaknesses. For a discussion of backache, see Ch. 23, *Aches, Pains, Nuisances, Worries.*

The Vertebrae

Although they will have features in common, no two of our 26 vertebrae are exactly alike in shape, size, or function. This is hardly surprising if we consider, for example, that the cervical vertebrae do not support ribs, while the *thoracic* vertebrae (upper trunk, or chest) do support them.

But for a sample vertebra, let us pick a rib-carrying vertebra, if for no other reason than that it lies about midway along the backbone. If viewed from above or below, a thoracic vertebra, like most of the others, would look like a roundish piece of bone with roughly scalloped edges on the side facing inward toward the chest and on the side facing outward toward the surface of the back, and would reveal several bony projections. These knobby portions of a vertebra—some of which you can feel as bumps along your backbone—are called *processes.* They serve as the vertebra's points of connection to muscles and tendons,

to ribs, and to the other vertebrae above and below.

A further conspicuous feature is a hole, more or less in the middle of the typical vertebra, through which passes the master nerve bundle of our bodies, the spinal cord, running from the base of the skull to the top of the pelvis. Thus, one of the important functions of the backbone is to provide flexible, protective tubing for the spinal cord.

Between the bones of one vertebra and the next is a piece of more resilient cartilage that acts as a cushion or shock absorber to prevent two vertebrae from scraping or bumping each other if the backbone gets a sudden jolt, or as the backbone twists and turns and bends. These pieces of cartilage are the intervertebral disks—infamous for pain and misery if they become ruptured or slipped disks.

Regions of the Backbone

The backbone can be divided into five regions, starting with the uppermost, or *cervical* region, which normally has seven vertebrae. Next down is the *thoracic* (chest) section, normally with 12 vertebrae. From each vertebra a rib extends to curl protectively around the chest area. Usually, the top ten ribs come all the way around the trunk and attach to the breastbone (or *sternum*); but the bottom two ribs do not reach the breastbone and are thus called floating ribs. The thoracic section also must support the shoulder girdle, consisting of the collarbones (*clavicles*) and shoulder blades (*scapulas*). At the end of each shoulder blade is a shoulder joint— actually three distinct joints working together—where the arm connects to the axial skeleton.

Below the thoracic vertebrae come the five vertebrae of the *lumbar* sec-

tion. This area gets a good deal of blame for back miseries: lower back pain often occurs around the area where the bottom thoracic vertebra joins the top lumbar vertebra. Furthermore, the lumbar region or small of the back is also a well-known site of back pain; indeed, from the word "lumbar" comes *lumbago,* medically an imprecise term, but popularly used to describe very real back pain.

Below the lumbar region are two vertebrae so completely different from the 24 above them—and even from each other—that it seems strange they are called vertebrae at all: the *sacrum* and the *coccyx.* These two vertebrae are both made up of several distinct vertebrae that are present at birth. The sacrum is a large bone that was once five vertebrae. The coccyx was originally four vertebrae—and, incidentally, is all that remains of man's tail in his evolution from the primates.

The Pelvic Girdle

The sacrum is the more important of these two strange-looking vertebrae. It is the backbone's connection to the *pelvic girdle,* or pelvis. On each side of the sacrum, connected by the sacroiliac joint, is a very large, curving bone called the *ilium,* tilting (when we stand) slightly forward and downward from the sacrum toward the front of the groin. We feel the top of the ilium as the top of the hip—a place mothers and fathers often find convenient for toting a toddler.

Fused at each side of the ilium and slanting toward the back is the *ischium,* the bone we sit on. The two *pubis* bones, also fused to the ilium, meet in front to complete the pelvic girdle. All the bones of the pelvis— ilium, ischium, and pubis—fuse together so as to form the hip joint (*acetabulum*), a deep socket into which the "ball" or upper end of the thigh-bone fits.

The Appendicular Skeleton

The bones of the appendages—arms, hands, and fingers; legs, feet, and toes—allow human beings to perform an astonishing array of complex movements, from pushing themselves through the physical rigors of the Olympic decathlon to creating an elaborate piece of needlework. The key points in the appendicular skeleton, as indeed, in the axial skeleton, are where the ends or edges of bones lie close together and must work with or against one another in order to achieve coordinated movement. These key points are the *joints*—not really bones at all but the non-bony spaces between bones.

The Joints

A typical joint consists of several different structures. First, there are the bones themselves—two, three, four, or more almost touching in the area of the joint—with their ends or edges shaped to fit in their respective niches. Between the bones of an appendage joint (as between the verte-

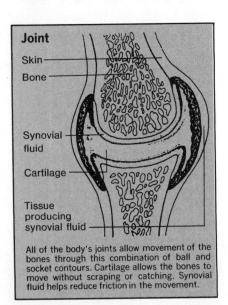

Joint

Skin
Bone

Synovial fluid

Cartilage

Tissue producing synovial fluid

All of the body's joints allow movement of the bones through this combination of ball and socket contours. Cartilage allows the bones to move without scraping or catching. Synovial fluid helps reduce friction in the movement.

brae of the back) is the smooth, resilient material called *cartilage* that allows the bones to move over one another without scraping or catching. At the joint, the bones, with their layer of cartilage between them, are held together by tough bonds of muscle. *Bursas,* tiny sacs containing a lubricating fluid, are also found at joints; they help to reduce the friction between a joint's moving parts.

The Hip and Knee

The hip joint must not only support the weight of the head and trunk, but must allow for movement of the leg and also play a part in the constant balancing required to maintain upright posture. Similar stresses and strains, often literally tending to tear the joint apart, are placed on every joint in the body.

The notoriety of athletes' bad knees attests to the forces battering at the knee joint, the largest in the human body. Sports involving leaping or sudden changes in direction, such as basketball, are especially hard on the knee. However, the fact that there are not more disabled sports heroes speaks well for the design of the knee joint. The same can be said of the ankle joint and the joints of the foot and toes.

The Shoulder, Elbow, and Wrist

The counterpart of the hip joint in the upper trunk is the shoulder joint. Free of weight-bearing responsibilities, the shoulder has a system of three interconnected joints that allow it and the arm far more versatile movements than the hip and leg.

The elbow connects the upper arm bone (*humerus*) with the two bones of the lower arm (*radius* and *ulna*). Like the knee, it is basically a hinge joint, which allows the lower arm to be

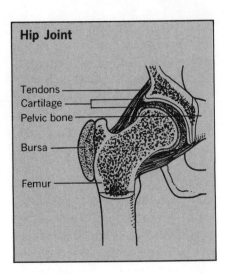

Hip Joint

Tendons
Cartilage
Pelvic bone

Bursa

Femur

raised and lowered. The elbow is also constructed to allow some rotation by the hand; likewise, the knee joint allows us to waggle the foot.

Of all our body parts, the wrist, hand, and fingers are perhaps the most elegantly and finely jointed—witness the performance of a concert pianist—and our ankles, feet, and toes probably the most subject to everyday misery.

Bone as Living Tissue

Our bones, like all our tissues, change as we grow up, mature, and finally grow old. There are changes in the chemical activity and composition of bone representative of each stage of life.

In young children, the ends and edges of bones are mainly cartilage, forming a growing surface on the bone that is gradually replaced by hard bone as full size is attained. The bones of a child are more pliable and less likely to break than those of a full-grown adult.

Similarly, as an adult ages, the bones turn from a resilient hardness to a more brittle hardness. This accounts for the much greater danger of broken bones in older people.

These changes with age are an indication of the great amount of chemical activity going on within bone. We sometimes forget that our bones are amply supplied and penetrated by blood vessels. There is a constant building up and breaking down, an interchange of materials between blood and bone.

The Composition of Bone

A living bone does not have a single uniform composition, but instead is composed of several different kinds of tissue. To begin with, there are actually two types of bone tissue in the same bone: compact and spongy. In addition, bone is sheathed in a tough membranous tissue called the *periosteum,* interlaced with blood vessels. Finally, within most of the larger and longer bones of the body, as well as in the interior of the skull bones and vertebrae, are two more kinds of tissue: red marrow and yellow marrow.

Marrow

Within the spongy bone areas, *red marrow* produces enormous numbers of red blood cells, at a rate of millions per minute. These are needed for growth as well as for replacement of red cells, which also die in enormous numbers. Children's bones contain greater proportions of red marrow than adults'. With age, *yellow marrow,* composed mainly of fat cells, begins to fill the interior bone cavities formerly occupied by red marrow.

Calcium

Bone also serves as a storage and distribution center for one of the most important elements in our body. Calcium, in the form of calcium phosphate, is the basic chemical of bone tissue, but this element also must always be present in the bloodstream at a certain level to ensure normal

heartbeat, blood clotting, and muscle contraction. When the calcium level in the blood is deficient, the bones release some calcium into the bloodstream; when the blood has a surplus of calcium, the bones reabsorb it.

Fractures

Like most other tissues, broken bone can repair itself, and it is a remarkable process to observe. It is a process, however, that will proceed even if the ends are not aligned or set—an important reason why any suspected fracture should be checked by a physician.

A break in a bone causes a sticky material to be deposited by the blood around the broken ends. This material begins the formation of a kind of protective, lumpy sleeve, called a *callus,* around the broken ends. Mainly cartilage, the callus hardens into spongy bone, normally within a month or two. Then, the spongy bone begins to be reduced in size by bone-dissolving cells produced in the marrow, while at the same time the spongy bone in the area of the break is beginning to be replaced by hard bone.

Depending on the particular bone involved and the severity of the fracture, the broken bone can be completely healed within four to ten months.

Potential Trouble Spots

Essentially there are two kinds of things that can go wrong with the skeletal system and cause trouble.

Mechanical Difficulties

A healthy bone's main mechanical functions—support, movement, protection—can be impaired. This can happen as a result of a physical injury resulting in a fracture or dislocation.

The stack of vertebrae called the backbone is vulnerable to a number of painful conditions from top to bottom, especially in the region of the lower back. Unfortunately, man seems to have evolved relatively quickly from a four-footed creature, and his backbone is not ideally suited for standing and walking on two feet. Back troubles become increasingly common with age.

Areas where bones interact are also very susceptible to injury because of the stresses and strains they undergo even in people who are not

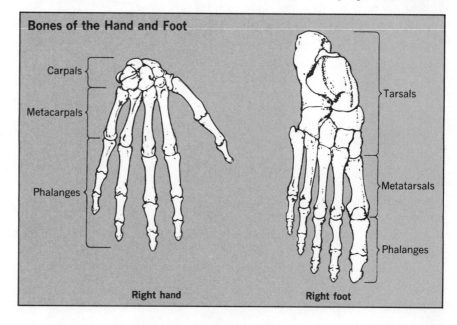

Bones of the Hand and Foot

Carpals

Metacarpals

Phalanges

Right hand

Tarsals

Metatarsals

Phalanges

Right foot

especially active. Normal wear and tear also takes its toll on our bones and joints; for example, the bones' structure or their alignment at a joint may be altered slightly with age, making one bone or another prone to slipping out of the joint causing a dislocation. In any case, it is not advisable to make the same demands on our skeletal system at 40 as we did at 20. Joints are also the site of arthritis.

Disease

Second, and generally more serious if untreated, the interior bone tissues themselves may become infected and diseased. This can lead as a secondary effect to impairment of the bones' mechanical functions. *Osteomyelitis,* for example, a bacterial infection of bony tissues, can destroy large portions of bone unless antibiotics are started at once.

Fortunately, disorders of the skeletal system generally reveal themselves early and clearly by pain. Any severe or lingering pain of the joints or bones should be reported to a physician. For example, some people may feel that aching feet are unavoidable—and a little undignified. But a foot is not meant to hurt, nor is any part of the skeletal system. Consulting a physician could prevent much present and future misery. See also Ch. 7, *Diseases of the Skeletal System.*

The Muscles

Some 600 muscles of all sizes and shapes are attached to the framework of the skeletal system. Altogether these muscles make up nearly half of a normal adult's weight. They hold the skeleton together and, on signals originating in the brain, empower its various parts to move. Everywhere throughout the skeletal system, muscles work together with bones to protect the body's vital organs and to support and move its parts.

Skeletal Muscle

Such muscles are called, collectively, *skeletal muscle*. They are also called *voluntary muscles* because, for the most part, we can choose when we want them to act and what we want them to do—drive a car, kick a football, turn a page, jump a brook, ride a bicycle. Skeletal muscle also goes by two other names, based on its appearance under a microscope—striped and striated.

Skeletal, voluntary, striped, striated—all refer to the same general type of muscle. To avoid confusion, the term used throughout this section is skeletal muscle.

Smooth Muscle

There are two other general types of muscle. One is called *smooth muscle* because, under the microscope, it lacks the clearly defined stripes of skeletal muscle. Smooth muscle has another name, *involuntary muscle,* so called because the brain does not voluntarily control its actions. Smooth muscle is responsible for movements such as the muscular action that moves food and waste along the

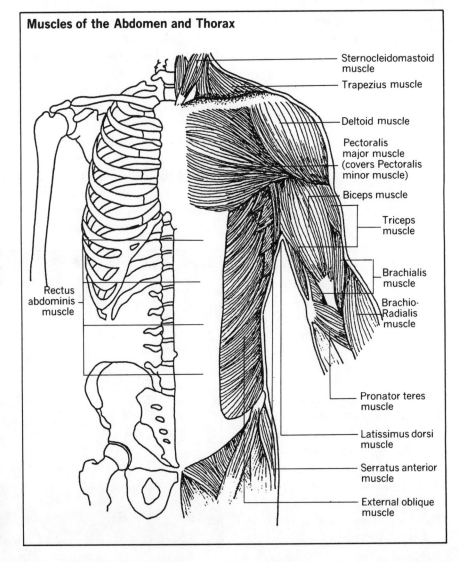

Muscles of the Abdomen and Thorax

Sternocleidomastoid muscle

Trapezius muscle

Deltoid muscle

Pectoralis major muscle (covers Pectoralis minor muscle)

Biceps muscle

Triceps muscle

Brachialis muscle

Brachio-Radialis muscle

Pronator teres muscle

Latissimus dorsi muscle

Serratus anterior muscle

External oblique muscle

Rectus abdominis muscle

digestive tract, or the contraction and dilation of the pupil of the eye, as well as countless other involuntary movements of the sense and internal organs—with the exception of the heart.

Cardiac Muscle

The third and last general type of muscle is confined to the heart area, and is called *cardiac muscle*. (Cardiac means having to do with the heart.) It is involved in the rhythmic beating and contractions of the heart, which are not under conscious control, and cardiac muscle is therefore termed involuntary.

Structure of the Muscles

Each of the three kinds of muscle shares certain structural similarities with one or both of the others. All are made up of bundles of varying numbers of hair-thin fibers. In skeletal and smooth muscles, these fibers are lined up side by side in the bundle, while in cardiac muscle the fibers tend more to crisscross over one another. Skeletal muscle and cardiac muscle are both striped, that is, they show darker and lighter bands crossing over a group of adjacent fibers, while smooth muscle lacks these distinct cross-bands.

Both involuntary muscle types, smooth and cardiac, are controlled by signals carried by the autonomic nervous system. Signals that result in movements of the skeletal muscles are carried by a different nerve network, the central nervous system. The individual fibers in a muscle bundle with a particular function all react simultaneously to a signal from the nervous system; there is no apparent time lag from fiber to fiber.

How the Skeletal Muscles Work

The great range and variety of functions served by skeletal muscles can be suggested by naming just four: the diaphragm, used in breathing; the muscles that make the eye wink; the deltoid muscle that gives the shoulder its shape; and the tongue.

As with the bones, the body tends to make its greatest demands on muscle tissue in the area of the joints and the backbone. A smoothly functioning joint requires that bone, cartilage, and muscle all be sound and able to work together effectively.

Tendons and Ligaments

We often hear the words tendon and ligament used in the description of the knee or another joint. These are actually two types of skeletal muscles, distinguished as to their function.

A *tendon* can be described as a tight cord of muscle tissue that attaches other skeletal muscle to bone. For example, the Achilles tendon running down the back of the calf, the strongest tendon in the body, connects the muscles of the calf with the bone of the heel. A *ligament* is a somewhat more elastic band of muscle fibers that attaches bone to bone.

A tendon is not always evident in the connection of muscle to bone. Various groups and shapes of muscle fibers may be similarly employed,

Muscles of the Back

- Trapezius muscle
- Infraspinatus muscle
- Deltoid muscle
- Rhomboid muscle
- Teres major muscle
- Triceps muscle
- Latissimus dorsi muscle (covers spinal erector muscle)
- External oblique muscle
- Internal oblique muscle
- Gluteus maximus muscle

Tendon

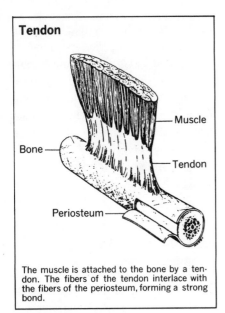

The muscle is attached to the bone by a tendon. The fibers of the tendon interlace with the fibers of the periosteum, forming a strong bond.

Muscles, Their Locations, and Exercises that Strengthen Them

Muscle	Location	Movement
Trapezius	Upper back and each side of neck	Shoulder-shrugging and upward-pulling movements
Deltoids	Shoulders	Arm raising and overhead pressing
Pectorals	Chest	Horizontal pressing and drawing arms across body
Latissimus dorsi	Wide back muscle stretching over back up to rear Deltoids	Pulling and rowing movements
Serratus	Jagged sawtooth muscles between Pectorals and lattissimus Dorsi	Pullover and Serratus leverage movements
Spinal erectors	Lower length of spinal column	Raising upper body from a bent-over position
Biceps	Front portion of upper arm	Arm bending and twisting
Forearms	Between wrist and elbow	Reverse-grip arm bending
Triceps	Back of upper arm	Pushing and straightening movements of upper arms
Rectus abdominals	Muscular area between sternum and pelvis	Sit-up, leg-raising, knee-in movements
Intercostals	Sides of waist, running diagonally to Serratus	Waist twisting
External oblique abdominals	Lower sides of waist	Waist twisting and bending
Buttocks	Muscular area covering seat	Lunging, stooping, leg raising
Leg biceps	Back of thighs	Raising lower leg to buttocks, bending forward and stretching
Frontal thighs	Front of thighs	Extending lower leg and knee bending
Calves	Lower leg between ankle and knee	Raising and lowering on toes

forming connective tissue without the formation of tendon.

Various associated tissues between or around skeletal muscles serve to reduce the wear and tear of friction in areas such as a joint, where muscle, bone, and cartilage may rub against one another. For example, the tendons that pass along the back of the hand from the wrist to the fingertips, as well as many other muscle groups throughout the body, are enclosed in lubricated sheaths. The muscle-sheathed *bursas,* lined inside with lubricating fluid, are also found in areas subject to friction, such as where a tendon passes closely over a bone.

Man's upright posture and two-legged locomotion subject the backbone to heavy stresses. It is buttressed, however, with scores of tightly packed bundles of muscle attached to either side of the spinal column.

Flexors and Extensors

Most of us probably first used the word "muscle" when, as children, we watched an older child or adult flex an arm and proudly display the bump of muscle between the crook of elbow and shoulder. This biceps muscle works together with the triceps muscle on the underside of the arm. The arm is bent at the elbow by contraction of the biceps, which makes this muscle get shorter and thicker; in this position, called *flexion,* the triceps muscle is relaxed. To return the arm to its normal straight position, called *extension,* the biceps relaxes and the triceps contracts. In this bit of muscle teamwork, the biceps, which bends the arm at the elbow joint, is called the *flexor,* while the triceps straightens the arm and is called the *extensor.* Similar flexor–extensor action can be observed at many body joints, including the fingers.

Smooth Muscle

Beginning about midway down the esophagus, layers of smooth muscle line the walls of the 25 feet of digestive tract, extending into the stomach and through the intestines. These muscles keep the stomach and intes-

Muscle Action in Forearm Movement

Biceps

Triceps

Muscles usually work in pairs to produce movement of a part of the body. Contraction of the biceps bends, or flexers, the arm. The biceps is a flexor muscle. Contraction of the triceps extends the arm. The triceps is an extensor muscle.

tinal walls continually in motion, constricting and relaxing to push food along. Smooth muscle also effects the opening and closing of important valves, called *sphincters,* along the digestive tract.

Trouble Spots

The functions and failures of the skeletal muscles are closely allied to those of the skeletal system. The same areas are vulnerable—joints and back—and the same rule holds: severe or persistent muscle pain is a cause to consult your physician.

Hernia

One type of disorder associated exclusively with a weakness or abnormality of muscle is a rupture or *hernia.* This is the protrusion of part of another organ through a gap in the protective muscle. A likely area for a hernia to appear is in the muscles lining the abdomen, although hernias may occur in any other part of the body where there is pressure against a muscle wall that is not as strong as it should be. Weight control and a sensible program of exercise—abdominal muscles being particularly liable to slackness—are good preventive measures against hernia.

All our muscles, in fact, benefit from regular exercise; but you don't have to exhaust yourself physically every day to reach and maintain the desirable plateau physicians describe as good muscle tone.

Atrophy of Muscle Tissue

Muscle tissues are likely to *atrophy* (shrink and weaken) if they are not used for too long a time. Thus, illness or injuries that cause paralysis or an extended period of immobility for the body or a part of it must be followed by a supervised program of physical therapy.   See also Ch. 8, *Diseases of the Muscles and Nervous System.*

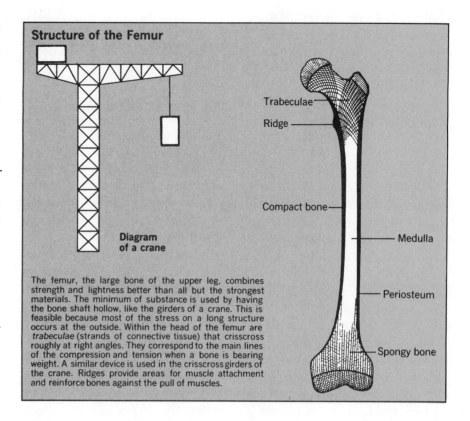

Structure of the Femur

Diagram of a crane

Trabeculae
Ridge
Compact bone
Medulla
Periosteum
Spongy bone

The femur, the large bone of the upper leg, combines strength and lightness better than all but the strongest materials. The minimum of substance is used by having the bone shaft hollow, like the girders of a crane. This is feasible because most of the stress on a long structure occurs at the outside. Within the head of the femur are *trabeculae* (strands of connective tissue) that crisscross roughly at right angles. They correspond to the main lines of the compression and tension when a bone is bearing weight. A similar device is used in the crisscross girders of the crane. Ridges provide areas for muscle attachment and reinforce bones against the pull of muscles.

Muscular Contraction

Tendon
Biceps
Triceps
Tendon
Becomes flexor
Becomes extensor

Skin, Hair, and Nails

Perhaps no other organ of the human body receives so much attention both from its owner and the eyes of others as the skin and its associated structures—hair and nails.

Vanity is hardly the issue. The simple facts are that skin is the last frontier of our internal selves, the final boundary between our inside and outside, and our principal first line of defense against the dangers of the outside world. It shows, not always clearly, evidence of some internal disorders; and it shows, often quite clearly, the evidence of external affronts—a bump, a cut, a chafe, an insect bite, or an angry reaction to the attack of germs.

In personal encounters, the unclothed portion of our skin is one of the first things other people observe, and—if we happen to have some unsightly scratch, rash, or blemish—the last thing by which we wish to be remembered. Of all our organs, the skin is the most likely candidate for a program of self-improvement.

The Organ Called Skin

It is always a little surprising to hear, for the first time, the skin referred to as a single organ. This is not to say it is a simple organ; on the contrary, it is an exceedingly complex and varied one. However, despite variations in appearance from part to part of the body, our entire outer wrapper (the more technical word is *integument*) is similarly constructed.

One might object: "But my nails and hair certainly look different from the skin on my nose!" This is perfectly true, but nails and hair are extensions of the skin, and wherever they occur are composed of similar tissues: the nail on a little toe is made of the same material as the hair.

Functions of the Skin

The skin has three main functions, and its different outward appearance on different parts of the body reflects to some extent which of these functions a certain area of skin primarily serves. The three main functions are protection (from germs or blows), temperature control (e.g., through perspiration, to aid in keeping the body's internal organs near our normal internal temperature of 98.6° F.), and perception. Nerve endings in the skin give us our sensations of touch, pain, heat, and cold. Associated with the skin's important role in temperature regulation is its function as an organ of excretion—the elimination, via perspiration, and subsequent evaporation of water and other substances. Skin is also the site of the body's natural production of vitamin D, stimulated by exposure to sunlight.

Anatomy of the Skin

Skin has three more or less distinct layers. The outermost is called the *epidermis;* the middle, the *dermis;* and the innermost, *subcutaneous* (under-skin) tissue. The epidermis may also be called *cuticle;* and the dermis either *corium* or *true skin.*

The Subcutaneous Layer

The subcutaneous layer is really a rather vague border zone between muscle and bone tissues on one side, and the dermis on the other, a kind of springy, fatty padding that gives bounce and a look of firmness to the skin above it. With age, the fatty cells of the subcutaneous layer are not continually replaced as they die, and this layer tends to thin out. The result is wrinkles, which form where the outer layers of skin lose their subcutaneous support, much like the slipcover of a cushion that has lost some of its stuffing.

Anatomy of the Skin

The epidermis has been lifted to show the papillae on the dermal layer. The pattern of these papillae creates the fingerprints.

Approximate depth of section shown

Sebaceous glands

Epidermis

Dermis

Subcutaneous tissue

Touch receptor

Sweat gland

Pressure receptor nerve ending

Hair follicle

Capillary tufts bring blood close to surface for cooling.

Erector pili muscle causes gooseflesh.

Nutrient blood vessel to hair follicle

The Dermis

The dermis is serviced by the multitude of tiny blood vessels and nerve fibers that reach it through the subcutaneous tissue. In addition, many special structures and tissues that enable the skin to perform its various functions are found in the dermis: *sebaceous* (skin oil) glands and sweat glands; minuscule muscles; and the roots of hairs encased in narrow pits called *follicles*.

The topmost layer of the dermis, interconnecting with the epidermis above it, resembles, under a microscope, nothing so much as a rugged, ridge-crossed landscape carved with valleys, caves, and tunnels. The basic forms of this microscopic terrain are cone-shaped hills called *papillae;* between 100 and 200 million of them are found in the dermis of an adult human being.

Because the dermal papillae serve as the bedrock for the surface layer of skin, the epidermis, we can understand why there is really no such thing as smooth skin; even the smoothest patch of a baby's skin appears ridged and cratered under a magnifying glass.

The distribution of papillae in the skin falls into certain distinctive patterns that are particularly conspicuous on the soles of babies' feet and on the fingertips, and give each of us our unique finger, toe, and footprints. The mathematical possibility of one person having the same fingerprints as another is thought to be about one in 25 billion. The papillae ridges on the fingertips also make it easier for us to pick up and handle such things as needles or pencils or buttons.

Finally, because there are relatively more papillae concentrated at the fingertips than on most other areas of the body, and because papillae are often associated with dense concentrations of nerve endings, the fingertips tend to be more responsive to touch sensations than other parts of the body.

The Epidermis

The bottom layer of the epidermis, its papillae fitted into the pockets of the layers of the dermis beneath it, is occupied by new young cells. These cells gradually mature and move upward. As they near the surface of the skin, they die, becoming tough, horny, lifeless tissue. This is the outmost layer of the epidermis, called the *stratum corneum* (horny layer), which we are continually shedding, usually unnoticed, as when we towel off after a bath, but sometimes very noticeably, as when we peel after a sunburn.

A suntan, incidentally, is caused by the presence of tiny grains of pigment, called *melanin*, in the bottom layers of epidermis. Sunlight stimulates the production of melanin, giving the skin a darker color. A suntan fades as the melanin granules move to the surface and are shed with dead skin cells.

Hair and Nails

Certainly the most noticeable of the specialized forms of skin are our hair and nails. What we see of them is really a dead tissue, called *keratin*, similar to the dead skin cells that are continually being shed by our bodies, but much more firmly packed together. However, hair and nails both originate in cells that are very much alive—as anyone who has plucked a group of hairs or suffered the pain of a torn-out nail knows very well. Growth occurs in this living region, with new cells pushing the dead, hard hair and nail stalks upward, then dying themselves and being replaced from below.

The bottom end or root of a hair is

Fingerprint

The pattern of ridges in a fingerprint reflects the contours of the papillae (conelike bumps) of the upper layer of the dermis, just below the epidermis.

lodged, as noted above, in a *follicle*, a hollow resembling a rounded bottle with a long, narrow neck slanting toward the skin's surface. Each follicle is supported by the little hummock of a papilla, and is serviced by tiny oil glands that lubricate the shaft (or neck) through which the hair pushes toward the surface.

The follicles of the long hairs of the scalp, groin, and armpits may be found deep in the subcutaneous layers of the skin; others are no deeper than the top layers of dermis. Attached to a follicle are microscopic muscle fibers that, if stimulated by cold or emotional factors, can contract around the follicle; the result is gooseflesh or sometimes even the sensation that our hair is standing on end.

A nail's living, growing part is found beneath the whitish half moon, or *lunula*, at its base. The lunula is sometimes obscured because a layer of epidermis (cuticle) has grown over it. Except at its very top (the part we can trim without pain), the nail is firmly attached to the ridged upper layer of the dermis, a region richly laced with tiny blood vessels.

Oil Glands

The skin's oil-producing (or *seba-*

ceous) glands are almost always associated with hair follicles, into which they seep their oils (or *sebum*). The oily substance works its way up toward the surface, lubricating both the hair and outer layers of epidermis, which need continual lubrication in order to stay soft and flexible. Also, skin oils serve as a kind of protective coat against painful drying and chapping.

Sweat Glands and Blood Vessels

While everybody is aware that the amount we perspire is related to the temperature around us, not everybody is aware that the countless tiny blood vessels in our skin—some 15 feet of them coursing beneath every square inch of skin—also react to changes in outside temperatures. Working together, and both controlled by an automatic "thermostat" in our brain, sweat glands and blood vessels have the all-important role of keeping our internal organs near their normal 98.6° Fahrenheit temperature.

The trick in maintaining an internal body temperature near normal is to conserve body heat when it is colder outside and to lose heat when it is warmer. Blood circulating near the surface of the skin is warmed (gains heat) or cooled (loses heat) according to the outside temperature.

The skin's myriad blood vessels constrict when the outside temperature is colder. This means that less blood can come into contact with the colder outside air, and therefore the overall temperature level of the blood remains warmer than if the blood vessels had not become constricted. On the other hand, when the body needs to lose heat—for example, during and after a vigorous tennis match—the skin's blood vessels dilate. This accounts for the "heat flush" or reddening of skin that light-skinned people

exhibit when very heated.

Sweat glands aid in temperature regulation by secreting moisture, which, evaporating on the skin's surface, cools the skin and therefore the blood flowing beneath it. Moisture that does not evaporate but remains as liquid on the skin or runs off in rivulets is not efficient in cooling. Humid air tends to prevent evaporation, while moving air or wind aids it. Sweat that evaporates as soon as it reaches the skin's surface usually goes unnoticed. Fresh sweat has no odor; but if it remains without evaporating, bacteria begin to give it the odor known medically as *bromhidrosis*.

There are some two million sweat glands in the skin. Each consists of a coiled, corkscrewlike tube that tunnels its way up to the surface of the skin from the dermis or from the deeper subcutaneous layer.

Potential Trouble Spots

All of us are very conscious of the condition of our skin and worry when something seems to be wrong with it. The temptations to worry too much, to overtreat, to take the advice of a well-meaning friend, to use the wrong (but heavily advertised) product are very great. Knowing about the properties of the skin and what medical knowledge has to say about skin problems can help to avoid mistakes in caring for it. See Ch. 21, *Skin and Hair.* For a discussion of adolescent skin problems, see also Ch. 3, *The Teens.*

The Nervous System and the Brain

Most of us have heard often

enough that the brain, acting as control center for a communication network we call our nervous system, is an incredible computer, weighing a mere three pounds. Its form and functions, however, are often described as being so much more intricate and complex than any existing or imagined computer that thorough knowledge of the brain seems very remote. This is certainly true. But it doesn't prevent us from knowing some general things about the brain and nervous system, or what its most significant parts are and how they work.

Basically, the nervous system has just two functions: first, getting information (impulses, signals, messages) from outside or inside the body to where it can be acted upon, usually in the brain; and secondly, feeding back information (for example, to the muscles) so that the indicated action can be taken. Thus, nerves can be divided by their function into two general types, each following a separate pathway. Those that receive information—for example, from our senses—and pass it along are called *sensory,* or *afferent* (inward-traveling). Those that relay information back, with a directive for action, are called *motor,* or *efferent* (outward-traveling).

The brain and the spinal cord can be considered as the basic unit of the *central nervous system.* All sensory and motor information comes or goes from this central core. The spinal cord is the master nerve tract (or nerve trunk) in our body and consists of millions of nerve fibers bundled together, somewhat like many small threads making up a large rope.

Like the spinal cord, all the lesser nerves, shown as single cords in a typical anatomical drawing, are made up of hundreds of thousands of individual fibers. Each fiber is part of a single nerve cell, or *neuron.* Neurons—there are 12 to 15 billion of them in our brain alone—are the basic structural units of the brain and nervous system, the tubes and transistors and circuits of which our personal computer is built.

The Brain

The appearance of the brain within the skull has been described as a huge gray walnut and a cauliflower. The inelegance of such descriptions is the least of many good reasons why we should be happy our brains are not exposed to public view.

Brain tissue—pinkish gray and white—is among the most delicate in our body, and the destruction of even a small part may mean lasting impairment or death. Its protection is vital and begins (if we are so fortunate) with a mat of hair on the top, back, and sides of our skull. Next comes the resilient layer of padding we call the scalp, and then the main line of defense—the rounded, bony helmet of skull.

The brain's armor does not stop with bone. Beneath are three strong, fibrous membranes called *meninges* that encase the brain in protective envelopes. Meninges also overlie the tissue of the spinal cord; infection or inflammation of these membranes by bacteria or viruses is called *cerebrospinal meningitis*.

Between two of the meninges is a region laced with veins and arteries and filled with *cerebrospinal fluid*. This fluid-filled space cushions the brain against sudden blows and collisions. The cerebrospinal fluid circulates not only about the brain but through the entire central nervous system. Incidentally, chemical analysis of this fluid, withdrawn by inserting a hypodermic needle between vertebrae of the spinal column (a spinal tap), can provide clues to the nature of brain and nervous system disorders.

The Cerebrum

What we usually mean by "brain" is that part of the brain called the *cerebrum*. It is the cerebrum that permits us all our distinctly human activities—thinking, speaking, reading, writing.

Only in man does the cerebrum reach such size, occupying the interior of our entire dome above the level of our eyes.

The surface of the cerebrum is wrinkled, furrowed, folded and infolded, convoluted, fissured—anything but smooth. This lavishly wrinkled outer layer of the cerebrum, about an eighth of an inch thick, is called the *cerebral cortex*. From its grayish color comes the term "gray matter" for brain tissue. There is a pattern among its wrinkles, marked out by wider, or deeper fissures, or furrows, running through the brain tissue. The most conspicuous fissure runs down the middle, front to back, dividing the cerebrum into two halves, the left hemisphere and the right hemisphere. The nerves from the left half of the body are served by the right hemisphere, and the right half of the body by the left hemisphere, so that damage to one side of the brain affects the other side of the body.

The Lobes of the Cerebrum

Smaller fissures crisscross the cerebrum and mark out various specific areas of function called *lobes*. The frontal lobes, one on the left hemisphere and one on the right in back of our eyes and extending upward behind the forehead, are perhaps the most talked about and the least understood by medical researchers. The specific functions of most other lobes in the cerebrum, such as the two occipital lobes (centers for seeing), the olfactory lobes (centers for smelling), and the temporal lobes (centers for hearing) are much better known.

The Brain Stem

The cerebrum, like a large flower obscuring part of its stalk, droops down

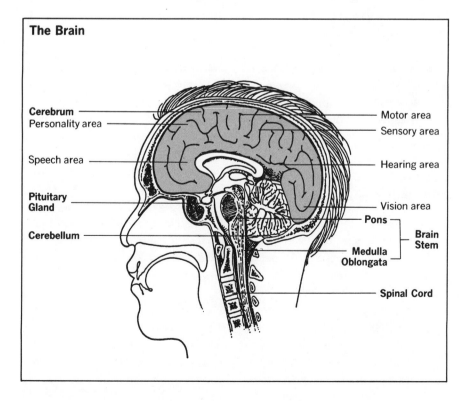

The Brain

Cerebrum
Personality area

Speech area

Pituitary Gland

Cerebellum

Motor area
Sensory area

Hearing area

Vision area
Pons
Brain Stem
Medulla Oblongata

Spinal Cord

The Brain and the Cranial Nerves

Cranial nerves

Eyeball

1. Olfactory: smell
2. Optic: vision
3. Oculomotor: muscle of eyes
4. Trochlear: muscle of eyes
5. Trigeminal: sense of touch in face
6. Abducens: muscle of eyes
7. Facial: muscles of face
8. Acoustic: hearing and balance
9. Glossopharyngeal: taste
10. Vagus: heart, lungs, abdomen
11. Hypoglossal: tongue muscles
12. Accessory: neck muscles, eyeball

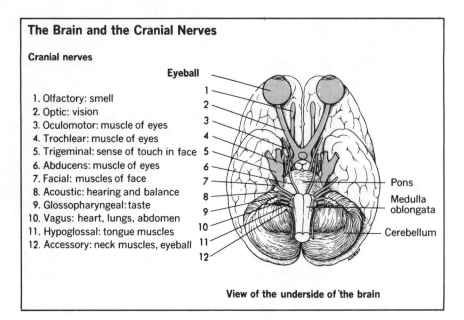

Pons

Medulla oblongata

Cerebellum

View of the underside of the brain

---

around the *brain stem.* Thus, while the brain stem originates just about in the middle of our skull, it does not emerge completely from the folds of the cerebral hemispheres until it reaches the back of the neck. Then it soon merges into the spinal cord.

Associated with this portion of the brain—roughly speaking, between the cerebrum and the spinal cord—are centers that take care of the countless necessary details involved in just plain existing, and structures (such as the *medulla oblongata* and the *pons*) that serve also as traffic control points for the billions of nerve impulses traveling to and from the cerebrum. The largest of these "lesser brains" is the *cerebellum,* whose two hemispheres straddle the brain stem at the back of the head.

The Cerebellum

The cerebellum is the site of balance and body and muscle coordination, allowing us, for example, to "rub the tummy and pat the head" simultaneously, or tap the foot and strum a guitar, or steer a car and operate the foot pedals. Such muscle-coordinated movements, though sometimes learned only by long repetition and practice, can become almost automatic—such as reaching for and flicking on the light switch as we move into a darkened room.

But many other activities and kinds of behavior regulated by the part of the brain below the cerebrum are more fully automatic: the control of eye movement and focusing, for example, as well as the timing of heartbeat, sleep, appetite, and metabolism; the arousal and decline of sexual drives; body temperature; the dilation and constriction of blood vessels; swallowing; and breathing. All these are mainly functions of the *autonomic nervous system,* as opposed to the more voluntary actions controlled by the *central nervous system.*

The Body's Nervous Systems

Simply speaking, the human body has only one nervous system, and that is all the nerve cells, nerve cords, nerve centers (both voluntary and involuntary) in the body. It is helpful, however, though quite arbitrary, to divide our nerves into the central and autonomic nervous systems. This division tends to obscure the countless interconnections and interplay between the two systems. For example, where do you place the control of breathing or blinking? Such actions are automatic except when we choose to regulate them.

The Central Nervous System

The central nervous system, as noted above, includes the brain and the spinal cord. It also includes all the nerves of conscious response and voluntary action that link up with the brain and spinal cord.

Twelve pairs of *cranial nerves* originate within the brain and emerge at its base. These include the very important nerves that connect with our sense organs, nerve bundles that control the facial and neck muscles, and the *vagus* (or tenth cranial nerve) that serves the heart, lungs, stomach, intestines, esophagus, larynx, liver, kidneys, spleen, and pancreas. The vagus nerve, although anatomically part of the central nervous system, controls bodily functions that are mainly automatic.

Spinal nerves branch out from the spinal cord as it snakes its way through the vertebrae of the spinal column. All the major nerve cords that wrap around the trunk and reach the arms and hands, legs and feet, originate from spinal nerves.

The cranial nerves and the spinal nerves, together with all those nerves lying outside the confines of the brain and spinal cord, are sometimes referred to as the *peripheral nervous system.* This term can be confusing, however, because it is also used to include all the nerves of the autonomic nervous system, next discussed.

The Autonomic Nervous System

The muscles served by the central nervous system are all of one general type (striated), while the muscles served by the autonomic system are called involuntary or smooth. The autonomic nerves regulate body activity without our conscious control—for example, as we sleep. They are rather elegantly divided into two categories: *sympathetic* and *parasympathetic* nervous systems. These are distinguishable primarily by their opposite effects on the body organs. For example, impulses along parasympathetic nerve trunks dilate blood vessels, slow the heartbeat rate, and increase stomach secretions, while the sympathetic system constricts blood vessels, increases rate of heartbeat, and inhibits stomach secretions.

The Neuron—What Nerves Are Made Of

A nerve cell is a grayish blob of tissue from which protrude several short gray fibers, *dendrites,* and one longer whitish fiber, an *axon.* Both the dendrites and the axon resemble ropes with their ends splayed and frayed. Dendrites register impulses coming into the central blob of the neuron (perhaps from a neighboring neuron's axon); an axon picks up the incoming impulses and carries them away.

Both units are equally important for normal nerve functioning, but the axon is far more showy as an anatom-

ical structure. All nerve cords are made up of the single strands of many axons, which may reach lengths of several feet. In other words, if we could stretch out certain neurons in our body—for example, those making up the sciatic nerve that runs from the small of the back to the toes—their axon "tails" would make them three or four feet long.

Myelin

A normal axon usually has a fatty coating of insulation called *myelin.* An axon severed into two pieces cannot grow together again; but if the myelin sheath is pretty much intact, a surgeon can sometimes restore nerve function by sewing the two ends together, or replace the nerve with one from another part of the body. The part of the severed axon connecting to the central portion usually remains alive in any case—which is why a person can often retain the sensation of feeling in an amputated part.

Certain serious and progressively disabling diseases involve the gradual loss (*demyelination*) of this coating, causing paralysis, numbness, or other loss of function in an organ; a demyelinated nerve fiber is not able to carry impulses to and from the brain. Two such diseases are multiple sclerosis and "Lou Gehrig's disease" (amyotrophic lateral sclerosis).

Effects of Aging

Once we reach maturity, the number of our nerve cells begins to decrease, because our bodies cannot manufacture new neurons to replace the ones that die in the normal process of living. (Other kinds of tissue are continually replenished with new cells.) This has some relation to senility, but the loss of a few million out of many billions of brain and nerve cells has

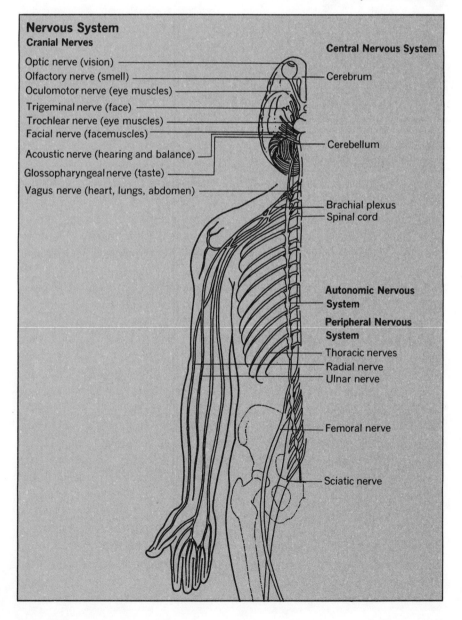

Nervous System
Cranial Nerves

Optic nerve (vision)
Olfactory nerve (smell)
Oculomotor nerve (eye muscles)
Trigeminal nerve (face)
Trochlear nerve (eye muscles)
Facial nerve (facemuscles)
Acoustic nerve (hearing and balance)
Glossopharyngeal nerve (taste)
Vagus nerve (heart, lungs, abdomen)

Central Nervous System

Cerebrum
Cerebellum
Brachial plexus
Spinal cord

Autonomic Nervous System

Peripheral Nervous System

Thoracic nerves
Radial nerve
Ulnar nerve
Femoral nerve
Sciatic nerve

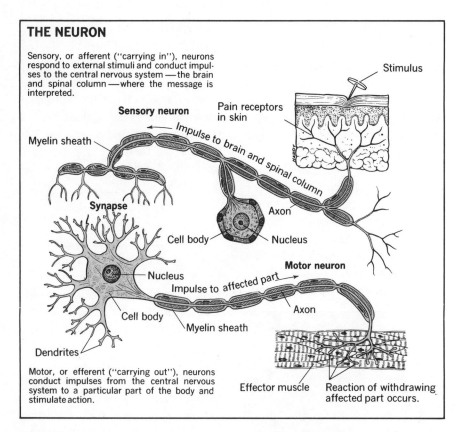

THE NEURON

Sensory, or afferent ("carrying in"), neurons respond to external stimuli and conduct impulses to the central nervous system — the brain and spinal column — where the message is interpreted.

Sensory neuron

Stimulus

Pain receptors in skin

Myelin sheath

Impulse to brain and spinal column

Synapse

Axon

Cell body

Nucleus

Nucleus

Motor neuron

Impulse to affected part

Cell body

Axon

Dendrites

Myelin sheath

Motor, or efferent ("carrying out"), neurons conduct impulses from the central nervous system to a particular part of the body and stimulate action.

Effector muscle

Reaction of withdrawing affected part occurs.

---

little effect on mental powers unless the losses are concentrated in one area.

Synapse, Ganglion, and Plexus

When a nerve impulse, traveling away from the neuron's central part, reaches the ends of an axon, it meets a gap that it must jump to get to the tentaclelike dendrites of the next neuron. This gap is called a *synapse*.

At certain points in the body a great many nerve cell bodies and branches are packed closely together, with a resulting profusion of interwoven axons, dendrites, and synapses. Such a concentration of nervous tissue is called a *ganglion*, or *plexus*. A blow or jolt to such an area can be extremely painful and even stupefying—affecting as it does a whole network of nerves—as anyone who has been hit in the solar plexus or learned the pressure points of karate knows.

The Movement of Impulses along Nerve Fibers

There is really no exact counterpart in the mechanical world for how an impulse moves along a nerve fiber and then jumps across a synapse to the next nerve. Nor is this movement completely understood by scientists. Suffice it to say that it is somewhat like an electrical current moving along in a chemical environment that allows the impulse to travel, in discreet little jumps, at a speed of about 200 miles per hour—quite slowly when we compare it to the speed of light or electricity: 186,000 miles per second. This speed serves us quite well in most situations, but there are times when we wish human beings' nerves could act more quickly—on the highway, for example, or when a cherished vase starts to topple off the mantelpiece.

One of the simplest and quickest kinds of reactions to an outside stimulus is one that bypasses the brain. We don't really think to pull our hand

away from a piping hot radiator. This is called a *spinal reflex*. What happens is that the sensory nerve endings in the finger pick up the "too hot" impulse from the radiator; the impulse then travels to the spinal cord where it activates the motor nerve pathway back to the burned finger, carrying the message, "Jerk your finger away!"

When to Suspect Trouble

Our entire existence as human beings depends so much on the normal functioning of our brain and nervous system that any real brain or nervous disorder or disease is a very serious matter. A sprained joint or cut foot can spell doom for an animal that depends on speed and mobility for survival; but the same injury is often not much more than a painful inconvenience to us. Impairment of our brain or nervous system is far more of a threat to our survival.

Multiple sclerosis and meningitis have been mentioned as serious disorders affecting the nerves, others are Parkinsonism, shingles, encephalitis, and brain tumors. The possible presence of one of these disorders is reason enough not to shrug off any of the following signs and symptoms: recurrent headaches, intense pain of unknown cause, tremors, numbness, loss of coordination, dizziness, blackouts, tics, cramps, visual difficulties, and loss of bowel and bladder control. Also, any person who has remained unconscious for more than a few minutes should be taken to a physician as soon as possible. This applies even when the person has regained consciousness and says he feels fine.

Our complex emotions, of course, are linked to the functioning of our brain and nervous system. A mind free of undue anxiety, guilt, and frustration functions better than a mind racked with worries and conflicts, and is a much more efficient and reliable leader of the body. See also Ch. 8, *Diseases of the Muscles and Nervous System.* For a discussion of mental and emotional health, see Ch. 36.

The Circulatory System, the Heart, and Blood

When the heart stops beating—that is to say, stops pumping blood—for longer than a couple of minutes, we stop living. But the heart, fortunately, is extremely sturdy. It is also simple in construction, capable of operating at a great many different speeds, in many cases self-repairing if damaged, and probably the one continuously operating automatic pump that we could, with any confidence, expect to last 70 years or longer.

These simple facts tend to be forgotten today, in what is probably the most heart-conscious era in history. True, heart disease, along with cancer, is statistically one of today's major killers. But we should remember two circumstances: not until about 50 years ago did deaths from heart disease begin to be accurately recognized and reported; second, with longer and longer life spans, it becomes more likely that a nonstop vital organ like the heart will simply wear out. Heart transplants, open heart surgery, and artificial heart parts—often reported sensationally in the public media—have also conditioned us to think of our hearts as terribly vulnerable, rather delicate, a bit inadequate to their tasks, and quite open to improvement.

Advances in heart surgery do, indeed, hold greater promise for per-

sons whose hearts had been considered, until now, irreversibly damaged or diseased. But the great attention accorded such miracles of medicine tends to obscure the humdrum, day-in-day-out, low-key drama performed for a lifetime by a healthy, uncomplaining heart.

The Heart and Circulatory Network

Perhaps the best way to put the heart in perspective is to place it where it belongs, at the hub of the body's circulatory system. This hollow, fist-sized lump of sinewy tissue is located behind the breastbone, centered just about at the vertical midline of our chest. It is connected into a closed system of flexible tubes, called blood vessels, ranging down from finger-thick to microscopically slender, that reach into every cavern, crevice, and outpost of our body—a network of some 70,000 miles.

The heart has essentially one function—to push blood, by pumping action, through this enormous network of blood vessels. We have about six quarts of blood in our body, pumped at the rate of about five ounces every time the heart beats (normally about 72 times a minute for an adult), which we feel as our pulse. The blood circulates and recirculates through the blood vessels, pushed along by the pumping of the heart.

Arteries and Veins

The blood vessels are generally described as *arterial,* referring to the *arteries* that carry blood away from the heart; or *venous,* referring to the *veins* through which blood seeps and flows back toward the heart to be re-pumped. A large artery such as the *aorta* branches into smaller arteries, and these eventually into still smaller vessels called *arterioles,* and the arterioles, finally, into the smallest

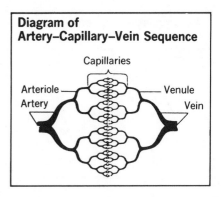

Diagram of Artery–Capillary–Vein Sequence

Capillaries

Arteriole
Artery

Venule
Vein

blood vessels, the *capillaries.* These in turn open onto other capillaries, which are the starting point for the return of blood to the heart.

The microscopic capillaries typically form a kind of cat's cradle connection, sometimes called a capillary bed, at the transition zone where arterial blood becomes venous blood. The returning blood moves from the capillaries to small veins called *venules* (the counterparts of arterioles) and through successively larger veins back to the heart.

Blood and Our Internal Fluid Environment

What makes this fairly rudimentary collection of plumbing so absolutely indispensable to life is the fluid it pumps—blood. If any part of the body—cell, tissue, or major organ—is denied circulating blood and the substances it carries with it for longer than a few minutes, that part will fail. It is the job of the heart and the blood vessels to get blood to all the body's far-flung tissues, where it both picks up and deposits substances.

Blood is really a kind of fluid tissue. About 80 percent of its volume is water, and blood's indispensable, life-sustaining power is owed in great part to its watery base, which permits it both to flow and to take up and carry materials in solution. All our tissues and organs have a kind of give-and-take arrangement with the circulating blood.

The Circulatory System

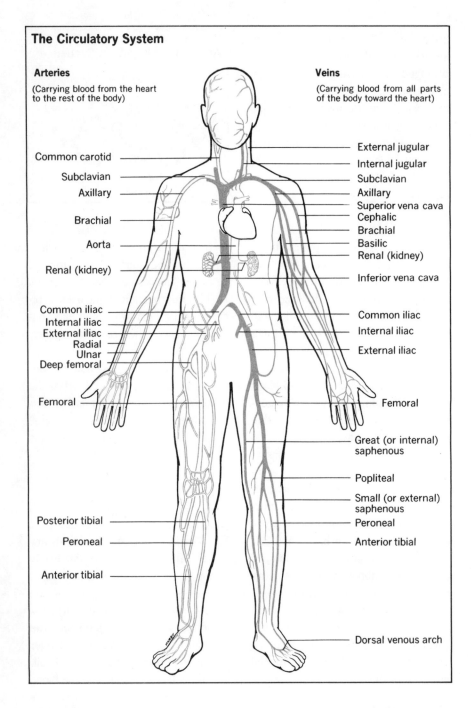

Arteries

(Carrying blood from the heart to the rest of the body)

Veins

(Carrying blood from all parts of the body toward the heart)

Common carotid

Subclavian

Axillary

Brachial

Aorta

Renal (kidney)

Common iliac
Internal iliac
External iliac
Radial
Ulnar
Deep femoral

Femoral

Posterior tibial

Peroneal

Anterior tibial

External jugular

Internal jugular

Subclavian

Axillary

Superior vena cava
Cephalic

Brachial

Basilic

Renal (kidney)

Inferior vena cava

Common iliac

Internal iliac

External iliac

Femoral

Great (or internal) saphenous

Popliteal

Small (or external) saphenous

Peroneal

Anterior tibial

Dorsal venous arch

Distributor of Nutrients

Food, or more accurately the nutrient molecules needed by cells, are also transported throughout the body by the blood. In the digestive tract, food is broken down into tiny submicroscopic pieces that can pass through the tract's walls (mainly along the small intestine) and be picked up by the blood for distribution around the body.

One of the specialized, small-volume transportation jobs handled by the blood is to pick up hormones from the endocrine glands and present these chemical messengers to the organs they affect.

Composition of Blood

Blood is a distinctive and recognizable type of tissue, but this does not mean it is a stable, uniform substance with a fixed proportion of ingredients. Quite the opposite is true; its composition is ever changing in response to the demands of other body systems. Other organs are constantly pouring substances into the blood, or removing things from it. Blood in one part of the body at a given moment may be vastly different in chemical makeup from blood in another part of the body.

Despite its changing makeup, blood does have certain basic components. A sample of blood left to stand for an hour or so separates into a clear, watery fluid with a yellowish tinge and a darker, more solid clump. The clear yellow liquid is called *plasma,* and accounts for about 55 percent of the volume of normal blood. The darker clump is made up mainly of the blood's most conspicuous and populous inhabitants, the red cells that give blood its color.

Plasma

It is the plasma that enables our blood

Carrier of Oxygen

Perhaps the most critical of these give-and-take transactions occurs in the lungs; it is this transaction that if interrupted by heartbeat stoppage for more than a few minutes causes death by oxygen starvation of vital tissues. Before a unit of blood is pumped out by the heart to the body, it picks up in the lungs the oxygen that we have inhaled and which every cell in the body needs to function. The blood then transports the oxygen, delivering it to other parts of the body. By the time a given unit of blood has made a tour of the blood vessels and returned to the lungs, it has given up most of its oxygen and is laden instead with carbon dioxide, the principal waste product of living processes. The venous blood releases its carbon dioxide, to be exhaled by the lungs.

to carry out most of the transportation tasks assigned it. Being over 90 percent water, the plasma has water's property of being able to carry substances both in solution and in suspension. (A substance in solution is one, like salt, that must be removed from water by chemical or physical action, such as boiling; while a substance in suspension—such as red blood cells within whole blood in a standing test tube—separates out more readily, particularly when its watery carrier has been contained and its flow stilled.)

Red Blood Cells

Red blood cells (or *erythrocytes*) numbering in the trillions are carried in suspension by the plasma. In turn, the red blood cells carry the single most important substance needed by the body's cells—oxygen. For such an important task, the red blood cell looks hardly adequate. As it matures, this cell loses its nucleus. Lacking a nucleus, it is sometimes not even called a cell but a red blood *corpuscle*. What gives red blood cells their special oxygen-carrying ability, and also their color, is their possession of a complex iron-protein substance called *hemoglobin*.

Hemoglobin

Molecules of hemoglobin have the property of loosely combining with oxygen where it is plentiful, as in the lungs. They can then hold on to oxygen until they reach an area where oxygen has been depleted by the demands of living processes. There— usually in the fine tubes of the capillaries—hemoglobin's hold on oxygen is challenged by the demands of other cells, and the red cells give up their oxygen. The hemoglobin of red cells develops an immediate affinity for carbon dioxide, the waste product of cell metabolism, and the red blood cells then carry this carbon dioxide back to the lungs for exhalation.

Hemoglobin's ability to carry oxygen is not unique. Water, and therefore plasma, also have this ability. Hemoglobin's specialness lies in how much oxygen it can carry. Hemoglobin increases by more than 50 times the oxygen-carrying capacity of our blood.

White Blood Cells

White blood cells have many different shapes and sizes, all going under the general scientific name of *leukocytes*. They are typically larger than red blood cells, but far less numerous. If we accept an estimate of 25 trillion as the number of living red blood cells in our body, then the number of white blood cells might be generously estimated at around 40 billion, a ratio of one white cell to about 600–700 reds.

According to their shape, size, and other characteristics, white blood cells have been divided into various categories such as lymphocytes, monocytes, and granulocytes. But as a group these blood cells are distinguished by their common propensity for attacking foreign bodies that invade our tissues, whether these invaders be sizable splinters or microscopic bacteria. White blood cells move in force to the site of an infection, do battle with the intruding agents, and frequently strew the area with the wreckage of the encounter— a collection of dismantled alien bacteria and dead white cells, which we know as pus.

Platelets

Platelets, also called *thrombocytes,* initiate some of the first steps in the complex biochemical process that leads to the clotting of blood. They thus help to spare us from bleeding to death from a slight injury. Platelets are the most rudimentary and diminutive of the major blood components. Like mature red blood cells, they lack nuclei, but are only one-quarter as big. By no stretch of the imagination can they be called blood cells. Rather, they are blood elements—bits of cell substance with a recognizable size and shape, circulating with the blood.

The Proportions of Blood Cells

All the several types of blood cells and subcells in a healthy body occur in proportions that, though never precisely fixed and unchanging, are recognized as having normal upper and lower limits. If a particular type of cell shows a sudden increase or decrease in population, so that its proportion relative to other blood cells shows a variation markedly outside its normal range, some infection, disease, or disorder must be suspected.

In addition to occurring in certain normal-range proportions, each type of cellular blood component has a typical shape, appearance, and set of chemical and physical properties. Variations from these norms occur in many diseases.

The analysis of blood samples (usually taken from the finger or arm) and their inspection under a microscope have proved invaluable in diagnosing illness and disease, often before a person feels any symptoms whatsoever. This is why a thorough medical checkup should always include taking a sample of your blood. It is then up to the physician to decide which of the dozens of tests should be made on your blood in the medical laboratory. One common test is a *blood count,* in which the number of a certain type of cell in a given unit of your blood can be estimated, and then compared to the normal number in the same amount of blood.

Blood Groups and Rh Factors

The identification of *blood groups* and *Rh factors* is another aspect of blood analysis. The four most common blood groups are called A, B, AB, and O, classifications based on chemical differences that may be incompatible if one group is mixed with another. Thus, it is absolutely essential before a person receives a blood transfusion to know both his own blood type and the type of the blood he is to be given. Blood group O is considered the safety for transfusion, and people with type O blood are sometimes called "universal donors." It is a wise practice to carry, along with your other important cards, a card giving your own blood type. The blood of a donor, however, is always *cross-matched* (checked for compatibility) with the blood of the person who is to receive it in order to avoid transfusion reactions.

Blood Cell Manufacture and Turnover

Most types of blood cells, both red and white, are manufactured in the red marrow of bones. The rate and quantity of total production is staggering; estimates range from one to five million red blood cells per second. This prodigious output is necessary because blood cells are disintegrating, having served their useful lives, in the same enormous numbers every second. The normal life span of a red blood cell is about four months, which means that four months from now every blood cell in your body will have died and been replaced with new cells.

The Liver As a Producer of Red Blood Cells

The red bone marrow is backed up by several other tissues that can, if called upon, turn out blood cells in quantity or serve as specialized producers of certain blood cells and blood elements. One such organ is the liver, which, before and after birth and into childhood, is a site of red blood cell production. In an emergency, such as severe internal hemorrhage, the liver sometimes reverts to its earlier function of manufacturing red cells. The liver also serves as a kind of salvage yard for the iron from dead red cells. It stores the iron for later combination into hemoglobin and passes off the rest of the red blood cell fragments as part of the bile pigments that empty into the duodenum of the small intestine.

The Spleen As a Producer of Blood Cells

Certain white blood cells, in particular the lymphocytes, are produced at a variety of locations in the body—for example, by the lymph nodes, by little clumps of tissue called *Peyer's patches* in the intestinal tract, and by the spleen.

The spleen plays a number of interesting secondary roles in blood cell production. Like the liver, it can be pressed into service as a manufacturer of red blood cells and serve as a salvage yard for iron reclaimed from worn-out red blood cells. A newborn baby is almost totally dependent on its spleen for the production of red blood cells, with a little help from the liver. In an adult, however, a damaged or diseased spleen can be surgically removed, with little or no apparent effect on the health or life span of the person, provided the patient's bone marrow is in good functioning order.

Movement of Blood Cells through the Capillaries

A blood cell must be able to slip through the microscopic, twisting and turning tunnels of the capillaries that mark the turn-about point in the blood cell's round-trip voyage from the heart. Blood cells, therefore, must be small (the point of a pin could hold dozens of red blood cells), and they must be jellylike in order to navigate the tight tortuous, capillary channels without either blocking the channel or breaking apart themselves. A red blood cell is further adapted to sneaking through the capillaries by its concave-disk shape, which allows it to bend and fold around itself. Nevertheless, so narrow are the passageways within some of the capillaries that blood cells must move through them in single file. If a substantial number of the cells are misshapen, as in sickle-cell anemia, they tend to move sluggishly or clog up the passageway—a condition that can have serious consequences. See also Ch. 9, *Diseases of the Circulatory System.*

Lymph and the Lymphatic System

Of all our body systems, perhaps the most ignored is the lymphatic system, although it forms a network throughout our body comparable to the blood vessels of our circulatory system.

Lymph is a whitish fluid that is derived from blood plasma. As plasma circulates through the body, some of it seeps through the walls of capillaries and other blood vessels. This leakage is of the utmost importance, because the leaked fluid, lymph, supplies the liquid environment around and between individual cells and tissues that is essential for their survival.

The presence of lymph requires a drainage system to keep the fluid moving. If there were no drainage system, two things could happen: the dammed-up lymph could create areas swollen with water in which cells would literally drown, or stagnant pools of lymph could become breeding

MUSCLES AND TENDONS

MUSCLES
1. Temporal
2. Mimetic muscles
3. Masseter (a muscle of mastication)
4. Infrahyoid muscles
5. Sternomastoid
6. Omohyoid
7. Deltoid
8. Pectoral muscles
9. Serratus anterior
10. External oblique
11. Rectus abdominus
12. Biceps brachii
13. Flexor digitorum superficialis
14. Gracilis (sublimis)

15. Adductor group
16. Sartorius
17. Rectus femoris
18. Quadriceps femoris
19. Vastus medialis
19a. Vastus lateralis
20. Dorsiflexors
21. Trapezius
22. Infraspinatus
23. Teres major
24. Triceps brachii
25. Latissimus dorsi
26. Rhomboideus major
27. Gluteus medius
28. Gluteus maximus

29. Digital extensors
30. Hamstring muscles
31. Gastrocnemius
32. Plantar flexors

TENDONS
33. Rectus sheath
34. Flexor retinaculum of carpal tunnel
35. Patellar tendon
36. Retinaculum of tarsal tunnel
37. Tendons of long digital extensors
38. Tendon of tibialis anterior
39. Lumbodorsal fascia
40. Fascia lata
41. Achilles

BONES AND LIGAMENTS

BONES
1. Skull
2. Mandible
3. Vertebrae
4. Clavicle
5. Scapula
6. Manubrium
7. Body of sternum
8. Xiphoid process
9. Ribs
10. Humerus
11. Radius
12. Ulna
13. Sacrum
14. Ilium
15. Coccyx
16. Femur
17. Patella
18. Tibia
19. Fibula
20. Carpals
21. Metacarpals
22. Phalanges
23. Metatarsals
24. Tarsals
25. Heel

LIGAMENTS AND JOINTS
26. Capsule of shoulder
27. Sternoclavicular
28. Capsule of elbow
29. Sacroiliac
30. Iliofemoral
31. Wrist
32. Capsule of knee
33. Ankle
34. Pubic symphysis
35. Intervertebral discs

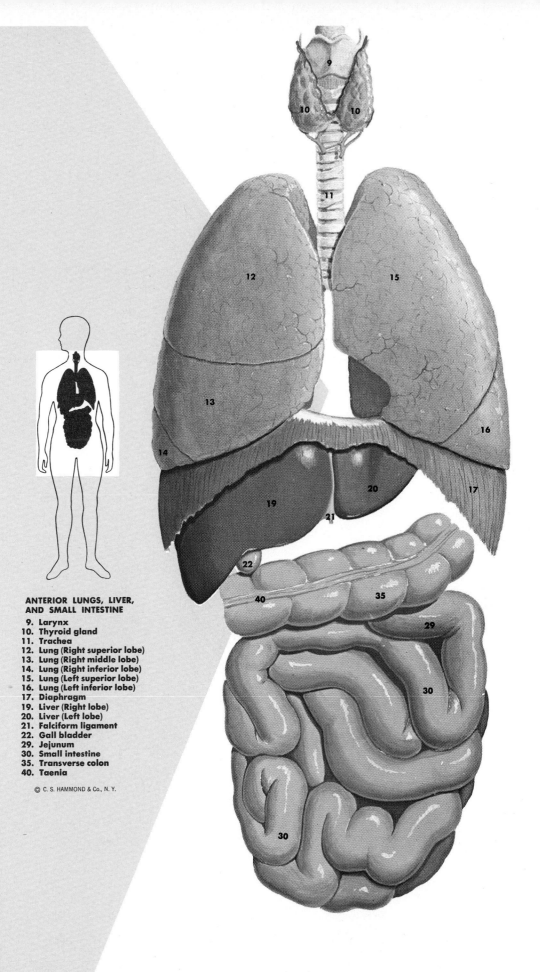

**ANTERIOR LUNGS, LIVER,
AND SMALL INTESTINE**

9. Larynx
10. Thyroid gland
11. Trachea
12. Lung (Right superior lobe)
13. Lung (Right middle lobe)
14. Lung (Right inferior lobe)
15. Lung (Left superior lobe)
16. Lung (Left inferior lobe)
17. Diaphragm
19. Liver (Right lobe)
20. Liver (Left lobe)
21. Falciform ligament
22. Gall bladder
29. Jejunum
30. Small intestine
35. Transverse colon
40. Taenia

© C. S. HAMMOND & Co., N. Y.

**POSTERIOR LUNGS, LIVER,
AND SMALL INTESTINE**

9. **Larynx**
10. **Thyroid gland**
11. **Trachea**
12. **Lung (Right superior lobe)**
13. **Lung (Right middle lobe)**
14. **Lung (Right inferior lobe)**
15. **Lung (Left superior lobe)**
16. **Lung (Left inferior lobe)**
17. **Diaphragm**
18. **Principal bronchi**
19. **Liver (Right lobe)**
20. **Liver (Left lobe)**
21. **Falciform ligament**
22. **Gall bladder**
29. **Jejunum**
30. **Small intestine**
31. **Ileum**
35. **Transverse colon**
40. **Taenia coli**
41. **Cystic duct**
42. **Portal vein**
43. **Hepatic artery**
44. **Hepatic vein**

ANTERIOR CIRCULATORY SYSTEM

17. **Diaphragm**
23. **Esophagus**
37. **Sigmoid colon**
38. **Rectum**
44. **Hepatic vein**
49. **Superior mesenteric artery**
53. **Common carotid artery.**
54. **Internal jugular vein**
55. **Subclavian artery**
56. **Subclavian vein**
57. **Aortic arch**
58. **Aorta**
60. **Heart**
61. **Pulmonary arteries**
63. **Superior vena cava**
64. **Inferior vena cava**
65. **Coronary arteries**
66. **Coeliac trunk**
68. **Inferior mesenteric artery**
69. **Renal artery**
70. **Renal vein**
71. **Common iliac artery**
72. **Common iliac vein**
73. **Femoral artery**
74. **Femoral vein**
75. **Internal iliac artery**
76. **Internal iliac vein**
77. **Kidneys (r. and l.)**
78. **Suprarenal glands (r. and l.)**
79. **Ureters (r. and l.)**

POSTERIOR CIRCULATORY SYSTEM

17. Diaphragm
23. Esophagus
37. Sigmoid colon
38. Rectum
53. Common carotid artery.
54. Internal jugular vein
55. Subclavian artery
56. Subclavian vein
57. Aortic arch
58. Aorta
60. Heart
61. Pulmonary arteries
62. Pulmonary veins
63. Superior vena cava
64. Inferior vena cava
69. Renal artery
70. Renal vein
71. Common iliac artery
72. Common iliac vein
73. Femoral artery
74. Femoral vein
75. Internal iliac artery
76. Internal iliac vein
77. Kidneys (r. and l.)
79. Ureters (r. and l.)

© C. S. HAMMOND & Co., N. Y.

**ANTERIOR INTERIOR
RIB CAGE AND SPINE**

5. **Ribs**
85. **Cervical vertebrae**
86. **Thoracic vertebrae**
87. **Lumbar vertebrae**
87a. **Transverse process of vertebra**
88. **Sacrum**
89. **Coccyx**
90. **Intervertebral discs**
91. **Scapula**
92. **Humerus**
93. **Head of humerus**
94. **Ilium**
95. **Femur**
96. **Head of femur**

© C. S. HAMMOND & Co., N. Y.

POSTERIOR RIB CAGE AND SPINE

5. Ribs
85. Cervical vertebrae
86. Thoracic vertebrae
87. Lumbar vertebrae
88. Sacrum
89. Coccyx
91. Scapula
92. Humerus
93. Head of humerus
94. Ilium
95. Femur
96. Head of femur

ANTERIOR CHEST CAVITY

1. Clavicle
2. Manubrium
3. Body of sternum
4. Xiphoid process
5. Rib
6. Floating rib
7. Cartilage
8. Anterior super-
   ior iliac spine

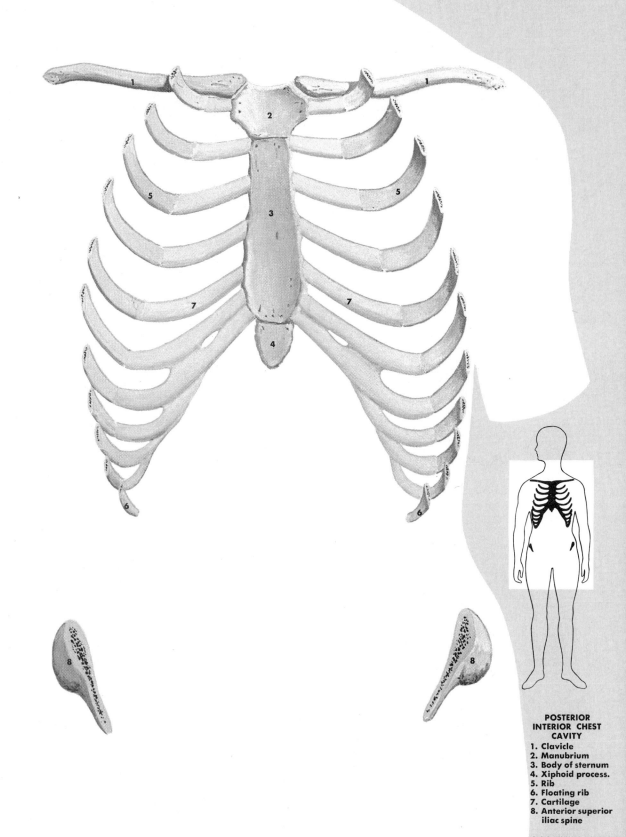

**POSTERIOR
INTERIOR CHEST
CAVITY**
1. Clavicle
2. Manubrium
3. Body of sternum
4. Xiphoid process.
5. Rib
6. Floating rib
7. Cartilage
8. Anterior superior
iliac spine

ANTERIOR STOMACH, COLON,
AND
ORGANS OF REPRODUCTION

23. Esophagus
24. Stomach (cardia)
25. Stomach (fundus)
26. Stomach (body)
27. Stomach (pylorus)
28. Duodenum
31. Ileum
32. Ileocolic junction
33. Caecum
34. Ascending colon
36. Descending colon
37. Sigmoid colon
39. Vermiform appendix
40. Taenia coli
45. Spleen
49. Superior mesenteric artery
50. Superior mesenteric vein
51. Pancreas (head)
52. Pancreas (tail)
80. Bladder
81. Urachus
82. Pubic symphysis
83. Inguinal ligament
100. Uterus
102. Vagina (cross section)
103. Fallopian tube
104. Ostium of fallopian tube
105. Ovary

POSTERIOR STOMACH, COLON, AND ORGANS OF REPRODUCTION

23. Esophagus
24. Stomach (cardia)
25. Stomach (fundus)
26. Stomach (body)
27. Stomach (pylorus)
28. Duodenum
31. Ileum
32. Ileocolic junction
33. Caecum
34. Ascending colon
36. Descending colon
37. Sigmoid colon
39. Vermiform appendix
40. Taenia coli
41. Cystic duct
41a. Common bile duct
42. Portal vein
43. Hepatic artery
45. Spleen
46. Splenic artery
47. Splenic vein
48. Inferior mesenteric vein
49. Superior mesenteric artery
50. Superior mesenteric vein
51. Pancreas (head)
51a. Pancreas (body)
52. Pancreas (tail)
80. Bladder
83. Inguinal ligament
100. Uterus
101. Cervix
102. Vagina (cross section)
103. Fallopian tube
104. Ostium of fallopian tube
105. Ovary

LACTATING BREAST

97. **Pectoralis major muscle**
117. **Areola**
118. **Nipple**
119. **Fat**
120. **Lactiferous (milk producing) glands and ducts**
120a. **Cross section of gland and duct**
121. **Tissue separating and supporting glandular tissue**

STRUCTURE OF THE MAMMARY GLANDS

The mammary glands are composed of three major elements:
1. Their skin covering and special structures (nipple, areola).
2. The lactiferous glands or functional units of the breast.
3. The supporting structures, the connective tissue "ligaments" and the fat tissue that makes up the mass of the breast.

The breast is supported by the "suspensory ligaments." These are anchored to the sheet of connective tissue surrounding the pectoralis major muscle, and extend in a complex network separated by the fat tissue outward to the skin. The lactiferous glands are buried in the supporting tissues and empty outward onto the surface of the nipple. These glands at first are very small and clustered just beneath the nipple and areola. In pregnancy they enlarge and push downward into the mass of the breast causing it to enlarge in turn. The enlargement continues through the period of breast feeding, following which the glands gradually grow smaller and the entire breast returns to normal size.

101. Cervix
108. Myometrium
109. Endometrium
111. Placenta
113. Amniotic sac
114. Umbilical cord
116. Fetus

THE FETUS AT 3 1/2 AND 6 MONTHS

Most of the definitive development of the fetus occurs during the first 3½ months, and the remaining 5½ months is primarily concerned with gradual increase in size and maturation of organs already begun. The fetus receives all of its nourishment through the placenta and umbilical cord. There is no direct contact between fetal and maternal blood in the placenta. During its entire development, the fetus floats in a fluid (amniotic fluid) contained within a sac (the amniotic sac) attached to the placenta. This sac is in turn surrounded by the uterine cavity, the endometrium and the muscle or myometrium of the uterus.

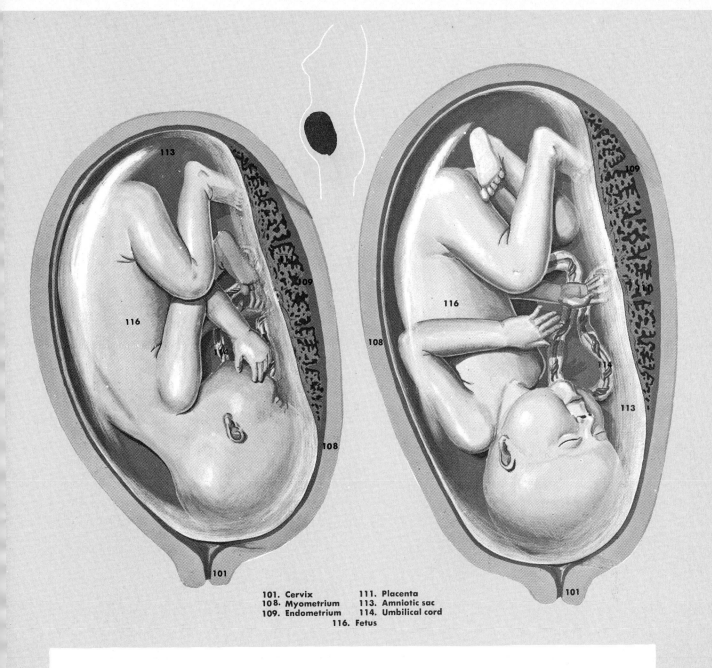

101. Cervix   111. Placenta
108. Myometrium   113. Amniotic sac
109. Endometrium   114. Umbilical cord
116. Fetus

THE FETUS AT 8 AND 9 MONTHS

Until birth, the fetus is surrounded by the amniotic sac and fluid, and attached to the placenta by the umbilical cord. The fetus continues to increase in size and the uterus stretches to accommodate it. Usually before the eighth month the fetus assumes a head-downward position. At birth, the amniotic sac ruptures, the fluid escapes, and the child is slowly pushed out of the uterine cavity by the contractions of the myometrium. Shortly after birth of the child, the placenta is similarly expelled having been detached from the endometrium.

PRINTED IN U.S.A

X-RAY OF THE HUMAN BODY
SHOWING THE
BONE STRUCTURE

grounds for infection.

As it moves through the vessels of the lymphatic system, lymph carries away from the tissues the bits and pieces of cells that have died and disintegrated, and also potentially harmful bacteria and viruses.

Lymph and Lymphocytes

Confusion often arises about the connection between the white blood cells called *lymphocytes* and the lymph itself. Lymph is not made up of lymphocytes, although it often carries

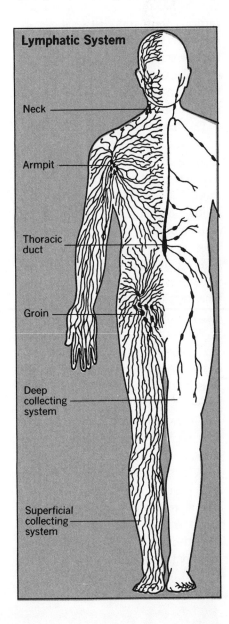

Lymphatic System

Neck

Armpit

Thoracic duct

Groin

Deep collecting system

Superficial collecting system

them; lymph is simply a watery vehicle moving through the lymphatic network. At certain points along this network, the vessels enlarge into clumpy structures called *lymph nodes* (or, misleadingly, lymph glands). Lymph nodes are major manufacturing sites for lymphocytes.

Lymph Nodes

Swollen glands are actually swollen lymph nodes, where a small army of lymphocytes is doing battle against invading bacteria or other harmful microscopic organisms. The lymph nodes, more than a hundred of them distributed around the body, serve as defense outposts against germs approaching the interior of the body. Those in the neck, groin, and armpits most frequently exhibit the pain and swelling that may accompany germ-fighting.

Circulation of Lymph

Lymph circulates without any help from the heart. From the spaces between cells, it diffuses into lymph capillaries which, like the venous capillaries, merge into larger and larger vessels moving inward toward the heart. The lymph moves—even upward from the legs and lower part of the body—because the muscles and movements of the body are constantly kneading and squeezing the lymph vessels. These vessels are equipped with valves that prevent back-flow. This is not so very different from the way venous blood makes its way back to the heart.

Eventually, master lymph vessels from the head, abdomen, and torso join in the thoracic lymph duct, which then empties into large neck veins that carry lymph and venous blood, mixed together, back to the heart.

The Heart at Work

The structure and performance of the heart, at first glance rather complicated, assume a magnificent simplicity once we observe that this pulsating knot of hollow, intertwining muscle uses only one beat to perform two distinct pumping jobs.

The heart has a right side (your right) and a left side (your left), divided by a tough wall of muscle called a *septum*. Each side has two chambers, an upper one called an *atrium* (or *auricle*), and a lower one called a *ventricle*.

How the Heart Pumps the Blood

Venous blood from the body flows into the right atrium via two large veins called the *superior vena cava* (bringing blood from the upper body) and the *inferior vena cava* (bringing blood from the lower part of the body). Where the blood enters the right atrium are valves that close when the atrium chamber is full.

Then, through a kind of trapdoor valve, blood is released from the right atrium into the right ventricle. When the right ventricle is full, and its outlet valve opens, the heart as a whole contracts—that is, pumps.

To the Lungs

The blood from the right ventricle is pumped to the lungs through the pulmonary artery to pick up oxygen. The trapdoor valve between the right atrium and ventricle has meanwhile closed, and venous blood again fills the right atrium.

Having picked up oxygen in the lungs, blood enters the left atrium through two pulmonary veins. (They are called veins despite the fact that they carry the most oxygen-rich blood, because they lead *to* the heart; just as the pulmonary artery carries the oxygen-poorest blood away from

How Blood Circulates through the Heart

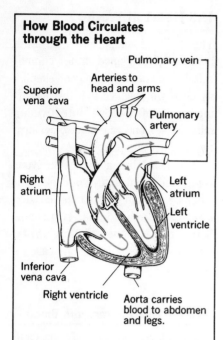

Blood from the head and arms enters the right atrium from the superior (i.e., upper) vena cava. Blood from the torso and legs enters from the inferior (i.e., lower) vena cava. The blood, controlled by a valve, passes to the right ventricle. It is then pumped into the pulmonary artery, which divides into two vessels, one leading to each lung. After being enriched with oxygen, the blood is brought back to the left atrium via the pulmonary veins, is admitted by a valve into the left ventricle, and is pumped through the aorta to be distributed to all parts of the body.

Both atria contract at the same time, forcing blood into the ventricles. Then both ventricles contract (while the atria relax), forcing blood into the great arteries. This period of contraction is called systole, and is followed by a period of relaxation called diastole.

the heart, to the lungs.) Like the right atrium, the left atrium serves as a holding reservoir and, when full, releases its contents into the left ventricle. A valve between left atrium and ventricle closes, and the heart pumps.

To the Body

Blood surges through an opening valve of the left ventricle into the aorta, the major artery that marks the beginning of blood's circulation throughout the body. The left ventricle, because it has the job of pumping blood to the entire body rather than just to the lungs, is slightly larger and more muscular than the right ventri-

cle. It is for this reason, incidentally, that the heart is commonly considered to be on our left. The organ as a whole, as noted earlier, is located at the center of the chest.

The Heart's Own Circulatory System

Heart tissue, like that of every other organ in the body, must be continually supplied with fresh, oxygen-rich blood, and used blood must be returned to the lungs for reoxygenation. The blood inside the heart cannot serve these needs. Thus the heart has its own circulation network, called *coronary arteries* and *veins,* to nourish its muscular tissues. There are two major arteries on the surface of the heart, branching and rebranching eventually into capillaries. Coronary veins then take blood back to the right atrium.

Structure of the Heart

The musculature of the heart is called cardiac muscle because it is different in appearance from the two other major types of muscle. The heart muscle is sometimes considered as one anatomical unit, called the *myocardium.* A tough outer layer of membranous tissue, called the *pericardium,* surrounds the myocardium. Lining the internal chambers and valves of the heart, on the walls of the atria and ventricles, is a tissue called the *endocardium.*

These tissues, like any others, are subject to infections and other disorders. An infection of the endocardium by bacteria is called *bacterial endocarditis.* (Disease of the valves is also called *endocarditis,* although it is a misnomer.) An interruption of the blood supply to the heart muscle is called a *myocardial infarction,* which results in the weakening or death of the portion of the myocardium whose blood supply is blocked. Fortunately,

in many cases, other blood vessels may eventually take over the job of supplying the blood-starved area of heart muscle.

Heartbeat

The rate at which the heart beats is controlled by both the autonomic nervous system and by hormones of the endocrine system. The precise means by which the chambers and valves of the heart are made to work in perfect coordination are not fully understood. It is known, however, that the heart has one or more natural cardiac pacemakers that send electrical waves through the heart, causing the opening and closing of valves and muscular contraction, or pumping, of the ventricles near the normal adult rate of about 72 times per minute.

One particular electrical impulse (there may be others) originates in a small area in the upper part of the right atrium called the *sinus node.* Because it is definitely known that the contraction of the heart is electrically activated, tiny battery-powered devices called *artificial pacemakers* have been developed that can take the place of a natural pacemaker whose function has been impaired by heart injury or disease. Through electrodes implanted in heart tissue, such devices supply the correct beat for a defective heart. The bulk of the device is usually worn outside the body or is implanted just under the skin.

The fact that both ventricles give their push at the same time is very significant. It allows the entire heart muscle to rest between contractions—a rest period that adds up to a little more than half of a person's lifetime. Without this rest period, it is more than likely that our hearts would wear out considerably sooner than they do.

Blood Pressure

A physician's taking of blood pressure is based upon the difference between the heart's action at its period of momentary rest and at the moment of maximum work (the contraction or push). The split-second of maximum work, at the peak of the ventricles' contraction, is called the *systole*. The split-second of peak relaxation, when blood from the atria is draining into and filling up the ventricles, is called the *diastole*.

Blood pressure measures the force with which blood is passing through a major artery, such as one in the arm, and this pressure varies between a higher *systolic* pressure, corresponding to the heart's systole, and a lower *diastolic* pressure, reflecting the heart's diastole, or resting phase. The device with which a physician takes your blood pressure, called a *sphygmomanometer*, registers these higher and lower figures in numbers equivalent to the number of millimeters the force of your arterial blood would raise a column of mercury. The higher systolic force (pressure) is given first, then the diastolic figure. For example, 125/80 is within the normal range of blood pressure. Readings that are above the normal range—and stay elevated over a period of time—indicate a person has high blood pressure, or hypertension.

Hypertension has no direct connection with nervous tension, although the two may be associated in the same person. What it does indicate is that a heart is working harder than the average heart to push blood through the system. In turn, this may indicate the presence of a circulatory problem that might eventually endanger health. See also Ch. 9, *Diseases of the Circulatory System* and Ch. 10, *Heart Disease.*

The Digestive System and the Liver

A physician once remarked that a great many people seem to spend about half their time getting food into their digestive tracts and the other half worrying about how that food is doing on its travels. The physician was exaggerating, but he made his point.

The digestive tract has essentially one purpose: to break down food, both solid and fluid, into a form that can be used by the body. The food is used as energy to fuel daily activities or to nourish the various tissues that are always in the process of wearing out and needing replacement.

A normally functioning digestive tract, dealing with a reasonable variety and quantity of food, is designed to extract the maximum benefit from what we eat. Urine and feces are the waste products—things from which our body has selected everything that is of use.

Our digestive system's efficiency and economy in getting food into our bodies, to be utilized in all our living processes, can be attributed basically to three facts.

First, although the straight-line distance from the mouth to the bottom of the trunk is only two or three feet, the distance along the intestinal tract is about 10 times as great—30 feet—a winding, twisting, looping passageway that has more than enough footage to accommodate a number of ingeniously constructed way stations, checkpoints, and traffic-control devices.

Second, from the moment food enters the mouth, it is subjected to both chemical and mechanical actions that begin to break it apart, leading eventually to its reduction to submicro-

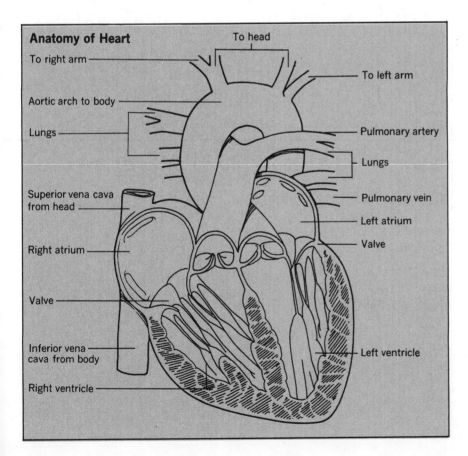

Anatomy of Heart

To head

To right arm

To left arm

Aortic arch to body

Lungs

Pulmonary artery

Lungs

Superior vena cava from head

Pulmonary vein

Left atrium

Right atrium

Valve

Valve

Inferior vena cava from body

Left ventricle

Right ventricle

scopic molecules that can be absorbed through the intestinal walls into the circulatory system.

Finally, each of the three main types of food—carbohydrates, fats, and proteins—receives special treatment that results in the body deriving maximum benefit from each.

Sensing the Right Kind of Food

Lips, eyes, and nose are generally given scant notice in discussions of the digestive process. But if we consider digestion to include selection of food and rejection of substances that might do us harm, then all three play very important roles.

The sensitive skin of our lips represents one of our first warning station that food may be harmful if taken into the mouth. It may tell us if a forkful of food is too hot or warn us of a concealed fishbone.

Our eyes, too, are important selection-rejection monitors for food. What else keeps us from sitting down to a crisp salad of poison ivy, or, less facetiously, popping a moldy piece of cake into our mouth?

As mammals' noses go, man's is a very inferior and insensitive organ. Nevertheless, we make good use of our sense of smell in the selection and enjoyment of foods. The nose adds to our enjoyment of favorite food and drink not only before they enter the mouth, but also after, because stimulation of the olfactory cells in the nasal passages combines with the stimulation of the taste cells on the tongue to produce the sensation-and-discrimination gradations of taste.

The Mouth: Saliva, Teeth, and Tongue

By the time food leaves the mouth and is pushed down into the gullet (or esophagus), it has already received a sampling of all the kinds of punishment and prodding that will be provided by the 30-foot tube that lies ahead of it. The chances are slim that any piece of food will end that journey in the same condition it started, but if it did it would have traveled those 30 tortuous feet at the rate of something less than two feet per hour. Normally, the elapsed time is between 17 and 25 hours.

As in the rest of the digestive tract, the mouth puts both chemical and mechanical apparatus to work on a bite of food. Saliva supplies the chemical action. Teeth and tongue, backed up by powerful sets of muscles, are the mashers, crushers, and prodders.

Saliva

The mere presence of food in our mouth—or even the smell, memory, or anticipation of it—sends signals to our brain, and our brain in turn sends messages back to a system of six salivary glands: one pair, called the *sublingual glands,* located under the tongue toward the front of the mouth; another pair, the *submaxillary* (or *submandibular*) glands, a bit behind and below them; and the largest, the *parotid glands,* tucked in the region where jaw meets neck behind the ear lobes.

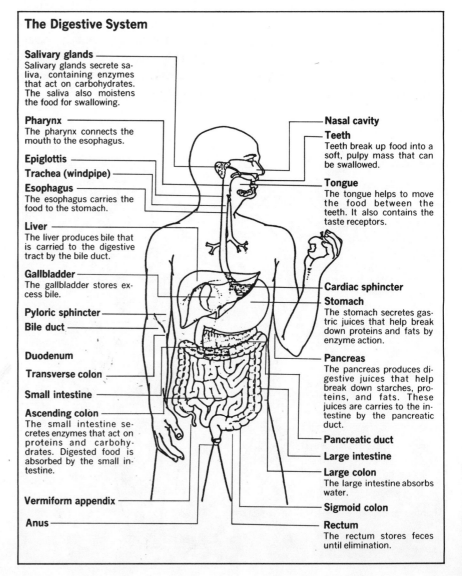

The Digestive System

Salivary glands
Salivary glands secrete saliva, containing enzymes that act on carbohydrates. The saliva also moistens the food for swallowing.

Pharynx
The pharynx connects the mouth to the esophagus.

Epiglottis

Trachea (windpipe)

Esophagus
The esophagus carries the food to the stomach.

Liver
The liver produces bile that is carried to the digestive tract by the bile duct.

Gallbladder
The gallbladder stores excess bile.

Pyloric sphincter

Bile duct

Duodenum

Transverse colon

Small intestine

Ascending colon
The small intestine secretes enzymes that act on proteins and carbohydrates. Digested food is absorbed by the small intestine.

Vermiform appendix

Anus

Nasal cavity

Teeth
Teeth break up food into a soft, pulpy mass that can be swallowed.

Tongue
The tongue helps to move the food between the teeth. It also contains the taste receptors.

Cardiac sphincter

Stomach
The stomach secretes gastric juices that help break down proteins and fats by enzyme action.

Pancreas
The pancreas produces digestive juices that help break down starches, proteins, and fats. These juices are carries to the intestine by the pancreatic duct.

Pancreatic duct

Large intestine

Large colon
The large intestine absorbs water.

Sigmoid colon

Rectum
The rectum stores feces until elimination.

Salivary Glands

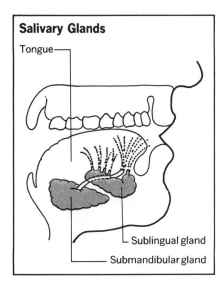

Tongue

Sublingual gland

Submandibular gland

Saliva is mainly composed of water, and water alone begins to soften up food so that it can pass more smoothly down the esophagus toward encounters with more powerful chemical agents.

There is also a very special substance in saliva, an enzyme called *ptyalin,* whose specific job is to begin the breakdown of one of the toughest kinds of food our digestive system has to handle—starches. Starch is a kind of carbohydrate, the group of foods from which we principally derive energy; but in order for the body to utilize carbohydrate, it must be broken down into simpler forms, which are called simply sugars. Ptyalin, then, begins the simplification of carbohydrate starch into carbohydrate sugar.

Saliva also does a favor or two for the dominating structures of the mouth—the tongue and teeth. Without its bathing action, the tongue's taste cells could not function up to par; and because it has a mild germicidal effect in addition to a simple rinsing action, saliva helps protect our mouth and teeth from bacterial infection.

Teeth

The role of the teeth in digestion can be summed up in one word: destruc-tion. What the wrecker's ball is to a standing building, our teeth are to a lump of solid food. They do the first, dramatic demolishing, leaving smaller fragments to be dealt with and disposed of in other ways.

Starting from the center of the mouth, we have two incisors on either side, top and bottom, followed by a canine, a couple of premolars, and three molars, the most backward of which (it never appears in some people) is the curiously named "wisdom" tooth, so called because it commonly appears as physical maturity is reached, at about 20 years of age.

Our teeth equip us for destroying chunks of food by a gamut of mechanical actions ranging from gripping and puncturing to grinding and pulverizing. The teeth in front—canines and incisors—do most of the gripping, ripping, and tearing, while the premolars and molars at the back of the jaws do the grinding.

The Tongue

The surface of the tongue is not smooth, but has a finely corrugated look and feel. This slightly sandpapery surface results from the presence of thousands of tiny papillae, little pyramid-shaped bumps. When we are young, the walls of a single papilla may contain up to 300 taste cells, or buds. As we get older, the maximum number of taste buds per papilla may decline to under 100.

There are four kinds of taste cells, distinguished by the type of taste message each sends to the brain: salty, sweet, sour, and bitter. Each of the four types is a narrow specialist in one type of taste. However, simultaneous or successive stimulation of all four types (combined almost always with information picked up by our sense of smell) can produce a tremendous variety of recognizable tastes—although perhaps not so many as some gourmets or wine-tasters might have us believe.

All four types of taste buds—salty, sweet, sour, and bitter—are found associated with papillae in all areas on the surface of the tongue; but there tend to be denser populations of one

The Transition from Breathing to Swallowing

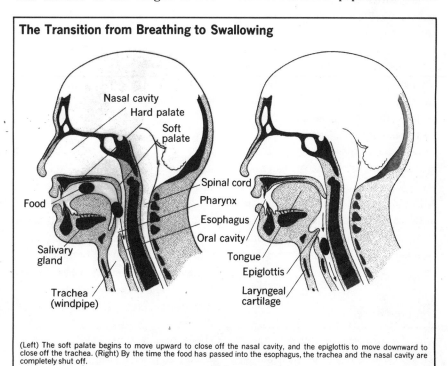

Nasal cavity
Hard palate
Soft palate
Spinal cord
Pharynx
Esophagus
Oral cavity
Food
Tongue
Salivary gland
Epiglottis
Laryngeal cartilage
Trachea (windpipe)

(Left) The soft palate begins to move upward to close off the nasal cavity, and the epiglottis to move downward to close off the trachea. (Right) By the time the food has passed into the esophagus, the trachea and the nasal cavity are completely shut off.

or the other kinds of taste cells in certain places. For example, salty and sweet cells predominate at the tip of the tongue and about halfway back along its sides; sour cells are more numerous all the way back along the sides; bitter buds are densest at the back of the tongue.

In addition to its tasting abilities, the tongue is a very versatile, flexible, and admirably shaped bundle of muscle. Not only can it flick out to moisten dry lips and ferret out and dislodge food particles in the oral cavity, but it also performs the first mechanical step in the all-important act of swallowing.

Swallowing

Swallow. You'll find that you feel the top of your tongue pressing up against the roof of your mouth (hard palate). You may never have thought about it consciously, but the pressing of the tongue against the hard palate prevents food from slipping to the front of your mouth—and also gives the food a good shove up and to the back of your mouth. At this point, the *soft palate* (from which the teardrop-shaped piece of tissue called the *uvula* hangs down) slips up to cover the passageway between mouth (oral cavity) and nasal cavity, nicely preventing the food from being misdirected toward your nose.

Once past the soft palate, the food is in the *pharynx*, a kind of anatomical traffic circle with two roads entering at the top, those from the mouth and nasal cavity, and two roads leading away from the bottom, the *trachea* (windpipe) and the *esophagus* or food tube.

The Epiglottis

A wedge of cartilage called the *epiglottis* protrudes from the trachea side, the side toward the front of the neck.

When we are breathing, the epiglottis is flattened up against the front wall of the pharynx, allowing free movement of air up and down the trachea. Simultaneously, the epiglottis helps to close off the entrance to the esophagus; a good part of the esophagus-closing work is done by a bundle of sinewy, elastic tissue we associate primarily with speech—the tissue of the vocal cords, otherwise known as the voice box or *larynx*. The laryngeal tissue is connected to the epiglottis above it, and supplies the epiglottis with most of its muscle for movement.

During the movement of a swallow, the larynx exerts an upward force against the epiglottis that serves to block off the trachea. At the same time, the larynx relaxes some of its pressure on the esophagus. Result: food enters the esophagus, where it is meant to go, and not the windpipe, which as we all know from having had something "go down the wrong way," produces an immediate fit of coughing.

Once we have swallowed, we lose almost completely the conscious ability to control the passage of food along the intestinal tract. Only when wastes reach the point of elimination do we begin to reassert some conscious control.

Peristalsis

The mechanical action called *peristalsis,* affected by muscles in the walls of all the organs of the gastrointestinal tract, first comes into play in the esophagus. Two layers of muscles intermesh in the intestinal walls: the inner layer encircles the esophagus in a series of rings; the outer layer stretches lengthwise along the tube. These two sets of muscles work in tandem to produce the basic action of persistalsis, called a *peristaltic wave.*

The alternative contraction and relaxation of the muscles—closing behind swallowed food and opening in front of it—combine to move both liquid and solid food (medical term, *bolus*) along the digestive tract. Gravity, in a sense, is left behind once food enters the esophagus. Because of peristalsis, we can swallow lying down or even standing on our heads; and astronauts are able to eat in near zero-gravity or under weightless conditions.

Peristalsis has another important function besides moving food through the body. The constricting and relaxing muscles serve also to knead, churn, and pummel the solid remains of the food left after our teeth have done their best.

Digestive Sphincters

If you think about it, the gastrointestinal tract has to be equipped with a number of gates that can open or shut, depending on the amount of food that is passing through. Otherwise, the food might push through so fast that little nourishment could be extracted from it: we would feel hungry one minute and glutted the next. The gastrointestinal tract is thus equipped at critical junctures with a number of muscular valves, or *sphincters,* which, usually under the direction of the autonomic nervous system, can regulate the movement of food through the digestive tube. Another function of a sphincter is to prevent backflow of partially digested food.

The muscles of a sphincter are often described as "pursestring muscles" because the way they draw together the sides of the digestive tube is roughly similar to drawing up the strings of a purse. The first of these pursestring valves occurs at the *cardia,* the opening where the esophagus meets the stomach, and is called the *cardiac sphincter,* from its location almost directly in front of the heart. (But there is no physical connection.)

Another important muscle ring is the *pyloric sphincter,* at the opening called the *pylorus,* located at the other end of the stomach, at the connection between stomach and small intestine. The release of waste from the rectum is controlled, partly voluntarily, by an *anal sphincter,* located at the *anus,* which marks the end of the tract.

The Stomach

About ten inches down the esophagus, the food we swallow must pass the cardiac sphincter. Then the food, by now fairly well diced and mashed, passes into the stomach.

Inelegant as it sounds, the stomach is best described as a rough, leather-skinned balloon. When empty, its skin shrivels around itself like a deflated balloon; but when "pumped up" by a hearty meal, the stomach becomes a plump, J-shaped bag about a foot long and six inches wide, holding about two quarts of food and drink.

The Passage of Food through the Stomach

Although its food-processing function tends to get more attention, the stomach's role as a storage reservoir is equally important. A moderate, well-rounded meal with a good blend of carbohydrates, proteins, and fats takes usually a minimum of three hours to pass out of the pyloric sphincter into the small intestine—more if the meal is heavy in fats and rich foods. Thus, a meal that might take us 15 minutes to eat, may take up to 20 times as long to pass from the stomach into the small intestine. This decelerating of food's rate of passage has two very significant re-

sults: first, it allows time for the food-processing activities within the stomach; and second, it releases food (in a mushy form called *chyme*) in small, well-spaced amounts that can be efficiently handled by the small intestine.

Although the stomach is not an absolutely essential organ—a person can live a full life with part or even all of it removed—it is a tremendous convenience. Without a stomach, frequent, carefully selected, well-chewed small feedings rather than "three square meals a day" are necessary so as not to overburden the small intestine, which can handle only a small quantity of food, well-mashed, at one time. If too much food goes directly to the small intestine, only so much nourishment (carbohydrates, proteins, fats) per meal can be supplied to the body, with the result that we would be weak from hunger after going a few hours without eating.

It will come as no surprise to know that the food processing done in the stomach is both mechanical and chemical. The three layers of crisscrossing muscles in the stomach walls are rarely still. They contract and relax continually, squeezing, pummeling, and mixing the stomach's contents into chyme. So active and relentless is the stomach's muscular activity that it actually "chews up" pieces of food that have been swallowed too hastily.

Stomach Chemicals

The various chemicals found in the stomach are produced and secreted into the stomach cavity by some 40 million gland cells that line the interior stomach walls. The constant wiggling and jouncing of the stomach helps to mix these chemicals thoroughly into the food. Each of the chemicals is secreted by a special type of cell and has a specific function. They include the digestive enzymes pepsin, rennin, and lipase; hydrochloric acid; and wa-

tery mucus.

A look at the special assignments of rennin, pepsin, hydrochloric acid, and mucus—and how they interact with and depend upon one another—provides a good glimpse into the elegant and complex chemical events that occur when the stomach encounters a swallow of food.

Rennin and Pepsin

Rennin, well known to cheesemakers, has essentially one task: to turn milk

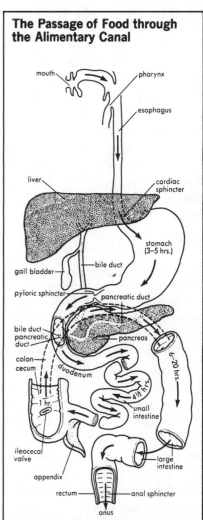

The Passage of Food through the Alimentary Canal

This drawing indicates the duration of each digestive process. Food enters the mouth and is passed through the pharynx and esophagus into the stomach, where it is partly digested. The small intestine completes digestion and absorbs digested food. The large intestine absorbs excess water. Indigestible residue collects in the rectum for later disposal.

into milk curds. But the curds are not ready to pass on to the small intestine until they are further dismantled by *pepsin*. Pepsin has other duties as well: one of them is to begin the breakdown of proteins. But pepsin can only begin to split up protein foods after they have been worked on by *hydrochloric acid*.

Hydrochloric Acid

Hydrochloric acid is a corrosive substance and, except in very dilute strengths, could quite literally eat away the lining of the stomach. (This is apparently what happens in cases of gastric ulcers.) Mucus secretions, with the help of fluids in the food itself, dilute the hydrochloric acid to a point where (in a normal stomach) it is rendered harmless. Even so, the normal, healthy condition inside our stomach is slightly acid. The slight acidity of the stomach serves to inhibit the growth of organisms such as bacteria.

The Small Intestine

By the time food-turned-chyme gets through the pyloric sphincter, it has already traveled about two-and-a-half feet: about 6 inches from lips to epiglottis; 10 or 12 inches down the esophagus; and about a foot through the stomach. But at this point it has actually traveled less than one-tenth of the gastrointestinal (GI) tract, and the longest stretch lies just ahead: the 20-plus feet of the small intestine, so named because of its relatively small one-to-two inch diameter. The preparation of food particles to pass through the walls of the GI tract is completed in the small intestine—almost completed, in fact, before the chyme has traveled the first foot of the small intestine. By the time it leaves the small intestine, chyme has

given up virtually all its nutrients. In other words, the process called *absorption* or *assimilation* has taken place: the nutrients have left the GI tract for other parts of the body via the circulating blood and lymph. What passes on to the large intestine is principally waste and water.

The small intestine is somewhat arbitrarily divided into three sections: the *duodenum,* the *jejunum,* and the *ileum.*

The Duodenum

Within this horseshoe loop, eight to ten inches long and about two inches in diameter, more chemical interactions are concentrated than in any other section of the GI tract. One of the first jobs in the duodenum is to neutralize the acidity of the chyme. The final steps of digestion, and the absorption of food through the intestinal lining, proceed best in a slightly alkaline environment.

The alkaline juices needed to neutralize the acidity of the chyme come mainly from the liver in the form of bile. Bile produced by the liver but not needed immediately in the duodenum is stored in concentrated form in the gallbladder, a pouchlike, three-inch-long organ. On signal from the autonomic nervous system, the membranous muscular walls of the gallbladder contract, squeezing concentrated, highly alkaline bile into a short duct that leads to the duodenum. Bile components are indispensable for the digestion and absorption of stubborn fatty materials.

Through a duct from the pancreas, a host of pancreatic enzymes, capable of splitting apart large, tough molecules of carbohydrate, protein, and fat, enters the duodenum. These digestive enzymes manufactured by the pancreas are the most powerful in the GI tract.

What triggers the production of

bile and pancreatic juice for the duodenum? Apparently, it is a two-step process involving hormones. When the stomach walls secrete hydrochloric acid on the arrival of food, hormones are released; they travel to the liver and pancreas with instructions to step up their production of digestive juices.

Still other strong enzymes are secreted by the walls of the duodenum and join the bile and pancreatic enzymes in the duodenum.

Thus, in the not quite foot-long tube of the duodenum, the final breakdown of food—digestion—reaches a dramatic climax. The nutrients in the food eaten some hours ago have almost all been reduced to molecules small enough to be absorbed through the intestinal walls into the bloodstream. Carbohydrates are reduced to simpler sugars; proteins to amino acids; and fats to fatty acids and glycerol.

Some absorption of these nutrients occurs in the duodenum, but the far greater proportion takes place in the next two, longer sections of the small intestine: the eight- to ten-foot jejunum and the twelve-foot ileum. Likewise, some oversize food molecules that get past the duodenum may be digested further along in their passage through the small intestine.

The Jejunum

As peristalsis pushes the nutrient broth out of the duodenum and into the first reaches of the jejunum, a gradual change in the appearance of the intestinal lining is evident. Greater and greater number of *villi*—microscopic, hairlike structures—sprout from the already bumpy walls of the intestinal lining into the GI tube.

The Villi

The villi (singular, *villus*) have the primary responsibility for absorbing amino acids (from protein), sugars (from carbohydrates), and fatty acids and glycerol (from fats) from the digested contents of the small intestine, and starting them on their way to other parts of the body. What the villi do not remove from the chyme—such as the cellulose fragments of fruits and vegetables—passes on to the large intestine in a thin, watery soup almost completely lacking in nutritional value.

Gland cells near the bottom of a villus secrete various enzymes, mucus, and other substances that perform digestive "mop-up operations" along the whole length of the small intestine.

The Ileum

In this third and final 12-foot section of the small intestine, villi line the walls in such profusion that the intestinal lining resembles, under moderate magnification, nothing so much as a plush, velvety carpet. The greatest numbers of the estimated five or six million villi in the small intestine are found along the lining of the ileum, making it the primary absorption site of the GI tract.

Also adding to the ileum's absorption efficiency is its gradually narrowing diameter (just one inch at its junction with the large intestine), which helps to keep the chyme always in close contact with the swishing villi. The end of the ileum is marked by the *ileocecal valve,* beyond which lies the first bulge of the large intestine, the *cecum.*

Principally because of vigorous peristaltic contractions and relaxations, the walls of the small intestine are always moving like the walls within some spasmodically flexing, nightmarish tunnel. Attached to the intestinal walls, the villi, too, are always in restless motion: waving and

thrashing, protracting and retracting, even growing thinner or fatter.

Although the entire distance through the small intestine, from the pyloric sphincter to the ileocecal valve at the junction with the large intestine, is only a bit over 20 feet, the villi give the small intestine's internal lining a relatively gigantic surface area—over 100 square feet. This is about five times the surface area of our body's skin. Of course, the greatly enlarged surface area gives the small intestine lining that much more space in which to absorb nutrients.

The small intestine is supported in the abdomen by a fan-shaped web of tissues called the *mesentery.* Attached at the back of the abdomen, the mesentery connects to the small intestine at various points, and yet allows it some freedom to squirm and sway—much like the V network of ropes that attaches either end of a hammock to a tree. Nerve fibers and blood vessels also reach the small intestine via the mesentery.

The Liver, Gallbladder, and Pancreas

These three organs all share a common function—sending digestive substances to the duodenum—although, except in the case of the gallbladder, it is not their only function. Lying outside the GI tract proper, they nevertheless are indispensable in the processes of digestion and absorption. Digestive fluids from all three converge like tributaries of a river at the common bile duct, and their flow from there into the duodenum is controlled by a sphincter muscle-ring separating the duodenum and common bile duct.

From the liver, bile drips into the *hepatic duct,* which soon meets the *cystic duct* arriving from the gallbladder. Converging, they form one duct,

the *common bile duct,* which meets the *pancreatic duct,* carrying enzymatic fluid from the pancreas. Like a smaller river meeting a larger one, the pancreatic duct loses its own name at this confluence and becomes part of the common bile duct, which empties on demand into the duodenum. When the sphincter of the bile duct is closed, bile from the liver is forced to back up into the cystic duct, and eventually into the gallbladder. There it is stored and concentrated until needed, when it flows back down the cystic duct.

The Liver

Four pounds of highly efficient chemical-processing tissues, the liver is the largest solid organ in the body. You can locate it by placing your left hand over your right, lowermost ribs; your hand then just about covers the area of the liver. More than any other organ, the liver enables our bodies to benefit from the food we eat. Without it, digestion would be impossible, and the conversion of food into living cells and energy practically nonexistent. Insofar as they affect our body's handling of food—all the many processes that go by the collective name of nutrition—the liver's functions can be roughly divided into those that break down food molecules and those that build up or reconstitute these nutrients into a form that the body can use or store efficiently.

Breaking Down Food Molecules

Bile, as we have seen, assists in the destruction of large food molecules in the small intestine, enabling absorption of nutrients by the villi. Bile acts to increase alkalinity, breaking down big fat molecules; stimulates peristalsis; and prevents food from putrefying within the digestive tract. Unusable portions of the bile, destined to be eliminated as waste, include excess cholesterol, fats, and various components of dead disintegrated cells. Pigments from dead cells in bile give feces its normal, dark, yellow-brown color. Other cell fragments in bile, especially iron from disintegrated red blood cells, are reclaimed from the intestines and eventually make their way via the bloodstream to other parts of the body, where they are built into new cells.

Reconstituting Nutrients

Oddly enough, the liver rebuilds some of the proteins and carbohydrates that the bile has just so effectively helped to break down in the digestive tract. But this is really not so strange as it sounds. The types of proteins and carbohydrates that can be used by man for cell-rebuilding and energy are usually somewhat different in fine structure from those in food. Thus, the liver receives the basic building blocks of proteins and carbohydrates—amino acids and sugars— and with them builds up molecules and cells that can be utilized by the human body. The amino acids and sugars reach the liver through the *portal vein,* which is the great collection tube for nutrient-carrying blood returning from capillaries along the stomach and small intestine.

Glycogen and Glucose

In the liver, sugars from the small intestine are converted into a special substance called *glycogen;* amino acids are made available as needed for building new cells to replace the cells that are always naturally dying in a healthy normal body. Glycogen, simply speaking, is the liver's solution to a difficult space and storage problem. The form of carbohydrate the body can use best is a sugar called *glucose,*

but the liver isn't large enough to store the necessary amount of glucose. The answer is glycogen, a tidy, compact sugar molecule that the liver can store in great quantities. When a call comes from any part of the body for glucose, the liver quickly converts some glycogen to glucose and releases it into the bloodstream. By this mechanism, healthy blood sugar levels are maintained.

The liver also builds up human fats from fatty acids and glycerol, packs them off to storage, then reverses the process when necessary by breaking down body fats into forms that can serve as fuel to be burned by the body for energy.

Other Functions

In addition to its functions closely related to digestion and nutrition, the liver also serves as a storehouse and processor of vitamins and minerals— it is, in fact, the manufacturer of vitamin A. It can remove many toxic substances from the blood and render their poisons harmless. It picks up spent red blood cells from the circulation and dismantles them; and it continually manufactures new blood elements.

The liver is also a manufacturing site for *cholesterol,* a substance belonging to the class of body chemicals called steroids. Above-normal levels of cholesterol in the blood have been linked to hardening of the arteries and heart disease; but cholesterol in the proper amounts is needed by almost every tissue in the body. Some brain and spinal tissues, for example, have cholesterol as one of their main structural components.

With all these vital chemical activities and more, the liver might be expected to be a most delicate and fragile organ. In a sense it is: minor liver damage from one cause or another is thought to be fairly common. But

what saves our lives (and us) is that we have a great deal more of it than we need for a normal healthy life. Before symptoms of a liver deficiency appear, more than 50 percent of the liver cells may be destroyed. Furthermore, the liver has a great capacity for regeneration, rebuilding diseased tissues with new liver cells.

The Gallbladder

Bile stored in the gallbladder is much more concentrated and thicker than bile that is fresh from the liver. This allows the three-inch gallbladder to store a great deal of bile components. But the thickening process can also create problems in the form of extremely painful gallstones, which are dried, crystallized bile. Fortunately, the entire gallbladder can be removed with little or no lasting ill effect. All that is missing is a small storage sac for bile.

The Pancreas

This manufacturer of powerful digestive enzymes, only six inches long, resembles a branchlet heavily laden with ripe berries. Its important role in digestion is often overshadowed by the fact that it also manufactures the hormone *insulin.* The pancreas cells that manufacture digestive enzymes are completely different from those that manufacture insulin. The latter are grouped into little clusters called the *islets of Langerhans,* which are discussed under *The Endocrine Glands* in this chapter.

The Large Intestine

The large intestine, also called the large bowel, is shaped like a great, lumpy, drooping question mark— arching, from its beginning at the ileocecal valve, over the folds of the small intestine, then curving down and descending past more coiled small intestine to the anus, which marks the end of the GI tract. From ileocecal valve to anus, the large intestine is five to six feet in length.

The junction between the ileum and the *cecum,* the first section of the large intestine, occurs very low in the abdomen, normally on the right-hand side. The cecum is a bowl-like receptacle at the bottom of the colon, the longest section of the large intestine.

Just below the entrance of the ileum, a dead-end tube dangles down from the cecum. This is the *appendix vermiformis* (Latin, "worm-shaped appendage") commonly known as the appendix. Three to six inches long and one-third inch in diameter, the appendix may get jammed with stray pieces of solid food, become infected, swell, and rupture, spewing infection into the abdominal cavity. This is why early diagnosis of *appendicitis* and removal (*appendectomy*) are critically important.

Sections of the Colon

The colon is divided into three sections by pronounced *flexures,* or bends, where the colon makes almost right-angle changes of direction. Above the bowl of the cecum, the *ascending colon* rises almost vertically for about a foot and a half.

Then there is a flexure in the colon, after which the *transverse colon* travels horizontally for a couple of feet along a line at navel height. At another flexure, the colon turns vertically down again, giving the name of *descending colon* to this approximately two feet of large intestine. At the end of the descending colon, the large intestine executes an S-shaped curve, the *sigmoid flexure,* after which the remaining several inches of large intestine are known as the *rectum.*

Some people confuse the terms rectum and anus: the rectum refers specifically to the last section of the large intestinal tube, between sigmoid flexure and the anal sphincters, while the anus refers only to the opening controlled by the outlet valves of the large intestine. These valves consist of two ringlike voluntary muscles called anal sphincters.

Any solid materials that pass into the large intestine through the ileocecal valve (which prevents backflow into the small intestine) are usually indigestible, such as cellulose, or substances that have been broken down in the body and blood in the normal process of cell death and renewal, such as some bile components. But what the cecum mainly receives is water.

Functions of the Large Intestine

The principal activity of the large intestine—other than as a channel for elimination of body wastes—is as a temporary storage area for water, which is then reabsorbed into the circulation through the walls of the colon. Villi are absent in the large intestine, and peristalsis is much less vigorous than in the small intestine.

As water is absorbed, the contents of the large intestine turn from a watery soup into the semisolid feces. Meanwhile, bacteria—which colonize the normal colon in countless millions—have begun to work on and decompose the remaining solid materials. These bacteria do no harm as long as they remain inside the large intestine, and the eliminated feces is heavily populated with them. Nerve endings in the large intestine signal the brain that it is time for a bowel movement.

The Peritoneum

Lining the entire abdominal cavity, as well as the digestive and other abdominal organs, is a thin, tough, lubricated membrane called the *peritoneum.* In addition to protecting and supporting the abdominal organs, the peritoneum permits these organs to slip and slide against each other without any harm from friction. The peritoneum also contains blood and lymph vessels that serve the digestive organs. See Ch. 11, *Diseases of the Digestive System.*

The Respiratory System and the Lungs

The heart, by its construction and shape, tells us a great deal about the lungs and respiration.

Interaction between Heart and Lungs

The heart is divided vertically by a wall called a septum into right (your right) and left parts. The right part is smaller than the left: its muscles only have to pump blood a few inches to the lungs, while the muscles of the left half have to pump blood to the whole body.

The function of the right half of our heart is to receive oxygen-poor blood from the veins of the body. Venous blood empties into the top-right chamber, or right atrium, of the heart, and the right ventricle pumps that oxygen-poor blood (via the pulmonary artery) to the lungs, where the blood, passing through minute capillaries, picks up oxygen.

From the lungs, the oxygen-rich blood flows back into the heart's left atrium via the pulmonary veins; and from the left atrium, the oxygen-rich blood drains into the left ventricle,

Interaction between Heart and Lungs

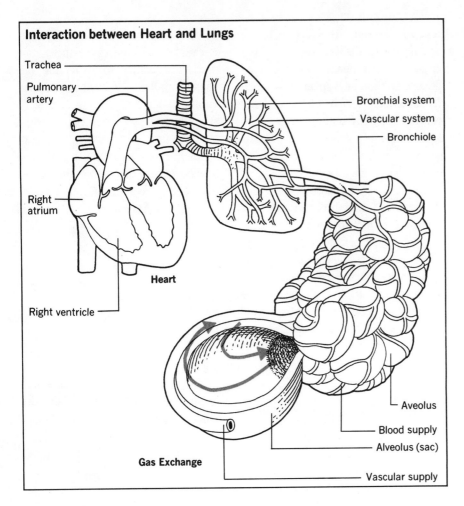

Trachea

Pulmonary artery

Bronchial system

Vascular system

Bronchiole

Right atrium

Heart

Right ventricle

Aveolus

Blood supply

Alveolus (sac)

Gas Exchange

Vascular supply

conditions, the carbon dioxide carried by the hemoglobin in our blood to the lungs diffuses (as tiny gaseous "bubbles") across both the wall of a capillary and the wall of an alveolus.

Once inside the sac of the alveolus, carbon dioxide is ready to be exhaled from the body by "breathing out." One indication of just how well this system works is the fact that the air we exhale has roughly 100 times more carbon dioxide than the air we breathe in.

At the same time that hemoglobin dumps carbon dioxide at the interface of the capillary and alveolus walls, it picks up the oxygen made available from inhaled fresh air that has reached the alveoli. The molecular oxygen bubbles cross the membranes in the same way—but in the opposite direction—as the carbon dioxide.

Hemoglobin in the capillaries picks up the oxygen and carries it via veins leading away from the lungs, to the left atrium of the heart.

Essential Role of Moisture

The alveolar membranes are supplied with a thin film of moisture that is absolutely indispensable to the exchange of gases in the lungs. As in so many of our body's reactions, our evolutionary descent from water-dwelling ancestors is revealed by the wet environment demanded if our lungs are to supply our body with oxygen.

from whence it is pumped via the aorta to the body.

The blood pumped to the lungs by the right ventricle is oxygen-poor blood; it has given up its oxygen to the cells that need it around the body. But this "used blood" is rich in something else—carbon dioxide. As the body's cells have taken oxygen, they have given up carbon dioxide to the circulating blood. For both oxygen and carbon dioxide, the "carrier" has been *hemoglobin,* a complex iron-protein substance that is part of our red blood cells.

Capillaries and Alveoli

The pulmonary artery carrying this lung-bound blood soon branches into smaller and smaller vessels, and eventually into microscopic capillaries that reach into every crook and crev-

ice of the lungs.

In the lungs, the walls of the capillaries touch the walls of equally microscopic structures called *alveoli* (singular, *alveolus*). The alveoli are the smallest air sacs of the lungs. These tiny, expandable air cells are the destination of every breath of air we take. Estimates of the total number of alveoli in both our lungs vary between 300 million and a billion—in any case, we normally have several hundred million of them.

Carbon Dioxide and Oxygen Exchange

Where they meet, the membranous walls of both a capillary and an alveolus are both about as thin as any living tissue can be—a thickness that is only the width of one cell. Under such

The Alveoli

Bronchiole

Pulmonary artery

Pulmonary vein

Cross section of alveolus

Capillaries on alveolus

The branches of the pulmonary tree terminate in the alveoli, grapelike clusters of air sacs covered by capillaries, where the gaseous exchange occurs.

Respiration at the One-Cell Level

Oxygen molecules, then, are carried to the body's cells by the hemoglobin of the arterial blood pumped by the heart's left ventricle. But how does a cell take oxygen from the blood and use it?

Exchange of Gases

The transfer of oxygen from blood to cell is accomplished in much the same way as the exhanges that take place in the lungs. The circulating arterial blood has a surplus of oxygen; the cells have a surplus of carbon dioxide. When the oxygen-rich blood reaches the finest capillaries, only the very thinnest membranous walls (of cell and capillary) separate it from the carbon-dioxide-rich cells. As in the lungs, both these gases (dissolved in water) diffuse through these thinnest of membranes: the oxygen into the cell, the carbon dioxide into the blood for eventual deposit in the alveoli, and exhalation.

Within the cell, the oxygen is needed so that food, the body's fuel, can be burned to produce energy. At the cellular level, the most convenient and common food is a fairly simple carbohydrate molecule called glucose.

Conversion of Carbohydrates into Energy

Energy is locked into a carbohydrate molecule such as glucose in the form of chemical bonds between its atoms. If one of these bonds is broken—say, a bond holding together a carbon and a hydrogen atom—a bit of pent-up energy is released as if, in a stale-mated tug of war, the rope suddenly broke and both teams went hurtling off a few feet in opposite directions. This is precisely the effect of respiration within a cell: the cell "breaks the ropes" holding together a carbo-hydrate molecule. The result is the release of energy—either as body heat or to power other activities within the cell.

It is useful—but a somewhat misleading oversimplification—to consider cellular respiration as a type of burning, or combustion. When a typical cell burns food, a carbohydrate molecule (glucose) together with molecules of oxygen are changed into carbon dioxide and water. During this change, chemical energy is released—energy that has been trapped, as we have seen, in the carbohydrate molecule. That complex, energy-rich molecule has been dismantled into the simpler molecules of carbon dioxide (CO_2) and water (H_2O). Oxygen is necessary here just as it is in fiery combustion. But the energy released here, instead of rushing out as heat and flame, is used to power the living activities of the cell.

This description of cellular respiration is all right in principle, but the trouble is this: if it all happened at once—if carbohydrate was so abruptly dismantled, split up at one stroke to water and carbon dioxide—such a great amount of energy would be released that the cell would simply burn itself up. As one biologist has said, the cell would be in exactly the same position as a wood furnace built of wood.

What protects the cell is its army of enzymes. These remarkable protein molecules combine briefly with energy-containing food molecules, causing them to break down bit by bit, so that energy is released gradually rather than all at once.

Carbon Dioxide— Precious Waste

In most of our minds, oxygen tends to be the hero of respiration and car-bon dioxide the villain or at least the undesirable waste gas. This isn't really a fair picture. While it is true that too much carbon dioxide would act as a poison in our body, it is also true that we must always have a certain amount of the gas dissolved in our tissues. If we did not, two potentially fatal events could occur. First, our blood chemistry, especially its delicate acid-alkali balance, would get completely out of control. Second—and something of a paradox—the body's whole automatic system of regulating breathing would be knocked out.

It is the level of carbon dioxide in the bloodstream that controls our breathing. This level is continuously being monitored by the autonomic nervous system, specifically by the lower brain's "breathing center" in the medulla at the top of the spinal cord. When the level of carbon dioxide in our body goes above a certain level, signals from the medulla force us to breathe. Almost everybody has played, "How long can you hold your breath?" and knows that, past a certain point, it becomes impossible *not* to breathe. When you are holding your breath, the unexhaled carbon dioxide rapidly builds up in your system until the breathing center is besieged with signals that say "Breathe!" And you do.

Our Big Breathing Muscle: The Diaphragm

What gets air into and out of our lungs? The answer may seem as obvious as breathing in and out. But except for those rare instances when we consciously regulate our breathing pattern—which physicians call "force breathing"—we do not decide when to inhale and when to exhale. And even when we do force-breathe, it is not primarily the action of opening the

Diaphragm

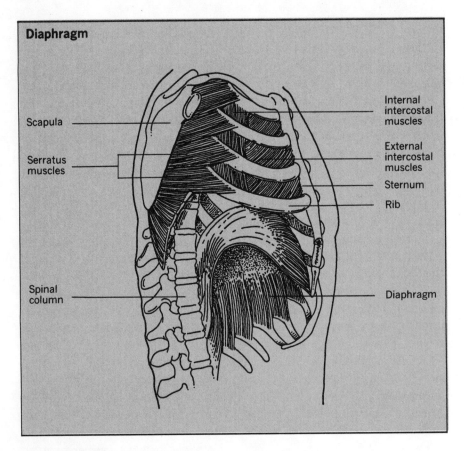

Scapula

Serratus
muscles

Spinal
column

Internal
intercostal
muscles

External
intercostal
muscles

Sternum

Rib

Diaphragm

mouth and gulping in air, then blowing it out, that gets air down the windpipe and into the alveoli of the lungs. The main work of inhaling and exhaling is done by the contraction and relaxation of the big helmet-shaped muscle on which the lungs rest and which marks the "floor" of the chest or thoracic cavity and the "ceiling" of the abdominal cavity. This muscle is the *diaphragm*.

It is the diaphragm that causes the lungs to swell and fill with fresh air, then partially collapse to expel used gases. The muscles and tendons of the sinewy diaphragm are attached at the back to the spinal column, at the front to the breastbone (*sternum*), and at the lower sides to the lower ribs.

The diaphragm contracts and relaxes on orders from the brain's breathing center, orders that are carried along the pathways of the autonomic nervous system. When the medulla sends messages to the

breathing muscles to contract, the diaphragm is pulled downward, enlarging the space filled by the lungs. This creates a temporary partial vacuum, into which air rushes, inflating and expanding the lungs. When the diaphragm relaxes, the lung space is reduced, pushing air out.

Other Breathing Muscles

The diaphragm muscle's leading role in breathing is supported by several other muscles that play minor parts. Among these are the *intercostal muscles* between the ribs that give the rib cage a slight push upward and outward, enlarging the thoracic cavity, and the *serratus muscles,* which are mainly muscular sheaths along the ribs, to which other muscles are attached.

The Trachea and the Lungs

The right lung (your right) is somewhat bigger than the left. The lungs

hang in the chest attached to the windpipe or *trachea.*

The Trachea

The trachea itself branches off at the back of the throat, or *pharynx,* where the epiglottis prevents food from entering the trachea and channels swallowed food along its proper route, the esophagus. The top part of the trachea forms the voice box or *larynx,* made up of vocal cords—actually two flaps of cartilage, muscle, and membranous tissue that protrude into the windpipe—whose vibrations in response to air exhaled from the lungs give us our voice.

Below the larynx, the trachea descends five or six inches to a spot just about directly behind your breastbone, where the first of many thousands of branchings into *bronchi, bronchioles,* and alveoli occurs. C-shaped rings of cartilage give the trachea both support and flexibility. Running your finger down the front of your neck, you can feel the bumps made by the cartilage rings.

Above the base of the trachea in midchest the lungs arch on either side like giant butterfly wings, then fall to fill out the bottom of each side of the thoracic cavity.

The Pleural Membranes

Both lungs are encased in moist, clinging, tissue-thin membrane called the *pleura,* which also lines the inside of the thoracic cavity where it comes into contact with the pleural coating of the lungs. The slippery pleural membranes hold tightly to each other, because there is an air lock or vacuum between them, but at the same time are free to slide over each other. The principle is the same as that illustrated by moistening the surfaces of two pieces of plate glass and placing the moistened surfaces together: the two pieces of glass will slide over each other but will resist being pried apart, because a partial vacuum exists between them.

The Pleural Cavity

The vacuum space between the pleura of the lung and the pleura of the thoracic cavity—although it is normally not a space at all—is called the *pleural cavity*. Each lung has its own pleural membrane: that of one lung does not interconnect with the other, so that one pleura may be injured without affecting the other.

It is extremely fortunate for us that the pleural linings both stick fast and can slide along each other's surfaces. Although the lungs are virtually without muscle, they are extremely elastic and in their natural condition are stretched fairly taut, held to the sides of the thoracic cavity by the suction of the pleura.

Collapsed Lung

Should this suction be broken and the pleural linings pull apart, the lung would shrink up like a deflated balloon. Such a condition, caused by the rush of outside air into the pleural cavity, is known medically as *pneumothorax* and causes a lung collapse. Violent injuries such as gun and stab wounds, various lung diseases, and obstructions of the breathing tubes can cause a lung or portion of a lung to collapse.

In the surgical procedure called *artificial pneumothorax,* a physician deliberately injects air between the pleural linings to collapse a portion of a lung. This is done to rest a lung in severe diseases such as tuberculosis, or to control heavy bleeding within the thoracic cavity.

Pleurisy

The intense chest pains called *pleurisy* are caused by inflammation of the pleura. The pleural linings lose their slipperiness and the increased friction stimulates pain receptors in the pleural lining of the chest. There are, however, no pain receptors in the lungs' pleural linings nor in the lungs themselves: this is why pain is not an early warning signal of lung cancer.

The Bronchi

Just behind the breastbone and just in front of the heart, the trachea divides into the right bronchus and the left bronchus, leading respectively to the right and left lungs. These are the primary two *bronchi* or *bronchial tubes*. Each is the main trunk of a bronchial tree that serves its respective lung.

Soon after leaving the trachea, each bronchus branches repeatedly into smaller tubes called *bronchioles,* which in turn branch into alveolar ducts, which terminate finally with the hundreds of millions of microscopic air sacs called alveoli, discussed at the beginning of this section. The alveoli are the site of the all-important exchange of carbon dioxide and oxygen.

Lobes and Segments

The larger right lung has three distinctive sections, or *lobes*—upper, middle, and lower. The left lung has only an upper and lower lobe. The lobes themselves are divided into smaller segments. Medically, these lobes and segments are important because they are somewhat independent of each other and can be damaged or removed surgically, as in operations for lung cancer, usually without damaging the function of adjacent, healthy segments or lobes.

The fact that a lung segment, lobe, or even an entire lung can be removed implies that we have plenty of reserve lung tissue, and this is indeed the case. When we are at rest, we use only about one-tenth of our total lung capacity. The total surface area exposed within our lungs to outside air is, amazingly, 600 square feet. This compares to a mere 20 square feet of skin surface. To appreciate the incredibly intricate, lacelike finery of the lungs' structure, we need only know that those 600 square feet of surface area are contained within two organs that together weigh only two-and-a-half pounds.

Oxygen Requirements

How much air do we breathe, and how much oxygen do we absorb into our body from the air? A normal, moderately active person breathes in and out (a complete respiration or breath cycle) about 18 times a minute; that is, the diaphragm contracts and relaxes 18 times a minute, or something over 25,000 times every day. At about four-fifths of a pint of air per breath cycle, this means that we inhale and exhale about 20,000 pints, or 10,000 quarts, or 2,500 gallons of air every day.

Only a very small proportion of this volume is oxygen that finds its way into our bloodstream: about a pint every minute in normal, quiet breathing, a little over 1,400 pints, or 700 quarts, or 175 gallons of oxygen every day. The amount of oxygen our lungs are capable of delivering to our body, however, varies tremendously: during sleep a person may need only a half-pint of oxygen per minute, half the average, while the lungs of a hard-driving athlete striving to break the mile record can deliver up to five quarts to the bloodstream—ten times the average.

At any given time, there are about two quarts of oxygen circulating in our blood. This is why a stoppage of breathing has an upper time limit of about four minutes before it causes irreversible damage or death. With our body needing about a pint of oxygen every minute for normal functioning, we have about four minutes before we use up the oxygen dissolved in our blood and other tissues.

Pollution Control— Filters, Cleaners, and Traps

Air pollution being what it is these days, it is fortunate that we have several natural devices that serve to filter out and wash away most of the impurities in the air we inhale.

Air gets into the lungs from outside about equally well via the nose or mouth. The mouth offers the advantage of getting more air in at a faster rate—absolutely a must if we have to push our body physically. But the nose has more and better equipment for cleaning air before it reaches the trachea. Via the mouth, air must only pass over a few mucous membranes and the tonsils, which can collect only so many germs and impurities.

Nose Filter System

Air taken in through the nose, however, first meets the "guard hairs" (*vibrissae*) of the nostrils, and then must circulate through the nasal cavity, a kind of cavern framed by elaborate scroll-shaped bones called *turbinates,* and lined with mucus-secreting membranes and waving, hairlike fibers called *cilia.* Foreign particles are caught by the cilia and carried away by the mucus, which drains slowly down the back of the throat.

It would be nice to be able to ascribe an important function to the eight *paranasal sinuses,* four on either side of the nose: the headache and discomfort of sinusitis might then be more bearable. But these "holes in the head" seem to exist simply to cause us trouble; for example—swell-

ing to close the nasal air passages, making it impossible to breathe, as recommended, through the nose.

Filter System beyond the Nose

The cleansing and filtering action started in the nose and mouth does not stop there, but is repeated wherever air travels along the air passages of the lungs. Cilia project inward from the walls of even the tiniest bronchioles of the lungs, and impurities are carried from the alveoli on films of mucus that move ever back toward the trachea for expulsion—as when we cough. See also Ch. 12, *Diseases of the Respiratory System* and Ch. 13, *Lung Disease.*

The Endocrine Glands

Technically speaking, a gland is any cell or organ in our bodies that secretes some substance. In this broad sense, our liver is a gland, because one of its many functions is to secrete bile. So too, is the placenta that encloses a developing baby and supplies it with chemicals that assure normal growth. Even the brain has been shown by modern research to secrete special substances. But lymph glands are not considered true glands and are more correctly called lymph nodes.

Physicians divide the glands into two categories. *Endocrine glands* are also known as *ductless glands,* because they release their secretions directly into the bloodstream. *Exocrine glands,* by contrast, usually release their substances through a duct or tube. Exocrine glands include the sebaceous and sweat glands of the skin; the mammary or milk glands; the mu-

cous glands, some of which moisten the digestive and respiratory tract; and the salivary glands, whose secretions soften food after it enters the mouth. The pancreas has both an endocrine and an exocrine function and structure.

Role of the Endocrine Glands

The *endocrine glands* have the all-important role of regulating our body's internal chemistry. The substances they secrete are complex compounds called *hormones,* or chemical messengers.

Together with the brain and nerves, the system of endocrine glands controls the body's activities. The nervous system, however, is tuned for rapid responses, enabling the body to make speedy adjustments to changing circumstances, internal and external. The endocrine glands, with some exceptions, like the adrenal, are more concerned with the body's reactions over a longer period of time—from season to season, as it were. They regulate such processes as growth, levels of metabolism, fertility, and pregnancy.

For a group of tissues that exercise awesome power over our body's well-being, the endocrine glands are surprisingly small and inconspicuous—all of them together would weigh less than half a pound. Nor are they placed with any particular prominence in our body. They tend to be little lumps of tissue attached to or tucked behind grander bodily structures. Their power comes from the hormones they release into the bloodstream.

Scientists have discovered the exact chemical makeup of a number of these complex substances, have extracted several in pure form from living tissue, and have succeeded in making a few synthetically in the lab-

Endocrine Glands

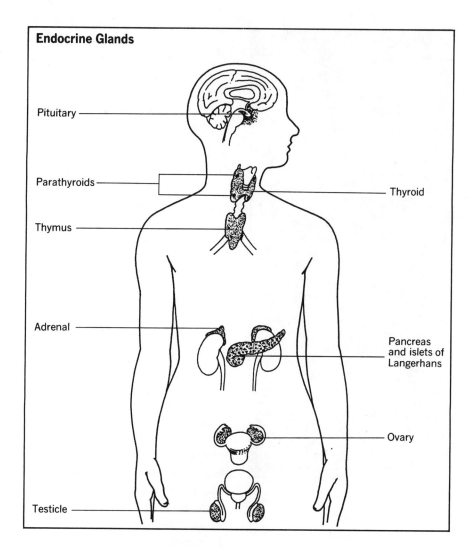

Pituitary

Parathyroids

Thymus

Adrenal

Testicle

Thyroid

Pancreas and islets of Langerhans

Ovary

oratory. This avenue of research, called *endocrinology,* has enabled physicians to treat persons suffering from certain endocrine gland disorders.

Hormones have been aptly described as chemical messengers. Their action, while still not completely understood, is that of catalysts. This means that the presence of a hormone (the name comes from a Greek word meaning "arouse to activity"), even in very small quantities, can affect the rate at which a chemical change occurs or otherwise stimulate a reaction, and without itself being affected. The hormone is a promoter, either of a positive or negative sort; it speeds up a process or slows it down.

The endocrine glands form an interdependent family. The functioning or malfunctioning of one can affect all the others.

The Pituitary—Master Gland

The *pituitary* is often called the master gland because the hormones it secretes play an active part in controlling the activities of all the other endocrine glands. This impressive power is wielded from two little bumps at the base of the brain, about midway between the ears at eye level. The two parts, or lobes, are connected by a tiny bridge of tissue, the three structures together being about the size of a small acorn. The lobe lying toward the front of the head is the *anterior lobe;* the one at the back, the *posterior lobe.* Each lobe is really an independent gland in itself, with its own quite distinct activities.

The Posterior Lobe and the Hypothalamus

The posterior lobe, so far as is known, does not make any of its own hormones, but serves as a storehouse for two hormones manufactured by the *hypothalamus,* located in the brain's cerebellum. The hypothalamus, apart from having a role in controlling the body's autonomic nervous system, also functions as an endocrine gland, secreting its own hormones, and as a connecting link between the brain's cerebral cortex and the pituitary gland.

The posterior lobe of the pituitary releases the two hormones it receives from the hypothalamus, called *vasopressin* and *oxytocin,* into the bloodstream. Vasopressin plays a role in the fluid balance of the body; oxytocin is thought to pace the onset and progress of labor during childbirth.

The Anterior Lobe

The anterior lobe secretes no less than six known hormones, five of which act as stimulators of hormone production by other endocrine glands. The sixth, identified as *somatotrophin*

The Pituitary Gland

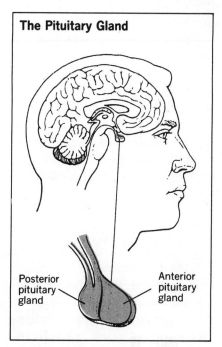

Posterior pituitary gland

Anterior pituitary gland

in medical textbooks, is more popularly known as the *growth-stimulating hormone* or simply as the growth hormone. It controls the rate of growth and multiplication of all the cells and tissues in our bodies—muscle, bone, and all our specialized organs.

Gigantism

In rare instances, during childhood, the pituitary releases too much or too little somatotrophin. If too much is secreted, the result is an overstimulation of growth processes, causing a disorder known as *gigantism*. Victims of this disorder have been known to grow nine feet tall and weigh 500 pounds.

Dwarfism

If too little somatotrophin is secreted, *dwarfism* results. This pituitary-type dwarf, of which Tom Thumb was one, is different from a dwarf suffering from a disorder of the thyroid (another endocrine gland, discussed below). The pituitary dwarf is usually well proportioned despite a miniature size, while the thyroid dwarf typically has short, deformed limbs.

Neither pituitary gigantism nor dwarfism affects basic intelligence. If oversecretion of somatotrophin occurs after full size has been reached—as, for example, because of a tumor affecting the pituitary, the condition known as *acromegaly* occurs. The bones enlarge abnormally, especially those of the hands, feet, and face.

Anterior Pituitary Hormones

Of the five anterior pituitary hormones that regulate other endocrine glands, one affects the adrenal glands, one the thyroid, and the remaining three the sex glands or gonads (the

Pituitary Gland

ACTH
TSH
FSH
LTH
FSH
LH

Vasopressin

Oxytocin

Posterior lobe   **Anterior lobe**

testicles in men and the ovaries in women). Each is identified by a set of initials derived from its full name, as follows:

- *ACTH,* the *a*drenocor*t*icotrophic *h*ormone, affects the production of hormones by the outer "bark" of the adrenal glands, called the *adrenal cortex.*

- *TSH,* the *t*hyroid-*s*timulating *h*ormone, also known as *thyrotrophin,* causes the thyroid gland to step up production of its hormone, *thyroxin.*

- *FSH,* the *f*ollicle-*s*timulating *h*ormone, spurs production in women of estrogen, a sex hormone produced by the ovaries; and in men, of sperm by the testicles. Follicle here refers to the *Graafian follicles* in the ovary, which contain developing female egg cells whose

growth is also stimulated by FSH. Graafian follicles have approximate counterparts in the male—tiny pouches (seminal vesicles) on either side of the prostate gland that store mature sperm cells.

- *LH,* the *l*uteinizing *h*ormone, transforms a Graafian follicle, after the follicle has released a ripened egg cell, into a kind of tissue called *corpus luteum.* The corpus luteum, in turn, produces *progesterone,* a hormone that prepares the mucous membrane lining the uterus (the endometrium) to receive a fertilized egg.

- *LTH,* the *l*actogenic *h*ormone, or *luteotrophin,* stimulates the mother's mammary glands to produce milk; LTH also joins with LH in promoting the production of progesterone by the sex glands.

The last three hormones mentioned—follicle-stimulating, luteinizing, and lactogenic—are sometimes called the *gonadotrophic* hormones because they all stimulate activity of the gonads.

The Adrenal Glands

Resting like skull caps on the top of both kidneys are the two identical *adrenal glands.* Each has two distinct parts, secreting different hormones.

Adrenaline

The central internal portion of an adrenal gland is called the *medulla.* Its most potent contribution to our body is the hormone *adrenaline* (also called *epinephrine*). This is the hormone that, almost instantaneously, pours into our bloodstream when we face a situation that calls for extraordinary physical reaction—or keeps us going past what we think to be our normal

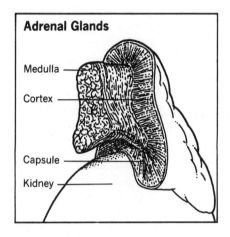

Adrenal Glands

Medulla

Cortex

Capsule

Kidney

limit of endurance.

A surge of adrenaline into the bloodstream stimulates our body to a whole array of alarm reactions—accelerating the conversion of stored foods into quick energy; raising the blood pressure; speeding up breathing; dilating the pupils of the eyes for more sensitive vision; and constricting the blood vessels, making them less vulnerable to bleeding.

Adrenaline provides a good example of the interdependence of the endocrine system. Its production stimulates the secretion of ACTH by the pituitary gland. And ACTH, as noted above, causes the adrenal cortex to accelerate production of its hormones. Some of these adrenal cortex hormones enable the body to call up the reserves of energy it does not normally need. For example, body proteins are not usually a source of quick energy, but in an emergency situation, the adrenal cortex hormones can convert them to energy-rich sugar compounds.

The Corticoids

There are some 30 different hormones, called the *corticoids,* manufactured in the adrenal cortex—the outer layer of the adrenal. A few of these influence male and female sexual characteristics, supplementing the hormones produced in the gonads. The others fall into two general cat-

egories: those that affect the body's metabolism (rate of energy use), and those that regulate the composition of blood and internal fluids. Without the latter hormones, for example, the kidneys could not maintain the water–salt balance that provides the most suitable environment for our cells and tissues at any given time.

Corticoids also influence the formation of antibodies against viruses, bacteria, and other disease-causing agents.

Extracts or laboratory preparations of corticoids, such as the well-known cortisone compounds, were found in the 1950s to be almost "miracle" medicines. They work dramatically to reduce pain, especially around joints, and hasten the healing of skin inflammations. Prolonged use, however, can cause serious side effects.

The Islets of Langerhans

Strewn at random throughout the pancreas are hundreds of thousands of tiny clusters of cells. Each of them, when seen under a powerful microscope, forms an "islet" of its own, similar to the other distinct islets, but markedly different from the pan-

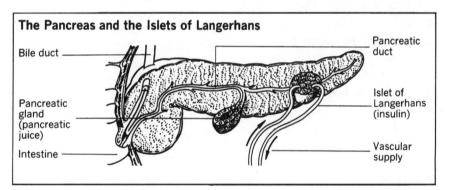

The Pancreas and the Islets of Langerhans

Bile duct

Pancreatic gland (pancreatic juice)

Intestine

Pancreatic duct

Islet of Langerhans (insulin)

Vascular supply

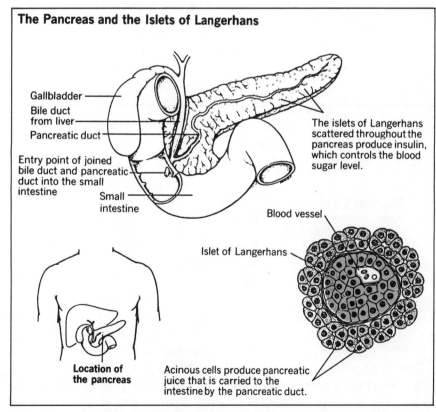

The Pancreas and the Islets of Langerhans

Gallbladder

Bile duct from liver

Pancreatic duct

Entry point of joined bile duct and pancreatic duct into the small intestine

Small intestine

The islets of Langerhans scattered throughout the pancreas produce insulin, which controls the blood sugar level.

Blood vessel

Islet of Langerhans

Location of the pancreas

Acinous cells produce pancreatic juice that is carried to the intestine by the pancreatic duct.

creatic tissue surrounding it. These are the *islets of Langerhans,* named after the German scientist who first reported their existence in 1869. Each of these little cell clumps—up to two million or more of them—is a microscopic endocrine gland.

They secrete the hormone *insulin,* and the disease that occurs if they are not functioning properly is *diabetes mellitus.*

Actually, the islets of Langerhans produce not only insulin, but also a related hormone called *glucagon.* Both regulate the amount of sugar (glucose) that is present in the bloodstream and the rate at which it is used by the body's cells and tissues. Glucose supplies the energy for life and living processes.

When insulin and glucagon are not in sufficient supply, the cells' ability to absorb and use blood sugar is restricted, and much of the sugar passes unutilized out of the body in urine. Because the body's ability to obtain energy from food is one of the very foundations of life, diabetes calls for the most careful treatment.

One of the great advances of twentieth century medicine has been the pharmaceutical manufacture of insulin and its wide availability to diabetics. With regulated doses of insulin, a diabetic can now lead a normal life. See Ch. 15, *Diabetes Mellitus* for a full discussion of this disease.

The Thyroid Gland

The *thyroid gland* folds around the front and either side of the trachea (windpipe), at the base of the neck, just below the larynx. It resembles a somewhat large, stocky butterfly facing downward toward the chest.

Thyroxin

The thyroid hormone, *thyroxin,* is a complex protein-type chemical con-

Thyroid Gland

Thyroid cartilage

Parathyroid

Thyroid

Trachea

taining, along with various other elements, a large percentage of iodine. Like a number of other hormones manufactured by the endocrine glands, thyroxin affects various steps in the body's metabolism—in particular, the rate at which our cells and tissues use inhaled oxygen to burn the food we eat.

Hypothyroidism

A thyroid that is not producing enough thyroxin tends to make a person feel drowsy and sluggish, put on weight (even though his appetite is poor), and in general make his everyday activities tiresome and wearying. This condition is called *hypothyroidism.*

Hyperthyroidism

Its opposite—caused by too much secretion of thyroxin—is *hyyperthyroidism.* A hyperthyroid person is jumpy, restless, and may eat hugely without gaining weight. The difference between the two extremes can be compared to environments regulated by two different thermostats, one set too high and the other set too low.

Although a normally functioning thyroid plays a significant part in making a person feel well, physicians to-

day are less willing than in former years to blame a defective thyroid alone for listlessness or jittery nerves. Thirty or forty years ago it was quite fashionable to prescribe thyroid pills (containing thyroid extract) almost as readily as vitamins or aspirin; but subsequent medical research, revealing the interdependence of many glands and other body systems, made thyroxin's reign as a cure-all a short one.

Of course, where physical discomfort or lethargy can be traced to an underfunctioning thyroid, thyroxin remains an invaluable medicine.

Goiter

One disorder of the thyroid gland—the sometimes massive swelling called *goiter*—is the direct result of a lack of iodine in the diet. The normal thyroid gland, in effect, collects iodine from the bloodstream, which is then synthesized into the chemical makeup of thyroxin. Lacking iodine, the thyroid gland enlarges, creating a goiter. The abnormal growth will stop if iodine is reintroduced into the person's diet. This is the reason why most commercial table salt is iodized—that is, a harmless bit of iodine compound has been added to it.

The Parathyroid Glands

Four small glands, each about the size of a small pea, cling to the base of the thyroid gland, two on each of the thyroid's lobes curving back of the trachea. These are the *parathyroids,* whose main role is to control the level of calcium—as well as other elements needed in carefully regulated amounts by the body—in the bloodstream and tissues. The parathyroids secrete two hormones: *parathormone* when blood calcium is too low; *calcitonin* when the calcium level is too high. These hormones work by controlling the interchange of calcium between bones and blood.

The most common symptom of defective parathyroids is *tetany*—a chronic or acute case of muscle spasms, which can be controlled by administration of synthetic parathyroidlike chemicals or concentrated vitamin D preparations.

The Gonads

The *gonads* refer to both the two male testicles and the two female ovaries.

There are four hormones secreted by the gonads: the female sex hormones, *estrogen* and *progesterone;* and the male hormones, *testosterone* and *androsterone.* Each sex merely has a predominance of one or the other pair of hormones. Men have some of the female hormones, and women some of the male hormones.

In both sexes, puberty is signaled by the release of the gonadotrophic hormones (or *gonadotrophins*) of the pituitary gland. These stimulate the production of sex hormones by the sex glands and the subsequent appearance of secondary sexual characteristics. In men, these include the enlargement of testicles and penis, growth of facial, axillary (armpit) and pubic hair, and enlargement of the larynx, resulting in deepening of the voice. Pubescent women also experi-

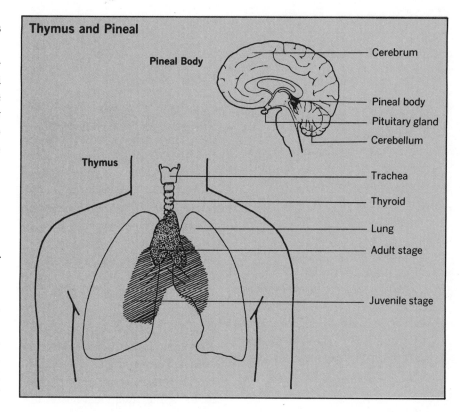

ence pubic and axillary hair growth, in addition to breast growth and changes in the genital tract that give it child-bearing capability.

Estrogen and progesterone control the cyclic changes within the uterus that involve the development, ripening, and discharge of the egg (ovulation) to be fertilized; the preparation of the lining of the uterus to receive a fertilized egg; and this lining's subsequent dismantling—all the complex biochemical events that occur as part of every woman's menstrual cycle.

The Thymus and Pineal Glands

These are the least known of the endocrine family; in fact, physicians do not know the function of one of them—the *pineal*—and are not even agreed that it is an endocrine gland. Situated near the hypothalamus, at the base of the brain, this tiny, pine-cone-shaped body has follicles that suggest a glandular function and some calcium-containing bits that medical researchers have descriptively dubbed "brain sand."

The *thymus,* only slightly better understood, has the intriguing characteristic of shrinking in size as a person grows up. It is located in the middle of the chest, about midway between the base of the neck and the breast line. There is some evidence that the secretions of the thymus play a role in the body's natural immunity defenses. See also Ch. 14, *Diseases of the Endocrine Glands.*

The Sense Organs

Once upon a time, a grade-school teacher would ask, "How many senses do we have?" And his pupils would confidently chorus back, "Five!" People who displayed a knack for predicting future events, or whose quick reactions seemed to give them a jump over most everybody else, were credited with having a "sixth sense."

Scientists now recognize about twice that number—12 or 13 or more. Man, of course, has not grown a number of new senses in addition to the traditional five: sight, hearing, touch, smell, and taste. What has happened is that scientists have discovered many more specific kinds of sense receptor cells. For example, whereas touch was formerly thought of as just one sense, it has now been divided into no less than five different senses, each having its own special kind of receptor cell in the skin.

We can talk with a little more justification of the five sense organs, the five anatomical structures we associate with our senses—the eyes, ears, nose, tongue, and skin. But here, too, it does seem to be oversimplifying things to thus equate the nose—having only a tiny patch of olfactory (sense of smell) receptor cells—with the marvelously complex arrangement of sensing structures that make up the eye. Moreover, the other sense organs are not nearly so specialized as the eye. For example, a good case could be made for the nose being more valuable as an air purifier than as an organ of smell, or for the tongue being more valuable as an aid in digestion than as a source of the taste sensation.

Suppose we accept the proposition that pain is one of the senses of the skin; how then do we explain a pain from inside our bodies—say, a stomachache or a deep muscle pain? The answer, of course, is that there are pain receptors in many other places besides the skin.

What Is a Sense?

A sense is a nerve pathway, one end of which (the receptor end) responds in a certain way to a certain condition affecting our bodies, and whose other end reaches to a part of our brain that informs our conscious mind of what has happened or is happening. A sense is thus distinguished from the body's countless other nerve pathways by the fact that our brain *consciously* registers its impulses, although the impulses themselves are no different from those of the autonomic nervous system.

While remaining aware of the limitations of the traditional list of five sense organs, let us now analyze what they can do and how they operate:

- The eye (vision): Nerve impulses to the brain are stimulated by light waves, from which the brain forms visual images.

- The ears (hearing): Nerve impulses to the brain are stimulated by sound waves, out of which the brain forms meaningful noise, such as speech. Deep within the ear, also, are structures that give us balance.

- The nose (olfaction): Nerve impulses to the brain are stimulated by airborne chemical substances, moistened within the nasal cavity, from which the brain elicits distinctive smells.

- The tongue (taste): Nerve impulses to the brain are stimulated (in presence of water) by chemical substances in food, from which the brain forms sensations of sweet, salty, sour, bitter, or combinations of these tastes.

- Skin (touch): Nerve impulses to the brain are stimulated by the presence of outside physical forces and changes in the physical environment, including varying temperatures, which the brain registers as feelings of contact, pressure, cold, heat, and pain. (Some medical texts add traction, as when the skin is pulled or pinched, as well as the sensation of tickle.)

The Eye

Rather than take a name-by-name anatomical tour of the eye, let's instead take just three programmed tours of the eye to explore:

- the transformation of light energy into vision;

- focusing, or how the structure of the eye prepares light for transformation into vision; and

- the supporting structures and service units of the eye.

Transforming Light Energy into Vision

If you could look through the opening in the front of your eye (the *pupil*), and see to the very back surface of your eye (as if you could see through the needle valve opening to the inside skin of a basketball), you would see your own *retina*. On your retina are located all the sense receptor cells that enable us to see. There are none anywhere else in the body.

Rods and Cones

A good argument can be made that man's vision is really *two* senses. For on the paper-thin retina are two quite anatomically distinct sense receptors (nerve endings) named, for their appearance under high magnification, *cones* and *rods*. The cones are concentrated at a tiny spot on the retina called the *fovea*.

If the focusing machinery of the eye (cornea, lens, etc.) is working just right, light rays from the outside have their sharpest focus on the fovea. Surrounding the fovea is a yellowish area called the *macula lutea* (Latin, "yellow spot"). Together, the fovea and macula lutea make a circle not much bigger than the head of a pin.

All our seeing of colors and fine details is accomplished by the cones of the fovea and the macula lutea. Beyond the yellowish circumference of the macula lutea, there are fewer and fewer cones: rods become the dominant structures on the retina. It has been estimated that there are something less than 10 million cones on the retina of each eye, but more than 10 times as many rods—100 million of them or more.

Although the tight circle of cones in each eye gives man his ability to do close, detailed work (including reading) and to discriminate colors, the cones are virtually useless in detecting objects that are a bit off center from our direct focus, and furthermore operate only in good lighting conditions or in response to bright light sources.

The rods compensate for the specialized limits of the cones. They take over completely in dim light, and also give us the ability to detect peripheral objects and movements—"out of the corner of the eye." Because the rods are not sensitive to colors, our seeing at night is almost completely in black-and-white.

You can give yourself an interesting demonstration of the interacting functions of your own cones and rods if you walk from bright, sunny daylight into a dimly lit theater. In the bright light, your cones have been picking out sharp images and colors. But once

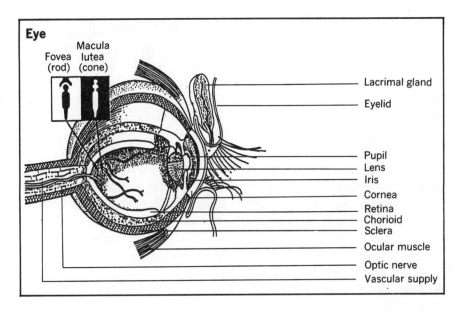

Eye

Fovea (rod)
Macula lutea (cone)

Lacrimal gland
Eyelid
Pupil
Lens
Iris
Cornea
Retina
Chorioid
Sclera
Ocular muscle
Optic nerve
Vascular supply

in dimness, the cones become inoperative. For a few moments, in fact, you may see almost nothing at all.

Visual Purple

The momentary interval after the cones stop working but before the rods begin to function is explained by a curious pigment present in the eye called *visual purple*. This substance is manufactured constantly by the rods, and must be present for the rods to respond to dim light—but it is destroyed when exposed to bright light. Thus, after entering a darkened room, it takes a few moments for visual purple to build up in the retina.

One of the principal constituents of visual purple is vitamin A, which is why this vitamin (present in carrots and other yellow produce) is said to increase our capacity to see in the dark.

The Optic Nerve

Every nerve ending is part of a larger unit, a neuron or nerve cell, and the sense receptors called rods and cones are no exception. Like all nerve cells, each rod and cone sports a long nerve fiber or *axon* leading away from the site of reception. In each eye, fibers serving the hundred-million-plus rods and cones all converge at a certain

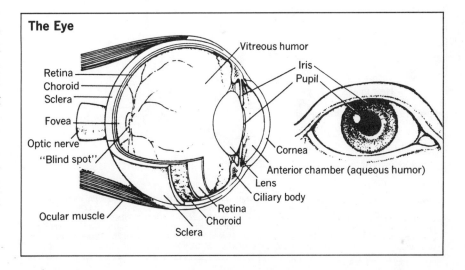

The Eye

Retina
Choroid
Sclera
Fovea
Optic nerve
"Blind spot"
Ocular muscle
Vitreous humor
Iris
Pupil
Cornea
Anterior chamber (aqueous humor)
Lens
Ciliary body
Retina
Choroid
Sclera

spot just behind the retina, forming the *optic nerve*. There are no rods and cones at the point where the optic nerve exits from behind the retina at the back of the eyeball: that is why everybody has a "blind spot" at that point. An image passing through that spot completely disappears.

From the retina, both optic nerves set a course almost directly through the middle of the brain. Right and left optic nerves converge, their individual fibers partially intertwining a short distance behind the eyes. Then this joint optic nerve trunk proceeds toward the rear of the head, where the *occipital lobes,* the brain's "centers for seeing," are located. Just before reaching the occipital lobes, the optic nerve splits again into thousands of smaller nerve bundles (called *visual radiations*) that disappear into the visual cortex or "outer bark" of the occipital lobes. Only at this point are the bits of light energy that have stimulated our rods and cones transformed into images that our brain can "see."

Focusing and Light Control

Lacking the structures of the retina and their connection to the brain via the optic nerve, we could not see. Lacking reasonably normal functioning of the cornea, lens, and iris, we do not see well.

Good vision depends upon the eye being able to bend incoming light rays in such a way that the image being observed falls directly on the retina—in other words, upon proper focusing. The bending or *refraction* of light rays is the joint work of two curves, transparent slivers of specialized tissue through which light passes on its way to the retina. These are the *cornea* and the *lens*. Broadly speaking, the degree of curvature and thickness of these two structures determines whether we see well or poorly, are nearsighted or farsighted.

The Cornea and Lens

The cornea, which does the major light-bending, has a virtually fixed

curvature and thickness. The lens puts the finishing touches on the focusing. Its thickness and curvature are adjustable—more or less without our conscious awareness—depending on whether we wish to focus on something nearer or farther away. The lens is made thicker or thinner, a process called *accommodation,* by the relaxing and contracting of tiny, attached *ciliary muscles*. Normally, these muscles do not have to work at all if we are looking at objects more than 20 feet away: but they often are overworked by a great deal of close work.

The Pupil and Iris

Effective focusing in various light conditions also depends upon the diameter of the hole through which light enters the eye. This hole is the *pupil*. Its diameter is controlled automatically—wider in dim light, narrower in bright light—by the muscles of the surrounding *iris*. The iris muscle contains pigment that gives our eyes color (brown, blue, green, etc.). The pupil, opening into the dark interior chamber of the eye, is black. A fully dilated (widened) pupil, as would occur in the dimmest light, illuminates over 15 times more retinal surface than the tiny "pinhole" pupil of an eye exposed to very bright light.

Structural Support and Protection of Eye

Two outer layers protect the eye. The tough outermost layer is the *sclera,* the white of the eye. Underlying the sclera is another layer, the *choroid,* which contains numerous tiny blood vessels that service the sclera and other structures on the eyeball. Both sclera and choroid have concentric openings that allow for the hole of the pupil. The cornea is really a specialized extension of the sclera,

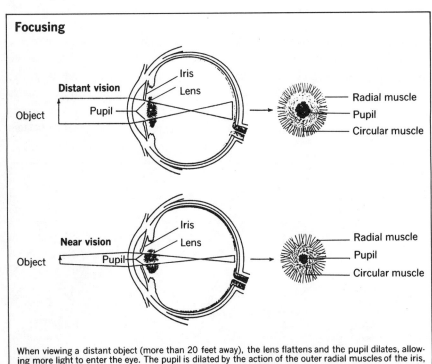

Focusing

Distant vision — Iris, Lens, Pupil — Object — Radial muscle, Pupil, Circular muscle

Near vision — Iris, Lens, Pupil — Object — Radial muscle, Pupil, Circular muscle

When viewing a distant object (more than 20 feet away), the lens flattens and the pupil dilates, allowing more light to enter the eye. The pupil is dilated by the action of the outer radial muscles of the iris, which contract and thus stretch the previously contracted circular muscles. When viewing a near object, the lens becomes more oval and the pupil contracts as more light enters the eye. This prevents overstimulation of the retina. The pupil is reduced in size by the contraction of the inner circular muscles, which serve to stretch the previously contracted radial muscles.

Muscles of the Eye

- Eyelid muscle
- Oblique muscles
- Superior muscle
- Inferior muscle
- Lateral muscle
- Medial muscle

and the iris of the choroid.

Two trapped reservoirs of fluid within the eye are important in maintaining the eye's shape as well as the frictionless operation of its moving parts. These two reservoirs contain fluids called the *aqueous humor* and *vitreous humor.* The tiny space between the cornea and lens, corresponding to the pupil, is called the anterior chamber and is filled with the clear, watery, aqueous humor. The larger interior space behind the lens is called the posterior chamber, and is filled with the vitreous humor.

Muscles for Movement of Eye

In addition to the tiny muscles within the eye that control the opening of the pupil and the shape of the lens, we also have a number of elegant muscles that control the movements of each eyeball, and make both eyeballs move together in unison.

The movements of each eyeball are affected by six muscles attached to its top, bottom, and sides. The teamwork between these muscles—some contracting while others relax—allows the eye to move from side to side, up and down, and at all intermediate angles (obliquely). One of our eyes is always a dominant or leading eye; that is, its movements are always followed by the other eye.

Our protective eyelids, of course, are controlled by opening and closing muscles that lie outside the eye proper. These muscles can function both voluntarily and involuntarily.

Lubrication and Hygiene of Eye

Without the moisture provided by tears, our eyeball would scrape excruciatingly on the inside lining (*conjunctiva*) of the eyelid. In addition to lubrication, tears also have a cleansing action, not only because they supply water for washing and rinsing but also because they contain a mild germicide called *lysozyme* that kills bacteria and other potentially harmful microbes.

Ciliary Muscle Contraction

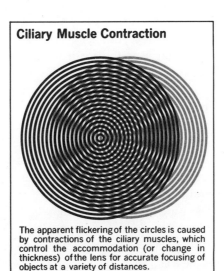

The apparent flickering of the circles is caused by contractions of the ciliary muscles, which control the accommodation (or change in thickness) of the lens for accurate focusing of objects at a variety of distances.

Tears are produced by the *lacrimal glands* above the eyeball, just under the eyebrow, a bit further toward the temple side than the nose side. They are discharged from several short ducts and spread over the surface of the eyeball by blinking. The *conjunctival sac* at the bottom inner (nose) side of the eye—visible in the mirror as a pinkish flap of tissue—serves as a collecting pool for tears; from there, they drain down a duct into the nasal cavity. This is why somebody who is crying also snuffles and must blow his nose.

There is another tiny drainage network in the eye, located at the interconnection of the cornea and iris, which serves to keep the fluid pressure of the space filled by the aqueous humor within normal limits. Drainage of this area is through microscopic conduits called the *canals of Schlemm.* Improper drainage can cause build-up of pressure, such as occurs in glaucoma, and impairment or loss of vision.

The Ear

Within the tunnels and chambers of the ear lie the two special types of sense receptors that give us, respectively, the sense of hearing and the sense of balance.

The Outer Ear

The *outer ear* includes that rather oddly shaped and folded piece of flesh and cartilage from which earrings are hung, and more important, the external *auditory canal,* a tunnel leading from the ear's opening to the *tympanic membrane,* or *eardrum.*

The Middle Ear

The *middle ear* includes the inner surface of the eardrum and the three

Ear

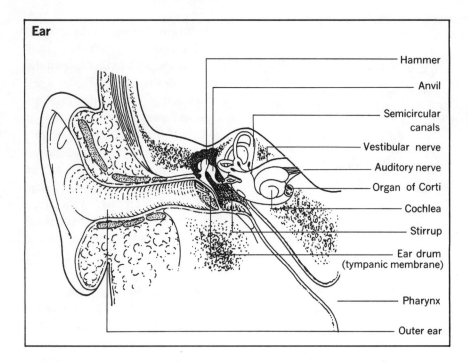

- Hammer
- Anvil
- Semicircular canals
- Vestibular nerve
- Auditory nerve
- Organ of Corti
- Cochlea
- Stirrup
- Ear drum (tympanic membrane)
- Pharynx
- Outer ear

tiny, bony *ossicles,* named long ago for their shape (apparently by some blacksmithing anatomist), *the hammer, the anvil,* and *the stirrup;* or in Latin: *the malleus, the incus,* and *the stapes.* These bones respond to the vibrations in the air that are the basis of sound, vibrate themselves, and transmit their vibrations to the inner ear, where the sense receptors for hearing are located, and the *auditory* (or *acoustic) nerve* to the brain begins.

The middle ear is connected to the back of the throat (pharynx) by the Eustachian tube. This tunnel between throat and middle ear makes the pressure on the inside of the eardrum, via the mouth, the same as the pressure of the atmosphere on the outside of the eardrum. (Thus yawning helps to equalize pressure.) Without it, or if the Eustachian tube becomes clogged, the taut membrane of the eardrum would always be in imminent danger of bursting.

The Inner Ear

The chambers of the *inner ear* are completely filled with fluid, which is jostled by the ossicles "knocking" on a thin membrane called the oval window, separating the middle from the inner ear. Another flexible membrane, the round window, serves to restrict the motion of the inner ear fluid when the movement is too stormy.

Organ of Hearing

Within the inner ear is a bony structure coiled like a snail shell about the size of a pea. This is the *cochlea,* the actual Latin word for snail or snail shell. Following the internal spiral of the cochlea is the *organ of Corti,* the true sense receptors for hearing.

The organ of Corti is made up of thousands of specialized nerve endings that are the individual sense receptors for sound. These are in the form of tiny hairs projecting up from the internal membrane lining the cochlea; they wave like stalks of underwater plants in response to the oscillating currents of the inner ear fluid. There are some 20,000 of these hairs within the cochlea, responsive to almost as many degrees of movement of the fluid. These thousands of nerve endings merge at the core of the

cochlea and exit from its floor as the nerve bundle of the *auditory nerve.*

Organ of Balance

The organ of balance, or equilibrium, is also behind the oval window that marks the beginning of the inner ear. The principal structure consists of three fluid-filled *semicircular canals* arranged, like the wheels of a gyroscope spinning on a perfectly flat plane or surface, at right angles to each other. When we are in a normal, upright position, the fluid in the canals is also in its normal resting state. But when we begin to tilt or turn or wobble, the fluid runs one way or another in one or more of the canals. This fluid movement is picked up by crested, hairlike nerve endings lining the inside of the canals and relayed as nerve impulses along the *vestibular nerve* to the brain. Then, the brain sends messages to the muscles that can restore our equilibrium.

The Semicircular Canals

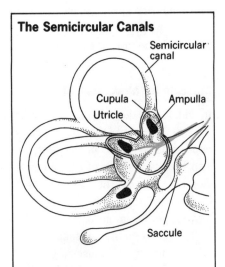

- Semicircular canal
- Cupula
- Ampulla
- Utricle
- Saccule

The semicircular canals are swollen at their bases into three ampullae in which receptors are located. When the head moves or accelerates, the fluid within the canals (endolymph), tends to move slower than the head, and the cupula is displaced. This is communicated to the hairlike nerve receptors. Soon the endolymph catches up to the head movement and the cupula returns to its normal position. When movement stops, the endolymph continues to move, the cupula is again displaced, and the nerve receptors are activated until the endolymph ceases to move.

The Ear and the Perception of Sound

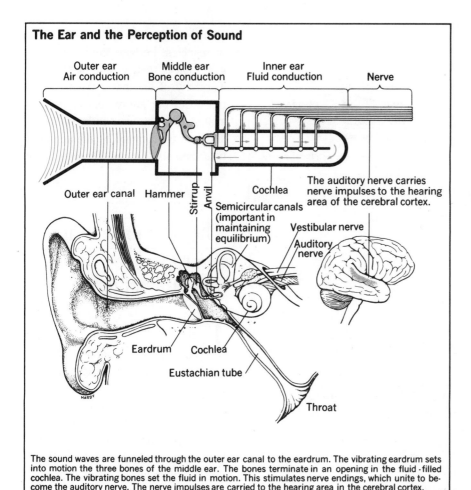

The sound waves are funneled through the outer ear canal to the eardrum. The vibrating eardrum sets into motion the three bones of the middle ear. The bones terminate in an opening in the fluid-filled cochlea. The vibrating bones set the fluid in motion. This stimulates nerve endings, which unite to become the auditory nerve. The nerve impulses are carried to the hearing area in the cerebral cortex.

The term *labyrinth* is sometimes used to refer collectively to the cochlea, semicircular canals and associated structures of the inner ear. The space or cavity within the labyrinth is called the *vestibule,* which gives its name to the vestibular nerve.

How We Hear

Just as our eye has certain special equipment—its focusing apparatus—to prepare light for the retina, so our ear has special equipment to prepare vibrations for reception by the organ of Corti.

This equipment consists of structures that amplify the vibrations reaching the ear, or, more rarely, damping (decreasing) the vibrations caused by very loud or very close occurrences.

Sound waves are really vibrations in the air that reach the eardrum at the narrow end of the funnel-shaped auditory canal. These vibrations set the membrane of the eardrum vibrating ever so slightly. Behind the eardrum, the first ossicle encountered is the hammer, which is attached to the eardrum by a projection descriptively called the hammer-handle.

From the eardrum, vibrations travel up the handle and set the hammer vibrating. The hammer, in turn, sets the anvil vibrating; and the anvil, the stirrup. The stirrup then knocks like an impatient caller on the oval window of the inner ear, and the then vibrating oval window stirs the fluids within the cochlea. This chain of events can account for a tremendous amplification of vibrations—so that we are literally able to "hear a pin drop."

Tiny muscles in the middle ear relax or tighten the eardrum and adjust to changing volumes of sound. For example, a muscle connecting the stirrup and the eardrum relaxes when the stirrup is vibrating violently in the presence of very loud noises. A lax eardrum is less likely to rupture and transmits fewer vibrations to the delicate mechanisms of the middle and inner ear than a taut one. Thus we have to some degree built-in, automatic protection against the assaults of noise pollution—but not nearly enough, according to physicians who are convinced that more and more cases of deafness are caused by the incessant battering of the modern world against our eardrums. Human eardrums are not made to withstand the sound of jet planes taking off, for example.

The Nose and Tongue

The sense receptors on the tongue and within the nasal cavity work very closely together to give us our sense of taste. These five kinds of receptors—the olfactory cell in the nose and the four special cells or taste buds on the tongue for discriminating salty, sweet, sour, and bitter tastes—also have a functional similarity. All are chemical detectors, and all require moisture in order to function. In the nose, airborne substances must first be moistened by mucus (from the olfactory glands) before they can stimulate olfactory cells. In the mouth, the saliva does the wetting.

The general number and distribution of the four types of taste receptors are described earlier in this chapter under "The Digestive System and the Liver." These nerve endings, numbering in the hundreds of thousands, merge into two nerve bundles traveling away from the tongue to the

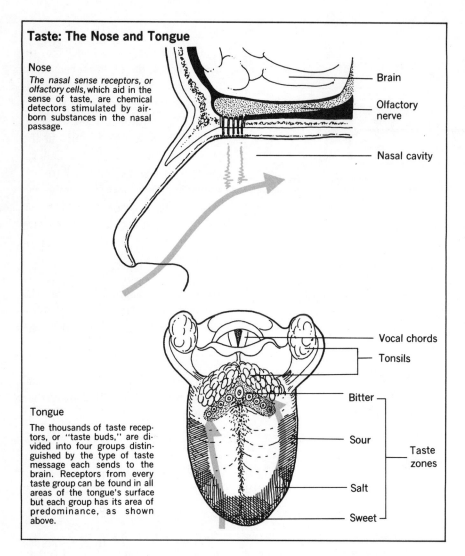

Taste: The Nose and Tongue

Nose
The nasal sense receptors, or olfactory cells, which aid in the sense of taste, are chemical detectors stimulated by air-born substances in the nasal passage.

— Brain

— Olfactory nerve

— Nasal cavity

Tongue
The thousands of taste receptors, or "taste buds," are divided into four groups distinguished by the type of taste message each sends to the brain. Receptors from every taste group can be found in all areas of the tongue's surface but each group has its area of predominance, as shown above.

— Vocal chords
— Tonsils

— Bitter
— Sour
— Salt
— Sweet

Taste zones

brain's "taste center." The receptors toward the rear of the tongue collect into the *glossopharyngeal nerve;* those at the front and middle are directed along the *lingual nerve.*

Our smell receptors are clustered in an area about a half-inch wide on ceiling of the nasal cavity. This is called, appropriately enough, the smell patch. The nerve endings pass upward through the sievelike *ethmoid bone,* separating the nasal cavity from the brain, and connect to the olfactory bulb, which is the "nose end" of the *olfactory nerve.* At the other end of the olfactory nerve is the "nose brain" or *rhinencephalon*—a tiny part of the cerebrum in man, but quite large in dogs and other mammals whose sense of smell is keener than man's.

Although man's sense of smell is probably his least used sense, it still has a quite remarkable sensitivity. With it we can detect some chemicals in concentrations as diluted as one part in 30 billion—for example, the active ingredient in skunk spray. Also, man's ability to smell smoke and to detect gas leaks and other warning scents has prevented many a tragedy.

Skin

The sensations stimulated by the various types of sense receptors in the skin are described at the outset of this section. It is worth noting, however, at the end of our tour of the sense organs that the senses associated

with the skin are really in a class by themselves. Perhaps the most telling indication of their unique place in the hierarchy of senses is the fact that practically our entire central nervous system is given over to handling the impulses transmitted by these receptors. See also Ch. 16, *Diseases of the Eye and Ear.*

The Urinogenital System and the Kidneys

In large part our good health depends on the quality of the body's internal environment. There is a kind of ecological principle at work within us—if one chain threatens to break, one system becomes polluted, one balance is tilted, then the whole environment is in imminent danger of collapsing. The major responsibility for keeping our internal environment clean and unclogged lies with our two kidneys. They are the filters and purifiers of body fluids: the body's pollution-control stations, its recycling plants, and its waste-disposal units.

The Kidneys

The kidneys are located just behind our abdominal cavity on either side of the spinal cord, their tops usually tucked just under the bottommost rib. Each of our kidneys is four to five inches long and weighs about half a pound. The right kidney is normally placed a bit below the left, to accommodate the bulky liver lying also on the right side above it. Neither kidney is fixed rigidly; both can shift position slightly. Lying outside the muscular sheath of the abdominal cavity, the kidneys are more vulnerable than most internal organs to outside blows, but good protection against all but the severest jolts is afforded by surrounding fatty cushions, the big back muscles, and the bone and musculature associated with the spinal column.

As it has with the lungs, the liver, and most other vital organs, nature has supplied us with a large reserve capacity of kidney tissue—a life-giving overabundance in the event of kidney disease or injury. Indeed, normal function of only one-half of one kidney can sustain a person's life.

The kidney's task of purifying our internal environment—that is, our circulating blood—is really a double task. Each kidney must purify the blood that passes through it, sending back into circulation only "clean blood"; and it must dispose of the impurities it has taken from the blood. The latter is accomplished by the urine draining down a tube, or *ureter,* leading from each of the two kidneys to one common urinary *bladder.* Urine is discharged from the bladder down another tube called the *urethra* to the external opening for urination.

How the Kidneys Process Body Fluids

Blood is brought to the kidney by a renal artery, is treated in the kidney's unique microscopic structures, and exists via the renal vein. (*Renal* means associated with the kidneys.) The sheer volume of blood processed by both our kidneys is prodigious: between 400 and 500 gallons are processed every day.

Internal Structure

Within each kidney are over a million microscopic units called *nephrons.* The nephron is the basic functional unit of the kidney—a little kidney in itself—and is really a superbly engineered and coordinated arrangement of many smaller structures, all working together.

Blood arriving at the kidney from the renal artery is quickly channeled into finer and finer vessels, until finally it flows into a kind of cat's cradle or "ball of wool" structure called a *glomerulus* (composed of intertwining, microscopic vessels called glomerular capillaries). The entire structure of the nephron is built around the microscopic glomerulus (Latin, "tiny ball"). Surrounding the glomerulus, like a hand lightly cupping a ball of wool, is another structure called *Bowman's capsule.* Fluid and dissolved materials filter out of the blood from the glomerular capillaries through the membranes into Bowman's capsule.

Substances in Bowman's Capsule

The fluids and dissolved materials filtering into Bowman's capsule are by no means all wastes and impurities. In fact, some of the substances must soon be reclaimed. Among the waste substances captured by Bowman's capsule and destined for excretion in urine are various nitrogen salts and other waste products of cellular metabolism, as well as actual or potential poisons that have entered or accumulated in the bloodstream. Nonwaste substances include needed sugars and salts, and water.

Reclaiming Essential Substances

Before we leave the glomerulus altogether behind, it should be noted that like any capillary bed, this small ball of blood vessels has not only an inflow from the renal artery but also outflow vessels leading eventually back to the renal vein.

From the cupped lips of Bowman's capsule, fluid and dissolved substances from the blood trickle into a single tube called a kidney *tubule.* The

---

The Anatomy of the Kidney

The cortex is the darker, outer part of the kidney. The medulla, the inner part, includes the renal pyramids and the straight tubules associated with them.

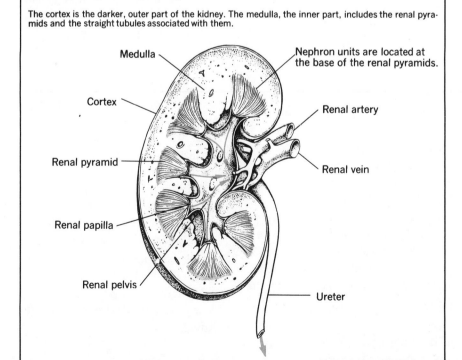

Medulla

Cortex

Renal pyramid

Renal papilla

Renal pelvis

Nephron units are located at the base of the renal pyramids.

Renal artery

Renal vein

Ureter

Urine is produced in the nephrons of the pyramids and drains by way of the papillae into the renal pelvis, which empties into the ureter. The ureter carries the urine to the bladder.

The Nephron

Bowman's capsule

Glomerulus

Proximal convoluted tubule

Renal artery

Renal vein

Distal convoluted tubule

Capillary network

Descending limb

Ascending limb

Collecting tubule

Loop of Henle

The nephron is a microscopic unit that filters out certain products from the blood. Useful products are reabsorbed by the capillary network. The waste product (urine) is carried to the collecting tubule and emptied into the renal pelvis.

outflow vessels from the glomerulus wind closely over and around the tubule, forming a capillary network around it. By this means the non-waste substances are reclaimed and returned to refresh the blood moving away from the nephron.

The tubule itself makes many twists and turns—including one hairpin turn so stunning that it has its own medical name—*Henle's loop.* So much twisting and turning gives the tubule a great deal more surface area than a simple, straight tube would have within the same space, thus increasing the amount of water and dissolved substances that can be recaptured by the encircling capillaries.

If there were no recapturing system in the kidneys, death would probably result from dehydration. Even if that could be avoided, the loss of essential salts and other substances would prove fatal in a short time.

The arithmetic of the situation goes something like this: every day, an estimated 42 gallons of fluid filter out of the glomeruli and into the two kidneys' approximately two and a half million tubules. Dissolved in this 42 gallons—representing about three times the body's weight—are about two-and-a-half pounds of common salt, just one of the many substances in the fluid that our body needs in sufficient amounts. The loss of either water or common salt at a rapid rate would prove fatal in a matter of hours.

But so efficient is the tubule-capillary recapturing system that only an average of less than two quarts of fluid, containing just one-third ounce of salt, pass daily out of the kidneys into the ureter and are excreted as urine. In other words, over 99 percent of both the water and common salt removed from the blood at Bowman's capsules is returned to the blood.

The Kidneys and Blood Pressure

A surprising insight into the critical role played by our kidneys in almost every body function is provided by the relation of blood pressure to kidney function. The blood in the glomerular capillaries must be at higher pressure than the fluid around them, so that the fluid and its dissolved substances can push through the capillary membranes toward Bowman's capsule. If blood pressure in the body falls too low (severe *hypotension*) the formation of urine ceases.

On the other hand, if a portion of the kidney is suffering from anemia due to some disorder, kidney cells secrete *pressor hormones,* which serve to elevate the blood pressure. Thus high blood pressure (*hypertension*) may be a sign of kidney disorder.

The Urinary Tract

From the ends of the million or so tubules in each kidney, urine drains into larger and larger collecting basins (called *calyces,* singular *calyx*) which drain in turn into the kidney's master urine reservoir, the *kidney pelvis.* Then, drop by drop, urine slides down each ureter to the urinary bladder.

Urine is held in the bladder by the contraction of two muscle rings, or *sphincters,* one located just inside the bladder before it meets the urethra, and the other encircling the urethra itself. When about a half-pint has accumulated, nerves convey the urge to urinate to the brain, and the person voluntarily causes the sphincters to relax, emptying the bladder. (In exceptional circumstances, the elastic-walled bladder can hold two or three quarts of urine.) Up to the point where the bladder drains, the male and female urinary tracts are very similar, but after the bladder, any similarity stops.

Female Urethra

The female's urethra, normally about

The Female Urinary System

- Kidney
- Ureter
- Bladder
- Urethra

The Male Urinary System

- Kidney
- Ureter
- Bladder
- Prostate gland
- Urethra

gynecologist and *obstetrician*.

However, all the distinctly male sex glands and organs are linked more or less directly into the eight- or nine-inch length of the male urethra.

The Genitals

The Female Reproductive System

As indicated above, the urinary and genital systems of women are dealt with by two different medical specialties. For this reason, the female genitals are discussed elsewhere. For a description and illustration of the female reproductive system, see Ch. 3, *The Teens.* For a description of infections of the female reproductive tract, see Ch. 25, *Women's Health.*

The Male Reproductive System

From its emergence below the bladder, the male urethra serves as a conduit for all the male sexual secretions.

Prostate Gland

Directly below the bladder outlet, the

one and a half inches long, is not much more than a short channel by which urine is eliminated from the bladder. Its very shortness often gives it an undesired significance, because it represents an easy upward invasion route for bacteria and other infection-causing microbes from the outside. Acute and painful inflammations of the urethra (*urethritis*) and bladder (*cystitis*) are thus common in women. These lower urinary tract infections, however, can usually be halted before spreading further up the urinary tract by the administration of any of several antimicrobial drugs. See Ch. 25, *Women's Health* for more information on these disorders.

Male Urethra

In contrast to the female, the male's urethra is involved with reproductive functions. So closely connected are the male's lower urinary tract and genital organs that his urethra (from bladder to the outside) is properly called the urinogenital (or genitouri-

nary) tract. This is the reason why the medical specialty known as *urology* deals with both the urinary and genital apparatus of men; but with only the urinary tract of women. The urologist's specialty does not extend to the female genital and childbearing organs, which are the concern of the

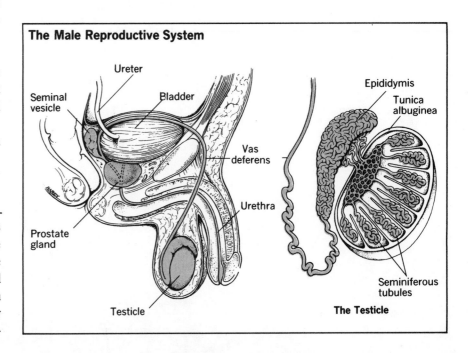

The Male Reproductive System

- Ureter
- Seminal vesicle
- Bladder
- Vas deferens
- Urethra
- Prostate gland
- Testicle

- Epididymis
- Tunica albuginea
- Seminiferous tubules

The Testicle

prostate gland completely enwraps the urethra. The prostate secretes substances into the urethra through ejaculatory ducts; these substances are essential in keeping alive the spermatozoa that arrive from their manufacturing sites in the *testicles* (or *testes*).

Testicles

The two testicles hang down within a wrinkled bag of skin called the *scrotum*. Although the vulnerable position of the testicles remains something of an evolutionary mystery, one clue is that the optimum production of spermatozoa takes place at a temperature some degrees lower than the normal internal body temperature.

Spermatozoa produced in the testicles travel upward toward the urethra through a seminal duct or tube called the *vas deferens* (one from each testicle). (These are the ducts, incidentally, that are tied and cut in the male sterilization procedure known as a vasectomy.) The sperm cells are then stored, until ejaculation, in little reservoirs called *seminal vesicles* which are situated on either side of the urethra in the area just above the prostate gland.

The portion of the male urethra from the bladder to where it emerges from the encircling prostate, having received the emission of both the prostate and the testicles, is called the prostatic or posterior urethra. The remainder, mainly consisting of the conduit running down the middle of the shaft of the penis, ending in the external opening called the *meatus,* is known as the anterior urethra. See also Ch. 17, *Diseases of the Urinogenital System.*

2

The First Dozen Years

Birth, Infancy, and Maturation

Before the Baby Arrives

When a husband and wife decide to have a baby they should both undergo complete physical examinations. This will make it possible to detect and treat abnormalities like diabetes and anemia that might affect the future pregnancy. A pregnant woman should have periodic checkups so that her physician can observe both her progress and that of the growing fetus. Such observation will help to assure a pregnancy and delivery that are free from troublesome complications.

What the Newborn Baby Looks Like

At birth the baby's skin is wrinkled or scaly, and may be covered by a cheesy substance called *vernix caseosa*. During the first two weeks the skin will become quite dry to the touch. The skin of white newborns is red, and sometimes turns yellow during the first few days. Black newborns often are not as dark as they might be later. Their skin becomes just as yellow as that of white babies, but the change is more difficult to observe.

The newborn's head is large in proportion to the rest of its body. The genitals too may seem large, especially in girls. Newborn girls may have swollen genitalia that is a result of *edema* (fluid in the tissues, causing puffiness), but the swelling is usually present for only a few days after birth.

The eyes, slate blue in color, can open and react to light, but are unable to focus. Noises produce a *startle response*, a complex involuntary reaction marked by a sudden, jerky, arm and leg movement. The newborn cries a great deal, sucks, and may sneeze.

The infant's stomach may look rather large and protuberant, and, of course, it has the stump of the umbilical cord dangling from it. The umbilical cord has been cut and tied near the navel, and will eventually fall off.

If you feel the front and back of the baby's head, you will notice one or two soft spots, called the *anterior* and *posterior fontanelles*. The posterior fontanelle usually closes at the baby's second month of life, and the anterior at 18 months or earlier.

You also may feel many different ridges in the baby's head. These are the borders of the different skull bones, which fuse as the baby gets older. They are present so that the skull can grow as the baby's brain and head continue to grow.

Soon after birth, you may detect a swelling on the baby's head just under the scalp. This is called *caput succedaneum*. It is nothing to worry about, as it dissolves a day or two after birth. Occasionally, another swelling known as *cephalhematoma* may also be present. This, too, disappears, within a few weeks.

The baby's weight will, of course, vary. Most full-term babies weigh between six and eight pounds. Babies of diabetic mothers are often heavier, and may weigh up to twelve pounds.

Some Advice to New Mothers

Unless the new father and mother are really prepared to change some of the conditioned patterns of their relationship, both can be in for a very difficult time. The father suddenly finds himself taking second place in his wife's attentions and affection. The new mother is tired physically and mentally. In-laws and other relatives may infringe on the couple's privacy and interfere with their right to make their own decisions. The new mother may find it hard to reconcile her maternal instinct with her desires as a woman and wife.

All of these problems can be minimized if the mother follows a few commonsense guidelines:

- The new baby is a shared responsibility. Do not shut your husband out of the experience of parenthood. Let him learn to feed the baby, diaper her, hold her, get acquainted with her. Make your husband feel just as important to the baby as you are, and just as important to you as he was before the baby was born.

- Arrange for some kind of assistance in your home, and don't wait until the day you bring the baby home to do it. Plan ahead. You will be physically and emotionally tired after childbirth, no matter how marvelous you may feel when you leave the hospital. During the hospital stay the baby was cared for by a trained staff. At home the burden will fall mainly on you, unless you take steps to get help. If you cannot get your mother or another relative to stay with you, engage a housekeeper or some other trained person. The investment will pay off for you, the baby, and your husband.

- If it is at all possible, arrange to have a separate area for the baby. It is best for a baby not to be kept in the parents' room. Parents must have privacy. If you do not have a bedroom for the baby, section off some spot where you can put a crib and a dressing table to hold the supplies you will need when you feed, change, bathe, and dress her.

- Don't make the baby the focus of attention 24 hours a day. If she fidgets and fusses at times, try not to get nervous. Don't run to her at every whimper so long as you know she has been fed, is dry, and nothing is really wrong. Relax. The baby will be very sensitive to your emotional responses, particularly when you hold her. Through your physical contact you will develop a kind of communication with your baby which she will sense when you pick her up or feed her.

- As important as it is for you and your husband to avoid overhandling the baby, it is more important that family and friends be made to follow a "hands off" policy except at your discretion. A new baby should not be subjected to excessive stimulation. For example, you

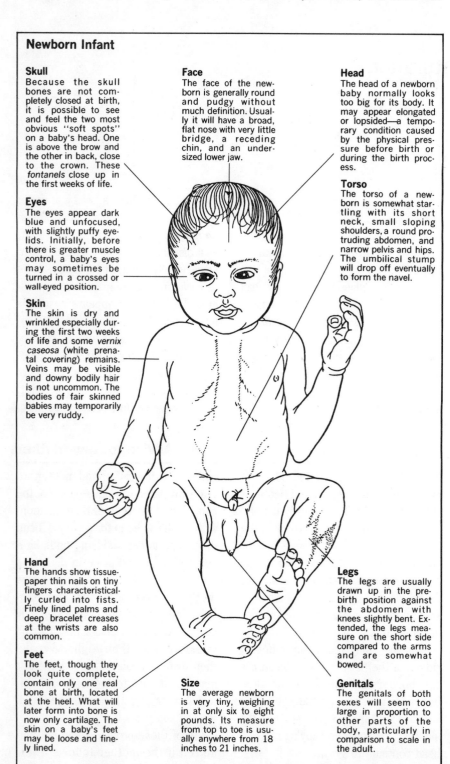

Newborn Infant

Skull
Because the skull bones are not completely closed at birth, it is possible to see and feel the two most obvious "soft spots" on a baby's head. One is above the brow and the other in back, close to the crown. These *fontanels* close up in the first weeks of life.

Eyes
The eyes appear dark blue and unfocused, with slightly puffy eyelids. Initially, before there is greater muscle control, a baby's eyes may sometimes be turned in a crossed or wall-eyed position.

Skin
The skin is dry and wrinkled especially during the first two weeks of life and some *vernix caseosa* (white prenatal covering) remains. Veins may be visible and downy bodily hair is not uncommon. The bodies of fair skinned babies may temporarily be very ruddy.

Hand
The hands show tissue-paper thin nails on tiny fingers characteristically curled into fists. Finely lined palms and deep bracelet creases at the wrists are also common.

Feet
The feet, though they look quite complete, contain only one real bone at birth, located at the heel. What will later form into bone is now only cartilage. The skin on a baby's feet may be loose and finely lined.

Face
The face of the newborn is generally round and pudgy without much definition. Usually it will have a broad, flat nose with very little bridge, a receding chin, and an undersized lower jaw.

Size
The average newborn is very tiny, weighing in at only six to eight pounds. Its measure from top to toe is usually anywhere from 18 inches to 21 inches.

Head
The head of a newborn baby normally looks too big for its body. It may appear elongated or lopsided—a temporary condition caused by the physical pressure before birth or during the birth process.

Torso
The torso of a newborn is somewhat startling with its short neck, small sloping shoulders, a round protruding abdomen, and narrow pelvis and hips. The umbilical stump will drop off eventually to form the navel.

Legs
The legs are usually drawn up in the pre-birth position against the abdomen with knees slightly bent. Extended, the legs measure on the short side compared to the arms and are somewhat bowed.

Genitals
The genitals of both sexes will seem too large in proportion to other parts of the body, particularly in comparison to scale in the adult.

may notice that if you pick her up and put her back in her crib, and then let someone else hold her a few minutes later, the baby may cry. If you slam a door, the baby's body reacts in the startle reflex, the involuntary reaction previously described. A baby needs a quiet, organized home, free from the kind of upsetting distraction that comes from being surrounded and fussed over by too many people. You and your husband must decide when you want the baby to have visitors and how those visitors are to behave. You must do this even if it causes hurt feelings among your friends and relatives. When the baby is a little older there will be time enough for friends and relatives to admire and play with her.

Feeding the Baby

One of the first questions a mother-to-be must ask herself is how she will feed her baby.

Breast-feeding is certainly the simplest method, and many women believe that a both mother and child get more emotional satisfaction from it than from bottle-feeding. It is also, obviously, less expensive.

Breast-Feeding

Almost any healthy woman who wants to breast-feed her baby can do so. All she needs is the desire and motivation. No special preparation is necessary except, perhaps, some stimulation of the breasts, as prescribed by her physician during pregnancy.

On the other hand, a variety of different factors might necessitate a change from breast to bottle-feeding. Although breast-feeding may be discontinued at any time, some mothers may feel a sense of failure or frustration at being unable to continue having

the intimate relationship that so many other mothers enjoy. No harm will come to the baby by being switched to a formula. Once started on a formula, however, it may be difficult to go back to breast-feeding on a regular basis. For a while, at least, the mother will have to stimulate her breasts artificially to increase their milk-producing capacity.

The First Few Days

When a mother first starts to breast-feed, she may be worried that she won't have sufficient milk for the baby. Her breasts are just beginning to fill up with a creamy, yellowish substance called *colostrum.* Transitional and then regular breast milk will not come in for three to five days or longer. Colostrum contains more protein and less fat than breast milk. Secretions of colostrum are small, but during this time the baby does not need very much fluid, and the colostrum will give her adequate nutrition.

Actually, it is important that the milk does not fill the breasts right away because engorgement would be so severe that the baby would not be able to suck well or strongly enough to empty them. During engorgement, the mother's breasts feel extremely tender and full. A good nursing brassiere will lift and support the breasts and alleviate the tender sensation during the one- or-two day period of the engorgement.

Some Advice to Nursing Mothers

If you do not have enough milk for the first few days, don't worry about it. Let the baby suck on your nipples for three, five, or even ten minutes. Don't keep her on your breasts for twenty or thirty minutes right from the beginning. Start with three minutes the first day, five minutes the

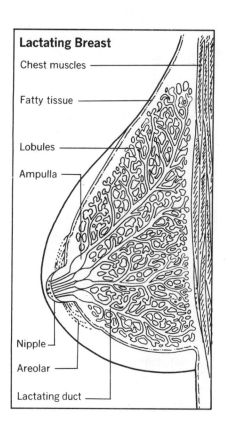

Lactating Breast
Chest muscles
Fatty tissue
Lobules
Ampulla
Nipple
Areolar
Lactating duct

second, and so on until you work up to fifteen or twenty minutes. In this way you will toughen your nipples so that your breasts will become accustomed to the baby's sucking. A bland cream may be used to massage the nipple area, particularly if the nipples become sore or cracked.

Be sure to use both breasts. By emptying the breasts, milk production is stimulated; thus an adequate milk supply is dependent upon using both breasts. To avoid any soreness or tenderness, use one breast longer than the other during each nursing period.

Let us assume, for example, that at the first feeding of the day you nurse the baby on the left breast for a long period, then on the right for a short period. During the next feeding the right breast will become the first one on which the baby nurses (for the long period), and the left will be nursed second (for the short period). After a few weeks you should be nursing the baby on the first breast for twenty minutes and on the other for ten minutes.

The Feeding Schedule

Depending on how often the baby wants to feed, you will be wise to adhere to a modified demand schedule. Don't watch the clock and feed the baby every four hours on the dot. You might feed at approximately every fourth hour, which means that you could start a second feeding early—at a three-hour interval—or late—at a five-hour interval. And, needless to say, never wake your baby up at night. She will awaken you.

Bottle-feeding

New parents have a choice between prepackaged formulas and the homemade variety. Either provides the same basic nutritional requirements.

The basic homemade formula for newborns consists of evaporated milk, water, and sugar or one of the sugar derivatives. Twice as much water as evaporated milk is used with one to two tablespoons of sweetening. A similar formula can be made with whole milk in somewhat different proportions. As the baby gets older, the formula will be changed from time to time by your physician.

If one formula does not agree with the baby, it will not help to put her on a similar formula; its ingredients are likely to be virtually the same. You must switch to a radically different formula, such as one containing no milk at all or no carbohydrates. It is up to your physician to advise you which modified formula to try.

As to how much formula should be given at each feeding, let the baby decide. If she is satisfied with two-and-a-half ounces, she is probably getting enough. If she wants up to four-and-a-half ounces, give it to her. The amount is not important as long as

your physician feels the baby is in good health.

A final thing to remember about feeding is this: whether you use breast or bottle, you must give your baby the love, warmth, and body contact that she needs. As you feed her, you are not only providing nutritional nourishment for her growing body but giving her emotional and mental food for her developing personality.

The First Six Months

It is extremely important that the baby have regular health supervision. Your baby's physician—whether pediatrician or general practitioner—will check the baby's height and weight on each visit, and make certain she is growing and gaining at a satisfactory rate. Often, the first sign of illness in a baby is a change in her height and weight pattern.

Although no two children develop at the same rate, it is possible to make certain generalizations about their development. See the charts in this chapter showing the growth rates for boys and girls.

By two months a baby often holds her head up when she lies on her stomach or when she is being held up. She recognizes large objects, and she knows her bottle or feeding position. She can probably smile.

Sometime during the second or third month, your physician will start a series of injections against diphtheria, whooping cough, and tetanus (called *DTP*), as well as oral immunizing agents against polio—the *Sabin vaccine*. See the chart in the "Alphabetic Guide to Child Care" under "Immunization" later in this chapter.

The Three-Month Mark

By three months most babies are eating some solids specially processed

for babies—fruits, cereals, vegetables, meats—in addition to having formula. They may, of course, still be entirely on breast milk. Your physician will also suggest the use of vitamin supplements, in the form of drops, which can be added to the baby's milk or solid food. All babies need vitamins A, C, and D. Occasionally, vitamin B is also prescribed. If fluorides are not present in your drinking water, they are often added to the baby's vitamins to retard tooth decay.

At Four Months

By four months the baby will look at moving objects. Do not be surprised if her eyes cross. This is a normal condition during early infancy, and may even persist for a year.

At about this time, the baby may also learn to turn over from front to back—an important milestone. Some babies may have developed bald or flat places on the back of the head from lying more or less in one position. At about this time the condition should begin to disappear.

The Second Six Months

At six months most babies smile when they are brought to the physician's office. At one year of age a visit to the physician is more likely to produce tears and screams. The friendly, sociable attitude of the six-month-old gives way to one in which strangers are shunned or mistrusted, and everyone other than mother may qualify as a stranger.

By the sixth month the baby may roll over when placed on her back. She may learn to crawl, sit, pull herself up, and even stand. By a year she may start to walk, although walking unaided does not often occur so soon.

At this stage the baby is full of life and activity. She won't lie still when you change her diaper, and often needs distraction. She cries if you put her down or leave her alone. Unless you are firm and resist running to her first whimper, you may set the stage for spoiling her as she gets older. Of course, if she continues to cry for any considerable length of time—not more than half an hour—make sure there is nothing wrong with her besides her displeasure at your not appearing like a genie because she screams or fusses.

Other Changes

Other changes occur at this age. Where before she had been a good sleeper, she may now not want to go to sleep or she may awaken at night. Let her know that you are nearby, but don't make a habit of playing with her in the middle of the night—not if you value your sleep.

If you should notice, as many parents do at about this time, that your baby seems to be left-handed, do not try to make her right-handed. Each of us inherits a preference for one hand or the other, and it is harmful to try to change it. In any case, you are not likely to know for sure which hand your child prefers until the second year of her life.

In this second six-month period, the baby will probably take some of her milk from a cup. Don't be surprised if she takes juices out of a cup but insists on taking milk from a bottle. If she tries to hold the bottle or cup herself, let her. Of course, it may be wise to keep a mop handy at first, but after few months her skills will improve. In any case, nonbreakable cups are recommended.

Diet and Teeth

The baby's diet is soon expanded to include pureed baby foods. You might even want to try the somewhat lumpier junior foods; as more of her teeth erupt, the baby will enjoy lumpier food more and more. Teething biscuits can be added to the diet, too. By the time she is one year old she will usually have six teeth (incisors), although, because no two children are alike, she may have none at all. By the end of the first year she will have lost some of her appetite, and her rapid weight gain will cease. This is entirely natural in a period when the outside world is taking more and more interest.

As she starts to move around she wants to investigate everything. Keep dangerous objects—detergents, poisons, and medicines, especially baby aspirin—out of her reach. Tell her "no" to emphasize the seriousness of certain prohibitions. She should understand what "no" means by the time she is one-year-old, and will also probably respond to other simple commands.

It is essential that your baby's health supervision be continued without interruption. During the second six months of life she will complete her protection against diphtheria, whooping cough, tetanus (DTP), and polio (Sabin), and be tested for exposure to tuberculosis (the tuberculin test).

Behavioral Development during Infancy

During a child's first year she needs a warm and loving emotional environment in the home. It is during this time that a child establishes what psychiatrists and psychologists call basic trust. That is, she learns to be a trusting individual who feels that her important needs—those of being cared for, fed, and comforted—will be met by other human beings, initially by her mother.

Emotional Needs

Such activities as holding and cuddling the infant, talking to her, and playing with her in an affectionate, relaxed way are important for her emotional growth. Experiments with animals have shown that if the infant animal does not get sufficient cuddling and physical contact from its mother during its early development, it is unable to perform adequately as an adult later in life. It has also been shown that infants growing up in an environment lacking warm, loving, close physical and emotional contact with a mother or a mother-substitute often fail to thrive and may even die.

Fondling and Sucking

During the first year, most of an infant's satisfactions and gratifications are through the skin's perception of being touched—through physical contact with her mother and other caring adults—and through the mouth, especially sucking. Infants have a great need to suck even when they are not hungry, and this sucking should be both allowed and encouraged.

Parents frequently worry that if they respond to a baby's crying by picking her up they will spoil her, and the baby will cry often in order to get attention. In general, it could be said that during its first year an infant cannot be spoiled. When an infant cries she usually does so because she is uncomfortable, hungry, sick, or needs some physical attention.

Social Responses

As she matures, one of a child's tasks is to begin to see herself as separate from the world around her. During early infancy, the infant does not see herself as an individual who is separate from her mother, from other adults, and from the rest of the world. But, gradually, some time within the first year of life, this feeling of separateness and individuality begins to emerge in the developing infant.

One of the important and gratifying events in the early months of a child's life is the smiling responses. For the first time the infant can respond in a social way to other human beings. It is often at this time that the infant's mother and father begin to think of her as a real person and an individual. Thus the smile could be considered one of the infant's first social communications.

Suspicion of Strangers

Somewhere around the age of eight months, an infant who has in the past without complaint allowed anyone to pick her up begins to distinguish her mother from other individuals. When picked up by another the infant usually cries, acts frightened, and, in general, looks unhappy. This response indicates that she can now tell her mother and other individuals apart—an important and normal step in an infant's development.

Fear of Separation

Some time later, usually around the age of one year, the infant begins to become fearful upon separation from her mother. When her mother walks out of the room or leaves the baby with a sitter, the child may respond with crying, fear, and anger. This again indicates that the infant can now tell her mother from strangers and does not like being separated from her. Although the response is normal and usually subsides within three to four months, parents should learn to leave the child in the hands of a competent sitter, and walk out without guilt or anger. The child must learn that separations are temporary and that parents do return.

The Second Year: The Toddler Stage

It is during the second year of a child's life that begins to develop independence and separateness from his mother. Beginning with his growing ability to walk, usually some time early in the second year (age 12 to 16 months), an infant starts to explore the world around him more actively. He experiments with greater and greater distances and increasing independence from his mother.

Toward the end of the second year, children frequently become quite independent, trying to do many things for themselves, and resenting their parents or other well-meaning adults doing things for them. Even if the child is not yet capable of performing the tasks he attempts, he should be encouraged in these early moves toward independence. It is also during the second year that speech begins to develop, with the child's first words usually being "ma ma," "da da," "milk," and the ever-present "no."

Developing Relationships with Mother and Father

It is in this phase of the child's life that he develops a real relationship with his mother. In most homes, mother is the loving, warm, secure comforter in his life, the giver of rewards and disciplinarian of his activities, the center of his life. During this period it is imperative that the child's father spend as much time with his son or daughter as possible, so that the child begins to recognize the difference between his relationship to his mother and father.

In some cases the father, because of the demands of business, may find it impossible to spend enough time with his family. This is an unfortunate fact, but one that can be dealt with positively, because it is the quality of

the time a father spends with his child rather than the quantity that is most important.

Testing Himself and the World around Him

The toddler is insatiably curious. He wants to explore and investigate everything. Take him outdoors as much as possible. Let him meet children of his own age so that he can play and learn the beginnings of social contact.

Physically, the toddler tries to do many things apart from walking, running, and climbing—including quite a few things that he can't do. He is easily frustrated and may have a short attention span. (Girls are better than boys in this respect.) Don't be impatient with your toddler; don't punish him for his clumsiness. He has a great many experiences ahead of him, and many skills to learn and develop.

You can now expect a negative reaction to your control. Obviously, you must set limits on your child's behavior—on what is acceptable and what is not, while still giving him the freedom to express his emotions and energies in vigorous physical play.

Make the rules easy to understand so that the child will not become confused about what is expected of him. And do not set up impossible standards.

The Third Year

The third year is extremely important. Children are usually toilet trained, show marked growth in their language abilities, and demonstrate a continuing and growing independence.

Negativism

From two to about three and perhaps beyond, a child is extremely negative.

When asked to do anything or when asked about anything, he often responds by saying, "No, no, no, no, no." This saying of the word "no" on the slightest provocation indicates a child's wish to become separate and independent from parents, to do what he wants to do when he wants to do it, and to be free from the control of others.

The child's desire for independence can be respected and encouraged by parents within limits, but this does not mean that a parent must give in to a child on every issue. A parent should try to determine what is really important and not make an issue over petty matters that can best be handled with relaxed good humor.

Language Development and Play

A rapid spurt in language development takes place at this time. A child may increase his vocabulary from about 50 words at the beginning of the third year to an almost countless vocabulary at the end of the third year. It is during this year, too, that children first show marked interest in imaginative play activities. Play, including making up stories, using toy trucks and cars, blocks, dolls, and toy furniture, is vital activity for children and should be encouraged by parents. It is through play that children express their feelings, often feelings that cannot be expressed in ordinary ways. The child also experiences what it feels like to be an adult by playing the role of physician, fire fighter, police officer, teacher, mother or father. In addition, during play children discharge tensions and learn to use their muscles and bodies.

Exploring the Body

From very early infancy, all children show a strong interest in their own and in other's bodies. During infancy this takes the form of playing with his own or his mother's body. A baby puts his fingers in his own mouth, in his mother's mouth, ears, eyes, and pats her on the tummy or on the breast. An infant also explores and touches his own body, including the genital region. This interest is normal and need not be discouraged.

Dental Development

The roots of all 20 primary teeth are complete at the child's third year of life. These teeth, which began erupting between 6 and 7 months of age, are called the *central incisors*. The primary teeth, the last of which usually fall out between the eleventh and thirteenth year, are smaller and whiter than the permanent teeth, of which there are 32. The first permanent tooth erupts between 7 and 8 years of age, while the last, the third molars, or *wisdom teeth*, erupt between the seventeenth and twenty-first year.

The Preschooler

This is the age when many children go to school for part of the day and begin learning how to get along with other children in play and in organized activities. They also begin to meet adults other than their parents.

First Separation from Mother

During the ages of three and four, the preschooler develops increasing interest in the world around him, in children his own age, and in himself. One of the key problems that the preschooler has to deal with is his impending separation from his mother when he becomes old enough to go to school. This can often be made less painful by arranging for the child to spend at first short and then increasingly longer periods of time away from his mother. By using baby-sitters both in the evening and during the day, by later having the child spend three or more half-days a week at a preschool, and lastly by enrolling him in kindergarten for either all day or half a day, five days a week, the mother can ease the child's adjustment to the world outside the home.

Although his first nearly full-time separation from mother is difficult for the child, it may be difficult for the mother as well. Mothers often feel that this initial separation from their child will eventually lead to their child's growing up and leaving home. Parents are often nostalgic and somewhat regretful about their children's first going off full time to school. The child's fearful anticipation of a strange situation can be eased by a mother's anticpating school with the child, talking with him about it and reassuring him regarding his fears of abandonment or separation.

Differences between Boys and Girls

A word might be mentioned here concerning differences between boys and girls. At the age of five most girls are ready to attend kindergarten; they can sit in their seats for long periods of time, pay attention to a teacher, and be interested in a task. Boys, because of their somewhat slower rate of maturity, are often less ready than girls for coping with a classroom situation at the age of five.

A child of five grows at a slower rate than in earlier years, but his body is nonetheless changing. The protruding abdomen and knock-knees of the toddler begin to disappear.

Television

Students of the medium suggest that television offers some worthwhile programs for the young child. At the same time, the experts warn that television watching can, over time, become addictive. A basically passive experience, it may also decrease the quality of family life and raise early obstacles to literacy and learning.

The parent's main task, insofar as television watching is concerned, is to find ways to use "the tube" to help the child develop. Parents can, for example, turn on programs that their child enjoys, that do not frighten or overexcite, and that the toddler can learn from. The television should not be used as an "electronic baby-sitter"; as much as possible, parents should watch when their child does. If a child is 18 months old or older the experts say parents should select the special programs they want their child to see. Television should not, finally, be used as a reward for being good. Such an approach can suggest the TV is more important than interesting games and other worthwhile activities.

Personal Hygiene

Good habits of cleanliness should be established. The child should know that hand-washing before meals is essential even when the hands look clean. He will learn this only if he sees parents do it. As he gets older he should select his own clean clothing and know that dirty clothing should be washed. A daily routine of washing or bathing should be set up, and the child should be encouraged to observe it.

School-Age Children: Parent–Child Relationships

Beginning around the age of four, boys show a decided preference for their mothers. A boy may, for example, tell his mother that when he grows up he would like to marry her

and kick father out of the house. At times he may even suggest that he would work to support her and that life would be much nicer if daddy were not around.

This interest in his mother is often expressed in what may be thought of as sexual ways. That is, the child of this age enjoys his mother's affection, including kissing, hugging, and close bodily contact. This wish to have mother all to himself and to have father out of the picture is called the *Oedipal complex* by psychiatrists and psychologists, after the ancient Greek tragedy, *Oedipus Rex*, in which Oedipus kills his father and marries a woman whom he later discovers to be his mother.

At about this same age, similar emotional developments take place in a girl. She will likely be somewhat seductive, coy, and coquettish with her father, and may talk about marrying father (or a man like father) and having mother out of the picture. This phase of emotional attachment between a girl and her father is called the *Electra complex* after the Greek play, *Electra*.

At these times, both the girl and the boy have a strong, although not always conscious, wish to displace the parent of the same sex and have the opposite-sexed parent all to themselves. Strong conflicts disturb children in this phase of development, for they also realize that they love and need the same-sexed parent to instruct them, to guide them, to provide for them, and to love them.

Identification

Both males and females eventually resolve these conflicts by abandoning their so-called sexual attachment to the opposite-sexed parent, forming a closer attachment to the same-sexed parent and trying to be like that parent. This is not a conscious decision,

but one that a child makes without realizing it. This process of *identification* with the parent of the same sex starts very early, perhaps as early as the second year, and continues through adolescence, but it is especially noticable from five to ten.

Much of the energy that had previously been utilized in loving the parent of the opposite sex is now spent in loving the parent of the same sex. The boy follows father around, wants to do whatever he does, and holds as his greatest ambition to be exactly like father when he grows up—even to marrying a woman like the one father did.

The girl during this same period spends the energy that was once expended in love for her father in an attempt to learn to be like mother and perhaps eventually to marry a man resembling in some way her father. This, however, does not mean that children do not continue to love the opposite-sexed parent; it means only that their primary attachment during these years is to the same-sexed parent. It is this process of identification with the same-sexed parent that facilitates the chief task of the school-age child from 5 or 6 to 11: the task of learning.

Six Years to Adolescence

The years from 6 to 11 have generally been regarded as quiet years as far as emotional development is concerned. Many of the tasks of earlier childhood have been completed, and the relatively stormy years of adolescence have not yet begun. A child's interests begin to turn more and more away from his family and to other children his own age, usually children of the same sex. At this stage, a child's interest in learning is broad and intense.

During this period children begin to be more and more individualistic. Some are solitary, others sociable; some are athletic, others not. One likes only other children, another prefers the company of adults. Some children have imaginary fears that disappear with age or when the fears are discussed with an adult who can explain how or why they originated.

Curiosity about Sex

The child's earlier curiosity about naked people may change to a concern about being clothed and being with people who are clothed. Questions about sex should be answered simply and truthfully.

Adolescence

Adolescence arrives anywhere from 9 to 14 years of age. A girl usually enters adolescence at 10, a boy at about 12.

In female children, there is growth of the breasts and nipples; the pelvis matures, and the external genitalia develop. Axillary (underarm) and pubic hair appear. On the average, girls have their first menstrual period around age thirteen, but it can occur between 10 and 16 years of age. Be sure to explain menstruation to your daughter before the beginning of adolescence.

In male children, the penis and testes develop. Facial, axillary, and pubic hair appear. The voice begins to deepen.

In both boys and girls, there is a rapid growth in height and weight which is related to sexual development. In general the average height of the adolescent is double what is was at age two. See Ch. 3, *The Teens.*

Alphabetic Guide to Child Care

The following Guide is an alphabetically arranged list of articles dealing with many of the problems that confront parents. It includes articles on physical disorders and ailments of childhood; behavioral and emotional problems; and on situations that occur normally in the life of almost every child which may cause tension or distress for parents, child, or both. It is hoped that having information about such normal developmental tensions will help to minimize them.

A note on the cross-references: Where a particular subject is covered elsewhere within this Guide, the reference is printed in small capital letters. (For example: See also TONSILLITIS.) References to sections in other chapters are printed in italic type along with the chapter number. (For example: See "Tonsils and Adenoids" in Ch. 20, *Surgery.*)

Abilities and Aptitudes

In families that place a high value on "performance," a child who has a special aptitude for dealing with animals may get less recognition than a sibling who is an athletic whiz; a mother who never went to college and wishes she had may encourage her daughter's intellectual gifts at the expense of any others.

Parents should make every effort not to foist their own unrealized fantasies onto their children. They should try to keep in mind that each child differs in aptitudes and abilities, and that these individual differences should be fostered, respected, and allowed to find expression.

Precocity

The emphasis on the competitive—not to mention showoff—aspects of any special talent rather than on the satisfaction of accomplishment for its own sake, is a tendency that some parents have to guard against. The most satisfactory approach to outstanding abilities of no matter what category is to recognize their existence as a fact and to keep them for becoming a burden to the child and an ego trip for the parent.

Sibling Rivalry

In large families, the relationship between brothers and sisters is sufficiently complicated by tensions between the oldest and next oldest and so on without introducing additional reasons for competitiveness. Sibling rivalry should not be further fostered by parents who favor the offspring with special abilities. Here is the defensive remark of a middle child (often neglected) in a family with four children: "Tommy is the smartest and Ann is the best swimmer and Jesse is the best at chess, but I'm the goodest." Is the ability to be good a special ability?

Accidents

See Ch. 31, *Medical Emergencies,* and "The Emergency Room" in Ch. 20, *Surgery.*

Adenoidectomy

See "Tonsils and Adenoids" in Ch. 20, *Surgery.*

Adenoids, Swollen

The adenoids are clusters of lymph tissue located behind the soft palate where the nasal passages join the throat. Along with the tonsils and lymphoid tissues elsewhere in the body, the adenoids are involved in warding off infection. When they themselves become inflamed because of bacterial or viral invasion, they become swollen. Swelling may also occur because of allergy.

Swollen adenoids may block the air passages sufficiently to cause mouth breathing, which in turn will not only give the child an "adenoidal" look, but will lead to more frequent upper respiratory infection, as well as to eventual malformation of the lower jawbone. Chronic swelling may also block the Eustachian tube, causing pain in the ear and increasing the possibility of ear infection as well as of intermittent hearing loss. The child's physician can keep track of the severity of such symptoms during periodic checkups and can evaluate the need for surgery. See also TONSILLITIS. For a description of adenoidectomy, see "Tonsils and Adenoids" in Ch. 20, *Surgery*.

Adopted Children

No matter what their individual differences about child rearing, all specialists agree that an adopted child should be told that she was adopted. It doesn't matter that the adoptive parents have come to feel that the child is completely their own. Biologically, she isn't, and it is her human right to find this out not from a neighbor or schoolmate but from the people she trusts as her parents. The fact of her adoption should be talked about naturally in the child's presence even before she can understand what it means. If she is being raised in a loving atmosphere and feels secure in the acceptance of her adoptive parents, she isn't likely to be upset by the reality of her situation.

When the child becomes curious about the circumstances of her adop-tion, or if she wants to know about her "real" mother and father, she should be given no more—and no less—information than the adoption agency provided originally. It isn't unusual for a couple to adopt a baby because they can't have one of their own, and then, because of some hormonal magic, for the woman to become pregnant. In families where this has occurred, the adopted child can be given the feeling that, whatever the advantages of the "natural" child, she was the chosen one.

A widow or divorcee who remarries when her children are still very young may be faced with the possibility that her second husband wants to legally adopt the offspring of her first marriage. Far-reaching consequences are involved in such a decision, and it should not be undertaken lightly. The problem should be discussed with a lawyer who can present the facts in a detached way so that the decision will cause the least anguish and fewest unpleasant consequences.

Aggressiveness

In the rough and tumble of play, some puppies are obviously more aggressive than others, and one of them is clearly determined to be top dog. The same is true of children, especially in any society where energy and enterprise are rewarded.

Aggressive tendencies are natural; the form they take is up to the civilizing efforts of the parents. It is they who have the responsibility of helping a child understand that bullying and bossiness are unacceptable. It seems that because of inheritance, body build, or temperament, some youngsters, whether male or female, are more clearly aggressive than others. It is especially for such children that healthy outlets must be provided for aggression—in the form of toys and playground activities when they are little, and in suitable physical and intellectual endeavors when they get older.

Guilt Feelings

Making a child feel guilty about the strength of his aggressive feelings or thwarting them constantly won't wipe out or destroy the feelings; they'll simply be turned inward, or take the form of nail-biting, or express themselves in some sneaky and antisocial way. Parents who are upset by children's play that simulates violence and who disapprove of toy guns should make their feelings clear without making the youngster feel like a monster because he enjoys them. Aggressiveness that expresses itself in violence and bloodshed—as it so often does in Westerns and in TV programs—should not be the day-in-day-out entertainment to which children are exposed no matter what the parental feelings are.

Boy/Girl Differences

As for a boy who doesn't seem aggressive enough to suit a parent's idea of what a boy should be, or a girl who seems too aggressive to conform to family notions about what "feminine" is all about: these stereotypes are being reexamined and discarded by many people because they are too confining and too rigid to permit the full development of a child's personality. It's no disgrace for a boy to cry, and it should be a source of pride to have a daughter who's determined to be the best math student in the fourth grade.

Allergies

See Ch. 24, *Allergies and Hypersensitivities*.

Allowance

See MONEY.

Ambitions

No matter how grandiose and unrealistic a child's ambitions might seem to parents who pride themselves on being practical, they should be taken seriously and permitted to thrive if the child is working to achieve them. Sometimes the clumsy little girl does become a ballet dancer against all odds, and the boy whose father was a day laborer does become a physician. Ambitions needn't be that exalted. The youngster who goes down to the firehouse with his father may indeed dream of being a fire fighter; the girl who loves looking after babies should be encouraged in her goal to be a pediatric nurse.

Lack of Ambition

What about the youngster who isn't ambitious about anything and who seems to have no goals, not even small ones? This passivity may be a reaction to overambitious parents who have given him the feeling that nothing he aspires to is good enough for them. Or it might result from his never having been made to feel worthwhile enough to have his thoughts about his future taken seriously. Many children who suffer from parental neglect or inadequate educational facilities may need some extra attention from an older person before ambition plays a role in their lives. No matter what the limitations of circumstance, it's rare to find a child who doesn't have some special skill, aptitude, or interest that can become the basis of ambitions for his future as an adult.

Anger

Anger is a feeling that everyone is familiar with. There are moments when even the most controlled and civilized adult experiences the kind of anger that might become blind rage. A child whose bike has been stolen has a right to her anger; a child whose baby brother has broken a valuable doll is justifiably angry. Some youngsters seem to be angry all the time because they feel they're always being pushed around by adults. (Many adults are always angry because they feel they're being pushed around by other adults.) Almost continuous anger seems especially common among some children of six, seven, and eight. Their theme song is "It isn't fair" and they get to be known as injustice-collectors, angry at their friends, siblings, teachers.

Means of Expressing Anger

When parents know that a child's anger comes from a healthy feeling of outrage or because of confusion, they should allow the anger to be expressed—in words or tears. But it does have to be made clear that smashing things in a fit of rage or having a tantrum is unacceptable. A child at the mercy of powerful feelings of rage can be frightened by them and should be helped to understand and control them. It's also a comfort to children to know that grown-ups get terribly angry from time to time, but that part of growing up consists in being able to handle one's feelings and in learning how to express them in the right way at the right time. Thus, a father who is in a rage with his boss will find ways of letting him know that he feels an injustice has been done rather than swallow his anger at work and let it out against his wife or children as soon as he comes home.

Animal Bites

See "Animal Bites" in Ch. 31, *Medical Emergencies.*

Anxiety

Children become chronically anxious when their parents constantly criticize them for failing to measure up to some unachievable standard of perfection. Likewise, parents become anxious about being parents when they criticize themselves for failing to measure up to some unachievable standard of perfection.

Anxiety is one of the most widespread and most debilitating stresses from which people of all ages suffer in the United States, chiefly because many Americans have been victimized by the notion that everybody can be everything. Thus, a parent will expect a little child to be good, bright, neat, polite, aggressive enough to complete adequately but not so aggressive that the other children don't like him, relaxed and cheerful at the same time that he's supposed to do all his chores and the homework and remember to be nice to his baby-sister. What child burdened with such expectations isn't going to feel anxious about fulfilling them so that he can gain his parents' love and approval?

Parents may waste emotional energy feeling anxiety because they think they're inadequate mothers or fathers, perhaps because they lose their tempers from time to time or because they're often too tired to play with their toddler and stick him in the playpen just to keep him out of trouble. A child will also be made chronically anxious if he's always being threatened with punishment, or if he's made to feel that he's bad when he's trying to be good but doesn't know how. The way to keep anxiety at a minimum is to have achievable goals. Is the child healthy, moderately well-behaved, cheerful, and inspiring no complaints from his teachers? Are you as a parent helping him to be healthy, moderately well-behaved, cheerful, and cause no trouble at school? No reason for anybody to be anxious.

Aptitudes

See ABILITIES AND APTITUDES.

Asthma

Asthma, also known as *bronchial asthma*, is a respiratory disturbance in which breathing becomes difficult and labored and is accompanied by a wheezing sound. It is a chronic disorder in which the bronchial tubes suddenly contract or go into spasm, thus cutting off the passage of air from the windpipe to the lungs. Spasms are accompanied by secretion of mucus into the air passages and a swelling of the bronchial tubes, causing the intake and outflow of air to be further obstructed. The disorder may be triggered by a variety of factors; in children it is associated chiefly with allergy and emotional stress. In some cases, asthma may accompany a bacterial or viral infection of the nose or throat.

The Asthma Attack

It can be very frightening to witness a child's first asthma attack, because judging from the sounds and the effort involved in breathing, the child seems to be suffocating. Call the child's pediatrician promptly. Until the physician can be consulted for emergency treatment, parents should try to be calm and reassuring. Immediate symptoms can be alleviated by prescribed medicines given orally or by injection, or by placing the child in a moist environment, such as in the bathroom with the shower turned on (but not *in* the shower). Otherwise, the child should be kept in bed in a humidified room. The condition itself should be carefully assessed by the physician to decide whether desensi-

tization to a particular food or pollen is necessary, whether a pet has to be given away, or whether the child's emotional needs are being neglected. Chronic asthma should not go untreated because frequent and acute attacks can affect general health. Medicines now available can sometimes prevent acute attacks if taken daily by inhalation when one is well.

Autism

See under MENTAL ILLNESS.

Baby-sitters

Families who can always count on a grandparent or an older child to look after the little ones in their absence are spared the complications and expense of hiring baby-sitters. However, many parents must rely on their own resources, especially when both parents work. In such situations the sitter has become an indispensable adjunct of the family.

Instruction in Baby-sitting

In some communities, parents have found it worthwhile to offer a free, informal course in baby-sitting to groups of teenage girls and boys. The course need consist of no more than two or three sessions and can be given by the parents themselves at a local community center. All aspects of the sitter's responsibilities and privileges should be covered. Does the sitter do the dinner dishes? May local phone calls be made? May the refrigerator be raided? The potential employees should be encouraged to ask all the questions they feel uncertain about, and after the course is over, a single sheet of paper summarizing the most important material can be prepared, reproduced in quantity, and distributed to everyone taking the course. The sheet should include a

list of hourly rates with all variants: base rate per hour; increase in rate after midnight; increase per number of children to be looked after, and so on. It might also be a good idea to include the names and telephone numbers of places where sitters can be obtained, such as nursing schools and coed colleges.

Cooperative Sitting

For families who want to get out occasionally but can't afford the extra expense of a sitter, a cooperative parents' pool is a good solution. Each month, one participating parent is responsible for keeping track of who had been sitting for whom, how many hours are owed and how many have been "paid for" and so on. The advantage of this arrangement is that mothers or fathers sit for each others' children and no money changes hands. If such a cooperative pool is worked out, remember that the more accurately the records of time asked for and given are kept, and the more businesslike the arrangements, the longer the system will work and the less friction there will be. Each group should decide for itself what the maximum number of participants should be, and as the group becomes too large to function efficiently, it can split into two separate pools.

Provide for Emergencies

Parents should always leave clear and explicit instructions about possible emergencies with baby-sitters and if possible should leave a telephone number where they can be reached. As the children become opinionated about hired sitters, their wishes should be taken into account. When your own youngsters begin to be hired as sitters themselves, you might keep track of where they're working and when they'll be escorted home.

Bedtime

From babyhood on, the routine of bedtime should be as relaxed as possible for both parent and child. Little babies love to be chanted to (even off-key) or talked to in a gentle tone of voice (even though they don't understand the words) or rocked a bit in their crib. Some little ones seem to resist and fight falling asleep: they fuss and whimper, and then, as though they had been bewitched in the middle of a cry—off they go, all of a sudden. Toddlers may want to hear the same story every night for months, or may cling to the bedtime bottle for quite a while after they've begun to use a cup in the daytime.

Keeping things peaceful at bedtime doesn't mean giving in to the child's pressures or whims. It generally involves keeping one's voice calm, pleasant, and firm: "It's bedtime, and you tell me which story to read to you tonight." The youngster who keeps calling out after having been tucked in—for water, for a last hug, for a last question, for a last trip to the bathroom—isn't determined to make a nuisance of herself; she's just a little scared and wants to make absolutely sure that you're still there. If the family tradition calls for prayers at bedtime, the tone should be cheerful. No child can be expected to relish, "And if I die before I wake I pray the Lord my soul to take" as an accompaniment to sleep.

In a crowded family where siblings share a bedroom, compromises have to be made about the bedtime hour: the younger ones may stay up a little later than they otherwise would, and the older ones may go to bed a little earlier—but they have the pleasure of each other's company. Adjustments in the bedtime hour should be made from time to time not because of a child's wheedling, but because you decide that the occasion calls for it.

Bedwetting

See "Bedwetting" in Ch. 17, *Disease of the Urinogenital System.*

Behavior Problems

See AGGRESSIVENESS, ANGER, DELINQUENCY, DESTRUCTIVENESS, DISHONESTY, DISOBEDIENCE.

Birthmarks

See "Pigment Disorders and Birthmarks" in Ch. 21, *Skin and Hair.*

Blindness

See HANDICAPPED CHILD.

Booster Shots

See IMMUNIZATION.

Boredom

Babies are usually too hungry or too sleepy—or too cranky—to be bored. Toddlers have so much to investigate around the house that boredom is not likely to be one of their problems. As a child gets older and complains about having nothing to do, you might get him involved in a household chore by saying, "Let's . . ." rather than "Why don't you" or "How would you like to." "Let's tidy the cans on the pantry shelf" or "Let's make some cookies" can make a three-year-old feel useful and interested.

Rainy Days

If you're too busy for a cooperative effort and there's a long rainy day ahead, provide for it in advance by keeping a "boredom box" in the closet and renewing its contents from time to time: wrappings saved from gifts; bits of material; boxes of various sizes; discarded magazines to be cut up; old clothes for dress-up activities, and the like.

Coping with Boredom Can be Productive

A child who is never allowed to be bored because his parents or older siblings feel that they have to entertain him or play with him is deprived of the possibility of calling on his own resources and learning how to amuse himself. The fact that an only child may have to live through stretches of boredom often contributes to his exploring his own abilities in a creative way. Sometimes just asking a child to "Tell *me* a story" can work wonders. Some parents solve the recurrent problem of boredom by organizing informal play groups of three or four children; others find a nursery school the best solution.

Convalescence

An older child who is recovering from an illness that has kept him out of school and isolated him from his friends may require some special project to work on in addition to catching up on his homework. A period of protracted convalescence is a good time to introduce a new hobby or craft such as model-making or clay sculpture that may solve the boredom problem for years to come.

Brain Damage

Brain damage refers to an organic defect of the brain—that is, tissue destruction—caused by an injury to the nervous system occurring before, during, or after birth. Such injury can be caused by toxic chemicals as well as by physical trauma. It can result in any of a variety of neurological disorders, such as cerebral palsy or other impairment of motor coordination, mental retardation, convulsive seizures, hyperkinesis, or perceptual difficulties.

Minimal Brain Damage

Minimal brain damage (or, more formally, *minimal brain dysfunction*) refers to a condition of some children who suffer from a motor or perceptual impairment that may affect their ability to learn or use language, interfere with memory, or make it difficult for them to control their attention. Some learning disabilities are attributed to minimal brain damage. See also DYSLEXIA.

Bribes

No child should be bribed into behaving properly except in an emergency. If she's given an ice-cream cone so that she'll stop having a tantrum in public, or if she gets a toy instead of a spanking when she carries on in a store, it will surely occur to her that she can blackmail her parents into getting whatever she wants—which ends up by her being rewarded for being naughty.

A child should not be bribed with money for doing the things that should be expected of her as a matter of course. As a member of the family, she can be counted on to help set and clear the table, and when she's a little older, to help with the dishes without being paid to do so. She should be expected to do as well as she can at school without being told that her allowance will be increased if her grades are better than her best friend's.

The line between a bribe and a reward is a delicate one and should be kept somewhat flexible if it is to be realistic. Certainly a youngster who has made extra efforts should be rewarded, but in some way that doesn't involve the handing over of money. Treating her and her friends to a special outing, or spending some extra time with her in a pursuit of her own choice is a way of showing that you appreciate the good job she's done—whether it's taking the reponsibility for cleaning up the garage or doing a series of complicated errands without complaining about them. See also MONEY.

Brothers and Sisters

Rivalry and jealousy and bickering are inevitable among brothers and sisters; companionship, a helping hand, and good times together are part of the picture too. Parents can keep resentments and quarrels at a minimum by not playing one child off against the other or by refraining from holding up one child as an example of virtue to another. In an atmosphere of equal recognition, brothers and sisters will love and respect each other most of the time and fight only occasionally. Special privileges granted on the basis of such distinctions as "Well, he's the oldest" or "She's the youngest" or exceptions made because "He's a boy" or "She's only a girl" can cause resentments that last a lifetime.

Burns

See "Burns" in Ch. 31, *Medical Emergencies.*

Camps

There seems to be no end to the diversity of camps available for summer enrollment. Most urban and suburban communities have day camps in which children may be accepted for certain minimum periods. They range from expensive groups that offer sightseeing trips, swiming instruction, and other special attractions to groups that cost very little and function more or less like day-care centers. "Sleepaway" camps run by organizations such as the Scouts and the 4-H Clubs are comparatively cheap and will register a child for a week rather than for a month or for the entire summer. Camps subsidized by community funds or private endowment are available for urban children from poor families.

Special Camps

The proliferation of special camps has been a blessing to the parents of handicapped children: those with diabetes, muscular dystrophy, learning disabilities, obesity, and other problems need no longer be deprived of a camping experience with their peers. In many cases, particularly for overweight youngsters, the summer experience can be a major health contribution.

In general, an effort should be made to choose a camp that suits the tastes and temperament of the child. A youngster who hates competitive sports is likely to have a miserable time in a camp that emphasizes team spirit. He may enjoy a place that offers lots of nature study, hiking, and animal care. A child eager to improve his swimming should go to a camp with better-than-average water sport facilities rather than one that concentrates on arts and crafts and offers only a nearby pond for all water activities. Information about camps that have official standing can be obtained by writing to The American Camping Association, 5000 State Rd., 67 N, Martinsdale, IN 46151.

Cancer

Rare as it may be and affecting only one child in about 7,000 each year, cancer still claims the lives of more children between the ages of one and fourteen than any other single disease. Among the cancers that more commonly affect children in their early years are the following: *acute lymphocytic leukemia,* in which white blood cells proliferate in the bone marrow in such great quantities that they disrupt normal blood production; *neuroblastoma,* which may occur in any part of the body but characteristically involves a tumorous growth in the sympathetic nerve tissues of the adrenal glands; *brain* or *spinal cord tumor; Hodgkin's disease,* or cancer of the lymph nodes; *Wilms' tumor,* a rare kidney cancer that accounts for about one-fifth of all childhood cancers; *retinoblastoma,* an eye tumor that is probably hereditary and is most frequently encountered in children under four; and *bone cancer* that may attack the long bones of the forearm and leg during the growing years. Many of these cancers can now be arrested, and some can be cured if symptoms are detected early enough. See Ch. 18, *Cancer,* for further information about cancer.

Early Symptoms

Early detection is best accomplished by calling to a physician's attention any of these symptoms that last for more than a few days: continued crying or pain for which there appears to be no explanation; intermittent nausea and vomiting; the development of lumps or swellings in or on any part of the child's body; stumbling or walking unsteadily; a loss of appetite and general lassitude; any marked change in bowel or bladder habits; any unexplained discharge of blood, whether in the stool or urine, or in heavy nosebleeds, or any marked slowness of bleeding to stop after an injury.

Celiac Disease

Celiac disease, officially known as *malabsorption syndrome,* is the designation for a group of congenital enzyme deficiencies in which certain nutriments are not properly absorbed from the intestinal tract. *Celiac* means having to do with the abdo-

men. Celiac disease is characterized by frothy, bulky, and foul-smelling stools containing undigested fats. Diarrhea may alternate with constipation, the child has severe stomach cramps, and the abdomen becomes conspicuously bloated. If the disease is untreated, anemia results, and the child's growth is impaired. Early symptoms should be brought to a physician's attention so that a correct diagnosis can be made based on laboratory investigation of the stools. Treatment consists of a special, gluten-free diet under a physician's continuing supervision. *Gluten* is a protein component of wheat and rye; special breads, cookies, etc., must therefore be used. If the diet is strictly adhered to, full recovery can be expected although it may take over a year.

Cerebral Palsy

Cerebral palsy is the general term for a group of abnormal conditions commonly associated with a brain disorder that causes the loss or impairment of muscle control. Approximately one child in about 7,000 suffers from some degree of this disability. Damage to the nervous system that results in cerebral palsy may have occurred before birth, during delivery, or in rare cases, as a consequence of accident, injury, or severe illness during infancy or childhood. Because symptoms vary widely, each individual case is assessed for proper treatment by a team of therapists under the supervision of a specialist, usually a pediatrician. One of the most important aspects of treatment involves parental understanding of the fact that it is essential that they help the child to help himself as much as possible. Guiding the youngster towards self-acceptance and independence requires the patience, persistence, and resource-

fulness of the entire family, and may require a certain amount of group therapy and counseling. For a discussion of symptoms and treatment, see "Cerebral Palsy" in Ch. 8, *Diseases of the Muscles and Nervous System.*

Cheating

See DISHONESTY.

Checkups

Medical and dental checkups are essential to everyone's health, but they are especially important for the growing child. An infant should be examined by a physician every month for the first six months, and less frequently after that. The pediatrician usually recommends a schedule for immunization and future checkups. If possible, parents should try to maintain continuity with the same physician so that when an illness occurs, the child sees the physician as an old friend rather than a threatening stranger. Continuity also gives the physician a total picture of the child in sickness and in health and enables him to diagnose variations from the normal with more accuracy. Parents who cannot afford the services of a private physician can be assured of good infant and child care at a local child-health station or at the well-baby clinic of a nearby hospital. Between checkups, it's a good idea for parents to keep a running list of questions or problems they would like to discuss with the doctor at the next visit.

Chicken Pox

Chicken pox cannot be prevented at this time. It does not usually cause any severe complications in a child, but it can be serious in an adult. It is highly infectious and spreads rapidly.

Chicken pox is caused by a virus. Its incubation period is two to three weeks. Symptoms include those of the common cold, a fever, general malaise, and a rash.

The rash, which may be either mild or severe, is different from that produced by measles or by rubella. The measles rash is red and blotchy. Chicken pox look like bunches of blisters close together. These blisters are filled with fluid, and there is a reddened area around each lesion. As new blisters appear, the older ones become encrusted. The rash may affect the mouth, nose, ears, vagina, penis, or scrotum. In an older child the symptoms may be more severe than in a younger one, and may be accompanied by headache and vomiting.

Treatment

The only way to treat chicken pox is symptomatically. The rash is very itchy, and an affected child must be prevented from scratching. Otherwise, he may develop a secondary infection and be left pitted and scarred.

Treatment involves the use of lotions, such as Calamine, which is applied locally to the pox to relieve the itching. If the child is old enough, it's a good idea to let him paint it on himself. Your physician may also prescribe medicine to be taken orally to help the child stop scratching the blisters. In a few days, the rash clears up, the lesions dry, and the crusts fall off.

Child Abuse and Neglect

Child abuse and neglect have been defined in various ways.

In 1962, Dr. C. Henry Kempe, chief pediatrician at the University of Colorado Medical Center, coined the term *battered child syndrome*. According to Dr. Kempe's definition, the victim of battering is "any child who

[has] received *nonaccidental* injury or injuries as a result of acts or omissions on the part of his parents or guardians." Under the Child Abuse Prevention and Treatment Act (Public Law 93-247), passed by Congress in 1974 and amended in 1978, child abuse and neglect are defined as

> the physical or mental injury, sexual abuse or exploitation, negligent treatment, or maltreatment of a child under the age of 18 by a person who is responsible for the child's welfare under circumstances which indicate that the child's health or welfare is harmed or threatened thereby.

Abuse and neglect clearly take many forms. *Physical abuse* may involve punching, scalding, suffocating, headcracking, and stomping. *Sexual abuse* can mean intercourse, incest, rape, sodomy, or impairing of a minor's morals (see SEXUAL ABUSE). *Physical neglect* occurs when parents or parent surrogates fail to provide the essentials of a normal life. These include food, clothing, shelter, care, and supervision. Under *emotional abuse or neglect* authorities include parental failure to provide love and proper direction, parental rejection, and deprivation of mothering.

Incidence

Figures on the incidence of child abuse and neglect are difficult to confirm. Many such cases are never reported. At least one agency, the National Center on Child Abuse and Neglect, a federal agency, has concluded that more than one million children are maltreated each year. Another estimate indicates that some 3,000 children die annually in New York City alone as a result of physical abuse.

Most of the abuse victims are three years old or younger. Some authorities believe that the cases of neglect are far more numerous than those of actual abuse.

Control

Approaches to control of the problem of child abuse and neglect have been both legislative and social. Laws passed by all 50 states require physicians and other professionals to report suspected cases of child abuse. In increasing numbers the states also require reports from nurses, teachers, counselors, social workers, clergymen, law enforcement officers, attorneys, and coroners. Some states provide for penalties, including fines up to $1,000 or prison sentences of as much as one year, for persons mandated to report but failing to do so.

Control measures have focused in addition on the rehabilitation of abusive parents and protection of abused children. The National Center on Child Abuse and Neglect, established in 1974 as part of the Children's Bureau of the federal Office of Child Development, receives funding that makes possible protective services for the short-term care of endangered children outside the home. The Center also provides counseling for parents, foster-care payments, and other services.

On the principle that the abusive parent must be treated if child abuse and neglect are to be controlled, various organizations have instituted parent-oriented programs. Parents Anonymous sponsors therapy sessions in which abusive parents can meet to help themselves and each other. "Helplines" operating in many communities offer aid and counseling to parents who have abused a child but are afraid to contact a social service or other agency. A number of other agencies and groups provide emergency, counseling, outreach, and related services to parents or parent surrogates. Some helplines have workers available to visit homes in life-threatening situations.

Other groups and agencies take a

multidisciplinary approach. Alliance, a division of Catholic Charities, brings together existing community agencies that work together in teams to treat child abuse and neglect cases. Hospital-based treatment programs may include a physician, nurse, social worker, and consulting psychiatrist. Lay therapists may visit homes under other programs, and "foster grandparents" over 65 years of age may be recruited to care for battered children who have been hospitalized.

Sources of Help

Persons seeking help or advice on abused and neglected children can look in their communities' yellow pages under the heading "Social Services Organizations." A number of organizations that offer assistance are listed in the SEXUAL ABUSE section. Others include:

- Parents Anonymous, 22330 Hawthorne Place, Ste. 208, Torrance, CA 90505; 800/421-0353.

- American Association for Protecting Children (a division of the American Humane Association), 9725 E. Hampden Ave., Denver, CO 80231; 303/695-0811.

- Parents without Partners, 7910 Woodmont Ave., Bethesda, MD 20814; 800/638-8078.

- Parents United, 840 Guadelupe Parkway, San Jose, CA 95110; 800/422-4453.

Circumcision

Circumcision is a surgical procedure in which the foreskin, or *prepuce*, that covers the cone-shaped tip of the male infant's penis is removed. The Book of Genesis speaks of circumcision as a religious rite. Once relatively common in the United States,

the procedure has become more rare. The American Academy of Pediatrics has stated that "routine circumcision of the newborn infant lacks medical justification."

Usually performed a few days after birth, the procedure takes only a few minutes and can be done in various ways. A scalpel may be used, for example. Possible complications include excessive bleeding, infection, and urinary obstruction resulting from contraction of the skin at the base of the foreskin. But complications are infrequent.

The parents of the newborn male infant should decide whether to have their son circumcised or not. They may first consult their obstetrician or pediatrician. Most decisions are made on the basis of family, religious, or cultural traditions. Many family health insurance policies today provide no coverage for the procedure.

Cleanliness and Neatness

Most healthy youngsters are too busy exploring the world or are too involved in what they're doing at the moment to be concerned about being neat and clean.

What is cleanliness all about anyway? Parents used to talk a lot about germs, and the germs are certainly still all around us in spite of the success of antibiotics in dealing with a large number of them. But there are the unconquerable viruses, and parasites, and worms, and children should thus be told in a factual way that habits of personal cleanliness are important for reasons of their own health and the health of the people around them. Coming to the table with freshly washed hands, keeping their bodies clean, washing their hands after using the toilet, covering their coughs and sneezes—these minimal practices should be instilled until they become habitual and no longer need to be dis-

cussed. Children do get dirty, but TV commercials have taught practically every one of them that getting their clothes clean is no big deal, so it's futile for parents to get worked up over stains.

As for neatness, the point of putting things where they belong is not merely for the sake of appearances, but for the more important reason that time won't be wasted and tempers lost in trying to find them when they're needed. The aesthetics of tidiness doesn't interest most children, but a functional reason that makes sense to them usually does. When it comes to looking neat, some children seem to accomplish that with no effort at all; others look like slobs until adolescence begins, when parents deprived of the use of the bathroom mirror may yearn for the good old untidy days of childhood.

Cleft Palate and Cleft Lip

A *cleft palate* is a split in the roof of the mouth sometimes extending to the lip and into the nose. The split is caused by the failure of the two sides of the face to unite properly during prenatal development. The condition occurs in about 1 out of 1,000 births and is sometimes associated with a foot or spine deformity. It is in no way related to mental retardation.

An infant born with a cleft palate cannot suck properly unless a special device, called an *obturator*, is inserted into the split to close it against the flow of air. Where this is undesireable, feeding may be done with a spoon or a dropper.

Because the condition eventually causes speech distortion, it should be corrected at about 18 months of age, before the child begins to talk. The surgery consists of reconstructing the tissue. Sometimes, even at this early age, the child may need some corrective speech therapy following the operation.

If the split occurs only in the lip, commonly called a *harelip*, surgery may be recommended when the infant weighs about 15 pounds, usually at the age of 12 to 15 months. When the operation is performed this early, there is no danger of speech impairment, and the result is only a thin scar.

Clothing

Children's clothing should fit comfortably so that it doesn't chafe or bind, especially in hot weather. In addition to allowing for freedom of movement, it should be sturdy and washable. In most communities, blue jeans and shirts seem to serve both sexes in all stages of growing up, starting with nursery school. In some few places, schools have more formal clothing codes, but it's a rare institution that still insists on white shirts and ties for elementary students. A youngster who occasionally enjoys wearing a dress shirt or a party dress can usually find one that's drip-dry and doesn't require ironing.

Many families economize on children's clothing by buying at rummage sales or thrift shops. (Not shoes!) If parents are proud of having found bargains, children will be pleased to wear them. Parental attitude also affects a child's feelings about hand-me-downs from within the family or from friends. There's no reason why children's clothing—and especially such expensive items as heavy outer coats—shouldn't be successively used as long as they fit properly.

Fashions and Status

Even sensible clothing can present problems of status that require tactful handling. Your eight-year-old son may announce that everyone in his class is wearing those fancy imported sneakers that cost as much as a pair of good shoes; or your ten-year-old daughter brings you the news that all her friends have expensive coats with a suede look or fur-trimmed collars. For families that can't afford or don't believe in acquiring such luxuries— and the majority can't—the facts are probably these: a few privileged youngsters may indeed be wearing such sneakers or such coats, and the majority have embarked on a concerted campaign of pressuring their parents into making the same expenditures. If your child is really conspicuous because he doesn't own an expensive garment that all his friends have, you must decide whether to make it clear to him that you spend money in different ways—say on family vacations or good dental care. On the other hand, you may decide to capitulate about the item of clothing and deprive the child (not yourself) of something else—perhaps his birthday present for the coming year. That's one way to teach a child a basic lesson about the inevitability of choice-making.

Clubfoot

Clubfoot is a bone deformity characterized by an inturning or outturning of the foot. An orthopedist must put the clubfoot and part of the leg into a cast to correct the condition. If casting does not cure the abnormality, orthopedic surgery may be necessary.

Occasionally, a benign and easily correctable condition involving a child's legs may have been produced by the position the baby was in while still in the uterus.

The mother can help to correct the condition by daily passive exercises of the baby's feet. She does this by turning the feet correctly for a few minutes every day. To maintain the corrected position, the application of plaster is sometimes necessary. Such a procedure requires the attention of an orthopedic surgeon.

Colic

During the first three or four months, many babies have occasional attacks of *colic*, a general term applied to infantile digestive discomfort. After feeding, the baby may cry out in pain and draw up her arms and legs. Her abdomen may feel hard. Apart from making sure the baby is as comfortable as can be, there's not much that can be done for colic. You must try not to let the baby's crying make you a nervous wreck, for your nervousness will be communicated to the baby, which will only create a vicious circle of increasing tension. Usually colic tapers off at about the third month. If the baby's colic attacks are very frequent or persistent, consult your pediatrician.

Color Blindness

Color blindness is a genetic inability to distinguish between certain colors, most commonly between red and green. This defect, which is characteristically male, is inherited through the mother. That is, a woman whose father was color blind can pass the trait to her son without herself suffering the defect. About 8 million people in the United States have the red/green form of color blindness which can neither be cured nor corrected. Many of them are scarcely aware of their deficiency. Parents who suspect that their child may have this minor disability can arrange for simple testing.

Common Cold

By recent count, there are about 150 different viruses that cause common cold symptoms, and because not a single one of them can be treated effectively by medicines, coping with a cold seems to be part of the human condition. Parents who are sniveling, sneezing, and coughing should ask the physician what precautions to take when handling the baby.

Young children with stuffy noses and breathing difficulties should be kept indoors, near a humidifier or steam kettle if the air is especially dry. Nose drops should not be given unless the physician says so. Older children may not want to miss school because of a cold. If they do go, they should be given lots of liquid when they get home and steered in the direction of an afternoon nap. Colds in and of themselves are unavoidable and not serious, but the proper precautions should be taken to prevent complications, such as an ear infection or a sore throat.

Competitiveness

See AGGRESSIVENESS.

Conscience

See GUILT AND CONSCIENCE.

Constipation

Parents who are anxious about the frequency of their own bowel movements or who are excessively refined in their attitudes towards defecation are pretty sure to transmit these feelings to their children unless they make some effort not to. Concerns of this kind are one sure way of constipating a child. Actually, if a child is eating a proper diet, getting enough exercise, and drinking a sufficiency of liquids, constipation is not likely to be a problem.

Frequency of Bowel Movements

Not everyone has a bowel movement every day. On the other hand, some people routinely have more than one movement a day. There is considerable variation among normal patterns of bowel movements. This should be borne in mind before parents conclude that their child is constipated. Children need to be assured that they are not necessarily abnormal if they deviate from the one-a-day pattern.

However, any abrupt change in the normal pattern of bowel movements should be noted, and if it persists contact a physician. Frequent small movements can be a sign of constipation.

A youngster on a light diet because of illness, or one who is dehydrated because of a fever, may suffer from mild constipation that will clear up when he recovers. If constipation becomes chronic, don't resort to enemas or laxatives on your own; discuss the problem with your physician who will want to check on other symptoms that might indicate an intestinal disorder.

Cradle Cap

This condition is marked by yellowish crusts on the baby's scalp. It is usually harmless, and can be taken care of by regular shampooing. Occasionally, a special soap as well as a very fine comb may be helpful.

Crib Death

See SUDDEN INFANT DEATH SYNDROME.

Crossed Eyes (Strabismus)

Do not be alarmed if your baby's eyes do not focus. Crossed eyes are a common condition that usually corrects itself somewhere between the ages of six and twelve months. If crossing of the eyes persists after one year, an ophthalmologist (eye specialist) should evaluate the baby's vision.

If a real problem does develop, one eye—or each eye alternately—may cross, turn outward, or focus below or above the other. Frequently the reason for "turning" is that there is a larger refractive error in one eye than in the other. Eyeglasses will often correct this condition.

Occasionally, eye muscle weakness is the cause of crossed eyes. This is most often true of premature children. The weakness of some muscles causes overaction of other muscles.

Eyeglasses will often prevent the need for eye surgery. Sometimes, however, surgery will be necessary to straighten the eyes. Either before or after surgery the eyes may need further attention in the form of eye drops, a patch to cover one eye, or glasses.

Croup

Croup, a most harassing and terrifying experience for new parents, is a spasm of the windpipe or trachea, especially involving the larynx. When such a spasm occurs, an affected child has great trouble in breathing and produces a cough that sounds like the bark of a dog. In some cases, the child can't breathe at all.

An attack of croup is an emergency. The younger the child, the more dangerous it is. You must get the baby's airway open. The best thing to do is to take the child into the bathroom, shut the door, and turn on the hot water of the shower full force, or of the bathtub and sink if you don't have a shower. The idea is to fill the room with hot steam in order to loosen the mucus plug in the baby's trachea, thus enabling him to cough up the mucus.

Get to your physician as soon as possible so that more effective treatment can begin. If the croup is viral in origin, antibiotics may not help; but when the infection is caused by bacteria, your physician will put the child on one of the antimicrobial agents. If your child is subject to croup, it is a good idea to invest in a hot or cold air vaporizer and use it whenever he has congestion resulting from a cold.

In a really severe emergency, when the windpipe closes completely, a *tracheostomy* must be performed so that the throat can be opened and an airway inserted. A tracheostomy should be performed in a hospital, but if for some reason it is performed elsewhere, the child should be hospitalized as quickly as possible.

Curiosity

If we weren't born curious, we'd never learn a thing. Even before a child can walk and talk, curiosity motivates a good part of her behavior: putting things into her mouth, poking at things, pointing at people, and as the natural urge to speak becomes stronger, holding things up or bringing them to mother or father in order to find out what they're called.

Respecting Curiosity

A parent who respects the child's curiosity will be attentive to it and satisfy it as part of the ongoing learning experience. It doesn't take any extra time when a toddler is sitting in your lap to say the words for the parts of your face (and hers) as she touches them, or the words for her articles of clothing as she tries to help put them on. Dealing with the "why" stage of curiosity is more complicated, especially because in many instances, the child is asking "Why?" for the sheer joy and sense of power of being able to do so.

Many parents who don't know anything about mechanics or astronomy have developed a sense of security by heading for the children's shelves at the local library and reading the simplest books on the subject that interest their preschool children so that they can answer some of their questions. Of course, no one can answer all the questions that a child might ask during an average day. Some should be answered by mother, some by father, and some will have to wait. There's no harm in telling a four-year-old child who wants to know why the wind makes a whistling sound that she'll find out about such things when she goes to school. That's a much better answer than "Don't ask so many questions." Questions should always be listened to even if the answers aren't readily available.

As the child reaches the age of eight and can do a certain amount of reading, it's a good idea to invest in a fairly simple encyclopedia. With such a source of information available, it's possible to respond to some questions with "Let's go find the answer together."

Each family must decide for itself where the line is to be drawn between legitimate curiosity and unacceptable snoopiness or nosiness as children get older and become interested in such matters as how rich the neighbors are, or "What were you and mommy fighting about when I was falling asleep last night?"

Cystic Fibrosis

Cystic fibrosis is an inherited disease in which the child cannot handle the normal secretions of the respiratory tract. There is a lack of ciliary action—the beating movement by the hairs of the cells lining the bronchial tubes of the lungs. Thick mucus collects at the base of the lungs, obstructing the smaller air passages and causing labored breathing and chronic cough.

Respiratory Complications

Bacteria multiply in the accumulated lung secretions, predisposing the patient to chronic bronchitis and other respiratory infections, such as pneumonia. Lung tissue changes can result eventually in severe, permanent damage to the lungs.

Digestive Complications

The abnormally thick, viscous mucus produced by the cystic fibrosis patient tends to obstruct the ducts or openings of the mucus-secreting glands. When such mucus obstructs the pancreas, it interferes with its ability to supply important digestive enzymes to the intestinal tract, thus leading to poor digestion and malabsorption of a number of important nutrients. A child with cystic fibrosis may therefore be poorly nourished in spite of an adequate diet.

Other Complications

Tissue changes in the lungs can restrict blood flow to the heart, leading to increased blood pressure and chronic heart strain. Loss of large amounts of salt through malfunctioning sweat glands can become a very serious problem for youngsters in hot weather, causing dehydration and heat exhaustion. Laboratory tests usually find an abnormally high concentration of salt in the sweat of cystic fibrosis patients. (Indeed, the skin of a cystic fibrosis patient is apt to taste salty.) Some tissues may show three times the normal concentration of sodium and twice the normal levels of potassium.

Treatment

There is no known cure for cystic fibrosis. Treatment includes the use of humidifiers and inhalation medication in the form of aerosols to loosen secretions. Another method used is *postural drainage*—lying facedown with the head lower than the feet to let gravity help loosen secretions. Antibiotics are used to control infections; special diets with reduced fat intake and added nutrients are prescribed to compensate for abnormal digestive function. Other medical techniques are utilized in individual cases to maintain normal heart and lung function.

Once considered strictly a disease of early childhood, an increasing number of cases of cystic fibrosis have been detected in recent years among adolescents and adults. Symptoms of the disease, including respiratory difficulty with chronic coughing, may resemble those of an allergic reaction.

How the Disease Is Inherited

Cystic fibrosis is transmitted to a child only when both parents are carriers of the trait. When only one parent carries the trait, however, some of the children can become carriers. Through marriage with other carriers, they may then become the parents of a child afflicted with the disorder.

Information on new treatment techniques, the location of treatment centers, and genetic counseling may be obtained from the national headquarters of the Cystic Fibrosis Foundation, 6000 Executive Blvd., Ste. 309, Rockville, MO 20852.

Daydreaming

See FANTASIES.

Deafness

Major advances have been made in recent years in educating and socializing incurably deaf children who are normal in all other ways. Starting with a proper assessment of the child's degree of deafness at the earliest possible time and the fitting of a hearing aid are two crucial considerations. The child's instruction in lipreading and the use of her own vocal equipment are professionally supervised, and the rest of the family is very much involved in the whole process. Nowadays an important advance in speech therapy is the use of a feedback system that make it possible for the youngster to be self-corrective. Parents seeking information about special schools and services, summer camps, and other facilities can write to the following agencies: Alexander Graham Bell Association for the Deaf, 3417 Volta Place, N.W., Washington, D.C. 20007; American Speech-Language-Hearing Association, 10801 Rockville Pike, Rockville, MO 20852. See also HEARING.

Death

Some children's first experience of death is the loss of a grandparent; others may have to confront the fact of death for the first time when a beloved pet dies. A child wants to know where people or animals go when they die. Parents should be as honest as possible in answering such questions and tell their offspring what they themselves truly believe. Those parents who believe that there is life after death should say so; those who do not should say that they do not. Whatever one's beliefs, there are better ways to phrase them than "Grandma is in heaven watching you" or "People who are naughty go to hell when they die."

Death of a Parent

A child who has to cope with the death of a parent may be so disoriented that his behavior will seem odd to the adults around him. He may pretend that the death never happened; others may protect themselves from the shock by burying their feelings and never talking about the dead parent. Still others may feel rage at having been abandoned. Many youngsters are overwhelmed by guilt, feeling that in some magic way they caused the death because from time to time they secretly wished it. In cases where the bereft child cannot cope with the loss, it may be advisable to provide some help in the form of psychiatric therapy.

Delinquency

Juvenile delinquents are minors who are guilty of breaking the law or who are engaged in associations and activities considered harmful to children's morals, such as running errands for gamblers, acting as a lookout during a robbery, or sniffing glue for kicks. Swiping a candy bar or a comic book at the age of ten doesn't define a child as a hardened delinquent, but where such behavior becomes chronic, it's a sign that something is wrong that needs to be corrected. With the guidance of a therapist, it may turn out that the child alone is not entirely responsible for his delinquent tendencies. See also DESTRUCTIVENESS, DISCIPLINE, DISHONESTY, DISOBEDIENCE.

Dental Care

The proper attitude toward dental care is best instilled not by lectures or warnings, but by example. Parents who themselves go regularly to the dentist for checkups, who take care of their teeth by keeping them clean with routine brushing and the use of dental floss, can do more for their child's dental health than those who depend on stern warnings to shape the attitudes of their children. Parents can hardly expect their offspring to be heroic about dental visits when they themselves scarcely ever go unless they have a toothache.

Start Early

Dental care can begin by having the toddler accompany the parent to the dentist so that his baby teeth can be inspected and he can be given a special toothbrush of his own with instructions about how to use it. In communities where the water supply is not fluoridated, the dentist may recommend an ongoing program of fluoride application to the teeth themselves. Some families find that a pediatric dentist who specializes in children's dentistry can deal with a frightened or anxious child more expertly than the family dentist. Other families use the services of the dental clinics that are part of the dental schools of large universities.

No matter who is in charge of the family's dental health, it is important that professional attention is given to the child's dental development at every stage: fillings for decay in the first teeth, routine cleanings and checkups, and preventive orthodontics where advisable. Another aspect of dental care involves keeping the consumption of sweets to a minimum, and making sure that the child's daily diet contains the proper nutrients for building healthy teeth. See also ORTHODONTICS. For full discussion, see Ch. 22, *Teeth and Gums*.

Destructiveness

"It was an accident!" is a common cry when a child destroys a valuable object because of carelessness. And it probably was an accident. Parents who don't want precious bric-a-brac or other delicate possessions broken had better put them out of the reach of curious and clumsy little fingers. Young children should not be punished because their toys always seem

to be destroyed; better to give them playthings that are sturdy and comparatively indestructible.

The child who is destructive unwittingly should not be spoken to in the same way as one would speak to a boy who willfully breaks his sister's doll or a girl who spitefully tears her brother's model-making manual. Destructiveness born of anger ("I was so furious, I smashed a dish") may happen rarely, but when it does, it should be commented on as an unsuitable way of dealing with the problem that caused the anger in the first place. When destructiveness gets out of hand or involves group activities amounting to vandalism, parental action should be taken with the guidance of a professional counselor.

Developmental Disability

Any disability that interferes with a child's normal development is a *developmental disability*. The term has been used more specifically, however, to refer to mental retardation, cerebral palsy, epilepsy, and autism.

Diabetes

No one knows why some children develop diabetes. Diabetes is a noncontagious disease that results from the body's inability to produce enough insulin for the normal metabolism of sugar. The diabetic child is thus improperly nourished because the sugar that should be incorporated into the tissues is excreted in the urine. Finding sugar in the urine facilitates early diagnosis. Also, because this disorder causes a disturbance in the metabolism of fat, there is an increase of fat in the blood, detectable in a routine blood count.

Early Signs

Parents who are themselves diabetic

will be alert to any symptoms in their offspring. The disease occurs more frequently in children where there is a family history of diabetes. However, because the disorder may occur in children where there is no previous family history of diabetes, alertness to the following signs is advisable: an abnormally frequent need to urinate; an excessive desire for fluids; itching of the genitals; general listlessness; frequent boils and carbuncles; slow healing of cuts and bruises.

If a diagnosis of diabetes is made by the physician, the child may be hospitalized for a few days for a series of definitive tests, and all the members of the family will be educated in the best way to supervise the child's diet and daily routine so that serious complications can be avoided. Professional guidance is also available to ensure that the youngster's emotional adjustment is a healthy one. For a full discussion see Ch. 15, *Diabetes Mellitus*.

Diaper Rash

See RASHES.

Diarrhea

Diarrhea, or loose and watery bowel movements, is common in babies because they are more sensitive to certain intestinal germs than older children. They may also be reacting to a change in their formula or to the roughage in a newly introduced fruit or vegetable. In older children, diarrhea may occur not only as a symptom of bacterial or viral infection, or because of food poisoning, but also as an allergic response, or because of overexcitement or anxiety.

Diarrhea in an infant should always be brought to a doctor's attention if it continues for more than 24 hours. The same holds true for an older child, especially when there are also symptoms of cramps, fever, or aches and pains in the joints. Persistent diarrhea from any cause, because it can lead to serious dehydration, especially in infants, requires prompt medical attention.

Diphtheria

Diphtheria is a severe and contagious bacterial infection, often fatal if untreated. Once one of the most threatening of all childhood diseases, there are now fewer than 1,000 cases a year in the United States because of widespread and effective immunization.

The first symptoms—fever, headache, nausea, and sore throat—may be confused with the onset of other disorders. However, there is a manifestation of diphtheria that is uniquely its own: patches of grayish yellow membrane form in the throat and grow together into one large membrane that interferes with swallowing and breathing. The diphtheria bacteria also produce a powerful toxin that can eventually cause irreversible damage to the heart and nerves. Diagnosis is usually verified by laboratory identification of the bacteria in a throat culture.

If diphtheria does occur, it is best treated in a hospital. The prompt prescription of antitoxin serum and antibiotics results in recovery in practically all cases. See IMMUNIZATION.

Discipline

There are no easy answers or sure guides to the discipline of children; but there are some basic principles that, if followed, can make life together more enjoyable and tolerable for parents and children alike. All children, whether they be normal, retarded, geniuses, sick, or well, need and want discipline in their daily lives, even though they will say, when asked, that they would rather do as they please. From time to time most parents have been jolted to realize that their only interactions with their children seem to be when they are nagging them to do something or reprimanding them for doing something wrong.

The Effect of Praise

One of the most important principles of discipline is that praise is more effective than punishment. As has been noted by many students of human behavior, children crave attention from their parents. To gain this attention, they will behave in any way necessary; if misbehavior is the only action that receives attention, the child misbehaves. Parents should make a point of being attentive to their children when they are behaving properly and should reinforce good behavior with praise. The result will usually be an increase in good behavior and a decrease in misbehavior.

Need for Consistency

Consistent discipline is important. Children should know what is expected of them and should know what the consequences of their misbehavior will be. Once a promise or threat is made, it should be carried out. Failure to carry out a threat encourages a repetition of the undesirable behavior. Failure to carry out a promise may cause the child to lose faith in the parent.

Discrimination

See PREJUDICE.

Dishonesty

Nobody is honest about everything all the time, and that goes for children as well as adults. It's unrealistic to expect a child never to lie about anything.

Parents Lie, Too

Many parents will lie in the presence of their children without realizing that they're doing it. "No, Mrs. Clark, I won't be able to pick the children up today because I have a bad cold." Your five-year-old girl looks you in the eye and says "Are you really sick, mommy?" Well, your explanation is likely to be just as lame as hers would be if you caught her out in a similar duplicity.

Little children like to make things up and can't be held strictly accountable for some of their tall stories when they're still at an age at which fact and fantasy are not clearly distinguished. A colorful exaggeration needn't call for an accusation of lying. It's better to respond with, "That's an interesting story," or "You're just imagining."

Lying and Punishment

As youngsters get older, they should feel secure enough to tell the truth about having been naughty, knowing that although they may be punished, they will get approval for having told the truth. Children shouldn't be so fearful of their parents that dishonesty is their only protection against a beating.

Cheating

Children who are pressured beyond their ability to perform are the ones likeliest to cheat; so are those for whom winning has been held up constantly as a transcendent value. A child who has been caught cheating at school is usually punished by the authorities. If the incident is discussed at home, the parents might reexamine their values before adding to the child's burdens. A youngster who cheats regularly at games will suffer the natural punishment of exclusion by his peers.

Stealing

Young children who embark on group enterprises of stealing "for fun"—whether it's taking candy from the corner market or shoplifting from a department store—needn't be viewed as case-hardened criminals unless the stealing becomes habitual. A nine-year-old who swipes a candy bar once or twice and regrets it belongs in a different category from one who is hired as a lookout for older delinquents. Children usually have respect for other people's property when they have property of their own that they value and don't want anyone else to take.

Disobedience

Father gets a parking ticket because he forgot about alternate sides of the street on Wednesdays; mother has a whipped cream dessert in spite of her physician's orders not to. Are mother and father disobedient? When Junior comes home from the playground at five instead of obeying orders to come home at four, is his disobedience any worse than theirs? Genuine forgetfulness, negligence, or occasional breaking of a rule is only human. Willful chronic disobedience is another matter.

Some children with a strong urge toward independence may test out many parental rules by disobeying them on purpose. A child who has been ordered not to spend any time with another child because the families are feuding, may, by flouting the order, be telling his parents that he has a right to choose his own friends.

Where disobedience affects a youngster's health or safety or morals, it's time for parental action, not necessarily in the form of punishment, but in taking stock of the situation to find out why the child won't obey.

Divorced Parents

See "Separation and Divorce" in Ch. 5, *The Middle Years.*

Dreams and Nightmares

Children go through periods of having "bad dreams" or nightmares that wake them up in the middle of the night in a state of terror and bewilderment. It won't do to say, "It's just a dream." To a young child who is just beginning to grasp the difference between what's real and what isn't, nightmare can be extremely threatening. If the child wants to describe the dream after she collects herself, she should be allowed to do so even at 3:00 A.M. She may amplify and exaggerate a little bit, but that's only to let you know that she's been very brave through it all. Parental patience is called for; with a certain amount of reassurance, the child can usually be led back to bed and to sleep.

Youngsters whose sleep is regularly interrupted by nightmares or who are in the grip of the same nightmare may be feeling anxious about a daytime activity or may be feeling guilty about some undiscovered naughtiness. A tactful chat can sometimes reveal what the trouble is so that it can be disposed of during waking hours.

Night Terrors

Some children may have occasional nightmares—often called *night terrors*—in which they scream or tremble in terror. They may sit up in bed while still asleep, or even walk

around. Their terror is certainly real, but the parents should remember that the cause of it is purely imaginary. Accordingly, they have no reason to be alarmed; in spite of the child's appearance, she is not in any danger, and no drastic action is called for.

Simply comfort the child, who frequently will be disoriented and confused in a half-awake state, until she can go back to sleep. She will probably have no recollection of the episode the next morning.

If night terrors occur only occasionally, there is no cause for concern, although it might be a good idea to check on the television shows your child is watching before bedtime. If there is a great deal of tension in the household, that could be a contributing cause. If night terrors are persistent or frequent, however, a physician should be consulted. See also SLEEPWALKING.

Dyslexia

Dyslexia is a condition in which an otherwise average or intelligent child suffers from a complex of motor-perceptual disabilities that interfere with the orderly processing and acquisition of language. The disability that results in an inhibition of symbol recognition essential for learning how to read, write, and spell is thought to originate in some form of brain circuitry malfunction that may have been caused by injury or by genetic defect. Recent researchers have established some connection between dyslexia and a faulty pathway between the lower brain—the cerebellum—and the inner ear, causing the dyslexic child to suffer from a mild and permanent form of motion sickness that interferes with learning.

Symptoms

The symptoms of dyslexia vary considerably and may include: garbled or disordered development of speech during the early years; an inability to learn the relationship between sounds and symbols for purposes of reading aloud; an inability to learn how to spell or how to organize written expression; confusion about serial order, as in naming the days of the week or in number concepts; unusual difficulty in doing simple repetitive tasks.

If a parent suspects that a child is suffering from dyslexia, a diagnosis should be made on the basis of tests administered by trained professionals. The child's pediatrician or the school guidance counselor should be consulted about where such tests are best given and assessed. Should the child be diagnosed as dyslexic, an appropriate remedial program or an accredited special school can help surmount some of the learning difficulties.

Earache

Earache is one of the most common complaints of childhood.

As Secondary Infection

Earache is often attributable to bacterial infection of the middle ear and should be treated promptly by a physician. Because the Eustachian tube that connects the back of the throat with the middle ear is shorter and wider in a child than in an adult, it affords easier entry to bacteria. Infections of the ear may thus occur as the result of a sore throat or a postnasal drip. Infectious mucus from the nose is often forced into the middle ear by way of the Eustachian tube because young children are inclined to sniff it back rather than to blow it out. And when a child is mastering the technique of noseblowing, he should be told that neither one nor both of the nostrils should be pressed closed

in the process. Rather, both nostrils should be blown out gently at the same time, and with the mouth open. If gentle blowing doesn't clear the nostrils, the nose should be wiped as necessary.

Recognizing Earache in an Infant

Earache in an infant may be combined with fever and the kind of crying associated with sharp pain. A toddler may indicate the source of discomfort by pulling at the earlobe. Until the pediatrician can prescribe proper medication, discomfort can be relieved by applying a heating pad to the involved ear and with aspirin.

Other Causes

Earache may also accompany teething or tooth infection, or it may be the result of pressure caused by water that has been trapped in the ear after swimming or bathing. In small children, an earache may be a sign that the youngster has stuffed a bean or a tiny plastic object so far into his ear that it won't come out as easily as it went in. If you suspect such an occurrence, avoid poking and prodding in an attempt to remove the object. The child should be taken to a physician or to a hospital so that the object can be removed with the proper instruments and the ear examined and treated for possible injury.

Consequences of Neglect of Earache

An earache should always be brought to a physician's attention without delay because untreated middle ear infections can lead to irreversible hearing loss. The leading cause of mild hearing loss in toddlers is believed to be *serous otitis media*, or serous infection of the middle ear. This condi-

tion is specifically an inflammation of the middle ear with an accumulation of fluid behind the eardrum. When the condition is chronic or improperly treated during the first three years, it may impair hearing permanently and as a consequence lead to a failure to develop normal language skills. Occasionally the physician may have to make a small opening in the eardrum to drain the fluid, a procedure known as a *myringotomy*. See also HEARING.

Eczema

See under RASHES.

Education

See SCHOOL.

Epilepsy

Epilepsy in childhood most commonly takes the form of petit mal or psychomotor episodes.

Petit Mal Seizures

Petit mal episodes are characterized by brief lapses of consciousness, sometimes occurring many times a day. The child does not fall down but simply stops what he is doing and may appear to stare absently.

Psychomotor Seizures

Psychomotor episodes are characterized by the performance of some activity during a brief lapse of consciousness. The child may walk around in circles, or sit down and get up in a purposeless way. During this type of seizure the child may babble nonsensically or chant the same word over and over. Such an attack may last no more than a few minutes, and when the child recovers he is likely to have no memory of its occurrence.

In many instances, parents who expect a certain amount of bizarre behavior from their youngsters may not realize that a form of epilepsy is the cause. Should such incidents occur frequently, they should be called to the attention of the physician who may think it advisable to have the child examined by a neurologist.

A parent witnessing a *grand mal* or convulsive epileptic seizure for the first time may be unduly alarmed and take measures that may harm the child rather than help. For a description of emergency measures during a grand mal seizure, see Ch. 31, *Medical Emergencies.* For a full discussion of epilepsy, see Ch. 8, *Diseases of the Muscles and Nervous System.*

Exercise

Some children seem to sit around a great deal; others are on the move from morning until bedtime. A youngster might be listless or lethargic because there's something the matter that needs to be investigated by a physician. This type of sitting around is quite different from playing with dolls for hours at a time or looking at picture books instead of running around. A young child who really cannot sit still at all may have a problem that needs diagnosing by a physician, too. Practically all children are found between these extremes.

Exercise as a Developmental Need

Toddlers must be allowed to get the exercise necessary for the development of their bodies. They shouldn't be confined in a playpen for most of the day. Three- and four-year-olds who don't go to a nursery school and have no play equipment in their backyard (if they have a backyard), should be taken whenever possible to a local park or playground that has swings, slides, seesaws, jungle gyms, or other devices that are safely designed and installed. Most schools have some kind of supervised gym activity or a free time for yard play, and if they don't, they should. If this scheduled exercise is insufficient for a nine- or ten-year-old, inquiries can be made about athletic facilities at a local YMCA, settlement house, church, or fraternal organization.

Choice of Activities

As children get a little older, they should be permitted to choose the exercise that appeals to them unless there's a good reason for its being forbidden. A girl who wants to join a sandlot baseball team shouldn't be forced to go to a ballet class, and a boy inspired by the dancing he's seen on TV shouldn't be discouraged if the family can afford the lessons. Exercise needn't be synonymous with competition unless the youngster wants it to be. See also "Physical Fitness" in Ch. 3, *The Teens.*

Eyeglasses

Now that infants and youngsters have periodic eye checkups with their physicians, and regular tests are given to all students, more children are wearing glasses than in former years. In addition to *strabismus* (crossed eyes), the three major eye problems encountered in children are *myopia* (nearsightedness), *hyperopia* (farsightedness), and *astigmatism.*

Myopia

The *myopic* or nearsighted child cannot see distant objects well but can see close objects clearly. A very young child so afflicted may stumble and fall easily. An older child attending school may make errors in copying because she has difficulty in making out the words and figures written on the chalkboard. She may be called a behavior problem or may even be said to be mentally retarded. Most cases of myopia can be helped with glasses.

Hyperopia

The *hyperopic* (also called *hypermetropic*) or farsighted eye is shorter from front to rear than the normal eye, and if not corrected will often hinder close work like reading. When a farsighted child reads she often complains of blurring of the printed page, sleepiness, and headache. Farsightedness is often associated with crossed eyes and is usually correctable with glasses.

Astigmatism

In *astigmatism* or distorted vision, there is an uneven curvature of the cornea or lens surface of the eye. This condition causes some light rays to focus further back than others and produces a blurred, distorted image on the retina.

Either a farsighted or nearsighted eye can be *astigmatic;* the abnormality can usually be corrected by properly prescribed eyeglasses.

Fantasies

Every normal child has fantasies, some highly pleasurable, some fearful and frightening. Young children sometimes have a hard time sorting out what they imagine from what's real; this may be especially true when a nightmare interferes with sleep. Many children quite consciously say, "Let's pretend" or "Let's make believe" when they embark on a dress-up activity; others simply and straightforwardly act out their fantasies by playing games of violence with toy guns. An only child may create a fantasy companion with whom she has conversations; a child who is encouraged to draw may give shape to her fantasies in pictures that mean a lot to her but not much to anyone else.

Daydreaming

Some children infuriate their energetic parents by sitting around and daydreaming (with one sock on and one off) instead of doing their chores. Whatever form fantasies may take, they are an inevitable part of growing up and should be respected, unless they become the equivalent of a narcotic escape from reality rather than a means of enriching it. When a child's fantasy life appears to be turning into a substitute for his real one, the time has come to consult a psychiatric authority.

Fatherhood

More and more fathers are finding themselves involved in child raising on an active basis rather than a passive one. As an increasing number of women take part- or full-time jobs even when children are very young, fathers have been taking over the care and feeding of their children on prearranged mornings, evenings, and weekends. Some men resent the responsibility; others enjoy it. But all who undertake it for the first time are surprised to discover how much time, energy, patience, resourcefulness, and thought are required in order to be a good mother. If the woman of the house is expected to be an attractive wife as well as a good mother, she needs some time to herself for her own development as a person.

Where child care is shared more than it used to be, mothers and fathers should agree on a consistent set of values: what's permitted and what

isn't; what's expected and what's unacceptable, etc. Otherwise the child may be confused by the demands of two conflicting authorities.

Estranged Parents

The part-time father who sees his child or children on a prearranged schedule following a separation or divorce shouldn't pack too many exciting experiences—and too many feelings—into every meeting with them. He, like the mother, should scrupulously avoid any disparagement of the other parent. He and the child will enjoy each other more, no matter what their age, if the hours together are comparatively calm and unhurried, and the projects for their time together are not overstimulating.

Fears and Phobias

Babies are fearful about being dropped, and they're frightened by a sudden loud noise. (You *can* make babies cry by saying, "Boo!" When they get older and catch on, they'll think it's fun to be scared.) Toddlers are taught to be afraid of a hot stove, and as children get a little older, they develop night fears that become bad dreams. Many parents transmit, deliberately or unknowingly, some of their fears to their children: fear of dogs, or thunder and lightning, or infection by germs.

Only a thin line separates sensible caution from anxiety. Where a threat of punishment is involved, an anxiety may develop that can last a lifetime. Parents should control the impulse to say such things as, "Don't eat that, it's going to make you sick" or "Don't climb so high, you're going to fall" or "Don't play in the mud; the germs will make you sick." Or, worse yet, "If you do that, the bogey man will get you" or "God will punish you."

Phobias

If fears are often legitimate and usually outgrown through reassuring experiences, phobias are deep-seated unconquerable fears. Many adults suffer from them; two of the most common are *claustrophobia*, the fear of being in an enclosed place, and *acrophobia*, the fear of heights. *Phobia* is a clinical term and shouldn't be used to describe a youngster's aversion to school at a particular time, or his apprehension about elevators and escalators. If parental reassurance can help a child overcome fears of this type, they need not be classed as phobias.

Fever

As every parent knows, babies can run very high fevers. In itself, a rectal temperature of 103° F or 104° F is not necessarily cause for alarm. (Normal rectal temperature is about ½° F to 1° F higher than the oral norm of 98.6° F.) Of course, you should take the immediate step of calling your pediatrician to find out what's causing the fever.

If a baby's fever climbs over 104° F, the baby may experience convulsions. To avoid this possibility, he may be bathed with cool water or with equal parts of water and alcohol. (The alcohol is not necessary.) If convulsions do occur, protect the baby from injuring himself by seeing that his head and body don't strike anything hard. The convulsion, though frightening, is usually brief and ends of its own accord. Get in touch with your physician without delay.

Although the mechanism that results in fever is not precisely understood, the elevation in temperature is almost always a sign that the child's normal body processes are being disturbed. A child old enough to talk can let you know that his throat is sore or that he has an earache.

Possible Causes

Fever is often the sign of the onset of an infectious disease such as measles or influenza; it usually accompanies severe sunburn; it may be a warning that the infection of a local cut is spreading through the rest of the body. When it comes suddenly and rises quickly, along with cramps or diarrhea, it may indicate a gastrointestinal infection or food poisoning. No matter what a child's age, if temperature by mouth rises above 101° F, a physician should be informed of the fever and accompanying symptoms.

Treatment

Until a diagnosis is made and treatment prescribed, the feverish youngster should be put to bed and kept on a diet of light foods and lots of liquids. If the elevated temperature is combined with stiff neck, aching joints, or headache, aspirin can be given for relief according to dose instructions indicated.

Fluoridation

Although it has been unequivocally established that fluoridated drinking water is the best safeguard against tooth decay, many parts of the United States continue to resist this public health measure, thus placing a special burden on the parents of preschool children. Families in such communities are strongly urged to consult their dentist or the closest dental clinic connected with a university's college of dentistry for advice on the appropriate measures to be taken to protect their children's teeth. A consultation of this nature is advisable as soon as the baby shows signs of teething, because the fluoride treatments should begin as early as possible.

In many areas where the water supply remains unfluoridated, programs in the public schools supply youngsters with fluoride tablets every day. Although this method of applying the chemical is less effective than its availability in the drinking water, it is a step in the right direction. Concerned parents can make an effort to initiate such programs where none exists by contacting state public health officials.

Foot Care

Unless the child's pediatrician indicates the need for corrective or orthopedic shoes, parents need have little concern for pigeon toes or bowed legs or flat feet. If a shoe salesman suggests remedial footwear, his suggestions should be discussed with a physician before complying with them. A good general rule to follow about the fit of shoes is that they should be about three-quarters of an inch longer than the foot itself. For a child whose feet have a tendency to perspire heavily, sweat socks made of cotton or wool are to be preferred to those made of synthetics. Blisters that form on the instep, heel, or any other part of the foot because of ill-fitting footwear must be treated promptly to avoid serious infection.

Friends

Everyone needs friends. Some children need only one; others seem to enjoy having several. A three-year-old who is just beginning to learn about sharing may be more relaxed playing with just one other child; a ten-year-old may like the hurly-burly of a group of friends to get together with when school is out.

Parents Please Stay Out

Parents should try to steer clear of squabbles between children. One day, Nancy and Harriet are best friends, the next, bitter enemies, because of some real or imagined outrage. Left to their own devices, the children will probably patch things up. If parents get involved, the situation gets magnified out of all proportion. It's not unusual in such situations for the two sets of parents to stop speaking to each other and the two little girls to go back to being best friends again.

Keeping Bad Company

What's to be done about "unsuitable" friends? Some parents may think a particular child is unacceptable because she's too aggressive or too foul-mouthed. If your child seems fond of her nonetheless, voice your opinions, but don't forbid the youngster from coming to the house. Any attempt to break up the friendship is likely to be resisted until your child learns from experience that your judgment was the right one. Children who are discouraged from bringing their friends home because they make a mess or make too much noise are actually deprived of feeling at home in their own house.

Friendships between girls and boys may begin in nursery school and continue for years afterward. Although the tone of the friendship may change, the closeness can be very valuable if it doesn't exclude other relationships.

Frostbite

See Ch. 31, *Medical Emergencies*.

Frustration

When infants want food, they want it now. Because frustration isn't something they can deal with, they cry until they get what they want. A toddler whose desire to stay in the playground is frustrated when his mother firmly leads him out may have a temper tantrum. A five-year-old who can't put a particular puzzle together may be so frustrated that he destroys it.

Practically all situations involving frustration are those in which a child (or person of any age) is trying to transcend arbitrary limitations, either his own or those imposed by circumstance. Parents can't eliminate the frustration factor from a child's life, but they can help him to cope with it. Suitable simple clothing is much less frustrating than garments with lots of buttons and buttonholes. Playthings can be a challenge, but not so complicated that they defeat a child's desire to learn. Too many strict rules frustrate a child's impulse to exercise his own judgment and to grow up by learning from his own mistakes.

An Only Child

An only child may be frustrated in his desire for attention when he starts to go to school. In this case, he may actually be spurred on to superior achievement so that he continues to get the attention he's been accustomed to at home. Or he may behave like a spoiled brat and get attention, but for the wrong reasons.

Some children learn that the desire for instant gratification is one of the chief characteristics of an infant, and so, with parental help and approval, develop the character traits of patience and self-discipline. Others become the kind of adult for whom frustration is so intolerable that it becomes an excuse for escape into drugs.

German Measles

See RUBELLA.

Gifted Child

See ABILITIES AND APTITUDES.

Grades

Many schools don't use a grading system for children under the age of ten. But no matter what the nature of the report and how elaborate it is, evaluation of the child is involved, and the evaluation is based on values, so the child is in fact being graded in a way after all. Some children are called more cooperative than others; some are said to try harder; some get along better with their peer group.

With or without grades, children usually know whether they're doing well or badly at school. If a youngster's accomplishments are falling short of her abilities, there may be temporary reasons for her underachievement. In some cases, underachievement is a child's way of saying "no" to too much pressure about grades; in other cases, something about the teacher or the classroom situation is interfering with the child's performance. If parents suspect such a case, they should arrange a parent-teacher conference to try to get to the bottom of the problem.

Grandparents

Children are fortunate when both sets of grandparents are easily accessible for visiting, treats, vacation trips, playing checkers, and baby-sitting. Parents and grandparents are lucky too, for family continuity is important to young and old alike.

Relationships between the generations have their difficulties, though. Tact may be essential in keeping a grandparent from spoiling a child, and a grandmother should resist the impulse to show how competent she is with the baby compared to her inexperienced daughter or daughter-in-law. Parents who are still working out

some of their own problems may take a rebellious tone toward the grandparent who moves into the household as a matter of economic necessity. Under these circumstances, the older generation should certainly expect consideration and politeness but should try not to impose its attitudes or child-rearing methods on its adult offspring—especially not in the presence of the children.

Growth Rates in Boys and Girls

See charts later in this chapter.

Guilt and Conscience

Children often feel as guilty about bad thoughts as they do about bad deeds. After being angry, a child may feel as badly about having had a fleeting wish to hurt his mother as he would have felt had he actually hurt her. A child should be helped to understand that his thoughts are his own, that his thoughts cannot harm anybody, and that he will not be punished for his thoughts. He should understand that it is only actions of certain kinds that cannot be allowed and that will result in a reprimand or punishment. In other words, a child should not be made to feel guilty for angry or aggressive thoughts toward other members of his family, but only for angry and aggressive acts.

A parent might say to a child, "I understand that you really disliked your brother when you hit him, in fact, even hated him and would have liked to hurt him. It's okay for you to be angry with him, but I am not going to let you hurt him." A clear distinction should be made between hostile feelings and hostile behavior.

Handicapped Child

Whether a handicap is hereditary or acquired, mental or physical, temporary or permanent, it is always a condition that prevents a child from participating fully on an equal footing in the activities of her own age group. But how fully she can participate and her attitude toward her disability are usually a reflection of the attitudes of her parents, teachers, and the community. Of primary importance is an assessment at the earliest possible age of the extent to which the handicap can be decreased or corrected.

Exactly how deaf is the deaf child? Can surgery repair a rheumatic heart? Is a defect of vision operable? Is the child with cerebral palsy mentally retarded or is the seeming mental malfunction a reversible effect of the physical condition? Parents should investigate all the available services offered by voluntary organizations and community groups that might help them and their child. See Ch. 36, *Voluntary Health Agencies.*

One promising development in recent years is the attempt to integrate handicapped children, whenever possible, into the mainstream of education rather than segregate them in special classes. School systems in various parts of the United States are placing deaf, blind, physically disabled, and emotionally disturbed youngsters into classrooms with their nonhandicapped peers and providing them with essential supportive services at various times during the school day. The experience of dealing with nonhandicapped children will provide them with a more realistic preparation for their adult lives.

Health Records

It may seem somewhat troublesome to keep orderly health records for every member of the family, but the accumulated information can be extremely helpful if it can be supplied at a moment's notice to a physician or a hospital. Chronologically arranged

Growth Rates in Boys*

*Adapted from National Center for Health Statistics *NCHS Growth Charts,* 1976. Monthly Vital Statistics Report. Vol. 25, No. 3, Supp. (HRA) 76-1120. Health Resources Administration, Rockville, Maryland, June, 1976. Data from The Fels Research Institute, Yellow Springs, Ohio. © 1976 Ross Laboratories

These charts indicate the rate of growth of boys and girls from birth to 36 months in the United States. In each chart the upper gray area indicates the range of growth in height from the 5th to 95th percentile, and the lower gray area indicates a similar range in weight. (If a boy or girl is in the 95th percentile in height, 95% of all other boys and girls are not as tall as he or she. If someone is in the 50th percentile in weight, half of other children weigh more and half weigh less. If one is in the 25th percentile

facts can also provide the material eventually needed by summer camps and school applications and insurance policies.

A notebook containing essential data about past illnesses, accidents, allergies, surgery, and other facts can

be extraordinarily helpful and time-saving in supplying a physician with a medical history that simplifies diagnosis and treatment. Such a notebook should have separate sections for immunizations and booster shots and their dates; annual weight and height

Growth Rates in Girls*

*Adapted from National Center for Health Statistics *NCHS Growth Charts*, 1976. Monthly Vital Statistics Report. Vol. 25, No. 3, Supp. (HRA) 76-1120. Health Resources Administration, Rockville, Maryland, June, 1976. Data from The Fels Research Institute, Yellow Springs, Ohio. © 1976 Ross Laboratories

of weight, 75% of other children weigh more and 25% weigh less. Thus, the percentile indicates how your child compares in height or weight with other children of the same sex and age in the United States.) Height, indicated at the left-hand side of each chart, is shown in inches and in centimeters. Weight, indicated at the right-hand side of each chart, is shown in kilograms and in pounds. The bottom and top lines of each chart indicate age in months.

progress; illnesses with dates and special notations; accidents with dates and any permanent consequences; hospitalization and reason; individual problems relating to allergies, hearing, vision, speech, and the like. Visits to physician and dentist should be recorded, and the blood type entered in a conspicuous place. If possible, parents should also provide a summary at the back of the notebook of their own major illnesses, disabilities, and surgical history.

Hearing

Approximately half of all adult hearing problems are thought to have originated in childhood. About five out of every hundred children reveal some hearing disability when screening tests are given. Total deafness among children is uncommon, and where it does exist, its symptoms become manifest to parents and physicians alike during infancy.

Partial Hearing Loss

Partial hearing disability, on the other hand, is common, and is likely to be overlooked until it may be too late to correct its consequences.

A physician begins to suspect a hearing problem when the mother of a young baby tells him that the child does not react to her voice, to noises, or to other auditory stimuli. As the child gets older, he may not speak properly. Because he has never heard speech, he cannot imitate its sound and may fail to develop normal language skills. Sometimes these children, like visually handicapped children, are mistakenly called mentally retarded or are classified as suffering from hyperkinesis or brain dysfunction. Often the undetected hearing disability stemmed from a middle ear infection that was treated inadequately or not treated at all.

Language Problems

A hearing loss of 15 decibels is considered sufficiently large to produce language problems for a very young child, causing a major handicap in the acquisition of language skills. Specialists therefore recommend that parents ask that their physician test a baby's hearing, especially during and after an ear infection. If a compensatory hearing aid is necessary, the baby should be supplied with one immediately. Speech will not develop normally—that is, the language function of the brain will be impaired—unless the essential sounds of language can be perceived during the first two years of life.

Just as glasses or surgery can help eye problems, simple hearing aids, the surgical removal of excessive lymphoid tissue blocking the Eustachian tube, or special instruction in lip reading can often help a hearing problem and open up a new world for the child afflicted with a hearing disability.

Heart Disease

See RHEUMATIC FEVER. See also "Congenital Heart Disease" in Ch. 10, *Heart Disease.*

Hernia

A *hernia* is a condition in which part of an organ protrudes through a weak spot or other abnormal opening in the wall of a body cavity. There are three types of hernias that may occur in children.

Umbilical Hernia

The most common is an *umbilical hernia*, in which there is a protrusion of some of the contents of the abdomen through an opening in the abdominal wall at the navel where the umbilical cord was attached. When the baby cries or strains, the protrusion becomes more obvious, and when the baby is at rest, the bulge recedes. An umbilical hernia usually disappears by the time a child reaches the second year. Because it represents no danger to any of the body functions, the condition need be no cause for concern. It is very common in non-Caucasian children.

Inguinal Hernia

The second most common type of hernia in childhood is known as an *indirect inguinal hernia*, occurring frequently in boys. At birth it may have the appearance of a marble located under the skin at the groin. In time, it may descend into the scrotum that encloses the testicles. This type of hernia is usually corrected by simple surgery that repairs the weakened musculature. The weak muscles are often present on both sides.

Hiatus Hernia

Another congenital hernia is known as a *hiatus hernia* (or *diaphragmatic hernia*) in which part of the stomach protrudes upward through the part of the esophagus that opens into the diaphragm. In some cases, this structural defect is self-healing. Surgical correction is advised only if the hernia interferes with respiration. See also Ch. 11, *Diseases of the Digestive System.*

Hobbies

Because hobbies are considered leisure-time activities, they don't usually develop until a child begins to go to school. His day is then separated into doing what he has to do—homework, household chores—and doing what he wants to do. Some youngsters get ideas about hobbies from their school friends, especially in the earlier grades where some form of "show and tell" is likely to be part of the group's activities.

Collecting

Such hobbies are often based on collecting: foreign stamps, seashells, baseball cards, minerals, dolls—the list is endless and often involves little expense. Whatever the trivia that's being collected, parents should refrain from criticism. Many children

have had the last word when their masses of comic books turned out to be valuable properties as the years went by.

Some youngsters choose their hobbies from among the pursuits that give pleasure to their parents or older siblings: crafts, boating, reading, sewing, fishing, drawing, tennis, chess. There are those children who don't seem to be able to settle on a hobby until they've tried and discarded several. Although parents should be patient about this, they certainly needn't rush out for a telescope or a chemistry set—or a silver flute!—at the slightest suggestion of their ten-year-old's enthusiasm. A child who thinks he'd like to try some experiments should be encouraged to use materials that are close at hand. A child who expresses interest in astronomy can be told to identify the constellations he can make out with the naked eye and with the help of a library book.

Homework

See RESPONSIBILITIES.

Hospitalization

Most children at some time in their first 15 years of life require at least one hospitalization, ranging in time from a few days to many months. This can be a frightening experience and may leave permanent emotional scars on a child. Parents can do many things to make the experience less harmful.

Preparing the child for the hospital stay may be the most important task for the parent. Authorities generally agree that parents should:

- Try to answer all the questions the child asks. If you have no answer, try to find one.

- Be as honest as possible. The child

will want to know why he or she has to go to the hospital, what will be done there, how long it will take, and whether it will hurt.

- Be reassuring. The child should know that he or she will receive good care and that the hospital visit will be temporary.

- Explain what the hospital is and what it is like—with wheeled carts, people in uniform, and so on.

- Using sheets as gowns, role-play to make it clear that under the gowns will be helping people.

- Let the child know when they will be in the hospital and how long they will stay.

Most hospitals today try to work with parents to make the child feel at home and to allay the child's fears. Many hospitals offer rooms so that parents can "room in"—and stay near the young patient. A playroom may be available. Hospital staff members may hold parent-nurse sessions to introduce mothers and fathers to the hospital's schedule, locations of facilities, and other details. Parents of a child who has to be hospitalized can, by learning as much as possible and cooperating with the staff, help alleviate a child's natural fears of separation, of mutilation, and of the strange new situation.

Fear of Separation

Hospitalization for an operation or an illness affects different children at different stages of their development in different ways. Very young children may be particularly worried about separations from their mothers. Parents can help with this fear by assuring the child that separation will not be permanent.

If at all possible, the child's mother or another member of the family should stay with the child during much of the hospital stay. During an extended hospitalization, of course, this may become difficult or impossible. Barring accidents, children should always be forewarned of a hospitalization; if they are not, they may feel they were deceived by their parents and lose trust in them.

Fear of Mutilation

Children of about 4 to 10 or 11 may be more worried about possible damage or mutilation of their bodies than about separations from their families. They often have fears that parts of their bodies may be cut out or that in some way they may be permanently harmed. They may feel that when they come back from the hospital they will not be the same as they were when they went in. Matter-of-fact reassurance by the parents can be most helpful in alleviating these fears.

Fear of the Strange

Both younger children and older children aged 10, 11, or 12 may fear the new or strange, such as the anesthetic that goes with an operation. The child should be allowed to talk out fears. Simple explanations usually help. A child can, for example, understand that when you get sick taking medicine can sometimes make you better. At other times an operation, or surgery, is the only thing that will help. In the hospital, physicians or nurses may have to make tests to find out what is wrong. One such test is the X ray, which is simply a "picture" of a part of the child's body.

The parent can prepare the child for the operating room and for the operation. Everything in this special place, for example, must be kept per-

fectly clean, so nurses and physicians wear long-sleeved gowns. They also wash carefully before the operation begins. They wear sterile gloves so that they can touch patients without passing on germs. They also wear masks, shoe coverings, and caps. They may make a small opening in the patient's skin so that they can take out or get rid of whatever is making the child sick. The physicians and nurses use stitches, or sutures, to pull the skin edges together and allow healing to begin. Some stitches may be under the skin; these simply melt, or dissolve, by themselves.

A dressing may be placed over the part of the child's body that was opened up. These pieces of soft cloth protect the skin opening and keep out germs. When the dressing comes off, a white scar may remain. The scar will not open up and it will not hurt. It will be a sign that the child was sick, got well, and came home.

Hostility

See ANGER.

Hyaline Membrane Disease

Hyaline membrane disease, now technically called the *respiratory distress syndrome,* is a disorder that affects approximately 50,000 newborn babies each year, and until recently was fatal for about half of them. The disorder occurs especially among premature infants, those born by caesarian section, and those with diabetic mothers. In premature infants, the immaturity of the lungs may result in a collapse of the air space within the lungs themselves when the first breath is exhaled. Each new breath then becomes a greater struggle, and with the spread of lung collapse, exhaustion and asphyxiation may occur.

A treatment known as *continuous positive airway pressure* is now being successfully used in many of the special hospital units equipped for newborns with disabilities. The therapy involves a pressure chamber that forces high-oxygen air into the lungs and keeps these air spaces open. The method has already prevented thousands of infant deaths. Newborns who need this assistance acquire the ability to breathe normally in about a week.

Hyperkinesis

Hyperkinesis is a behavioral disorder diagnosed in a large number of schoolchildren—more often boys than girls—who are unable to concentrate and who are overactive and excitable. These characteristics cause them to become disruptive in the classroom as well as disturbing to their families. There are indications that this disorder manifests itself in infancy, when the physician might describe an excessively fretful and restless baby as *hypertonic*, and prescribe medication to calm him down.

For reasons not yet understood, it has been found that the symptoms of hyperkinesis often respond to antidepressants or stimulants, and as a result, a significant number of otherwise unmanageable youngsters are being treated medically. Although the medication enables them to conform to classroom situations, it may have the negative effect of appetite loss; to avoid sleep difficulties, the medication is never given in the evening.

Hyperkinesis appears to run in families, although there is some evidence that imperceptible brain damage may be one of its causes. Parents of a clinically hyperkinetic child—not one who is simply rambunctious—should seek advice about proper treatment from the psychiatric and neurological staffs of the nearest teaching hospital or from specialists recommended by the family physician.

Imagination

See FANTASIES.

Immunization

Recently developed vaccines against measles, mumps, and rubella (German measles) should eventually wipe out these diseases in the same way that smallpox has been eliminated practically everywhere in the world. Routine immunization follows a schedule of shots administered with minor variations by most pediatricians and child care clinics. Severe reactions are rare, but should they occur, they should be reported to the physician promptly.

Keeping Records

Records should be kept of the child's immunization history so that booster shots can be given at proper intervals. Because families move from one place to another, changing physicians as they relocate, it saves a great deal of time and trouble if immunization data is written down rather than committed to memory. See HEALTH RECORDS.

DTP Injections

DTP stands for diphtheria, tetanus, and pertussis (or whooping cough). DTP injections are usually given in the muscles of the mid-thigh or upper arm, at intervals of one month, sometimes longer. To prevent fever or other severe reactions, the two- to five-month-old baby should receive one grain of baby aspirin within a few hours after the injection. If she nevertheless develops fever or has other severe reactions, your physician may have to give lower doses, and therefore give more than three injections. Very rarely is a severe reaction reported with smaller doses of the vaccine. If there is such a reaction, no further injections of pertussis vaccine will be given.

Occasionally, redness or a lump appears at the site of the injection. This is a local reaction. It is harmless and will disappear within a few weeks. If it does not, consult your physician.

It is recommended that a booster or recall shot be given at one-and-a-half and at three years of age. Another recall injection of only TD (tetanus-diphtheria toxoid) is given at six years and at twelve years.

DTP Reactions

Adverse reactions to the DTP vaccine have been reported in a few cases. The reactions ranged from permanent neurological damage to such mild symptoms as persistent crying and unusual sleepiness. Crying may be high-pitched and may continue as long as three hours or more. Sleepiness may resemble a shocklike state. Some children may run temperatures of 105° F or higher. In cases of suspected adverse reactions to DTP or any other vaccine, a pediatrician or family physician should be called immediately.

Parents may want to discuss their children's medical histories with their family physicians or pediatricians before taking a child in for an inoculaton. The American Academy of Pediatrics suggests that children with personal histories of convulsions or allergic reactions to DTP or other vaccines should not be given the DTP vaccine. The same is true of children born prematurely.

Independence

Many parents feel that the most memorable moment in a child's progress towards independence comes when he takes his first steps alone. Upright and walking! Most children accomplish this by going independently from the secure arms of one adult to the waiting arms of another. As youngsters move toward greater independence, they will do so with confidence if they can start out from a secure foundation of rules and limits, and return to the security of acceptance and understanding should they come to grief.

The Toddler Stage

The toddler relishes the independence of being able to explore the house or the playground but he won't go very far before he returns to check in with the person in charge of him so that he can start out all over again. He voices his independence, too: "no" to naps; "no" to outings; "no" to

a bath. This is the phase during which parents must be wary of asking "Would you like to" or "Do you want to" instead of just proceeding with the business at hand. Patience is required for the self-assertive fumblings and clumsy efforts at self-feeding and putting clothes on. Assistance should be subtle and tactful, not hurried and bossy: "Baby do, daddy help," is the general idea.

School Age

As the child moves into the larger arena of school and friendships, "I'm not a baby any more" may become a complaint if he wants more freedom than he's permitted to have. At this stage, he begins to learn that responsibility goes hand-in-hand with freedom and independence. Old enough

to ride the bike farther and farther from home means taking on the responsibility of keeping it in good repair and obeying all the traffic rules.

Influenza

See "The Common Cold, Influenza, and Other Viral Infections" in Ch. 12, *Diseases of the Respiratory System.*

Insect Stings and Bites

When a child is bitten or stung by an insect, he often complains about the pain or the itching, but with the application of a lotion or salve to relieve discomfort and a bandage to prevent infection, the incident is soon forgotten. There are times, however, when a sting or a bite may require emergency treatment.

It has been estimated that about four children out of every 1,000 have serious allergic reactions to the sting of a hornet, wasp, bee, yellow jacket, or the fire ant. A child who has sustained multiple stings, or whose body, tongue, or face begins to swell because of a single sting should be taken to the hospital immediately. Tests can clearly distinguish between those children who are highly sensitive to stings and those who are not.

Preventive Measures

A physician should be consulted about the advisability of testing youngsters who are going off to camp for the first time or who are planning long hikes. Rather than curtail the activities of a child who turns out to have an acute sensitivity, it may make sense to plan a series of desensitization treatments against the particular venom. For children who are very allergic to insect stings, an emergency kit containing adrenaline is now available and should always be carried.

Recommended Schedule for Active Immunization of Normal Infants and Children

Recommended Age	Vaccine[a]	Comments
2 months	DTP, OPV	Can be initiated earlier in areas of high incidence
4 months	DTP, OPV	2-month interval desired for OPV to avoid interference
6 months	DTP	OPV optional for areas where polio might be imported (e.g., some areas of southwestern United States)
12 months	TB test	May be given simultaneously with MMR at 15 months (see text)
15 months	Measles, Mumps, Rubella; DPT, OPV	MMR preferred
24 months	Hemophilus b polysaccharide vaccine	
24 months	Hemophilus b	Hemophilus b polysaccharide vaccine for Hemophilus influenzae type b
4–6 years[b]	DTP, OPV	

[a] *DTP*—diphtheria and tetanus toxoids with pertussis vaccine. *OPV*—oral, attenuated poliovirus vaccine contains poliovirus types 1, 2, and 3. *Tuberculin test*—mantoux (intradermal PPD) preferred. Frequency of tests depends on local epidemiology. The Committee recommends annual or biennial testing unless local circumstances dictate less frequent or no testing (see tuberculosis for complete discussion. *MMR*—live measles, mumps, and rubella viruses in a combined vaccine (see text for discussion of single vaccines versus combination). *Td*—adult tetanus toxoid (full dose) and diphtheria toxoid (reduced dose) combination.

[b] Up to the seventh birthday.

Mosquitoes

Every effort should be made to eradicate mosquitoes by eliminating their breeding places. A mosquito bite can be a serious threat to a child's health because these insects transmit several diseases. Where mosquitoes are a problem, infants and children should be protected against them by screens, netting, and the application of repellents.

Ticks

Families that travel and those that have pets should guard against the possibility of infection by disease-bearing ticks. A species of tick known as *Ixodes dammini* can transmit an illness called Lyme disease while another common tick may carry Rocky Mountain spotted fever.

Rashes may appear as symptoms of infection by either tick. The Lyme disease rash may be circular and hot to the touch. It may have a diameter as wide as 28 inches. Untreated in either children or adults, Lyme disease may trigger chills, fever, general feelings of malaise, fatigue, and attacks of arthritis that may last weeks or months to years. Heart and nerve abnormalities may appear. Penicillin is used to bring Lyme disease under control in pregnant women and children.

Less prevalent than Lyme disease, Rocky Mountain spotted fever usually produces a rash on the soles of the feet and the palms of the hands. Prompt medical attention is essential to prevent possible complications. See ROCKY MOUNTAIN SPOTTED FEVER and LYME DISEASE under RASHES.

Intelligence and IQ

Intelligence is a quality, not a quantity. It therefore cannot be measured as precisely as height or weight; nor can it be exemplified as definitely as mechanical skill or athletic ability or musical talent. Although child development authorities and educators may disagree about how to assess intelligence, they generally agree on the following premise: no matter what is inherited and what is instilled by experience, children function best in later life if their earliest years of nurture bring out and develop their inborn capacities.

Encouragement and Enrichment

Beginning with proper prenatal diet and care, a healthy baby is born, and from then on, her intellectual capacities are shaped by experience. Loving and attentive parents give her the self-confidence to explore and learn. She is encouraged to express herself in language. She is exposed to a variety of experiences that will stimulate her curiosity and interest: plants, drawing materials, pets, picture books, outings to the beach. Her efforts to use her intelligence by asking questions are respected and encouraged rather than minimized and ignored.

IQ Tests

Once a child gets to school her capabilities may or may not be measured by a standard IQ test. Such tests, which have been abandoned in some states, assess specific areas of intelligence and are graded according to a statistical norm. Newer techniques for measuring intelligence are designed to compensate for a cultural bias that some authorities believe exists in the standard tests.

Jealousy

See ABILITIES AND APTITUDES, BROTHERS AND SISTERS, NEW BABY.

Kidney Diseases

For a discussion of kidney diseases, see Ch. 17, *Diseases of the Urinogenital System*, and Ch. 18, *Cancer*.

Learning

See CURIOSITY, INTELLIGENCE AND IQ, READING, SCHOOLS.

Lead Poisoning

Lead poisoning in children is usually associated with the ingestion of paint and plaster flakes containing high levels of lead. This is a problem in city slums where old buildings are being leveled, or in cases where youngsters manage to gnaw on repainted cribs and other furniture originally covered with lead-base paint. In addition to this traditional source of poisoning, however, the daily exposure to exhaust fumes of leaded gasoline is causing an increasing number of children to have an excessively high level of lead in their blood. Suburban areas adjacent to heavily traveled superhighways are particularly susceptible to this problem. Those parts of the city regularly jammed with buses and cars are also unhealthy.

Lead poisoning is a serious danger to the health of approximately half a million children in the United States. Irreversible brain damage and anemia can occur if the condition becomes chronic; convulsions and death may occur in an acute case. To lessen such hazards, legislation now requires new cars to use only lead-free gasoline.

Learning Disability

A child with a learning disability is one who, though otherwise normal, cannot acquire certain skills or assimilate certain kinds of knowledge at the same rate as most other children. Obviously, almost every child lags behind her peers at one time or another in certain subjects; but the difficulties of a learning disabled child are far more severe. A 16-year-old who suffers from a learning disability may, for example, be capable only of third- or fourth-grade math while functioning at her own grade level in other subjects. Some learning disabilities are attributed to minimal brain damage, but in most cases the cause is unknown. See also DYSLEXIA.

Leukemia

See CANCER.

Lying

See DISHONESTY.

Malnutrition

Poor nutrition or undernourishment can occur not only as a result of a faulty diet, but also because a child may have a metabolic defect that prevents her body from making proper use of a particular essential nutrient. Temporary malnutrition may also accompany a long illness in which the child's appetite wanes.

Although malnutrition is usually associated with poverty and child neglect, it can also occur because of ignorance, carelessness, or fanaticism. Children have been found to be malnourished by parents following a macrobiotic diet or a faddish type of vegetarianism. Using vitamins as a substitute for food can also cause certain types of undernourishment.

Older children, especially girls approaching puberty, may embark on starvation diets in an attempt to ward off inevitable body changes and end up seriously malnourished. The general signs of malnutrition are increasing physical weakness, vague and unfocused behavior, as well as the particular symptoms associated with ane-

mia and vitamin deficiencies. See also Ch. 27, *Nutrition and Weight Control.*

Manners

Decent manners are most easily instilled in children not by scoldings, lectures, nagging, or punishments, but by setting a good example. In a family where consideration of each person's feelings is naturally taken into account, adults say "Please" and "Thank you" to each other and to their children. Thus even the youngest child gets the idea that part of growing up is to be polite to the people around him. If good manners begin at home, they're less likely to be forgotten in public.

Measles

Measles is by far the most dangerous of the common childhood diseases because of its possible complications, such as meningitis, encephalitis, and severe secondary staphylococcus infection. Fortunately, widespread protection is available in the live measles vaccine, which should be given to every child over one year of age.

Symptoms

Measles, a highly contagious disease caused by a virus, has an incubation period of one to two weeks. The most noticeable symptom is the rash that begins on the head and face within a few days after the onset of the disease, and gradually erupts all over the body, blending into big red patches. Other symptoms include fever up to 104° F or higher, a severe cough, sore throat, stuffy nose, inflammation of the *conjunctiva* (the mucous membrane on the inner part of the eyelid and extending over the front of the eyeball), sensitivity of the eyes to light, enlarged lymph nodes, and a generalized sick feeling.

Any child who has contracted measles should be seen by a physician and watched carefully for possible complications. Moreover, if he is of school age, the school should be promptly notified. This, of course, is true for any contagious disease.

Treatment

Measles can be treated only symptomatically. During the incubation period, an injection of gamma globulin will lessen the severity of the disease, or occasionally prevent it. If there are other children at home besides the affected one, they should also receive gamma globulin injections. Antibiotics are of no help unless there is a secondary bacterial infection.

All parents should make certain that their children are vaccinated against this potentially serious disease. See IMMUNIZATION.

Medication

New parents can save themselves time and trouble by getting into the habit of writing down a physician's instructions about medication when the child requires it. Although dosages are usually clearly indicated on labels prepared by the pharmacist according to the prescription, the physician may add comments about how or when to change the dosage.

How to Give Medicines to Children

As for administering medication, a calm and assured approach and a minimum of fuss are more effective than wheedling and urging. A very young child may need to be distracted by cheerful conversation as the spoon goes into her mouth; an older child can be given some factual information about the medication and what it will do. No matter what the youngster's age, parents should never trick or fool her about what she's being given, nor should candied medicine be used under any circumstances. Setting up this type of confusion in a young mind can lead to an overdose of "candy" serious enough to require emergency hospitalization.

Overusing Medication

As a child gets older, she will become increasingly conscious of the medication her parents take. Families that are constantly swallowing one or another kind of pill—diet pills, sleeping pills, tranquilizers—might give some thought to their attitude towards drugs and how these attitudes are affecting their children. Generally, it's a good idea to refrain from medicating a child unless the pediatrician recommends it.

Old Medicines

Once the illness for which a particular medication has been prescribed is definitely over, the remains of the bottle or the leftover capsules should be flushed down the toilet. Old, outdated pills can be dangerous. For safety's sake, parents should review the contents of the medicine cabinet on a regular basis and get rid of any medications left over from a previous illness. Basic medications that are essential for occasional emergencies should be reviewed for continuing effectiveness. Some of these might have a limited shelf life and be completely ineffective should they be needed.

Meningitis

Meningitis is an inflammation of the *meninges*, the thin membranes that cover the spinal cord and the brain. The inflammation, which may be caused by a virus or by bacteria, is more common among children than adults, and may occur in epidemics. This is especially true if the infectious agent is meningococcal (*meningococcal meningitis*), because the meningococcal bacteria are also found in the throat and are transmitted by coughing, sneezing, and talking. This type occurs mostly in young adults. Another type of meningitis that commonly occurs among young children during the spring and summer is caused by such organisms as the mumps virus and the coxsackievirus.

Symptoms

Whatever the cause, the symptoms are generally the same: headache, fever, vomiting, and stiff neck. If untreated, the child may go into delirium and convulsions. Drowsiness and blurred vision may also occur, and if the disease develops in an infant, the pressure on the brain caused by the inflamed meninges will create a bulge on the soft spot (fontanelle) of the baby's head. No time should be lost in calling the physician about any of these symptoms.

Meningitis was almost always fatal before the availability of antibiotics, and although it is no longer the threat it once was, it must be treated promptly if irreversible consequences are to be avoided.

Mental Illness

Behind the search for the causes and treatment of mental illness in children is the current research in the relationship between that mysterious entity called the mind and that palpable physical organism called the brain. Parents of children diagnosed as mentally ill are themselves caught up in this distinction, often preferring to call their youngsters "emotionally disturbed." It is now estimated that about one-and-a-half million youngsters under 18 require some kind of treatment for mental illness, and this figure does not include the one million children diagnosed as hyperkinetic. The two most serious forms of childhood mental illness are autism and schizophrenia.

Autism

The term "early infantile autism" was coined in the 1940s to describe babies and young children who show unpredictable deviations in development. Some never learn to speak; others refuse to look anyone directly in the eye. Autistic children may have one or two extraordinary skills and be incapable of remembering their own names. In spite of a tendency on the part of a few specialists to ascribe autism to a rejecting mother's refusal to love the infant, most authorities now describe this mysterious disorder as an organic condition caused by neurological rather than by psychological abnormalities. The same conclusions are more or less being reached about schizophrenia.

Schizophrenia

In schizophrenia, a child is likely to exhibit any of the following symptoms: confused speech and thinking; lack of emotional responsiveness; withdrawal into fantasy; and, occasionally, hallucinations. There are indications that genetic inheritance plays some role in this disorder, and that environmental influences are also involved.

Studies suggest that symptoms originate in abnormalities of brain chemistry that may be corrected by the proper medication. Over the past twenty years, many special schools, both day schools and residential ones, have been established for training autistic and schizophrenic children. The most successful enlist the cooperation of parents as cotherapists. The National Society for Children and Adults with Autism was organized to initiate schools, offer counseling to parents, and foster research. The Society operates a National Information and Referral Service that can be addressed at 1234 Massachusetts Ave., NW, Ste. 1017, Washington, DC 20005. See also HYPERKINESIS.

Mental Retardation

An estimated six million people in the United States are in some degree mentally retarded—almost three percent of the population. Mental retardation occurs among all nationalities, races, and religions, and among the children of those in the highest social and economic groups as well as the lowest.

What Is Mental Retardation?

Mental retardation is a developmental disability in which the individual's rate of development as a child is consistently slower than average. Learning cannot be acquired at the usual rate, and the child encounters difficulties in social adjustment.

Degrees of Mental Retardation

Mentally retarded children (and adults) are classified into four categories depending upon the degree of retardation.

Mildly retarded children—those with IQs roughly between 50 and 70—belong to by far the largest category; nearly 90 percent of all retarded people fall into this group. IQ scores by themselves can be misleading, but they are a convenient guide to probable learning and development patterns if understood properly—that

is, simply as one of the criteria by which the degree of a child's disability can be estimated. The retardation of mildly retarded children is usually not apparent until they are of school age. With special educational help, such children can achieve satisfying progress in school and, as adults, will be capable with proper training of handling any of a wide variety of regular jobs. They may be indistinguishable from nonretarded people and can be expected to take their places in the life of their community.

Moderately retarded children—those with IQs somewhat below 50—belong to a group that comprises about 6 percent of all retarded people in the United States. The retardation of these children is usually apparent before they begin school, often during the child's first year, in the form of delayed developmental landmarks—for example, late sitting, late standing, late walking, and delayed talking. Many children with Down's syndrome (Mongolism) fall into this group. These children require a more sheltered environment than the mildly retarded, but can be trained as adults to do productive, satisfying work.

Severely and profoundly retarded children often have other handicaps, such as impaired motor coordination or defective vision or hearing. The great majority of these children can be taught to care for their basic needs, and many can do useful work under supervision.

Causes

There are numerous causes of mental retardation. Some cases are specifically caused by congenital factors (conditions existing at or before birth). Among these are the following: deprivation of oxygen to the brain of a baby during the birth process; the mother's contraction of rubella (Ger-

man measles) during the first three months of pregnancy; complications resulting from Rh factor blood incompatibility between mother and baby; a grossly inadequate prenatal diet of the mother; syphilis; hydrocephalus (accumulation of spinal fluid in the brain); or any other pressure or injury to the brain of the fetus.

Some forms of retardation result from hereditary factors, the genetic makeup of the parents. Down's syndrome and phenylketonuria (PKU) fall in this category.

Mental retardation can also occur as a result of disease. Inflammation of the brain is a possible complication of measles—now wholly preventable by the administration of the measles vaccine. Other causes are brain injuries that result from a severe blow to the head, as from a fall. Some of these injuries are deliberately inflicted, usually by parents. (See CHILD ABUSE AND NEGLECT.) Among environmental hazards, lead and mercury poisoning are of particular importance. Lead-based paint chips have been eaten by unattended children. (See LEAD POISONING.)

If retardation is suspected by parents, medical advice should be sought immediately and a thorough evaluation of the child conducted. Some types of retardation can be greatly benefited by medical and educational treatment. It should be emphasized that all retarded children can learn and that many can be helped to the extent that they can become productive citizens. Parents would like further information about mental retardation or who are in need of counseling should write to the Association for Retarded Citizens, P.O. Box 6109, Arlington, Texas 76011. See also HANDICAPPED CHILD.

Minimal Brain Damage

See under BRAIN DAMAGE.

Money

Money may not be the root of all evil, but it certainly is the cause of a lot of family quarrels. To communicate to children the value of money and how to use it, spend it, save it, borrow it, lend it, and earn it, parents should try to clarify their own attitudes and settle their own differences.

Young children hear money talked about all the time: "We can't afford it," "That's a bargain," "That's a waste of money." What does it all mean to a preschooler?

The Weekly Allowance

The best way for a child to get first-hand experience in dealing with "I need" and "I want" in terms of cash on hand is to give her a weekly allowance. There isn't any point in doing this until she has mastered addition and subtraction. If the prospect of getting an allowance is motivation for improving her number skills at school, so much the better. The amount of the allowance should be calculated in terms of what it's supposed to cover. These details should be spelled out so that there's no confusion about who is responsible for paying for what. As the child gets older, the amount is adjusted for increasing needs—social occasions such as a ten-year-old might enjoy when she and her friends stop for an ice-cream cone on the way home from school.

Saving

If the family feels that a child should be required to save part of her allowance, a piggy bank and a brief talk about the virtues of saving are essential. Some children get so anxious about money that they turn into misers. When this occurs, it may be advisable to point out that the money is not meant to be hoarded but to be spent on needs and treats. Children who receive birthday or other special presents in the form of money from relatives can open a bank account and learn about interest accrual. Although the money is rightfully theirs, they might be encouraged to consult the family before they spend it all on a passing enthusiasm.

Mumps

Mumps, a mild disorder in most children, is caused by a virus and has an incubation period of from two to three weeks. The most familiar symptom is swollen glands involving the jaw. The glands usually affected are the *parotid glands*—large salivary glands below and slightly in front of the ear—although other glands may be affected, too. Other symptoms include fever and a general sick feeling. No rash is present. Mumps lasts about five days; then the swelling disappears.

In an adolescent boy, the disease sometimes causes an inflammation of the testes (called *orchitis*) and may be very painful. In addition, if it involves both testes, there is a possibility— fortunately only a very slight one— that sterility will result.

In older children mumps occasionally produces the complication called *mumps meningoencephalitis*. The signs of this more serious disease are headache, fever, and extreme debilitation. Finally, there may be an inflammation of the pancreas, which can cause severe abdominal pain and vomiting.

Because mumps is now preventable, every boy and girl should be given the mumps vaccine. Boys should be given the vaccine before puberty.

Muscular Dystrophy

See Ch. 8, *Diseases of the Muscles and Nervous System.*

Nausea and Vomiting

Nausea, the signal that vomiting may occur, is often described as feeling sick to the stomach. The feeling is experienced when irritated nerve endings in the stomach and elsewhere send messages to the vomiting reflex in the brain. When the nerve irritation is acute, vomiting occurs.

Physical Causes

Although nausea and vomiting are usually associated with a child's upset stomach or the sudden onset of a high fever and an acute infection, many youngsters feel nauseated and throw up because of motion sickness in a car or plane, or as the result of severe pain occasioned by a bad fall or other accident. A physician should always be consulted when nausea and vomiting are accompanied by fever, cramps, or diarrhea. For the child who feels sick in a moving vehicle, the physician can prescribe suitable medication. For a youngster who has swallowed a toxic substance, vomiting must often be induced. See Ch. 31, *Medical Emergencies*, for further information on poisoning.

Emotional Stress

Chronic nausea may result from emotional stress. A child who doesn't want to go to school because of some threatening situation, or who is always too anxious before a test because of pressures to do well, or who is fearful about some athletic challenge but ashamed to admit it—children under these pressures are likely to develop symptoms of nausea. However, instead of dismissing the recurrence of nausea and vomiting as typical of an oversensitive child, parents should try to find out the source of the problem and, if necessary, arrange some family therapy sessions with the child.

Nervous Habits

Nervous habits both express and release inner tension, and because growing up isn't an easy process, it's inevitable that most children have one or another way of dealing with their fears, anxieties, and emotional pressures. There's no point in parental scolding or ridicule or punishment, because any of these approaches simply adds yet another pressure to those that exist already. After all, most adults have nervous habits too—whether it's smoking, or picking at a cuticle, or tooth-grinding—and no amount of nagging is likely to put a stop to any of them.

Some nervous habits can be unhealthy, and some can be socially unacceptable but essentially harmless. All are unconscious, and most eventually disappear with age. Among the habits that may need looking into in order to decide that they have no basis in a physical disorder are squinting and throat-clearing. Hair-twirling and foot-shaking can be entirely ignored. Nail-biting may persist for years, or it may yield to vanity or the comments of friends.

Thumb-sucking, abandoned at two, may recur at three because of the arrival of a new baby or because of the stresses of going to nursery school. Many school-age children continue to suck their thumbs when they're going to sleep. There's no need to worry about this habit unless the dentist notices the beginning of an orthodontic problem, in which case, the dentist and not you should discuss it with the child. Nose-picking in public is almost always abandoned when a child enters school. If a big fuss has been made about it, he may continue the habit at home as a gesture of defiance—or because it really is unconscious. When done in private, it's completely harmless.

Masturbation bothers many parents more than it should. In and of itself, there's no harm in it, but as a chronic expression of anxiety, it might be dealt with tactfully and indirectly by trying to get to the source of the tension rather than by punishing or humiliating the child.

New Baby

It's a good idea for parents to talk about the anticipated arrival of a new baby with their child or children before the pregnancy is really obvious. Conversations can be casual, and questions should be answered simply and factually. If any basic changes are to be made—especially if a child is to be shifted to a bed so that the new arrival can have the crib—this transition should be accomplished before the infant appears. Adults should refrain from asking such questions as "Would you like a little brother or a little sister?" or "Isn't it wonderful that there's going to be a new baby in the family?" Preparations made in advance of going to the hospital should, if possible, consider whether the child would prefer to stay at home or with a relative during mother's absence. When the baby is brought home and well-wishers arrive with presents, it's comforting for the first-born to sit in mother's or daddy's lap while visitors coo over the infant in the crib. Thoughtful baby-present givers will always include a little present for the baby's older siblings, too. Parents should do their best to make baby's big brother or sister feel that the new baby is his or hers no less than mother's or father's. See also ABILITIES AND APTITUDES, BROTHERS AND SISTERS.

Nightmares

See DREAMS AND NIGHTMARES.

Night Terrors

See DREAMS AND NIGHTMARES.

Nosebleeds

Children are likely to have nosebleeds more often than adults, and they are usually no cause for alarm. A small blood vessel near the nostril may be injured by energetic noseblowing, the presence of a foreign object, or by an accidental blow or an intentional wallop.

Apply Pressure

A minor nosebleed is most effectively stopped by applying pressure over the bleeding area. A child old enough to follow instructions should be told to sit down, hold the head slightly forward, and compress the soft portion of the nose between thumb and forefinger, maintaining the pressure for about five minutes and breathing through the mouth. Application of an ice pack to the outside of the nose is usually helpful. Fingers should be withdrawn very slowly in order not to disturb the clot that should have formed.

Packing the Nostril

If this method doesn't stop the bleeding, a small twist of sterile cotton can be inserted gently into the nostril so that some of it protrudes. Light pressure should be applied once again for five minutes and the cotton allowed to remain in place for a while. Should the bleeding continue in spite of these measures, the child should be taken to a hospital emergency clinic.

Orthodontics

Orthodontics is the branch of dentistry that specializes in the correction of *malocclusion* (an improper alignment of the upper and lower teeth at the point where they meet) or to irregularity of tooth positioning. Emphasis is now being placed on the prevention of malocclusion before it can occur. General practitioners of dentistry, *pedodontists* (specialists in children's dentistry), and orthodontists now believe that the need for expensive, time-consuming, and emotionally unsettling orthodontics can sometimes be avoided by beginning treatment as early as the age of four.

The positioning of the permanent teeth is the result not only of inheritance, but of other variables, such as lip-biting and thumb-sucking. Premature loss or partial disintegration of primary teeth also has a strong influence on whether the permanent teeth will be properly positioned.

Preventive Orthodontics

By the time the child is five, an X ray will show exactly how all the permanent teeth are situated in the gums. In some cases, it may be possible to guide these teeth as they erupt. If potential overcrowding and eventual crookedness are indicated, some baby teeth may be pulled to make room for the permanent ones. Normal positioning may also be accomplished by establishing a different balance of muscular forces.

Corrective Appliances

Corrective orthodontics uses many different types of appliances for the repositioning of permanent teeth, all of which operate on the same principle of applying pressure to the bone. Widening the arch of the upper jaw, for example, is accomplished by the use of a screw appliance fixed to the upper teeth so that the two halves of the hard palate are slightly separated along the middle suture, permitting new bone to fill in the space. Specialists point out that a bonus of this orthodontic correction is increased respiratory ease for youngsters who

were formerly mouth-breathers.

Parents who have been advised by the family dentist that an orthodontic consultation is advisable for a child, and who are concerned about the eventual economic burden that prolonged treatment might represent, should get a second opinion from the clinical staff of a dental school associated with a university. See also DENTAL CARE.

Overeating

It's simple enough to define overeating as putting more food into the stomach than the body needs for good nutrition, but that doesn't shed much light on why certain children do so. Parents need only indulge in some honest introspection and they are likely to remember times when they overate—or drank too much—because they were anxious about something or because they felt lonely or neglected or angry. These feelings may lead to compulsive overeating in children, too.

There are also those parents for whom plumpness is a sign of well-being. Without thinking of the permanent harm they might be doing, they overfeed their children; from an early age such children get in the habit of eating too much as a way of gaining parental approval. It's not unusual for girls about to enter puberty either to starve themselves or to stuff themselves; either impulse is an expression of fears about sexuality that are gradually eased if the family atmosphere is relaxed and understanding.

What to Do and What Not to Do

The least effective way of dealing with chronic overeating is parental nagging or teasing. Punishment in the form of cutting down a child's allowance or

withholding permission to attend a birthday party will very likely only make the child more anxious and angrier. In most cases, a pattern of overeating has to be changed by the child and not by the parent. However, where the problem is the result of overt or hidden pressure on the child to overeat, parents will have to change their notions of good eating habits, health, and attractive appearance. See also Ch. 27, *Nutrition and Weight Control*.

Pacifiers

Some parents can't stand the sound of a baby's crying; others can't stand the sight of a baby sucking on a pacifier. Whatever the preference, what the baby needs during the early months is satisfaction for the sucking impulse. For most babies, this need seems to taper off at about six months; with those babies in whom the need remains strong, the thumb seems to be a convenient substitute for the pacifier. Whatever decision is arrived at between you and your physician, the important thing to keep in mind is that the pacifier is no substitute for holding and cuddling the baby when she wants comforting, and that sometimes a parent is more dependent on a pacifier than the baby is.

If pacifiers are used regularly, more than one should be available, and they should be inspected periodically to make sure that bits and pieces of rubber haven't been chewed so loose that they may be swallowed and lodge in the windpipe.

Pets

Rural children usually have their own pet animals even if the animals aren't allowed in the house. Suburban families are likely to own a dog that's a pet as well as a discouragement to prowlers. It's the city child who may have to wage a persistent campaign before his parents capitulate to the idea of a pet. Yet even the smallest apartment can accommodate a pet bird or a small fish tank; a cat and a litter box won't cause extra crowding. Of course, dogs offer the greatest companionship but also impose the greatest responsibility; they do have to be housebroken and walked in all weathers at least twice a day. If a child brings a stray animal home, the dog or cat must be checked by a vet before it becomes a household member. Once a youngster can read, the acquisition of a pet hamster or a guinea pig or a pair of gerbils will provide the incentive for trips to the library for books on care and feeding.

Choosing a Dog

When a dog is to be the choice, it's often cheaper and more satisfactory to select one from the litter of a healthy dog you know than to buy one in a pet shop or from a commercial kennel. The breed chosen should be suitable in terms of size, temperament, and cost of feeding. Relative advantages and disadvantages should be checked out at the library by the child whose responsibility the pet will be.

For an only child, a pet animal is almost a must, not only for companionship, but so that there's a being in the house who's smaller and more helpless than she is. In families where allergies are a problem, the physician should be consulted about the type of pet that will cause the least discomfort to a vulnerable member of the household.

Pica

Pica is the technical term for an abnormal desire to eat substances that are not fit for food, such as clay,

earth, plaster and the like. This tendency is not to be confused with the tendency of babies and toddlers to put unsuitable things into their mouth. Pica is habitual and compulsive, and may result in serious disabilities. Because the phenomenon is especially conspicuous among poor and neglected children, some authorities associate it with nutritional deficiency, others with unsatisfied emotional needs. Signs of pica should be brought to the attention of a physician or a social service agency that can provide guidance on how the child's circumstances should be altered even if the total environment cannot be changed. See also LEAD POISONING.

Pills

See MEDICATION.

Pinworms or Threadworms

See Ch. 11, *Diseases of the Digestive System.*

PKU

PKU stands for *phenylketonuria*, an inherited metabolic defect. Approximately one baby in 10,000 is born with this disease, in which the body is incapable of producing certain enzymes that are essential for the metabolic conversion of the amino acid phenylalanine. The disorder causes the amino acid and some of its by-products to accumulate in the bloodstream to a dangerous degree. If the condition goes undetected and untreated, irreversible brain damage and mental retardation are the result.

PKU babies are characteristically blond and blue-eyed, with sensitive skin and faulty muscle coordination. In many parts of the United States, state laws require that three days after birth, all babies be given the blood test that detects the presence

of PKU so that treatment can begin at once if necessary. Supervised treatment usually continues for several years, and in some communities is available at special therapy centers. Parents or prospective parents who would like to find out whether any member of the family is a carrier of the recessive gene that transmits the PKU disorder can arrange for diagnostic testing and genetic counseling based on the results.

Play

See FANTASIES, TOYS.

Pneumonia

See "Pneumonia" in Ch. 12, *Diseases of the Respiratory System.*

Poisons and Poisoning

Every year, hundreds of thousands of children swallow some poisonous substance—in too many cases with fatal results—because of parental carelessness, or because the child hasn't been given clear and unequivocal instructions about the difference between "candy" and medicine. Poisoning because of the ingestion of sugar-coated aspirin is a continuing problem; iron-containing multiple vitamins that seem to be a gourmet treat to some children also present a problem because iron in excess doses is a stomach irritant.

Safety Measures

Toddlers can do themselves damage because they're curious about everything, and their sense of taste isn't all that discriminating. Thus it's an absolute necessity to see that all household cleansers and strong chemicals are kept on high shelves rather than on the floor. Many bottles containing medicines come with safety caps that presumably cannot be opened by children—for instance, because pressure must be applied—but can be opened by adults. The experience of many parents, however, is that whereas their children can often open such caps, *they* frequently have a great deal of difficulty. Suffice it to say that the perfect childproof bottle cap has yet to be designed.

Because it's practically impossible for anyone except an expert to know what substances are poisonous to children in what amounts, or which seeds of which plants are harmful if swallowed, many authorities feel strongly that parents should immediately call the closest Poison Control Center for first-aid information rather than try to cope with antidotes or emetics on their own. The Centers are available by phone on a 24-hour-a-day basis. See Ch. 31, *Medical Emergencies*, to find the Poison Control Center nearest you. Make a note of the telephone number and make sure it's available to baby-sitters as well as to all responsible family members.

Poliomyelitis

Until the Salk vaccine was developed in the 1950s, there was no protection against polio (or, as it was then popularly called, *infantile paralysis*). The disease caused paralysis of the extremities and could cause death by paralyzing the muscles used in breathing.

The Salk vaccine utilizes doses of killed virus and is given by injection. Although it is still widely used in many parts of the world, in the United States the Sabin live virus vaccine, which is given orally, has virtually supplanted it. Repeated series of booster shots are unnecessary because the immunity persists for years.

It is advisable that a child receive three doses of the Sabin vaccine, six to eight weeks apart, starting at about the age of two months. One method employs *trivalent* vaccine, in which each dose contains three kinds of vaccine—to give protection against three strains of polio. Three separate doses are necessary, however, to insure full protection. The other method employs *monovalent* vaccines, in which each dose insures protection against a different type of polio.

Posture

"Stand up straight" is an order that many parents issue to their children with the regularity of drill sergeants. Actually, most youngsters tend to slump and have a potbellied look until they're about nine years old. This inelegant posture is not necessarily the sign of any disorder.

Youngsters who are regularly checked by a physician and given a good bill of health are not in any danger of developing a permanent curvature of the spine because they slouch. However, certain kinds of chronically poor posture may be an expression of some disorder that should be checked. Among these are flat feet, nearsightedness or astigmatism, or a hearing loss.

Emotional problems may also be expressed in a child's bearing. Anxiety can lead to carrying one shoulder higher than the other as if warding off a blow. Shyness or insecurity may cause a hangdog stance. For pubescent girls, embarrassment about burgeoning breasts may result in a round-shouldered slump. Some of these causes of poor posture should be discussed with a physician; others may be temporary and shouldn't be turned into major problems by incessant and unproductive nagging. A better corrective is participation in a dancing class or an exercise class. Sports such as ice-skating and bicycle-riding are good posture correctives, too.

Prejudice

The A student (female) who avoids studying mathematics because "girls aren't supposed to be good in math" and the black boy who goes out for the track team even though he'd rather be in the science club "because blacks are better at sports than at brainwork" have unconsciously accepted the prejudiced views of other people about them. What a waste for themselves and society!

Children who are raised in an atmosphere of contempt for and fear and mistrust of Catholics, Jews, Italians, blacks, women, men, are likely to spend the better part of their lives alternating between apprehension and arrogance. It's difficult to believe that adults can have a prejudice such as, "All Orientals are sneaky," which is supposed to describe millions of human beings, or "She's only a girl," which makes a judgment about one-half of the human race.

Being the Object of Discrimination

Parents who have themselves been discriminated against have to prepare their children for the reality of discrimination and how to cope with it. A child raised in an atmosphere of love and respect will have enough self-esteem to refuse to accept anyone else's false notions about him.

Privacy

Every child has a right to a certain amount of privacy even when he's very young. If, for instance, a parent or older child doesn't allow anyone into the bathroom when he's using it, a four- or five-year-old should be given the same option. When children share the same room, or even the same furniture, each one should have a drawer of his own and a shelf of his own for his things. Respecting his private property will lead him to respect other people's. A youngster does like the privacy of playing with his friends without having a parent hovering around all the time, and he certainly doesn't want anyone listening in on his phone conversations by the time he's nine or ten.

Parents have a right to privacy, too! Children should be led to understand—pleasantly but firmly—that some adult conversations are private and not meant for their ears. They should also be taught that when an older member of the family is behind a closed door, it's rude to barge in without knocking.

Puberty

See Ch. 3, *The Teens.*

Punishment

Severe physical punishment should be avoided. Ideally, punishment should be carried out because it has an instructional value for the child rather than because it helps a parent relieve his or her feelings of anger or frustration. Severe physical punishments—for example, the use of sticks, belts, or hard blows to the body—are extremely frightening and may even be permanently injurious to the child. Frequently, this kind of discipline can evoke even further anger on the part of the child and lead to further misbehavior.

Duration

Punishments should not be long and drawn out, but should be as immediate as possible and last only a reasonable length of time. For example, withdrawal of television privileges for a month for a seven-year-old's misbehavior would be excessively long, because at the end of the month it would be difficult for her to remember what she had done that was wrong. Excessively long punishments are also difficult to enforce. If possible, a punishment should be related to the misbehavior for which the child is receiving the punishment.

Immediacy

Punishment "when father gets home" or a day later frequently has little meaning for the child and is unlikely to help her stop misbehaving. Rewards for good behavior should also be immediate; affection and approval for most children are often more powerful rewards than candy and money. See also DISCIPLINE.

Radio, Record Player, and TV

Music hath charms not only to soothe the savage breast but also to lift the spirits and provide entertainment.

However, children who have their own transistor radios should be informed that playing them in public at a level audible to another person is against the law in most places, and if they're listening to music with earphones, the sound should be kept low enough not to damage their ears. Countless young people of the 60s have grown to adulthood with a permanent hearing disability because of chronic exposure to dangerously high sound levels.

The child who has a stereo or a cassette deck of his own should be permitted to express his own tastes in the music he buys with his own allowance. If the family installation is an expensive one, a young child should be permitted to use it only when he demonstrates the proper respect for the delicacy of the mechanism.

Television Time

As for the problem of how much time should be spent watching television: if as soon as the toddler's eyes can focus on the screen, TV is used as a pacifier, the child is likely to get the idea that the way to please mommy is to be glued to the screen as often as possible.

Rashes

Rashes of one kind or another are among the most common occurrences of childhood. Whether it's the discomfort of diaper rash soon after birth, the childhood markings of chicken pox, or a case of poison ivy, most skin eruptions aren't too serious and are usually of brief duration.

The First Six Months

Skin rashes are especially common during the first six months. They may result from overheating or overdressing, or to the use of detergents, powders, perfumes, and oils which cause *contact dermatitis*. In addition, certain foods may make the baby break out in facial rashes. Prolonged contact with wet diapers causes *diaper rash*, from the ammonia produced by urine.

Skin rashes can usually be prevented or controlled by:

- Control of temperature
- Proper clothing
- Avoidance of irritating perfumes, powders, and detergents in laundering baby clothes
- Avoidance, in certain circumstances, of milk or other foods, as suggested by your physician
- Avoidance of rubber pants over diapers
- Applications of ointments to rashy areas

If a disturbing skin condition persists or gets worse, your physician will check for special infections like impetigo or fungus, and, should they exist, recommend proper treatment. During the early years, most children develop the characteristic rashes of the contagious childhood diseases, and at these times, a physician's care is usually essential for the prevention of complications.

Eczema

Some children suffer from intermittent eczema that has a tendency to run in families. Eczema can be extremely uncomfortable, because the more it itches, the more it is scratched, and the more it's scratched, the more it itches. This cycle may be triggered by an allergy to a particular food or pollen; it may be a contact dermatitis caused by a particular fabric, or it might flare up because of emotional tension created by family arguments or anxiety about schoolwork. Eczema should be treated by the family physician who may be able to discover its source and prevent further attacks.

Other Allergic Rashes

Other rashes that are essentially allergic in origin are those resulting from contact with poison ivy, oak, or sumac. For information about these and other skin conditions, including hives, see "Disorders of the Skin," in Ch. 21, *Skin and Hair*.

The discomfort of many rashes can be eased by ointments or salves. Plain cornstarch is helpful for prickly heat. Rashes that are bacterial in origin, such as impetigo, or parasitic, have to be treated by a physician with antibiotic or fungicidal preparations.

Roseola

Among the more common rashes of early childhood is the one known as *roseola infantum*. It is believed to be caused by a virus. It begins with a high fever that subsides in a few days. There are no other specific signs of illness, and the end of the disorder—when the fever is usually gone—is signaled by the appearance of a body rash of red spots that disappear overnight. The one aspect of roseola that requires medical attention is the fever. Because high temperature can produce convulsions in infants and babies, efforts should be made to reduce it by sponging and aspirin. Antibiotics are not indicated unless there's some sign of a secondary infection.

Pityriasis Rosea

A long-lasting rash thought to be viral in origin is *pityriasis rosea*, easily identifiable because the onset of this infection is preceded by one large raised red scaly eruption known as the herald patch. The rash itself appears symmetrically and in clusters on the trunk, arms, and legs, and in some children on the hands and feet as well as the face. Unfortunately, this rash may last for more than a month. There is no treatment for it, and, although it leaves without a trace and almost never recurs, it can cause severe itching that should be eased with a salve or ointment. Soap is very irritating and should be avoided.

Rocky Mountain Spotted Fever

Among the diseases caused by organisms known as rickettsiae and transmitted to people by the animal ticks that are infected with them is *Rocky Mountain spotted fever*, also called *tick fever*. In addition to rising temperature, headache, nausea, and malaise,

this disease produces a characteristic rash that starts on the ankles, lower legs, and wrists, and then spreads to the rest of the body. Children who wander about in the woods during the summer or whose pets run loose in tick-infested areas should be watched for the presence of a tick on the skin and the ensuing rash. Rocky Mountain spotted fever is a serious disease against which youngsters should be protected by wearing the proper clothing.

Lyme Disease

A rash may be the first visible symptom of Lyme disease, which had been reported in 34 American states by the late 1980s. Caused by a tick-carried bacterium, the disease can produce symptoms similar to those of arthritis, multiple sclerosis, and heart disease. The initial rash can extend over an area 28 inches across. Antibiotics including tetracycline and penicillin may be used in treatment. The risk of infection may be reduced by frequent inspections of skin areas and prompt removal of the pinhead-sized ticks. If not embedded, ticks can be brushed off; if embedded, they can be lifted out with a tweezers. The skin should be washed carefully with an antiseptic such as rubbing alcohol.

Reading

Children who see their parents reading or who've heard an older sibling say, "Don't interrupt me when I'm reading" are much more likely to want to learn how to read than those who have never seen an older person absorbed in a book or magazine.

Reading Difficulties

No matter how much the world changes, the child who can't read easily is handicapped. Where a true reading problem exists, parents should confer with the school about a practical solution. If a learning disability appears to be the explanation, tutoring or a special class may be essential. See DYSLEXIA.

Reading for Information

Many youngsters who don't see the point in reading for pleasure when there are so many other things they'd prefer to do may dash off to the library if they want information about horses or sailing ships or sewing. Families who would like their youngsters to read more than they do have the responsibility of providing a quiet corner, a decent reading light, and an occasional hour of uninterrupted leisure and privacy. Parents who object to their ten-year-old daughter's habit of "always having her nose in a book" instead of "getting some fresh air and exercise" should withhold their criticism unless the physician recommends a change in the child's activities.

Responsibility

Most young children enjoy being given responsibilities suitable to their age and capabilities because it makes them feel grown up. Too few responsibilities and they think they're being treated like babies; too many, and they're likely to look for ways of shirking them.

The style and tone with which responsibilities are assigned have a lot to do with how cheerfully they're executed. A three-year-old can be assigned the responsibility of putting his toys away; a four-year-old can be trusted to help clear the table after dinner, and a five-year-old can be allowed to help with the new baby. Parents can provide a good example by shouldering their own responsibilities cheerfully. See also INDEPENDENCE.

Retardation

See MENTAL RETARDATION.

Rheumatic Fever

Once called growing pains, rheumatic fever is actually a disease of the connective tissues, a secondary manifestation of a primary infection by streptococcus bacteria of the throat or tonsils. Its chief symptoms are pains and tenderness in the joints and sore throat.

Rheumatic fever may be mild enough to escape attention or it may be disabling for a period of months. The insidious aspect of the disease is that it may damage the child's heart in such a way that tissue is permanently scarred and function is impaired in the form of a heart murmur. Acuteness of symptoms varies. Any time from a week to a month after the occurrence of strep throat, the child may complain of feeling tired and achy. Fever usually accompanies the fatigue, and pains in the joints may precede swelling and the development of nodules under the skin in the areas of the wrists, elbows, knees, and vertebrae. The pediatrician can usually detect an abnormal heart finding. The sooner treatment begins, however, the less likely the risk of permanent heart damage.

Close supervision of the affected child may be essential over a long period. Antibiotics, aspirin, hormones (cortisone), and other medicines control the course of the disease and protect the child from its potentially disabling effects. See also "Rheumatic Fever and Rheumatic Heart Disease" in Ch. 10, *Heart Diseases*.

Roseola Infantum

See under RASHES.

Rubella (German Measles)

Rubella was once thought of as a be-nign disease. Then it was discovered that it could have serious consequences if it were contracted by a woman during the first three months of her pregnancy. The virus that causes rubella is transmitted from the infected woman to her unborn baby, and has been linked to birth defects of the heart, eye, ear, and liver, and to mental retardation.

In addition, a baby who has been exposed to the disease in utero may infect others even though he himself is not affected by it and shows no symptoms. (In fact, most babies are immune to rubella during their first year.) The rubella virus is highly contagious and spreads rapidly.

The incubation period for rubella is two to three weeks. Symptoms include earache, swollen glands behind the ears, a low-grade fever, and a usually mild, blotchy rash that erupts over the body but lasts only a few days.

Most children are only mildly affected by rubella and require little treatment except rest. However, a pregnant woman who comes in contact with the child can contract it. It is, therefore, of great importance that all children over one year of age be immunized with the vaccine that prevents rubella. Any woman of child-bearing age who might be pregnant should *not* be given the vaccine, because the effects of the vaccine on an unborn fetus are not known.

Runaways

In growing numbers children and youth ran away from home in the early and middle 1980s. The runaways left home for various reasons. Some were escaping physical or sexual abuse while many others had severe long-term psychological and other problems. A smaller percentage faced temporary or less severe home or school difficulties. Other reasons include "status criminal offense problems"—minor violations of the law that would not be violations at all if committed by an adult—and "poor communication" with parents. Truancy is an example of a status offense. Many children who leave home are not technically "runaways." Professionals call these children *throwaways* because they have in fact been thrown out of the parents' home.

Social service professionals believe many young persons leave home to escape from "dysfunctional families." In such families, parental separation or divorce, poverty, unemployment, and high mobility have, separately or in combination, made the home ineffective as a nurturing environment. The young person may become labeled as a "failure" or "troublemaker"; and a lack of warmth may characterize parent–child relations. In other cases delinquency among a youngster's friends may exert a powerful influence.

The runaways represent diverse age and economic groups. They come from a variety of racial backgrounds. A large proportion are in the 15 to 16 age group. But runaways range in age from 10 or younger to 18.

Parents faced with the fact that a child has run away have to make difficult choices. The child who stays away overnight or for two or more nights has usually not traveled more than 10 miles from home. He or she is usually staying with friends. Only about one in five ventures more than 50 miles from home. The parent or parents of a runaway, considering such facts and not wishing simply to wait, can:

- Look for the youngster themselves. Recommended by many social workers as a logical first step, such a search may involve calls to relatives or the child's friends, checks on favorite haunts, and "driving around" in areas that the young person knows and frequents.

- Report the runaway to police. A "first impulse" alternative, calling the police may not be in the child's best interest. For one thing, the police, especially in large cities, are swamped with such reports. Parental searches actually succeed in finding runaways more frequently than police do. As a second consideration, once reported to police the youngster may be drawn into the juvenile-justice system. In some states, that could result in incarceration with adult offenders or delinquent juveniles. Other states provide that a runaway cannot be held—or cannot be held more than a brief, specified period.

- Contact a local branch of the National Network of Runaway and Youth Services. A private, nonprofit organization with more than 500 community-based shelter programs, the Network serves runaway, homeless, and other "problem" young people. It offers shelter and hotline services 24 hours a day, seven days a week. While not a search operation, the Network also provides crisis and long-term individual and family counseling, outreach, advocacy, referrals for medical, legal, and mental health assistance, and followup services.

- Contact the National Communications System. Supported by the U.S. Department of Health and Human Services, the system operates a nationwide toll-free telephone hotline. Services provided center on referral and crisis intervention aid.

Some national or local services have been established primarily to help runaways obtain clothing, shelter, and food. These organizations also try to mediate between parents and children and to bring families together. Three such groups operate the Runaway Hotline (800/231-6946), the National Runaway Switchboard (800/621-4000), and the National Center for Missing and Exploited Children (800/843-5678).

What happens after a child returns home may determine whether he or she will run away again. Family counselors suggest that parents remain calm. No matter how stressful the runaway incident may have been, parents should try to accept their child as a person. Many runaways, counselors say, are "testing the waters," or experimenting, or seeking a sense of self and identity. If the family can discuss what has happened, the problems that caused the young person to run away may be resolved.

In difficult situations, counseling may be necessary. More and more parents are turning also to inpatient psychiatric services. Usually, these parents have tried other solutions before turning to psychiatry. Contributing to the trend toward hospitalization and professional treatment is the increasing availability of insurance to cover the expected costs.

Safety

See "Accident Prevention" in Ch. 36, *Voluntary Health Agencies*.

Scarlet Fever

Scarlet fever used to be a disease that everyone dreaded. It is highly contagious, and can result in severe aftereffects like rheumatic fever, or the kidney disease known as nephritis.

It is now known that scarlet fever is simply a streptococcal infection—a strain of a specific organism that also causes a diffuse red rash. It can be dealt with quite simply by your physician, the usual treatment being a ten-day course of penicillin, which cures the streptococcal infection and prevents most complications.

Schizophrenia

See under MENTAL ILLNESS.

School

In the United States, an elementary school is a place where children are taught not only how to read, write, handle numbers, and correlate sets of facts; they are also taught how to get along with children different from themselves, how to express themselves creatively, and how to become responsible citizens of a democratic society. If the reality of education falls short of these goals, parents are supposed to exert influence on the proper authorities to see that they are in fact accomplished.

Nursery School

For a child, leaving the protection of the family if only for a half-day in a nearby nursery school is a big step forward. The step is likely to be taken with eagerness if parents present the school as a pleasurable place to be, and not as a dumping ground for a youngster who's in the way of a new baby or a working mother.

Elementary School

The elementary grades represent a major change in many different ways, but most importantly because new authority figures begin to displace parents as the source of all wisdom. Adults and older siblings can help a child make a happy and productive adjustment to school by talking about it with interest and respect. Wherever possible, one or another parent should be present at parent-teacher meetings and participate in the activities of the child's group, such as class trips, visiting days, and the like.

Homework

When youngsters come home with school assignments that they find baffling, parents should feel free to ask the teacher for clearer instructions. If the child is at fault through inattention or ignorance, it might be pointed out to her that whether or not she gets a good education depends on how hard she's ready to work and not how efficiently the teacher can spoon-feed her.

Private Schools

Some families feel that the local public school is not the best place for their children to learn during the lower grades. Alternative private schools, whether denominational, discriminatory, or for gifted children, may have advantages that are less apparent to the child than to the parents, especially if attendance isolates the youngster from her friends in the neighborhood.

Staying Home from School

It's not unusual for a child to avoid going to school once in a while by saying she's sick. She may actually need a rest from the routine every few months. This is quite different from truly getting sick at the thought of facing school. A child who is nauseated in the morning, or who throws up, or who has a stomachache at breakfast, is probably experiencing feelings of anger, resentment, or anxiety beyond her ability to cope with them. Whatever it is in the school situation that's worrying her, she should be given the opportunity to talk about what's going on and the reassurance that efforts will be made to help straighten things out.

For children with disabilities, special facilities are often provided within the structure of the local school so that they can spend at least part of their day with their own age group.

Sex Education

Children need and deserve to have access to correct information about sexual functioning. If there is a natural openness in a family about questions of all types, children first start asking questions about sex when they are three or four; it is then that parents can begin describing sexual functioning to their children.

Questions about Body Parts

The first questions about sex usually have to do with the functioning of body parts. For example, children want to know where urine comes from, what happens to food when they eat it, where feces come from, and where babies come from. Explanations should be given in a straightforward, unembarrassed manner. Children should not be overloaded with information that they do not understand, but parents should be willing to answer questions to the best of their ability.

With older children, particularly 11- and 12-year-olds, it is often helpful for sexual questions to be answered by the parent of the same sex. Reading a book on sexual development together with the child can be a good experience for both parent and child. Parents frequently wonder if sex education may not lead children to engage in experimentation. Most of the evidence on this question indicates that children are more likely to experiment sexually when they are ignorant than when their questions about sex are reasonably and accurately answered.

Sexual Abuse and Incest

Of all the forms of child abuse (see CHILD ABUSE), sexual abuse, including incest, is the most common. Estimates of the number of sexual assaults on children in the United States range as high as five million annually. As many as 80 percent of these assaults occur within families. In many cases the adults reside outside the family but are closely acquainted with their victims.

Child sexual abuse takes many forms. While tens of thousands of children and young people are sexually attacked or molested, thousands of others are filmed, photographed, or otherwise exploited for the private recreational purposes of abusers. An estimated 50,000 children disappear annually; most of them are never found. Experts say many of these lost children are forced into a kind of sex-slavery, becoming victims of the "kiddie porn" (child pornography) trade. Within the home, sexual abuse may include rape, inappropriate fondling, exhibitionism, sexual intercourse, sodomy, and other acts.

Who are the victims of child sexual abuse? They are both males and females; they range in age from a few months to 16 years or older. The mean age at which a child experiences sexual abuse is nine. The victims represent all socioeconomic groups, all races, all geographic regions.

Protecting Your Children

Parents have the delicate task of maintaining a loving, touching family relationship while also teaching their child or children to recognize and re-

---

> **Safety Tips for Parents**
>
> 1. Know your children's friends.
> 2. Never leave your child unattended.
> 3. Be involved in your child's activities.
> 4. Listen when your child tells you he or she does not want to be with someone.
> 5. Pay attention when someone shows greater than normal interest in your child.
> 6. Have your child fingerprinted and know where to locate dental records.
> 7. Be sensitive to changes in your child's behavior or attitudes.
> 8. Take a photograph of your child each year (4 times each year if under age 2).
> 9. Be prepared to describe your children accurately—including clothing, visible identifying marks, or special characteristics.
> 10. Develop a set procedure should you and your child become separated while away from home.
> 11. Do not buy items that visibly display your child's name.
> 12. Be sure your child's school or day-care center will not release your child to anyone other than you or someone you officially designate.
> 13. Instruct the school to contact you immediately if your child is absent or if someone other than you arrives to pick up him or her without advance notice from you.

---

ject "bad touches." Parents do not want to instill in their child fear, hysteria, or paranoia. But they should want their child to know how to escape or avoid abuse within or outside the home. Without dwelling on the details of what *could* happen, show what a bad touch involves—generally, a pinch, hard slap, or a touch in a body area normally covered by a bathing suit. One exception, of course, is a physician's examination. Parental approval makes such an examination acceptable.

Children can and should learn to say "no" to an adult, psychologists tell us. Having said "no," whether the would-be abuser is a friend, relative, or stranger, your child should leave the scene quickly. Then he or she should report the incident to a parent. "Be sure to emphasize that if someone asks them not to tell that they should immediately tell," advises one authority. Parents should make it clear that they will not be mad if they receive such a report.

Parents need to instruct children periodically in the ways to respond appropriately to abusers' approaches. But then they have to listen if the child wants to talk. Children have to be sure both of the parents' love and their willingness to pay attention.

Symptoms to Watch For

A child encountering molestation or sexual abuse of any kind is undergoing an emotionally stressful experience. But the young person may be too shy to reveal what has happened. If a parent suspects that a son or daughter has been molested, one authority suggests, asking directly if anything has happened.

What symptoms might cause suspicion? As published in "Child Protection Alert," a publication of the American Christian Voice Foundation, there are at least 25 symptoms that you should watch for:

1. Explicit (sometimes bizarre) sexual knowledge

2. Precocious sexually related experimentation or speech

3. Toilet training relapses

4. Smearing of feces or urine

5. Gagging and unexplained vomiting

6. Speech problems

7. Regressive behavior

8. Masturbation

9. Withdrawal from normal human contact

10. Stomach and head pains

11. Bedwetting

12. Suicidal depression and/or self-destructive tendencies

13. Excessive fear of selected individuals or locations

14. Loss of appetite

15. Unexplained bruises or injuries in genital areas

16. Blood spotting or unexplained substances on underwear

17. Abrupt or radical behavioral or attitude changes

18. Lack of self-esteem or self-worth

19. Ulcers, colitis, anorexia, or other stress related disorders

20. Alcohol or drug abuse

21. Frequent nightmares

22. Excessive passivity

23. Vaginal or urinary tract infections

24. Infections of the mouth, gums, or throat. (Be vigilant for venereal diseases of the anus or throat. Incidences are no longer uncommon in children.)

25. Unexplained gifts, extra money, or the presence of pornography in your child's possession

Sources of Help

Where does a parent seek help once it's certain that molestation or abuse has occurred? The recommended first stage is to notify the police or local rape crisis center, or (where incest is the crime) the state child protection agency. To avoid adding to your child's stress, parents should *not* confront the offender while the child is present. Make sure the young victim has a complete physical examination if only to reassure the boy or girl that no permanent physical damage has been done. Depending on need, you may also want to ensure that the child gets counseling. Resource centers that provide diverse kinds of aid include:

- CHILD HELP National Child Abuse hotline: 800/422-4453

- Child Find hotline: 800/931-5005

- National Center for Missing and Exploited Children: 800/843-5678 or 202/634-9821

- The Adam Walsh Child Resource Center: 305/475-4848

- SLAM (Society's League against Child Molestation): 801/328-3000

- National Crime Information Center (F.B.I.): 202/324-3000

- National Runaway Switchboard: 800/621-4000

Sibling Rivalry

See ABILITIES AND APTITUDES, BROTHERS AND SISTERS, NEW BABY.

Sickle-cell Anemia

See Ch. 9, *Diseases of the Circulatory System.*

Sisters and Brothers

See BROTHERS AND SISTERS.

Sleep

See BEDTIME, DREAMS AND NIGHTMARES, SLEEPWALKING.

Sleepwalking

Sleepwalking may be distressing to the parent who witnesses it, but it usually does the child no harm. If the child seems to be about to do something dangerous, it's a good idea to wake her up with a few reassuring remarks and guide her back to bed. In most sleepwalking incidents, the child goes back to bed by herself and gets up the next day without the slightest recollection of her nighttime prowl. Parents shouldn't tease or scold or make the child feel peculiar about walking in her sleep. It can be ignored unless it continues over a long period, and then it might be mentioned to your physician.

Smallpox

Smallpox has been eradicated everywhere in the world. Vaccination against smallpox has therefore been discontinued in the United States.

Smoking

Young children who see older children in the family or at home smoking cigarettes are going to equate smoking with being grown up even if their parents don't smoke. A ten-year-old who sneaks off to experiment with a cigarette shouldn't be treated like a criminal, but he should be told that he is harming himself. Parents who smoke and wish they didn't should concentrate on their own efforts to stop and hope that their offspring get the message. In any event, it might help to emphasize how hard it is to stop smoking once one has acquired the habit.

Sore Throat

"It hurts when I swallow" is a common complaint of childhood. It may be connected with a cold or tonsillitis, but if there is tenderness at the sides of the neck and a rise in temperature, the physician should be called promptly so that tests can be made to see whether the child has strep throat. Often a throat culture is necessary. A streptococcus throat infection that is undiagnosed and untreated can have serious consequences. See also TONSILLITIS.

Speech Defects

Among the more common speech defects are *lisping* (the substitution of *th* for *s* and *z* sounds); *lallation* (the inability to pronounce *l* or *r* correctly), and stuttering. Although many children do outgrow their speech disabilities, a considerable number do not. There are about two million adult stutterers in the United States.

Therapy

Corrective therapy should be undertaken without too much delay. In the case of stuttering, it is generally agreed that psychological factors play a considerable role in creating and perpetuating the problem. When professional efforts are made to correct it, they almost always involve some family therapy sessions. There have been many advances in the techniques used by speech pathologists, including the audiovisual devices and feed-back systems that promote self-correction. A list of certified speech pathologists can be obtained from the American Speech-Language-Hearing Association, 10801 Rockville Pike, Rockville, MD 20852.

Stealing

See DISHONESTY.

Stepchildren

See Ch. 5, *The Middle Years*. See also ADOPTED CHILDREN.

Stomachache

A wide variety of disorders begins with some kind of abdominal pain, but in most cases, a stomachache is temporary and unaccompanied by any other symptoms. Digestive upsets are frequent in infancy, becoming rarer as the baby approaches the fourth month. See COLIC.

After the baby's first year, a stomachache may signal the onset of a cold or some other infection. The physician should be called if any of the following conditions occurs:

- When the stomach pain is accompanied by fever, vomiting, or diarrhea

- If moderate pain lasts for a considerable time—several hours, for example

- If the pain is obviously acute—the child is doubled over

- If the location of the pain shifts from one place to another

Never give a child a laxative or an enema except on a physician's orders.

A youngster who complains regularly of stomachaches without any other symptoms, and who might also complain of headaches or constipation shouldn't be dismissed as a worrier. The problem should be discussed with your physician so that an investigation can be made of possible causes. In many cases, constipation is the source of stomach pain. When the constipation is cleared up, the stomach pains cease.

Stomach pain may also be of psychosomatic origin, in children as well as in adults. If the pain cannot be explained after a physical examination and tests have been made, parents should consider how they can lighten some of the stresses and tensions in the child's life.

Strabismus

See CROSSED EYES.

Stuttering

See SPEECH DEFECTS.

Sudden Infant Death Syndrome

Sudden Infant Death Syndrome, sometimes referred to as SIDS and generally known as *crib death*, claims about 10,000 babies every year. It is the chief single cause of fatalities in infants, usually occurring between the ages of one month and six months. Although there are a number of plausible theories being investigated, its cause remains unknown. In some cases, autopsies indicate a hidden infection or an unsuspected abnormality, but in 80 percent of the deaths, no obvious explanation can be found. One cause appears to be an inherited heart irregularity, and another is respiratory distress, discussed under HYALINE MEMBRANE DISEASE. Improved hospital facilities for the care of premature babies who are considered to be at higher risk than those born at full term, as well as prenatal tests and ultrasonic alarm systems that monitor breathing are expected to reduce the number of SIDS victims.

Parents of infant SIDS victims often suffer intensely, apart from their natural grief, from feelings of guilt, as if they were somehow careless or negligent. They must be reassured that they could not possibly have foreseen the susceptibility of their child to this affliction and that there is therefore no way they could have averted its tragic result. They will have suffered enough without the wholly unwarranted feeling that they were somehow responsible.

Swallowed Objects

Babies in a crib or playpen can certainly be depended on to put anything within reach into their mouths, so it's a good idea to make sure that surfaces are cleared of anything that would cause a crisis if it were swallowed. Plastic toys and rattles should be inspected for loose parts. Pins, buttons, and small change should be kept in drawers. It's no serious matter if a child swallows a cherry stone or a plum pit or a small button, because these are not likely to cause problems in their passage through the digestive system. They will be disposed of in regular bowel movements.

Emergencies

Emergencies occur when the object is stuck in the windpipe or when it goes into the bronchial passage. If it is in the windpipe and isn't coughed up right away, use the first aid maneuver for "Obstruction in the Windpipe," Ch. 31, *Medical Emergencies* without delay. If is doesn't work the first time, do it again—and again. You must clear the windpipe. If all efforts fail, rush the child to a hospital.

Swearing

Sooner or later most children learn swear words, either from hearing their parents use them or from their peers. Young children may use curse words without knowing what they mean or without appreciating how offensive they may be.

Nowadays it is virtually impossible for children to avoid hearing words in everyday use that were strictly taboo when their parents were growing up. However jolting it may be to hear foul words issuing from their angelic-looking children, parents should be neither surprised nor unduly upset if this happens occasionally, especially if they themselves use curse words. They might well point out to the child, however, that many people object strongly to such language, and if they want to be treated courteously by adults, they had better watch their language.

Swimming

Every child should learn to swim, and the earlier the better. Families fortunate enough to have their own large pools can accomplish this in their own backyards; others may spend summers near a suitable body of water.

Although there's nothing like the ocean for water play, it's not a good place to try to teach a small child how to swim. There are too many extraneous hazards, such as undertow, waves, and unexpected depths. Many communities have outdoor public pools; most large cities have indoor and outdoor pools where professional instruction is available. Even when a child can swim moderately well, she should not be allowed to do so alone, and she shouldn't be allowed to go out in a boat by herself either. Rubber floats, rafts, and the like shouldn't be made available to youngsters until they can swim. A nonswimmer depending on such a device is in trouble if it should drift away from her in deep water.

Talking

The ability to speak is part of the human heritage. How soon and how clearly a child begins to do so depends on several factors. First and foremost is the ability to hear.

Hearing and Speech

Any illness or infection in infancy that has caused even a small hearing loss will interfere with the baby's perception of sounds. This in turn will prevent the normal development of those parts of the brain that govern the imitative aspect of speech.

A Stimulating Environment

How much attention and stimulation the baby gets from his environment and the people around him will have a great effect on how much he tries to say and the age at which he begins to say it. Being listened to and automatically corrected instead of being ignored or teased is the indispensable feedback process that enriches the learning of language. The clarity of the child's speech depends to a large extent on the examples before him; what his ears hear his brain will order his vocal equipment to imitate. Parents who want a child to outgrow baby talk should avoid responding to the baby in kind. Normal adult speech should become the norm toward which the child is constantly striving. See also HEARING, SPEECH DEFECTS, SWEARING.

Tantrums

See ANGER, FRUSTRATION.

Teething

Babies of four to six months drool a great deal and put their fingers in their mouth. These habits, and the telltale small bumps you may detect on the baby's gums, are the signs of teething. But they don't necessarily mean that the first tooth is about to erupt. That may not happen until he is nearly one year old, although it usually happens earlier.

Teething may or may not be painful. If the baby does fret, medication is available to alleviate the pain. (A little whisky rubbed on the gums is a home remedy that often helps.)

Television

See RADIO, RECORD PLAYER, AND TV.

Tetanus

Tetanus (also called *lockjaw* because it causes spasms of the jaw) can occur at any age as the result of contamination of a simple wound. The causative organism is usually found in soil, street dust, or feces.

The disease is preventable by immunization. The triple vaccine DTP should be started at two to three

months of age. See also IMMUNIZA-
TION.

When a child suffers a puncture wound, dog bite, or other wound that may be contaminated, ask your physician to give the child a booster dose of tetanus toxoid if she has not had a shot within one year.

Tick Fever

See "Rocky Mountain Spotted Fever" under RASHES.

Toilet Training

During the toddler stage parents begin to teach their child how to control his bowel and urinary functions.

When to Start

A simple question parents always ask is, "How do I know when my child is ready to be toilet trained?"

Generally, children do not have muscular control over their bowel movements and urination until about the age of two, so attempting to toilet-train a child much before this is usually wasted effort. If it is accomplished, the result is usually a training of the parents rather than of the infant. Toilet training should usually take place some time between the age of two and three and one-half.

A child is emotionally ready when he understands what is meant by toilet training and is willing to perform toilet functions without expressing fear of them. This may occur at any age, but is perhaps most apt to start between the ages of 18 and 24 months. With a first child it is usually later than with a second or third child, because the first child has no siblings to emulate. But a first child should be trained, usually, by the time he is three. Training the child to stay dry through the long night hours may take even longer.

Resistance to Toilet Training

Early toilet training—training that is begun during a child's first year—may work, but as a child develops and asserts his personality and independence, he will resent any insistence on manipulating the control of his bodily functions. He may get even by refusing to empty his bowels when put on the potty. Worse yet, if another baby has entered the scene, the early-trained child may develop constipation, or may revert to wetting and having bowel movements in his training pants.

When you feel the child is ready for training, establish the fact that going to the bathroom is a normal part of daily life. If the child expresses fear, don't struggle with him. Don't fight about it. Take him right off the potty and let him know that you are not concerned or displeased. A genuine complication can arise if the child connects his fear of toilet functions with your displeasure at his failures.

Training can usually be facilitated by praise from the parents for putting the bowel movement and the urine in the proper place, rather than by punishment. Excessive punishment or the threat of it usually results in anger on the child's part and increasing stubbornness and resistances to toilet training. Praise immediately following the proper performance of the act is far more effective in encouraging compliance with the parents' goals.

Tonsillectomy

See "Tonsils and Adenoids" in Ch. 20, *Surgery.*

Tonsillitis

The tonsils are two masses of soft spongy tissue that are partly embedded in the mucous membrane of the back of the throat. Bacterial or viral infection of this tissue is known as tonsillitis. It used to be considered advisable to remove the tonsils if they became enlarged—which they normally do in the process of filtering out mild infections.

Nowadays, an occasional bout of tonsillitis isn't considered sufficient reason for surgical removal of the tonsils, especially because they're likely to be less prone to infection as the child gets older. However, even a mild case of tonsillitis should be called to a physician's attention. Acute symptoms such as swollen tonsils, sudden high fever, swollen neck glands, and severe pain when swallowing must be treated promptly since they might be an indication of a strep throat. The proper antibiotics are always effective in controlling this infection so that it doesn't turn into rheumatic fever or involve the kidneys. Tonsillitis caused by a virus usually responds to aspirin, bed rest, and a soft diet. See also ADENOIDS. For a description of tonsillectomy, see "Tonsils and Adenoids" in Ch. 20, *Surgery.*

Toys

Grandma is put out because the beautiful doll she brought to her 2-year-old granddaughter has been promptly discarded in favor of the parts of the percolator. Those parts are something to put together and separate; they have interesting shapes; they clink when they touch and make a nice sound. That's what toys are about, especially to younger children. In selecting them, look for sturdiness and versatility. Smoothly sanded wooden blocks are wonderful toys that stimulate the imagination, encourage putting things together creatively, and can last not only from older to younger child but from one generation to another.

Simplicity and Suitability

Suitability of a toy is important: the right object for the age and circumstance. A good strong pail and shovel and a few cookie molds taken to the beach make more sense than a complicated plastic toy with parts that will get lost in the sand. Water toys that float in the tub make the bath that much more interesting and less threatening to very little children.

Use Your Imagination

Where there's not much money available for spending on playthings, the results can be more satisfactory to the child if you use your imagination—you can be sure she'll use hers. Pots and pans are great toys for toddlers, especially if there's a collection of smaller items, such as lids and little plastic containers to go with them. A roasting pan with a cord tied to the handle at one end becomes a sturdy pulltoy.

Never throw anything away until you've considered its adaptability as a toy: empty spools of thread, large buttons, plastic juice containers or milk cartons with the tops cut off, bits of twine, and especially the corrugated cardboard cartons that groceries are delivered in. As children get older, toys can be constructed of odds and ends according to instruction books available in the local library. The communal effort of putting them together can be a special rainy-day activity.

Tuberculosis

See Ch. 12, *Diseases of the Respiratory System*.

Twins and Triplets

Multiple births may be *identical*—that is, the result of the splitting of a single egg fertilized by a single sperm—or they may be *fraternal*, which means that they developed from different eggs fertilized by different sperm. Most multiple births are fraternal; except for their birthdays, most twins and triplets are no more alike than other brothers and sisters of the same family.

Although there is no ready explanation for the occurrence of multiple births, the tendency is thought to be genetically determined through the mother. Twins occur about once in every 86 births, triplets once in every 8,000. Multiple births can be anticipated by a physician at least a month before delivery. They usually arrive about two weeks early, and if they give any indications of prematurity, they receive special hospital attention.

Typhoid Fever

See Ch. 11, *Diseases of the Digestive System*.

Urinary Infections

Urinary infections of either viral or bacterial origin are more common among girls than boys, especially during the preschool years. Such an infection is sometimes the explanation for a fever unaccompanied by other symptoms. Any inflammation that creates a burning sensation during urination should be cultured and treated promptly because it can spread from the bladder to the kidneys and create a major problem.

Girls can be spared frequent infection if tactful suggestions are made at an early age about their toilet routines. Fecal matter is high in bacterial content, so little girls should learn to wipe their bottoms from front to back. This procedure reduces the possibility of contaminating the urethra after a bowel movement.

Vaporizer

A vaporizer is a device similar to a humidifier that moistens the air with steam and thus alleviates some of the discomfort of respiratory congestion. During the winter months when heated interiors are likely to be especially dry and when colds are more common, children and grown-ups can benefit from moist air that keeps the throat and nasal and bronchial passages from feeling like sandpaper. Medication shouldn't be added to a vaporizer except at the physician's recommendation. If the device is used near a child's bed throughout the night, it should be placed on a surface high enough to prevent bumping into it accidentally should the child wake up in the middle of the night to go to the bathroom.

Vomiting

See NAUSEA AND VOMITING.

Warts

See Ch. 21, *Skin and Hair*.

Whooping Cough

Whooping cough (also called *pertussis*), like diphtheria a bacterial disease, occurs more frequently than diphtheria because immunity to it wears off, especially in the older child in whom the disease may appear as a severe bronchitis.

Whooping cough can be very serious in young babies because it can cause them to choke and be unable to catch their breath. If your child does contract whooping cough, call your physician immediately. He or she may give a specific drug against the organism that causes the disease as well as a specific antitoxin against the poison that the bacillus releases.

It is advisable to immunize children against whooping cough as early as possible. The effective triple vaccine known as DTP provides immunization not only against whooping cough, but against diphtheria and tetanus as well.

Worms and Parasites

See Ch. 11, *Diseases of the Digestive System*.

3

The Teens

Puberty and Growth

The bridge between childhood and adulthood is a period of growth and change called puberty. There seems to be no standard pattern for the physical changes of puberty. Two boys of the same age who have been nearly identical throughout childhood may appear to set off along entirely different paths of physical development as they enter the teenage years. One may quickly shoot up to a height of five feet eight inches within a couple of years while his companion lags for a while at preteen size, then begins growing into a six-footer. One may develop a heavy beard in his early high-school years while the other boy will have no use for a razor until he is in college. However, both boys are normal youngsters, and each will eventually attain all of the physical attributes of adulthood.

Similarly, one girl may begin menstruating in her 11th year while a classmate will not experience her first menstruation until she is 16. One girl may need a bra while still in grammar school but her friend will fret about a small bustline for many years. But both girls can look forward to normal womanhood. Each has an individual pattern of development, and if there

is any rule of thumb about puberty it is that each youngster has his or her own time schedule for the transformation into a mature man or woman.

Puberty: Changes in Girls

The physical changes that occur in the female body during puberty probably are more dramatic than those associated with a boy progressing into manhood. One definite milestone for the girl is her first *menstruation,* commonly regarded as the first sign of puberty. Actually, the first menstruation, known as the *menarche,* is only one of several signs of puberty, along with the slimming of the waist, gradual broadening of the hips, the development of breasts, the appearance of hair about the genitals and in the armpits, and a change in the rate of growth.

The Menarche

The age at which a girl first experiences menstruation generally varies over a period of ten years and depends upon the structural development of the youngster, her physical

condition, the environment, and hereditary factors. Menarche can occur as early as the age of 7, and most physicians would not be overly concerned if a girl did not begin to menstruate until she was approaching 17. The age range of 9 to 16 usually is considered normal. The median age for the start of menstruation is around 13½ years, which means that 50 percent of all females are younger than 13 years and 6 months when they reach the menarche, and half are on the older side of that age when they first menstruate. In general, the pubertal experiences of a girl follow a pattern like that of her mother and sisters; if the mother began menstruating at an early age, the chances are that her daughters will also.

If the girl has not reached the menarche by the age of 18, she should be examined by a *gynecologist,* a physician who specializes in problems related to the female reproductive system. A medical examination also should be arranged for any girl who experiences menstruation before she reaches the age of eight or nine years.

When menarche occurs on the early side of childhood, the condition

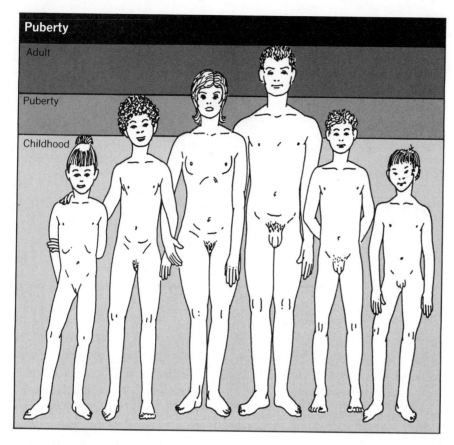

Puberty
Adult
Puberty
Childhood

tropical and arctic climates seem to be related to early menarche. The first menstrual periods also are likely to occur during the school year, September to June, rather than during the summer vacation.

The First Menstrual Cycles

The first menstrual cycles tend to be very irregular and have been known to be as short as 7 days and as long as 37 weeks. Even when regularity becomes established, the adolescent menstrual cycle usually is longer than the average for adult women. The typical menstrual cycle of a young girl may be about 33 days, compared to an average of 28 days for an adult woman. About three years elapse before the menstrual cycles become regular. In the meantime, irregular menstrual patterns can be considered as normal for girls during puberty.

The first menstrual cycles also are *anovulatory*. In other words, the young girl's ovaries have not matured sufficiently to produce an *ovum*, or egg cell, that can be fertilized by the sperm of a male. There are, of course, the exceptions that make newspaper headlines when a little girl gives birth to a baby. But anovulatory menstruation generally is the rule for the first few months after the menarche.

Delayed Puberty

Delayed puberty probably causes as much anguish as precocious puberty. The last girl in a group of childhood chums to develop breasts and experience the menarche may feel more self-conscious than the first girl in the class to menstruate. If the signs that usually precede menarche have not appeared by the age of 17 or 18, a medical examination should be considered, even though the girl may be a late-late-bloomer at the other end of

is sometimes called *precocious puberty*. The child may suddenly begin menstruating before her mother has told her what to expect, a situation that can prove embarrassing to both child and parents. It may first be detected by a teacher at school; occasionally, a young girl may be aware of bleeding from the vagina but because of fear or false modesty does not report the event to her mother or teacher. For this reason, parents should be alert for changes associated with early puberty and be prepared to explain the facts of life to their children. Also, in the case of precocious puberty, parents should arrange for medical consultation to be certain the bleeding actually is the result of first menstruation and not the effects of an injury or tumor.

Growth Spurt before Menarche

During the year or two preceding the menarche there is a growth spurt of two or three inches. This is because of the hormone changes of puberty. The *hormones* are chemical messengers secreted by glands in various parts of the body and carried rapidly through the bloodstream to organs or other glands where they trigger reactions. The spurt in growth preceding menarche results from the secretion of a growth hormone that is produced by the pituitary gland, and androgen, a hormone secreted by the adrenal glands. They produce rapid growth of the bones and muscles during puberty. The girl who is first among her classmates to menstruate often is larger than those who are of the same age but have not yet reached the menarche.

From numerous research studies of the menarche, it has been learned that poor nutrition and psychological stress sometimes delay the onset of menstruation, that girls reared in cities tend to menstruate earlier, and that climate is a factor, although both the spectrum from the 7- or 8-year-old child who has menstruated.

The absence of menstruation after a girl is 18 can be the result of a wide variety of factors. The cause sometimes can be as simple as an *imperforate hymen,* a membrane that blocks the opening of the vagina. It can be the result of a congenital malformation of the reproductive organs, such as imperfect development of the ovaries. Accidents, exposure to carbon monoxide gas, or diseases like rheumatic fever or encephalitis in earlier years can result in brain damage that would inhibit the start of menstruation. The relationship between emotional upset and delayed menarche was vividly demonstrated during World War II when some girls who suffered psychological traumas also experienced very late signs of puberty.

Preparing Your Daughter for Menstruation

A mother's main responsibility is to convince her daughter at the beginning of puberty that menstruation is a perfectly normal body function. The mother should explain the proper use of sanitary napkins or tampons and encourage her daughter to keep records of her menstrual periods on a calendar.

The mother also should explain that menstruation usually is not a valid reason to stay in bed or avoid school or work. The girl should be advised that bathing and swimming should not be postponed because of menstruation. There are many old wives' tales about menstruation that are not true. But there may be some truth to stories that loss of menstrual blood can be weakening, particularly if the girl's diet does not replace the body stores of iron which may be lowered during menstrual flow. Iron is a key element of the red blood cell, and if iron-rich

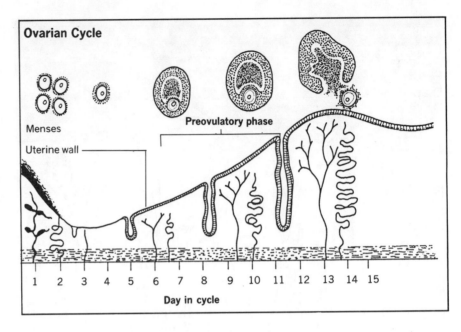

Ovarian Cycle

Menses

Uterine wall

Preovulatory phase

1 2 3 4 5 6 7 8 9 10 11 12 13 14 15

Day in cycle

foods are not included in the meals of women during their years of menstruation they can eventually suffer a form of iron-deficiency anemia.

Hormone Activity: Becoming a Woman

Although the sex hormones are the key to what makes girls grow into women and boys into men, both sexes appear to receive secretions of male and female sex hormones in approximately equal amounts for about the first ten years of life. But as puberty approaches, the adrenal glands of girls seem to increase production of a female sex hormone, *estrogen.* Meanwhile, a nerve center in the hypothalamus area of the brain stimulates the pituitary gland, the master gland of the body, to secrete another kind of hormone, *gonadotropin.* Gonadotropin in turn activates a *follicle-stimulating hormone* that causes a maturation of the ovaries, which are part of the original equipment girls are born with but which remain dormant until the start of puberty.

During the second decade of life, the hormone activity stimulates the development of body tissues that not only grow in size but give a girl more womanly contours. However, the fully mature contours of a woman usually do not appear until after the ovaries are functioning and still another female sex hormone, *progesterone,* has been introduced in the system. The ovaries, uterus, Fallopian tubes, and vagina gradually mature as the menarche draws near.

Puberty: Changes in Boys

The appearance of male sexual characteristics during puberty is also influenced by hormonal changes. But the manifestation of male puberty is somewhat more subtle. The pituitary gland in a boy also secretes a gonadotropic hormone that stimulates maturation of *gonads.* In the male, the gonads are the *testicles,* the source of *sperm.* But whereas maturation of the ovaries in females leads to the menarche, there is no obvious sign in the boy that *spermatozoa* are being produced.

However, the secondary sexual characteristics, such as the growth of a beard and pubic hair, the spurt of growth of bones and muscles, the increase in size of the sex organs, and the deepening of the voice, are all indications of puberty. The changes in a boy's characteristics during puberty are usually spread over a period of two years, beginning with an increase in the size of the penis and testicles and reaching completion with the production of spermatozoa in the testicles. During the two-year period there usually is a noticeable increase in the chest size of a boy, with the broad shoulders of manhood appearing during the peak of bone and muscle growth. Generally, the appearance of pubic and facial hair, as well as hair in the armpits, follows the growth of the shoulder and chest area and precedes the change in voice.

The Testicles

The testicles are contained in a walnut-size sac of skin called the *scrotum*. It is held outside the body by a design of nature in order to maintain a temperature for spermatozoa production that is less than internal body temperature. Muscle fibers in the scrotum hold the testicles closer to the body for warmth in cold weather and relax to allow the sperm-producing organ to be farther away from the body when surrounding temperatures are warm.

In some cases, one or both testicles do not descend from the abdomen during the male child's early years. The result is that the undescended testicle or testicles will not produce sperm. An *incompletely descended testicle* always lies somewhere along the normal path to the scrotum. An *ectopic* testicle has deviated from that path and lies somewhere near the inguinal canal, at the junction of the thigh and the lower part of the abdomen. In a third departure from normal

development, a *retractile testicle* has stopped short of the scrotum. It can be manipulated into the normal position or may descend to that position at puberty.

The danger of malignant change—of tumor development—usually warrants surgical removal of the incompletely descended and the ectopic testicle. A testicle trapped in the inguinal region may become inflamed because of the pressure of larger body parts in the area. In some cases, physicians are able to assist the descent into the scrotum through administration of hormones or by surgery. At some point during puberty, a medical examination should include a check on the condition of the testes.

Genital Size

Many boys are as sensitive about the size of their genitals as girls are about breast size. In the case of an empty scrotum because of undescended testicles, it is possible to have the scrotum injected with silicone plastic for cosmetic or psychological reasons so the sac appears less flaccid or larger. The size of the penis may become the

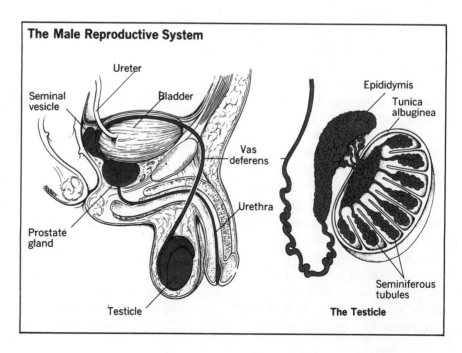

The Male Reproductive System

subject of discussion in the school shower room. If a boy appears sensitive about the subject, he should be assured that there is a wide variation in normal sizes and that like ears, noses, and other body parts the dimensions have little to do with function.

Nocturnal Emission

Another cause for concern by adolescent boys is the *nocturnal emission.* The nocturnal emission, sometimes called a *wet dream,* is the automatic expulsion of *semen* through the penis while the young man is asleep. The semen is secreted by the *prostate gland,* the *seminal vesicle,* and other glands that open into the *urethra.* The opalescent white fluid carries spermatozoa during intercourse and if the young male does not engage in sexual intercourse or does not masturbate, the semen simply accumulates until it overflows during a nocturnal emission. It is a harmless, normal occurrence.

Bone Growth

As the growth spurt subsides in the late teens, the *cartilage plates,* or *epiphyses,* in the long bones of the body close. Until the growth plates become filled in with calcium deposits, each long bone is in effect three bones—a central shaft separated from the ends by the cartilage growth plates. The growth plates are not completely replaced by bone until a female is about 20 and a male 23 years old. But the rate of growth begins to taper off as sexual maturity is achieved. After that, young women tend to retain fatty tissue and young men gain in muscle mass. It is a time to begin weight watching so that the hazards of obese adult life can be avoided. But the ravenous appetites developed

during the period of rapid body growth and intense physical activity can easily evolve into bad eating habits during the teen years.

Skin and Hair Problems

Hereditary influences may determine many of the physical and psychological traits that an individual first becomes aware of in the teen years. Because of the various crossovers of the 23 sets of *chromosomes* and the nearly infinite combinations of *genes,* it is not always easy to predict how a child is going to appear as a young adult. But some features, such as hair color and eye color, usually can be identified with one or both parents; other traits may seem to be those of uncles, aunts, or grandparents. Heredity and hormones frequently are involved in the distribution of hair on the body and the oiliness of the skin, both of which can cause concern to teenagers who are plagued by an overabundance or lack of these cosmetic traits. An example of hereditary influences on hair patterns can be seen in early baldness. A receding hairline is not a trait of the parents but rather an influence of the genetic makeup of a grandparent—the trait skips a generation.

Removal of Excess Hair

While not much can be done about baldness that is hereditary, there are ways of handling the problems of excess hair. If a woman has excess hair on her face, arms, and legs, it can be removed by shaving, with wax, by electrolysis, or depilatories. Shaving is the most direct but not always the most satisfactory method of hair removal because it is intended only as a temporary measure. An alternate shortcut is bleaching with diluted hydrogen peroxide; the hair is still there

but it is not as noticeable. Another method involves the use of hot wax spread on the skin and allowed to harden. When it is removed quickly, the hair is pulled away.

Depilatories are chemicals that destroy the hair at the skin line. Both hot wax and depilatories have longer-lasting effects than shaving, but they must be repeated at intervals of several weeks.

Depilatories, too, can produce unpleasant allergenic reactions. The only permanent method of removing excess hair is *electrolysis,* which is a time-consuming technique. Each hair root has to be burned out individually with an electric current. Electrolysis is recommended only for small areas and because of the time and expense involved would not be feasible for removing excess hair from regions other than the face.

Acne

There is some evidence that *acne* is partly hereditary. But it is such a common problem among teenagers— it has been estimated that up to 90 percent of all youngsters endure some degree of acne—that it must have been inherited from a mutual ancestor like Adam or Eve. In fact, one of the deterrents to effective control of the skin disorder is that acne is so common that it is neglected by many youngsters. Waiting to outgrow acne can be a serious mistake, because the pimples, blemishes, blackheads, and boils that make life miserable for so many teenagers can be eliminated or considerably reduced. They can also cause scarring. A physician should be consulted in cases of severe or especially persistent acne.

Overactive Oil Glands

Acne is not a serious threat to the life of a youngster, but it can be seriously disfiguring at a time of life when most young people are sensitive about their appearance. It can occur at any time from puberty into early adulthood, and it is caused by poor adjustment of the skin to secretions of sebaceous glands. The imbalance resulting from hormones in the bloodstream will correct itself eventually. But to prevent permanent scarring, a program of simple skin care must be followed faithfully.

Acne is caused by oil glands in the skin that become overly active at puberty. The glands become clogged, with the result that blackheads or pimples appear. The solution is to wash the skin frequently and thoroughly to remove the oils and to clear the plugged oil glands. The color of blackheads, by the way, is not caused by dirt but rather by a chemical change in the secretions of the oil glands.

Skin Care

The face should be washed several times a day with hot water and soap. The skin should be rinsed twice after washing, first with warm water, then with cold. Each time the face should be dried thoroughly with a clean towel. At bedtime, the face should be given a massage with soapsuds and water, rinsed, and patted dry with a clean towel. Any medication prescribed by a physician should be applied after the final washing of the day. Careless handling of blemishes, such as squeezing blackheads or picking pimples, can result in scarring. Teenagers also should avoid such habits as supporting the face with the hands or unconsciously rubbing the face.

Other Precautions

Young women should not use cold creams or cosmetics unless they have been approved by a physician. Young men who shave must be careful to avoid cutting pimples. A physician also should be consulted about how diet can help control acne. Although the skin disorder is not a dietary disease, there is some evidence that certain foods tend to aggravate it. However, there is a lack of agreement among physicians as to whether chocolate, carbonated beverages, nuts, sweets, and other specific snack items may be the culprits. And there always is the possibility that because each youngster develops along an individual path, a food item that causes one teenager's face to break out with blemishes will not affect a sibling or classmate in the same way.

Diet

A survey by the Food and Nutrition Board of the National Research Council recently showed that 40 percent of boys between 13 and 19 years of age and 60 percent of the girls in the same age group subsisted on diets that were substandard. Generally, the young people surveyed had abandoned the eating routines of their families. They habitually skipped breakfast and failed to make up the nutritional loss during other meals.

Perhaps in rebellion against parental control and to assert their independence, they tended to gather with their friends at candy stores and snack shops. They purchased items that could be held in the hand during informal rap sessions—chocolate bars and cans of soda. The economic standards for the quickie street-corner meals were based on what could be obtained with money from allowances and after-school jobs. The snack habit persisted through the potato chip and carbonated beverage evening routine before a TV set. Their idea of a good meal included a side dish of French fries, a food lacking in almost everything except calories.

Calories and Nutrition

Calories are not all bad. Young people burn hundreds of them daily through dancing, working, athletic competition, and other activities. A typical male teenager may burn up to 3,600 calories a day; a teenage girl can easily handle 2,500 calories daily—and calories are easy to come by in snack foods. For example, a chocolate milk shake at 520 calories, two doughnuts, totaling 270 calories, a chocolate candy bar at 150 calories, a can of soda at 100 calories, and a handful of potato chips at 10 calories each will easily provide half the daily energy requirements for a busy high-school girl. Adding French fries, at 15 calories each, and more cans of soda plus other snacks will bring the total up close to the 2,500-calorie level.

However, there is more to nutrition than snacking on calorie-rich foods. An individual obviously can fill up on high-energy goodies but suffer from malnutrition by disregarding the body's normal requirements of proteins, vitamins, and minerals. Also, calories have an insidious way of becoming excess weight. A calorie is a unit of energy, and the human body requires a certain amount of energy each day in order to sustain life and permit the muscle activity of work or play. To maintain the proper balance between foods consumed and energy used in work and play, the teenager, like the adult, must estimate the calories in his meals and check the results regularly by stepping on the bathroom scale.

People in their teens should develop the habit of weighing themselves at least once a week, recording the weight so it can be compared with previous readings. The weight check should occur at the same hour each time, and the same scale should be used. Also, the same type of clothing should be worn each time the weight is checked. If an overweight or underweight youngster can find a companion to challenge in a race toward optimum weight, the competition will be an added inducement.

Calcium and Phosphorus

Among the important minerals in teenage diets are calcium and phosphorus. Milk is the most easily available source of calcium and phosphorus, which are required for the development of strong bones during the period of life in which the body is still growing. Calcium also is required for the effective contraction of muscle tissues and is vital for normal heart function. The recommended daily intake of milk for teenagers is four eight-ounce glasses. It can be served as fluid whole milk, as skim milk, buttermilk, evaporated milk, or as nonfat dry milk. Cheese or ice cream can be substituted for part of the fluid milk allowance. One cup of ice cream is equivalent in calcium to one-half cup of milk. A one-inch cube of cheddar cheese is equal to two-thirds of a cup of milk, which also is equivalent in calcium to one cup, or eight ounces, of cottage cheese. Cream cheese can be substituted for milk in a two-to-one ratio; that is, two ounces of cream cheese are equal to one ounce of milk.

Iron

Iron is needed for the formation of *hemoglobin*, the substance that gives red blood cells their red coloration and is responsible for the transport of oxygen and carbon dioxide in the bloodstream. Hemoglobin has such an affinity for oxygen that without it humans would require 60 times as much

blood to transport oxygen from the lungs to tissues throughout the body. Studies indicate that girls are five times as likely to need additional supplies of iron in their diets because of blood loss through menstruation. Recommended sources of iron are liver, heart, kidney, liver sausage, meat, shellfish, egg yolk, dark molasses, bread, beans and other legumes. If basic food lists seem drab and boring, the teenager might think of the iron sources in terms of a peanut butter sandwich or two hamburgers; either choice would provide the daily iron needs for a girl. Other minerals that are important to a teenager's diet include the following:

- Sulfur is needed by the body for hair, skin, nails, and cartilage, and is available by eating nearly any protein-rich foods.

- Sodium is required for muscle activity and normal body fluid balance, and can be obtained by using ordinary table salt on foods.

- Iodine is needed for normal thyroid control of body metabolism and is supplied in the form of iodized table salt.

- Potassium is a tonic for the nervous system and the muscles and is available in adequate amounts in most kinds of meats, as well as bananas, orange juice, and milk.

- Magnesium collaborates chemically with calcium and phosphorus for normal muscle and nerve function, and is found in most forms of protein.

Weight Problems

Teens who are seriously overweight or who are contemplating radical weight reduction programs should be examined by a physician. Otherwise,

unfair comparisons with other persons of the same age and height may lead to wrong conclusions about the need to gain or lose weight. The weight–height standards are based on averages, and there are many youngsters who are above or below the average but quite healthy and normal. Good examples of misinterpretation of weight–height tables can be found among beefy football players who have been rejected by military recruiters because they weighed more than other fellows of the same height.

Another reason for a medical exam is to check the possibility of disease as the cause of the weight problem. The exam will also indicate whether the youngster has some other disorder that could be aggravated by a sudden weight loss.

Achieving optimum weight is only one step toward proper physical conditioning. A youngster who has been able to avoid physical activity by living in an elevator apartment, riding a bus to school, and watching TV after school hours instead of working or playing could be right on the button as far as weight for his age and height are concerned, but his muscular development and heart and lung capacity could be at the same time at a very low ebb.

Anorexia Nervosa

A psychological disorder that in extreme cases results in death, anorexia nervosa appears most commonly among teenage girls. The victims starve themselves in an exaggerated effort to lose weight. Medical experts believe that true anorectics weigh 25 percent or more less than the norm for their height and weight.

Anorectics may show other common symptoms. Many have been high achievers in school, and many are sports enthusiasts. An anorectic may alternate periods of strict fasting and periods of food binges, or develop rituals around eating. Where binges become "gorge and purge" sessions—stretches of overeating followed by self-induced vomiting—anorectics may also have a disorder called *bulimia*. But bulimia may afflict otherwise normal persons. Anorectics may weigh themselves several times a day and avoid eating even when they are hungry. Some avoid social situations that may call for eating. Most, according to experts, are unusually preoccupied with their appearance or bodily "image" as a result of personality or ego problems or deficiencies. Adolescent girls who are anorectic frequently suffer from amenorrhea, cessation or delay of menstruation.

Treatment of anorexia nervosa may be a lengthy, costly process. Psychiatric counseling is usually a part of such treatment. Physically, treatment seeks to build a normal relationship between *norepinephrine,* a body chemical that carries messages about food, and the *hypothalamus,* the part of the brain that directs eating behavior.

Physical Fitness

Good physical conditioning is as important as weight control during the teen years. Everybody cannot be an athletic champion, but almost anyone can improve his heart, lungs, and muscles so that he can cope more effectively with the stresses of young adult life. Physical conditioning can be accomplished with little or no exercise equipment. It can be programed for city living or country living, in a gymnasium or in an apartment. All that really is required is a little time each day plus a great deal of determination and patience. It is important for young people to understand the major health role of daily exercise. Although many school physical education programs are excellent, some still remain inadequate, and in many cases students are only going through the motions of calisthenic routines and are not really benefiting from the effort.

Exercise Goals for Teenage Boys

One of the goals of physical conditioning for teenage boys is muscle development. When muscles are not used they atrophy, or shrink in size. A muscle that has been immobilized because of an injury may shrivel to one-fourth its normal size. Some of the muscle fibers are replaced by non-elastic fibrous tissue. On the other hand, muscles that are exercised regularly and vigorously will grow in size and strength. Exercise causes an increase in the number of individual muscle fibers as well as an increase in the number of blood capillaries supplying the muscle tissue. A fringe benefit is that muscles become more efficient as they grow in size from exercise. In other words, the muscles can perform more work with less wasted effort.

In addition to muscle development, which every exercise program should provide, physical conditioning should include optimum cardiopulmonary development. This means increased heart activity and greater oxygen consumption and is the basis for the popular aerobics workouts. *Aerobic* means, literally, with oxygen. A goal of aerobics training is to achieve a steady state of exercising in which breathing is heavier than normal. In the steady state, the heart, lungs, and muscles work together as an efficient machine at an activity level that is more demanding of the body than the resting state. Jogging, running, and rapid walking are examples of aerobic exercises. They can be practiced with no special equipment.

The individual goals for physical fitness should be kept within sensible limits to avoid injury or impaired health. The maximum level of performance can be determined by the appearance of the panting and puffing that occurs when exercise exceeds the normal ability of the lungs to supply oxygen to the muscles. A youngster who is not in good physical condition may huff and puff after walking up a flight of stairs, whereas a classmate in top condition might run a mile without showing signs of excessive breathing.

There are many fine exercise programs which teenagers can follow, such as those published by the U.S. Air Force and the President's Council on Physical Fitness.

Exercise Goals for Teenage Girls

The young girl of today can be as involved in sports and the working world as the male, and the general guidelines for masculine conditioning apply to young women as well. Girls should follow exercise programs that develop muscular strength and the endurance provided by a sound cardiovascular system. Regular exercise causes the heartbeat to grow stronger and steadier and breathing to become deeper. As the flow of blood through the tissues is improved, waste products of the cells are removed more efficiently and complexion problems are reduced. Another benefit is that the body uses energy more efficiently in both physical and mental tasks; coordination is improved. Girls should not worry about developing bulging muscles when they follow a regular, well-balanced exercise routine that includes workouts for the hips and thighs, waist, bustline, calves, and ankles.

Care of the Teeth

During the teen years, careful supervision by the dentist and cooperation from the teenager are especially necessary. The poor eating habits of many teenagers are reflected in their cavity rate, which is usually higher during adolescence than in later life.

If a young person is conscientious about oral care, he can avoid not only a high cavity rate, but also bad breath and the unpleasant appearance of food particles left on the teeth. These problems are really caused by the same thing—*dental plaque.* For more information on this subject, see Ch. 22, *The Teeth and Gums.*

Need for Frequent Checkups

During the adolescent period, the dentist will often recommend more frequent checkups than in the past. Small cavities are treated before they become deeper and infect the pulp, the inner chamber of the tooth, containing nerves and blood vessels. Should the pulp become infected, the tooth must have special treatment, usually a root canal process, or be extracted.

The dentist also treats tooth decay, or *caries,* more popularly known as cavities, to prevent their spread. While they are not thought to be contagious, cavities begin as a break in the tooth surface, which later enlarges. Food debris can become lodged in the cavity, be attacked by bacteria, and cause a cavity on the next tooth. The only way to avoid such a problem is to have the affected tooth treated immediately.

Front teeth often decay for the first time during this period. They are restored with a silicate or plastic filling close in color to the tooth rather than silver or gold, which would be unattractive. Unfortunately, these materials are not permanent and will need to be replaced in time. As a result, neglect of diet and oral cleanliness by an adolescent may mean that

he may need many replacement fillings in the same cavity over his lifetime.

Orthodontic Treatment

The development and growth of teeth is completed during the adolescent period. When oral growth is improper, the adolescent needs treatment by an *orthodontist,* a dental specialist who treats abnormalities of the bite and alignment of teeth and jaws. Correction of such conditions as buck teeth, which mar a person's appearance, is a major reason for orthodontic treatment. But there are also major health reasons for orthodontic care. If teeth, for example, come together improperly, efficient chewing of food is impossible. The digestive system is strained because chunks of improperly chewed food pass through it. Orthodontic treatment will, therefore, result in lifelong better health and appearance. For more information, see Ch. 22, *The Teeth and Gums.*

Stimulants and Alcohol

Initial exposure to caffeine, tobacco, drugs, and alcohol usually occurs during adolescence. Teenagers should be fully educated regarding their physical effects and potential danger. They should learn how to use them, if at all, sensibly and in moderation, and to resist peer-group pressures.

Caffeine

Caffeine, which is naturally present in coffee and tea and is used in many carbonated beverages and medications, stimulates the central nervous system to overcome fatigue and drowsiness. It also affects a part of the nervous system that controls respiration so that more oxygen is

pumped through the lungs. In large amounts, caffeine can increase the pulse rate, but there are few long-range effects because the substance is broken down by the body tissues within a few hours and excreted. Because of the action of caffeine in stimulating an increased intake of oxygen, it sometimes is used to combat the effects of such nervous system depressants as alcohol.

Nicotine

Nicotine is one of nearly 200 substances in tobacco. It affects the human physiology by stimulating the adrenal glands to increase the flow of adrenaline. The blood vessels become constricted and the skin temperature drops, producing effects not unlike exposure to cold temperatures. When comparatively large amounts of nicotine are absorbed by the body, the pulse becomes rapid and the smoker has symptoms of dizziness, faintness, and sometimes nausea and diarrhea. The release of adrenaline, triggered by nicotine, will produce temporary relief from fatigue by increasing the flow of sugar in the blood. However, the effect is transient, and the feeling of fatigue will return again after the increased blood sugar has been expended.

Other Properties of Tobacco

The nicotine in tobacco can be absorbed simply by contact with the mucous membranes of the mouth; the tobacco does not have to be smoked to get the nicotine effects. Burning tobacco produces a myriad of substances found in the smoke of many plant materials when they are dried and burned. More than 50 different compounds are known to occur in concentrations of one microgram or more in each puff of tobacco smoke. Again, laboratory tests have demonstrated that the substances in burning tobacco do not have to be inhaled; most of the chemical compounds can be absorbed through the mucous membranes while a puff of smoke is held in the mouth for a few seconds. At least ten of the substances in tobacco smoke have been shown to produce cancer in animals. Other chemicals in tobacco tars are known as *cocarcinogens;* although they do not produce cancer themselves, they react with other substances to produce cancers.

Smoking and Disease

The relationship among tobacco smoking and cancer, heart disease, and emphysema-bronchitis is well established, even if some of the cause and effect links are missing. Large-scale studies of the death rates of smokers and nonsmokers have been carried on for more than 20 years. One group, consisting of nearly a quarter-million war veterans, yielded results indicating that smokers are from 10 to 16 times as likely to die of lung cancer as nonsmokers. (The higher ratio is for heavy smokers.) Similar results have been obtained from studies of smokers and nonsmokers with heart disease and lung ailments.

Buerger's Disease

One of the possible, although rare, effects of smoking is the aggravation of symptoms of a particularly insidious circulatory disorder known as *Buerger's disease.* As noted above, one of the effects of nicotine is a drop in skin temperatures. Smoking a single cigarette can cause the temperature of the fingers and toes to drop as much as 15 degrees Fahrenheit; the average is a little more than a 5-degree drop. The temperature change re-

sults from constriction of the blood vessels at the extremities. Blood clots may develop in the vessels that have been constricted, cutting off the flow of blood to the tissues of the area. When there is numbness or pain in the extremities, the condition should receive swift medical attention to prevent serious consequences.

Carbon Monoxide Accumulation

Another little publicized effect of smoking is the accumulation of carbon monoxide in the blood. Carbon monoxide is one of the lethal gases emitted in automobile exhaust. It is also produced by burning plant materials such as tobacco. It is a dangerous gas because of its strong affinity for the hemoglobin of red blood cells. Unlike oxygen and carbon dioxide, which become temporarily attached, then released, from the hemoglobin molecule, carbon monoxide becomes permanently locked into the red blood cell chemistry so that the cells are no longer effective for their normal function of transporting oxygen to the body tissues. With the oxygen-carrying capacity of part of the red blood cells wiped out, brain cells and other tissues suffer a mild oxygen starvation and the results are a form of intoxication.

A strong whiff of carbon monoxide can be fatal. Smokers, of course, do not get that much of the substance into their blood, but they do pick up enough carbon monoxide to render up to eight percent of their red blood cells ineffective. Experiments at Indiana University show that pack-a-day smokers have the same level of carbon monoxide in their blood as subjects who inhale an atmosphere of one-fourth of one percent carbon monoxide. That level of carbon monoxide increases the shortness of breath during exercise by approxi-

mately 15 percent, and, the study shows, about three weeks of abstinence from smoking are required to permit the oxygen-carrying capacity of the blood to return to normal. It is the carbon monoxide of burning plant materials that produces most of the "high" associated with the smoking of many substances.

Alcohol

Alcohol usually is not considered a potentially dangerous drug because it is easily available at cocktail lounges and liquor stores and is served generously at parties. Alcohol has been used by man for thousands of years, at times as a sedative and anesthetic, and when used in moderation has the effect of a mild tranquilizer and appetite stimulant. But when consumed in excess amounts, alcoholic beverages can produce both psychological and physical dependence. It can produce illusions of being a pick-me-up, but studies indicate that this is due to a letdown of inhibitions and the weakening of some functions of the central nervous system, particularly in the cerebral cortex.

Parents and teachers share an important responsibility to educate young people about the use and misuse of alcohol. Like marihuana, the effects of alcohol on human beings are not thoroughly understood. Some users develop a tissue tolerance for alcohol so that their body tissues require increasing amounts. When alcohol is withdrawn from such users, they develop tremors, convulsions, and even hallucinations. However, there are many varied reactions to the use of alcohol, and an individual may react differently to alcoholic drinks at different times. See Ch. 29, *Substance Abuse.*

Drugs

During the 1960s there was an alarming increase in drug use among teenagers—a problem that deservedly received nationwide attention. Education concerning the hazards and occasional tragedies accompanying drug use is imperative.

Marihuana

Marihuana affects the central nervous system, including the brain, after it enters the bloodstream. According to some researchers, the substance accumulates in the liver. Some of the effects of marihuana are not unlike those of tobacco. The rate of the heartbeat is increased, body temperature drops, and blood sugar levels are altered. The drug user also feels dehydrated, the appetite is stimulated, coordination of movements becomes difficult, there are feelings of drowsiness or unsteadiness, and the eyes may become reddish. Taken in higher strengths, marihuana can cause hallucinations or distortions of perception.

Varying Effects

Scientists are uncertain about the pathways of the drug in the central nervous system and its effects on other body systems. The drug's effects seem to vary widely, not only among individual users but also according to the social setting and the amount and strength of the marihuana used. The effects, which usually begin within 15 minutes after the smoke is inhaled and may continue for several hours, vary from depression to excitement and talkativeness. Some users claim to experience time distortions and errors in distance perception. But others sharing the same marihuana cigarette may experience no effects at all.

Although marihuana is not addictive, in that users do not develop a physical dependence upon the substance and withdrawal of the drug produces no ill effects, there are dangerous results from the use of marihuana. Marihuana users find it hard to make decisions that require clear thinking, some users develop psychotic reactions or an emotional disorder called "acute marihuana panic," and there is some evidence that the active ingredient is transmitted by expectant mothers to their unborn children.

Hallucinogens

Marihuana sometimes is described as a *hallucinogen* because of visual hallucinations, illusions, and delusions reported by users after they have inhaled the smoke from a large number of "joints" or "sticks" of the drug. But marihuana should not be confused with the true hallucinogenic drugs such as *mescaline* and *LSD* (lysergic acid diethylamide) which are known by doctors as *psychomimetic* drugs because they mimic psychoses.

LSD and Mescaline

LSD and mescaline have marked effects on perception and thought processes. Teenagers usually become involved with the use of LSD because they are curious about its effects; they may have heard about its purported "mind-bending" properties and expect to gain great personal insights from its use. Instead of great insight, however, the user finds anxiety, depression, confusion, and frightening hallucinations. The use of LSD is complicated by the reappearance of hallucinations after the individual has quit using the drug; the very possibility of repeated hallucinations causes a sense of terror.

Morphine and Heroin

Besides the hallucinogenic drugs, there are *opium* derivatives, *morphine* and *heroin*. Morphine is one of the most effective pain relievers known and is one of the most valuable drugs available to the physician. Morphine and heroin depress the body systems to produce drowsiness, sleep, and a reduction in physical activity. They are true narcotics, and their appeal is in their ability to produce a sense of euphoria by reducing the individual's sensitivity to both psychological and physical stimuli.

Addictive Properties

A great danger lies in the ability of the body tissues to develop a physical dependence on morphine and its derivative cousin, heroin. The degree to which heroin's "desirable" effects are felt depends in part on how the user takes it. *Sniffing* is the mildest form of abuse, followed by *skin-popping*—subcutaneous injection—and then by *mainlining*—injecting directly into a vein, which is the method used by almost all those dependent on heroin.

The body adjusts to the level of the first doses so that increasingly larger injections of the drug are required to produce the same feelings of euphoria. The ability of the body to adjust to the increasingly larger doses is called *tolerance*. And with tolerance goes *physical dependence,* which means that when heroin or morphine is withdrawn from the user he experiences a violent sickness marked by tremors, sweating and chills, vomiting and diarrhea, and sharp abdominal pains. Another shot of heroin or morphine temporarily ends the withdrawal symptoms. But the user, now dependent upon the drug, must continue regular doses or face another bout of the withdrawal sickness. Heroin has no value as a medicine and is available only through illicit channels at a high price. The heroin addict usually is unable to hold a job because of effects of the drug and often turns to crime in order to finance his daily supply of the narcotic.

Shortened Life Span

The health of a narcotics addict declines so that his life span is shortened by 15 to 20 years. He usually is in continual trouble with the law because of the severe penalties for illegal possession of narcotics. If he sells narcotics, as many heroin addicts are driven to do to get enough money to support their habit, the punishment is even more severe.

Amphetamines and Barbiturates

Other commonly abused drugs are *amphetamines*, also known as *uppers* or *pep pills*, and *barbiturates*, sometimes called *downers* or *goof balls*. Amphetamines are used by physicians to curb the appetite when weight reduction of patients is needed and to relieve mild cases of depression. However, some physicians doubt that amphetamines should be used as a weight-control medication because of the risks involved; other experts have questioned whether the drugs are actually effective for that purpose.

Amphetamines stimulate the heart rate, increase the blood pressure, cause rapid breathing, dilate the pupils of the eyes, and produce other effects such as dryness of the mouth, sweating, headache, and diarrhea. Ordinarily, amphetamines are swallowed as tablets, but a more extreme form of amphetamine abuse involves the injection of the drug, usually Methedrine, directly into the vein.

Dangers of Amphetamines

The danger in the use of amphetamines is that they induce a person to do things beyond his physical endurance, cause mental disorders that require hospitalization, and, in large doses, can result in death. Although they do not produce the kind of physical dependence observed in the use of narcotics, amphetamine withdrawal for a heavy user can result in a deep and suicidal depression.

Barbiturates

Barbiturates are sedatives used by physicians to treat high blood pressure, epilepsy, and insomnia, and to relax patients being prepared for surgery. They slow the heart rate and breathing, lower blood pressure, and mildly depress the action of nerves and muscles.

Dangers of Barbiturates

Barbiturates are highly dangerous when taken without medical advice. They distort perception and slow down reaction and response time, contributing to the chances of accidents. Barbiturates are a leading cause of accidental poison deaths because they make the mind foggy and the user forgets how many pills he has taken, thus leading to overdosage. They also cause physical dependence with withdrawal symptoms that range from cramps and nausea to convulsions and death. See also Ch. 29, *Substance Abuse.*

Adolescent Suicide

Suicides among teenage boys and girls increased greatly in number during the middle 1980s. Health experts termed the phenomenon an "epidemic of self-destruction." In some areas suicides or suicide attempts took place in clusters. Often, groups of close friends were involved. In some cases of cluster suicides or attempts, it appeared that a suicidal attitude was contagious.

Suicide became the second leading cause of death among adolescents. In the nearly 30 years beginning in the late 1950s, the suicide rate among teenagers tripled. Preadolescents also began to take their own lives more frequently: public health personnel reported suicides among children as young as three.

Risk Factors

As educators, social workers, psychiatrists, and others became involved in community efforts to prevent teenage suicides, a number of "risk factors"—signs of an intent to take one's life—were isolated. Changes in a teenager's behavior, whether in peer relationships, school activities, or academic performance, were said to be primary indicators. So were emotional shifts, particularly toward anger or irritability. Depression and withdrawal, experts said, might accompany the emotional changes. Sadness, changes in eating and sleeping habits, and preoccupation with death were other signs.

Young people considering suicide showed other symptoms. Many reported headaches, stomachaches, and other ailments. Some talked about taking their own lives. A young person who had lost a close friend through suicide was at unusual risk, according to studies. Family histories of suicide and parental depression were cited as indirectly contributing factors.

Parent Involvement

For parents concerned about the possibility of a child's or teen's suicide, such clues are only clues. The parent still has the task of trying to resolve the potential suicide. Authorities make the following suggestions.

Act at Once

Where a preadolescent or adolescent gives clear signals—usually risk factors appearing in combination—that suicide might be contemplated, parents should seek help immediately. Local suicide hotlines or suicide prevention centers should be contacted; counseling may have to be started.

School Help

Many schools cooperate in efforts to prevent suicides. The schools may sponsor group meetings at which students talk out their feelings about suicide, and such meetings may be appropriate as a first or second step. A representative of the community crisis or prevention center normally takes part in such meetings. Many schools have special counselors, psychologists, and others who can serve as direct lines to sources of help.

Out-of-School Contacts

Group meetings provide all teenage participants with the names and locations of out-of-school contact persons who may be able to help them in a crisis. Most crisis agencies operate 24 hours a day, seven days a week, providing aid during the "danger hours" between late afternoon and midnight. Parents may want also to contact clergy, trusted friends or relatives, or others.

Peer Support

Where possible, peer support should be mobilized in the effort to prevent a suicide. Many young people, especially the friends of a depressed or otherwise suicidal teenager, can help—and will do so rather than hear later that a suicide has taken place. But parents should, according to experts, remember that a youngster

with high status among his or her peers may influence those peers. Committing suicide, the high-status young person may convince others that "life isn't worth it." Surviving boy- or girlfriends are especially at risk.

Social and Sexual Maturation

The Prospect of Adulthood

As a youngster passes from childhood into adolescence, it is the psychological adjustments rather than the physical changes that are most likely to produce difficulties. The emotional problems, of course, are related to the hormonal activity of the developing body. However, the conflicts that frequently are upsetting to both the adolescent and other members of his family are the result of adjustments that must be made between the young person and the society in which he must live.

In certain primitive cultures, for example, the boy becomes an "instant adult" by undergoing puberty rites. There may be no restrictions on sex play between boys and girls; the girl does not have to be concerned about dating procedures because her parents select her husband. There is no question about economic independence; the young couple becomes a part of the economic unit of the parents.

In our own culture, the teenager must continually adjust to a complex set of rules and regulations. He frequently may feel that he must accept the responsibilities of adulthood before he is entitled to the privileges of being treated as an adult. Childhood

is only a step behind, but he has learned to suppress or ignore childhood relationships. He can easily forget the point of view of children and even resent the ability of his parents to recall the "cute" incidents of his earlier years. At the same time, he may be startled by the suggestion that within a few short years he and his teenage friends will face the selection of a career, marriage, establishment of a home, and a lifetime of responsibilities he may feel ill-prepared to assume.

Future Outlook for Girls

For a girl, the future is somewhat more complex than it was for her mother at the same stage of life. In her mother's day, a teenage girl might look forward to a brief period of work as a secretary, store clerk, or factory hand between the day of her high-school graduation and her wedding day. After the wedding, there followed a couple of decades or more of being a housewife and mother. Today's teenage girl can still follow the pattern of her mother's life. Or she can plan a lifetime professional career as a physician, lawyer, or scientist. She can compete with men as a business executive, writer, or politician, and she can schedule marriage and motherhood to complement rather than compete with career goals.

Future Outlook for Boys

The adolescent boy also has a wider choice of goals. He may or may not follow in his father's footsteps. If he decides to join a family business venture, the chances are that he will go to college and contribute a working knowledge of computer techniques or tax laws to the accumulated experience and business contacts his father acquired by starting as an apprentice and working for many years.

Advanced Education

The educational requirements for the jobs of tomorrow place an added strain on the pace of growing into adulthood. Although going steady may begin at an earlier age for both sexes, marriage may have to be postponed until the boy and girl have completed college or even gone to a university in pursuit of an advanced degree. An alternative is marriage and the start of a family while the boy and girl are still in college and dependent economically upon their parents.

Need for Independence

Just as natural as the boy–girl relationships of the teen years are the needs for independence and privacy. Sometimes a youngster feels it necessary to demonstrate a mind of his own by taking independent action, although such action could be considered as rebellion against parental authority. A recent survey showed that a girl may go steady with a boy not because she really likes the boy that much but to prove she is capable of handling a relationship that her parents have criticized. Carried to a sometimes tragic extreme is the compulsion of a boy or girl to marry a person the parents dislike in order to demonstrate so-called independence. The wise parent will avoid efforts to force a young person into a position in which the alternatives are a surrender to the will of the parents or an action such as a premature marriage that might have unfortunate consequences.

Conflicts between Parent and Teenager

Some conflicts between the generations are avoidable. The parents may be protective and slow to cut the apron strings because they love their children and want to prevent them from becoming involved in unhappy situations. The teenager resents the overprotective actions of the parents, regarding them as evidence that they do not trust their own children.

What parents should try to make clear to their children is that they are offering their years of experience as guidelines. Teenagers should value the counsel of more experienced members of the family; they should cooperate by listening to the adult viewpoint. If, after serious consideration of the parents' point of view, the youngster still wants to make his own decision in the matter, it should be understood that he may have to accept the responsibility for the consequences. A keystone in the training for adulthood is the concept that being an adult entails more than just privileges and the authority to make decisions; along with decision-making goes a responsibility to the family and society for the consequences of one's decisions.

Few parents, of course, would refuse to bail out a teenage son or daughter in real trouble. And even when a youngster is rebellious enough to leave home, he should know that the door will always be open to him when he decides to return. Again, limiting the options available to a teenager can lead to a snowballing of bad decisions and resulting complications.

In many cases, the conflicts between parents and teenagers derive from the illusion that a younger child has more freedom of choice. A small child may actually seem to have a freer choice of friends he can bring into his home and the games he can play with them. But there are always limitations to a child's choices, and parents are more understanding of the bad choices by attributing mistakes to the fact that "he's only a child."

Older youngsters become involved in situations in which the decisions are more important. A boy and girl at the age of five can "play house" together in an atmosphere of innocence. However, the same boy and girl could hardly suggest to their parents that they intended to play house at the age of 15. If the boy and girl, although next-door neighbors, are of different social or ethnic backgrounds, they may become aware of parental prejudices in addition to new rules of propriety as they grow into their teenage years.

Decisions of the teen years can involve the use of tobacco, alcohol, owning an automobile, handling of money, overnight trips with friends, association with friends who use drugs illegally, and relationships with members of the opposite sex. The consequences of all alternatives should be outlined for the adolescent.

Search for Identity

Part of the youngster's struggle for independence will involve what sometimes is described as a search for identity. A child accepts without much questioning that he is a member of a certain family and lives in a certain neighborhood. But as he grows older, he becomes aware of his status in the family as well as the status of his family in society. A seven-year-old could not care less about the background of his family or that of his second-grade friends. As he becomes a teenager he learns that such subjects may be matters of concern to parents and their circle of friends. He may imitate the attitudes of his family or disregard them, perhaps inviting criticism that he is rebellious.

More important to the youngster, however, is a growing concern about his position and role in life and where it may lead. He is still in the so-called formative years and is sensitive to countless influences in the world about him. Teenagers become concerned with approaching education and career decisions. It is natural for them to identify with older members in the family, teachers, and celebrities.

Need for Privacy

For the teenage girl, party invitations, dances, and diaries are important and an increasing amount of privacy is required. Even if she must share a room with a sister, there should be a part of the room that is her territory. She should have personal belongings that are not shared by a parent or sibling. If she has her own room, everything in the room probably will be regarded as her property. Even her mother should respect her privacy by knocking on the door and getting permission to enter her private world.

Although sometimes less sensitive about such matters, boys also are likely to insist on a certain amount of privacy as they grow older. They may share a room with a brother but they need trunks or other containers with locks in which they can keep personal possessions. Proof that such desire for privacy is not a passing fad for young men is found in their adult compulsion for private offices and a den or workshop area at home.

Contacts with Older Friends

Young teenagers, through part-time jobs as babysitters or errand boys, usually come in contact with young adults outside the family circle for the first time. The young adults may accept the teenagers as peers, which is flattering to the youngsters, who may in turn admire and imitate the young adults. If the teenager has been able to identify closely with his family's sense of propriety, the contacts can be a good social experience. But if the

youngster has not been able to identify effectively with his parents and family members, he may be vulnerable to misguiding influences. Because of the urge for adult status, the teenager may find a premature outlet for testing his abilities to live the adult life in the company of young adults. He (or she) can absorb a lot of information—and misinformation—about sex, alcohol, drugs, and other subjects.

Teenagers certainly should not be cautioned against contacts with all young adults, but they should also have a reliable older person aside from their parents with whom they can discuss matters they would not discuss with a mother or father. The alternate adult might be a clergyman, the family physician, a teacher, or even a favorite aunt or uncle. Such an arrangement provides the youngster with a means of learning a bit more about life in an independent manner and from a different point of view than could be obtained within his own immediate family circle.

Relationships with the Opposite Sex

First teenage contacts with the opposite sex tend to be awkward and sometimes embarrassing despite the best efforts and intentions of parents. The meetings may be at school dances or movie dates, perhaps in the presence of a chaperon who is a teacher or parent.

Overcoming Insecurity

Some youngsters will feel more secure than others in social gatherings; those who feel insecure may not participate at all when such opportunities first arise. As the youngsters grow older, however, they find that more and more of their friends are dating

or going to dances or parties to meet members of the opposite sex.

Some boys or girls who feel insecure may find that they are more gregarious or less ill-at-ease if they fortify themselves with a couple of drinks of an alcoholic beverage, or with drugs, before they join their friends. Youngsters who feel the need for stimulants or depressants in order to enjoy parties usually can be helped with psychological counseling to overcome their fears of inadequacy.

Young people should be assured that getting together at parties of mixed sexes is a natural thing to do. It has been going on for generations and although an individual youngster may feel ill-at-ease at his first few dances or parties, he probably will survive. As the boy or girl attends more parties the chances increase that he or she will meet a person of the opposite sex who is particularly attractive. If the feeling is mutual, the acquaintanceship may develop into more or less steady dating.

Going Steady

Steady dating, which leads to a formal engagement and marriage in many cases, should not be encouraged at an early age or before a young person has had an opportunity to date a number of prospective partners. At the same time, it should not be discouraged to the point of producing a rebellious reaction. As was pointed out earlier, some girls admit going steady with a boy for no other reason than to demonstrate their independence of judgment.

Controlling the Sexual Impulse

Teenagers who spend a lot of time together at parties, in their homes, or at recreational meetings such as beach outings are likely to be physically attracted to each other. It may begin with kissing, dancing, holding hands, or simply a natural urge to neck or pet. In more primitive societies, the couple might simply indulge in sexual intercourse without any concern for the possible consequences. But in our own society, young people are expected to control their natural urges.

Influence of the Mass Media

Complicating sincere efforts of a teenager to make the right decisions in relations with the opposite sex is the constant exposure of youngsters to movies, magazine articles, books, and other media suggesting that sexual relations between unmarried couples are not only acceptable but a common practice. Compared to the image of young love as displayed in movie promotion advertising, a teenage boy and girl may believe that a few ardent hugs and kisses in a secluded spot may be as innocent as making a plate of fudge together in the girl's kitchen.

Some girls, but not all, are as easily aroused as boys by close bodily contact with the opposite sex. Physical contact for most boys arouses sexual desire, partly because of the physiological makeup of the male.

The Sex Drive in Boys

Males are so constituted that during periods of abstinence from intercourse, their sperm builds up. During periods of sperm buildup, the male sex drive increases in strength. There are no standards or averages for the male sex drive; instead there is a wide variety of sexual appetites and abilities.

A girl who cuddles too closely to a boy may trigger a response she did not expect and may not want. Depending upon the boy and the status of his sex drive at that time, he might accept the girl's approaches as a suggestion that she is willing to have intercourse or is at least interested in petting. If the girl is simply being friendly, the results can be embarrassing to one or both of the youngsters. If the boy is the type who likes to discuss the details of his dates with friends, the girl may discover a sudden and unwelcome change in attitude by other boys of the group.

Walking hand-in-hand, or with an arm around the waist, and kissing that is not too passionate, usually are acceptable ways for young teenagers to display affection. And there are activities such as hiking or bicycle riding that afford a boy and girl a chance to be together and apart from the rest of the world. There also are picnics, ball games, movies, and concerts that permit togetherness without setting the stage for hard-to-control sexual impulses.

Masturbation

Another manifestation of the natural sex drives of young persons is masturbation. Discouraged by the rules and standards of society from fulfilling sex urges in the same manner as married couples, teenagers discover they can find sexual satisfaction in masturbation. Despite the stories that warn of physical or mental decay for youngsters who masturbate, the practice is not harmful unless the parents make an issue of it.

If there are dangers in masturbation, they are likely to be the isolation and loneliness associated with the practice and the confusion and anxiety that can result if the young person feels guilty or is punished or criticized for masturbating. Masturbation is such a natural reaction that most youngsters discover it by themselves even if the subject is never discussed by friends or family members. But for many young people, masturbation may violate religious or other beliefs or values. These youngsters may want to discuss the practice with a physician, understanding clergy, or some other trusted person.

Sex Education

Because boys and girls in their teens may be capable of producing children and are known to have strong sexual urges, they should be provided with authoritative information about human reproduction and birth control. It is up to the parents to make decisions regarding the proper sources of such information, how much information should be given, and at what age.

One of the reasons for the popularity of sex education in the schools is that teachers can get the parents off the hook by explaining the facts of life to youngsters. However, by forfeiting their prerogative to explain sex and human reproduction to their own children, parents must depend upon the teacher to make an acceptable presentation to the youngsters. The likely alternative is that youngsters will obtain a considerable amount of misinformation from friends and acquaintances at street-corner seminars or by experimentation.

In the days when the majority of the population lived on farms or near rural areas, children learned a few things about sex and reproduction simply by working with farm animals. They learned that cats produced kittens, dogs produced puppies, cows produced calves, and so on. This on-the-job type of sex education also provided farm youngsters with a smattering of genetics, because cross-breeding strains of animals frequently had economic consequences. It was not too difficult for the rural youngsters to relate their barnyard education to human experience.

Children enrolled in sex education

classes in the urban areas of America today receive similar information—dogs have puppies, cats have kittens, etc.—by watching movies and reading books. However, the lessons may be superficial or incomplete, depending upon the teacher and the prescribed curriculum. For example, the children in one eastern school were taught that the baby develops in the mother's abdomen, which led some youngsters to believe the baby lived in the mother's stomach until born. "Why isn't the baby digested by the stomach acid?" asked one confused girl. And when asked how the baby gets out when it's time to be born, the teacher told the students that such questions should be answered by their parents. The point here is that parents should establish some rapport with their children to be sure they are learning a practical set of facts about adult love, sex, and reproduction, including the possible emotional and physical consequences of premarital sexual intercourse.

Although parents may find it difficult or embarrassing to explain the facts of life to their own children, it is one of the most important contributions that can be made to a maturing youngster. At the present time, at least one out of six teenage girls in the United States will have an unwanted pregnancy. Obviously, thousands of parents and teachers are not providing adequate instruction in sex education subjects.

The Male Reproductive System

Any instruction in the facts of life should begin by use of the proper names for the body parts involved. In the male, the external sex organs are the *penis* and the *testicles,* or *testes.* The penis contains a tiny tube, the *urethra,* through which urine is eliminated. Much of the fleshy part of the

penis is composed of spongy tissue. When the penis is stimulated sexually, the spongy areas become filled with blood, which makes the penis larger and firm, a condition called an *erection.* The testicles contain male *sperm cells,* also called *spermatozoa.*

The sperm travel up tubules inside the abdomen to a storage organ, or reservoir, the *seminal vesicle.* The sperm storage area also contains a thick white fluid called *semen* that is secreted by glands that open into the urethra. One of the glands, the *prostate,* serves partly as a control valve to prevent urine from mixing with the semen, since both are discharged through the urethra. The semen, containing millions of sperm, empties periodically in a more or less automatic action, being squeezed out of the seminal vesicle by pulsating contractions. The contractions and ejection of semen are called *ejaculation.* During the sex act, or *intercourse,* with a female, the semen is ejaculated into the woman's vagina.

The Female Reproductive System

The *vagina* is the proper name for the tubular female sex organ. At the end of the vagina is an opening, called the *cervix,* which leads into the *uterus.* The uterus, or *womb,* is shaped somewhat like an upside-down pear. When a baby develops within the mother's abdomen, it grows inside the uterus. The uterus also is the source of the bloody discharge that occurs periodically during the fertile years of women. When the blood is discharged it is called *menstruation,* or the menstrual period. The menstrual blood passes out through the vagina, which stretches to become the *birth canal* when a baby is being born. The urethra of a female empties outside the vagina.

The Menstrual Cycle and Conception

Unlike the male reproductive organs, which produce perhaps millions of spermatozoa each day, the female reproductive system ordinarily releases only one germ cell, called an *ovum* or egg, at a time. An ovum is released at an average frequency of once every 28 days. It should always be remembered that the 28-day figure is only an average; the actual time may vary considerably for reasons that are only partly known. The cycles are more likely to be irregular for teenage girls than for mature women. An ovum is released from one of the two *ovaries,* or sex glands, comparable in function to the male testicles, located on either side of the uterus. The ovum, or egg, is transported from the ovary to the uterus through a *Fallopian tube.*

If the ovum encounters male sperm during its passage from the ovary to the uterus, there is a good chance that fertilization, or *conception,* will occur through a union of a spermatozoon and the egg. The fertilized ovum, called a *zygote,* soon divides into a cluster of human tissue cells that become the embryo of a baby. For further information about pregnancy, see under Ch. 4, *The Beginning of a Family.*

During the time that the egg is maturing in the ovary and passing into the uterus after its release, the membrane lining of the uterus becomes thicker because it accumulates blood and nutrients. If the ovum is fertilized, it finds a spot in the membrane where it becomes attached and develops rapidly into an embryo, gaining its nourishment from the blood and nutrient-enriched lining of the uterus. If the ovum is not fertilized, it passes through the uterus, and the blood-rich membrane sloughs off. The blood and some of the cells of the membrane become the discharged material of menstruation. The unfertilized ovum could pass through undetected because it is nearly microscopic.

After menstruation has begun, the female reproductive cycle starts over again. The lining of the uterus once more builds up its supply of blood and nutrients to support a fertilized ovum. Ordinarily, the next ovum will be released about 14 days after a menstrual period begins. If a female does not have intercourse, or avoids intercourse during the time the ovum is released, or in some other manner is able to prevent sperm from reaching an ovum, she will not become pregnant but will experience a menstrual period at intervals that average around 28 days.

When fertilization of an ovum occurs, menstruation ceases and no further egg cells are released until the outcome of the pregnancy has been determined. In other words, the cycles of ovulation and menstruation start anew after the baby is born or the pregnancy has been terminated.

Contraception

The first rule of birth control is that no method is guaranteed to be 100 percent effective. Sexual intercourse nearly always is accompanied by some risk of pregnancy, and the teenagers who try to beat the odds should be willing to take the responsibility for the results. Teenagers should be provided with the basic facts of birth control as soon as they are capable of producing children themselves. But the emphasis should be on the relative unreliability of the techniques which do not require a visit to a physician's office. Many birth control devices and substances can be purchased without a physician's prescription. But if young men and women were aware of their chances of effecting a pregnancy while using

such methods, they probably would have second thoughts about taking the risk. See under "Marriage and Parenthood" in Ch. 4, *The Beginning of a Family,* for a full discussion of birth control methods.

Venereal Disease

Equally important in the education of teenagers is a knowledge of the hazards of venereal disease. A poster prepared for a New York campaign against venereal disease carried the words "If your son is old enough to shave, he's old enough to get syphilis." The American Social Health Association estimates that 300,000 teenagers each year become infected with one or more forms of venereal disease. Most insidious has been the recent increase in gonorrhea, partly because girls who carry the infection may show no symptoms. A girl may have a slight but seemingly unimportant vaginal discharge. She may not be aware that she has gonorrhea until she is contacted by health officials after her boyfriend has reported to a physician for treatment. For more information on venereal disease, see Ch. 17, *Diseases of the Urinogenital System.*

Two reasons for the rising incidence of gonorrhea after it was once thought to be virtually eliminated by antibiotics are that condoms, once used as a mechanical barrier by males, have become less popular since teenage girls have obtained the use of oral contraceptives, and that new strains of the bacteria are resistant to the antibiotics. Some boys delay treatment when they realize they are infected with VD; they believe it makes them appear "tough" to be able to go without medical treatment even when it endangers their health. Because of rebelliousness, young-

sters may have a venereal disease and either refuse to tell their parents or boast about it, depending upon which approach they think will make them appear independent.

It is a bitter irony for many parents to realize that their children might carry the spirit of independence and privacy into areas that could endanger their health, for untreated syphilis can result in blindness, insanity, and heart disease. Such grave consequences can be avoided in most cases by establishing effective channels of communication between parents and teenagers, or between teenagers and another responsible adult.

The Generation Gap

Despite the attention devoted in recent years to the so-called generation gap, the gap is nothing new to the process of evolving from childhood to adulthood. Every generation has had its generation gap—a period in which the fledgling adult tests his ability to make his own way in the world. In previous eras youngsters were considered old enough to take on an adult role when they were big enough physically. A boy left home to become a farm hand or a factory apprentice. A girl would leave home to become a live-in maid with another family. Sometimes the generation gap was masked by great social upheavals such as a war or a wave of emigration. The fictional hero of many romantic stories was a young man who left home to make his own way in the world, discovering in the process a girl who wanted to be rescued from her environment. With a few jet-age variations the adolescent boys and girls of today experience the same emotional struggles as nature develops their minds and bodies toward becoming another generation of adults.

4

The Beginning of a Family

Infertility, Pregnancy, and Childbirth

The decision of a young couple to begin a family is usually a happy event, with overtones of great responsibility for the parents-to-be. Although parenthood does bring fulfillment, happiness, and great rewards, it can also involve anxiety and heavy responsibility. Therefore, the decision to have a child should not be made lightly. Before increasing the family unit and thereby complicating it, the husband and wife should have a strong, good marriage, one based on love, understanding, and the ability to compromise and share.

Infertility

Once the decision to have a child has been made, a new set of problems can arise. Though the majority of women are able to conceive within a year after ceasing all methods of birth control, a large number of couples are faced with the problem of infertility. Old census reports and records show that in the early 1800s about one in six marriages was childless—the same proportion as today. However, because of improved medical and surgical techniques, the modern woman

has a much better chance of overcoming a condition of infertility. For a description of the female reproductive organs and of the processes of conception and fertilization, see "Social and Sexual Maturation" in Ch. 3, *The Teens*. For a full treatment of women's health concerns other than those relating to pregnancy and childbirth, see Ch. 25, *Women's Health*.

Strain and Fatigue

There are many causes of infertility, and an equal number of cures. Nervous strain and mental fatigue can interfere with reproductive capacity, as can fatigue from physical work. If a woman has worries or fears about financial security or other matters, she may fail to conceive. It is believed that nervous tension can suppress human ovulation cycles through the relationship of the hypothalamus, a part of the brain, and the pituitary gland, which controls the flow of sex hormones. Recommended treatment for a wife under strain might include a vacation, a temporary interruption in her business or professional goals, or a reorganization of her living pattern to

relieve tension.

A similar tension problem can challenge the potential fatherhood of the husband. He may appear to lose his sex drive or suffer from impotency because of stress related to his job. The solution may be a second honeymoon to remove the couple from a stressful environment, or a willingness to accept a lower standard of living until financial security is truly established. Keeping up with the Joneses may put an extra car in the garage, but the penalty might be an empty crib in the nursery.

Timing Ovulation

Occasionally, the reason for infertility may be something as basic as timing. Because of misinformation or misapplication of the correct information, husbands and wives may time their intercourse so the husband's sperm does not enter the female reproductive organs during the 24 hours or so of the menstrual cycle in which the ovum is most likely to become fertilized. The wife's menstrual cycle must be watched with extreme care so that the time of ovulation can be judged.

Ovulation takes place 14 days before menstruation. In women with a 28-day cycle, ovulation would occur approximately 14 days after the previous period. Women with longer cycles ovulate later in the cycle. For a more accurate method of calculating ovulation, see "Basal Body Temperature" later in this chapter.

If the couple is in the habit of having rather frequent intercourse, including at the time of ovulation, they should abstain for a few days before the expected day of ovulation so the sperm count in the husband can build up to a higher level. Then, at the time of ovulation, the couple should have intercourse at least twice with an interval of six to eight hours between. For further assurance of success, the wife should lie on her back with her legs flexed following intercourse so that a pool of sperm will remain near the cervix.

Reproductive Incompatibility

Still another factor that can interfere with normal fertility is that of reproductive incompatibility, or an immune reaction, between sperm and ovum. This reaction between the male and female cells is similar to an allergic one and may happen in one of two ways. In the more complicated case of reaction between the sperm and the egg cell, the ovum may treat the sperm as a bit of foreign tissue, which it will reject. There is at present no foolproof remedy for this problem, but medical scientists are investigating it.

In the second type of situation, there can be an incompatible reaction between the acid environment of the female reproductive tract and the alkaline male sperm. Although the lining of the vagina usually is acid, it normally becomes alkaline at the time of ovulation to facilitate the survival of the sperm on its way to the cervix. But in some cases, the vagina remains acid enough to kill or immobilize the sperm. In cases of couples unable to have children for this reason, chemicals can be introduced into the vagina to neutralize its acidity.

The Fertility Examination

Although it has been popular for centuries to hold the female partner responsible for childless marriages, the male is just as likely to be the infertile one. But the ego of the man is often such that he may refuse to admit that he is infertile until it has been proved that the wife is indeed capable of bearing children. The easiest way to check out the causes of infertility is to submit to a series of tests by a physician.

The physician giving the tests may be a general practitioner or a specialist. There are two types of specialists who concentrate on the female reproductive system—the *gynecologist* and the *obstetrician*. The gynecologist is a physician who specializes in the care and treatment of women, especially of the reproductive organs; an obstetrician specializes in the birth process. Because the areas of responsibility frequently overlap, the same physician often handles both specialties and is referred to as an *Ob-Gyn* physician.

Fertility examinations usually require a series of at least four visits by the wife over a period of about three months, and a similar series of visits by the husband. Both husband and wife usually attend the first meeting, when the physician explains some of the common causes of infertility and outlines the rules for the tests to be performed.

Next, the physician schedules separate conferences with the marital partners so that he can obtain information that husband and wife might be reluctant to discuss in each other's presence. This discussion might touch upon possible venereal diseases of earlier years, previous marital experiences, possible illegitimate pregnancies, and so on. The medical records also will include information about general health, diet, surgery, or diseases such as mumps (which might affect fertility), sex interests and practices, family histories of miscarriages or abnormal children, and contraceptive methods used.

Basal Body Temperature

The physician will often suggest that the wife begin the BBT, or basal body temperature charts. Using a special thermometer, the BBT is taken each morning at the same hour, before getting out of bed or having a first cigarette, which would alter the results. The BBT record is a remarkably accurate way of determining the day of ovulation, because ovulation causes a sudden rise in temperature. If there is no sudden rise in temperature during the menstrual cycle, it is an indication that no ovum was released by the ovary. If the temperature rises to indicate ovulation and remains elevated for more than two weeks, it suggests that a pregnancy has begun. There are factors that can distort the readings, such as a fever or a mistake in reading the thermometer, but in general the BBT charts provide a reliable guide to the fertility cycles of the female partner.

Semen Exam

On the second visit to the physician, the husband is usually asked to bring a sample of semen in a corked bottle. The husband is generally advised to avoid intercourse for at least 48 hours before collecting the semen. The glass container of semen must be protected from heat and cold, and for this reason should be carried in a paper

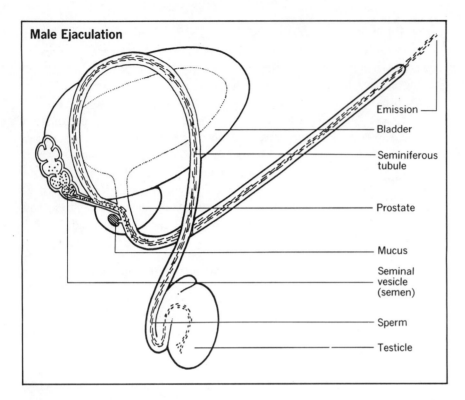

Male Ejaculation

Emission
Bladder
Seminiferous tubule
Prostate
Mucus
Seminal vesicle (semen)
Sperm
Testicle

bag to help insulate it from external temperature variations. A condom should not be used to collect or carry the semen because most rubber prophylactics contain chemicals that are harmful to spermatozoa.

The sperm examination should be made within an hour or so after it is collected so the spermatozoa will be nearly as alive and healthy as they are at the time of intercourse. If for some reason the results are not conclusive, the husband will be asked to bring another sample of semen when he accompanies his wife on her third visit, which will be scheduled about four weeks later.

During the second visit, both husband and wife may be given physical examinations, with emphasis on the pelvic and genital areas. Laboratory tests of blood and urine are made, and the examining physician may decide to make a study of thyroid function.

Tubal Insufflation

The physician generally tries to schedule the third visit to coincide with the 12th day of the wife's menstrual cycle. The examination at that time may include a *tubal insufflation* test. Also known as *Rubin's test,* tubal insufflation involves the injection of carbon dioxide gas, or sometimes ordinary air, into the uterus. Normally, the gas passes up through the uterus and Fallopian tubes and exits into the abdominal cavity. This would be a sign that the tubes are not obstructed. A pressure gauge shows a drop in pressure as the gas passes into the ab-

dominal cavity, and the physician may listen through a stethoscope for sounds of gas escaping through the tubes. The tubes are very narrow, and even a mild infection or scar tissue from a past infection can block them. Sometimes, forcing gas through the tubes is all that is needed to open them again so that chances of pregnancy will be enhanced.

A fourth visit, scheduled about four weeks after the third, should occur just before normal ovulation time. The couple may be instructed to perform intercourse about six hours before the visit. The tubal insufflation test may be repeated if the results of the earlier test were not satisfactory. In addition, a study of the cervical mucus may be made. In this study, the mucus is stretched into thin fibers or strands, which is possible only at the time of ovulation. During most of the reproductive cycle, the mucus is thick, dense, and jellylike. But the presence of estrogen hormones at the time of ovulation changes the mucus so that it makes a fibrous, fernlike pattern when placed on a glass slide.

The cervical mucus is also studied for the presence of active sperm. By using a high-power microscope, the examining physician can tell whether the cervical secretions are hostile to sperm. This would be the case if an

The Female Reproductive System

Fallopian tube
Fimbria
Ovary
Uterus
Cervix
Vagina

Ovum discharged from ovary moves toward open end of the Fallopian tube

Location of the reproductive organs

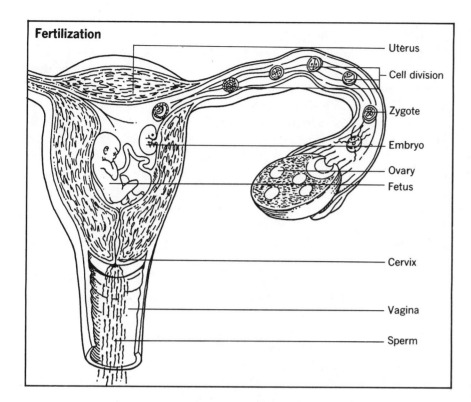

Fertilization

- Uterus
- Cell division
- Zygote
- Embryo
- Ovary
- Fetus
- Cervix
- Vagina
- Sperm

adequate number of sperm are present, but are inactive or dead. The tests can be verified by placing a bit of semen on a microscope slide next to a sample of cervical mucus.

Hysterogram

If the tests up to this point have not revealed the cause of infertility, the physician (or a recommended radiologist) can inject a special oil into the uterus and tubes and follow its path through the reproductive organs by an X-ray procedure called a *hysterogram*. If there is an obstruction or even a kink in the tubes that might interfere with the movement of an ovum, it should appear in the X-ray photographs, and the physician can then treat the problem accordingly.

Fibroids

The hysterogram may also reveal the presence of *fibroids*, benign tumors composed of fibrous tissue that usually attach themselves to the walls of the uterus. Fibroids come in varying sizes—from smaller than a pea to larger than a fist—and are present in varying degrees in about 30 percent of all women. Depending on where they occur, they may block conception, in which case they can be removed by surgery.

Other Procedures

Depending on what cause of infertility is suspected, the physician may recommend that the wife undergo a *culdoscopy, peritoneoscopy,* or *laparotomy.* The culdoscopy and peritoneoscopy require only a local anesthetic and a brief hospital stay. In the culdoscopy procedure, tubes are used to examine the pelvic organs without making a surgical incision. In the peritoneoscopy, a small incision is made just below the umbilicus. A laparotomy refers to any procedure involving an incision in the abdominal wall. Depending on the nature of the problem, a laparotomy and, to a lesser extent, the other two procedures, allow the

gynecologist latitude to make some on-the-spot corrections.

The physician may also decide to do an examination of tissue cells from the vagina or the testicles of the husband in an effort to find out what is causing infertility.

In general, the chances of success in the treatment of infertility vary with the severity of the abnormality and the length of time the disorder has gone untreated. Most minor problems can be treated by surgery, restoring normal hormone balance, proper diet, psychotherapy, or other methods, such as a change in the techniques or frequency of intercourse.

Reproductive Technology

The science of *reproductive technology* offers other ways of achieving fertilization and parenthood. In all cases the new methods require that a third party enter, at least indirectly, into the reproductive relationship. The following techniques range from the very simple to the very complex.

In vitro fertilization (IVF) is the process that produces test-tube babies. A physician removes an egg from the women's ovary and places it in a shallow dish filled with a special nutritional "bath." Some of the husband's sperm is added to the bath. If the egg becomes fertilized it is allowed to grow for a few days, then implanted in the woman's uterus to complete the gestation process.

Artificial insemination by donor (AID) is the injection by syringe of a donor's sperm into the woman's vagina. Injection takes place shortly before the woman is scheduled to ovulate. In such cases the husband's sperm, for one reason or another, cannot be used.

Surrogate motherhood occurs when a woman carries to term and delivers a child for another woman. The surrogate mother is first inseminated with the sperm of a husband whose wife cannot, for health or physical reasons, conceive and bear the child. After delivery, the surrogate mother signs for adoption by the husband and wife.

Egg donation involves removal of an egg from one woman for implantation in another. In some cases the transferred egg can be fertilized by the husband's sperm in natural intercourse. Following gestation, the baby is delivered through normal childbirth or caesarian section.

In *artificial embryonation* (AE) an infertile wife agrees to carry to term the embryo developed briefly in another woman's womb. In artificial embryonation, the childless couple form an agreement with the second woman, who is then inseminated with the husband's sperm. The embryo is allowed to develop for four or five days; physicians then try to flush out the growing embryo for implantation in the wife.

Embryo adoption (EA) is a procedure similar to artificial embryonation. But in EA the sperm of a donor, not that of the husband, is used to fertilize the volunteer "mother." Again the embryo is flushed out after a few days; the embryo is then implanted in the wife for gestation and delivery.

Many couples have specific personal reasons for using one of these methods of reproducing. The wife may, for a variety of physical reasons, be unable to conceive or carry a child. One spouse or the other may have inherited genetic defects that the couple do not want to pass on to their children. Two such defects are Huntington's chorea and hemophilia, for example.

The Expectant Mother

In most marriages there is no problem of infertility. A majority of women between the ages of 20 and 25 become pregnant during the first year of marriage. And that includes a substantial number who have tried to prevent conception with various birth control methods. The fertility prospects usually continue to be satisfactory for women up to the age of 35, but the chances decline for women in their late 30s.

When pregnancy does occur, it should be regarded as a natural process rather than a confining illness. Although some of the bodily functions are altered by approaching motherhood, it should be remembered that women have been bearing children for thousands of years, and the chances for a safe and successful delivery were never better than today.

The expectant mother can look forward to hearing a variety of old wives' tales about the hazards of pregnancy from well-meaning friends. But unless there are complications, there is no reason for anxiety. And many of the complications can be prevented or corrected with good medical care. The woman preparing for motherhood generally can relax and enjoy the state of pregnancy if she follows basic rules of health and hygiene.

Drugs and Cigarettes

Many obstetricians recommend that women refrain from taking any medications, including patent medicines such as cold remedies, during the first three months of pregnancy unless the medicine is essential for the preservation of the mother's health. There are a number of chemical substances in drugs which may or may not affect the development of the embryo. An example of the unfortunate results of drug use during the early months of pregnancy was that of thalidomide, used by a number of women in 1961–1962. The drug was one of the safest sedatives ever developed. But when used by pregnant women, thalidomide caused physically deformed babies.

Should an expectant mother smoke? A study of more than 16,000 pregnancies shows that mothers who smoke cigarettes are more likely to have stillborn babies, premature babies, and babies who are below average in weight than nonsmoking mothers. Other researchers have found that cigarette smoking stimulates contractions of the uterus, which could lead to premature birth. Mothers who smoke are also more likely to have spontaneous abortions or miscarriages.

Diet and Digestion

Acute dietary deficiencies also can affect the development of an unborn child. As the fetus develops, its growth rate is tremendous—the weight gain is as high as 650 percent per month after the unborn child has passed the third month in its mother's uterus. All of the nutrients needed for fetal growth must be taken from the mother's own diet and transmitted through the placenta. If the food eaten by the mother is not sufficient to sustain both mother and child, it is frequently the child who suffers.

This does not mean, however, that an expectant mother should eat double-sized meals because she has to feed two bodies. Obesity can be nearly as great a hazard to normal pregnancy as not eating enough. Overweight women should curb their food intake with such dietary shortcuts as drinking skim milk and eliminating as many fats and carbohydrates as possible. Meals should include a high level of proteins and all the essential minerals and vitamins. The number of total calories should not be less than 1,800 per day, unless the physician recommends otherwise.

The rule of thumb on weight gain for a pregnant woman is that she should be about 20 pounds heavier at the end of the nine months than she was before conception. The rate of gain is important. It should be held to around one pound per month during the first three months, and between two and three pounds per month during the last six months.

Throughout the pregnancy, cravings for such foods as strawberries, ice cream, pickles, or whatever are usually caused by psychological reasons rather than physical ones. However, if the food items craved are nutritious and low in calories, there is nothing wrong with satisfying the whim. Pickles, incidentally, are lower in calories and richer in vitamin C, iron, and other nutrients than most other snack foods.

Heartburn

Many mothers experience heartburn during pregnancy, and investigators have found that the treatment should be related to the length of time the mother has been carrying the unborn child. Heartburn during the first trimester, or three-month period, is usually due to anxiety and tension. If the symptoms are severe, the physician may prescribe antacids or tranquilizers. Heartburn during the last six months is usually due to the crowding of the enlarged uterus within the abdomen, which lessens stomach capacity. The solution in such cases is to eat a number of smaller meals during the day rather than three large ones. Expectant mothers with heartburn should also use additional pillows so they sleep with the head and shoulders higher than the rest of the body, avoid tight clothing that squeezes the abdominal area, and not stoop or bend over after eating.

Morning Sickness

Morning sickness, characterized by nausea and vomiting, is one of the most common complaints of mothers-to-be. Although it is unpleasant, morning sickness rarely becomes so serious that special medical treatment is needed. While friends and relatives may try to convince the expectant mother that the sick feeling is all in her mind—and she certainly may feel some anxiety about her pregnancy—there is good evidence that there is also a physical cause. The level of gastric acid in the pregnant woman's stomach declines during the first trimester of pregnancy. Also, stomach activity during that period is at a low ebb, and digestion is one to two hours slower after a meal than before pregnancy.

In most cases of morning sickness, the mother is unable to hold down her breakfast. The feeling of nausea usually subsides by lunch time, and does not appear again until the following morning. For the majority of women, the feeling fades away entirely by the 12th week. If it continues into the last two trimesters, the condition may not be related to the pregnancy.

Food for periods of morning sickness should include crackers and dry toast, lemonade or soft drinks served at cold temperatures, and hot soup, tea, or coffee. Items to be avoided are greasy foods and liquids that are only lukewarm.

Toxemia of Pregnancy

The expectant mother should visit her physician as often as recommended and follow instructions carefully. She should report any signs of puffiness of the hands and face, headaches, or visual disturbances that she experiences. Such signs and symptoms, especially in the last trimester of pregnancy, suggest *toxemia*. It is one of the most serious complications

of pregnancy, and it affects about five percent of all expectant mothers.

Toxemia of pregnancy is a catchall term that covers *hypertension,* or abnormally high blood pressure, and *edema,* or swelling of tissues due to fluid accumulation. Other symptoms are weight gain, *proteinuria,* or excretion of protein, and, in severe cases—when the disorder is sometimes called *eclampsia*—convulsions and loss of consciousness. Toxemia in late pregnancy is called *preeclampsia.*

Weight gain can amount to more than two pounds a week and may be due almost entirely to fluid retention. Proteinuria usually does not appear until after high blood pressure and weight gain have appeared. But even these clinical signs may develop before the mother-to-be knows that she has toxemia. As the problem progresses, she may have visual disturbances, puffy eyelids, headaches, and abdominal pains. When the latter symptoms occur the disease is rather well established.

The cause of toxemia is believed to be a failure of the mother's body to adjust to the metabolic and physiological stresses of pregnancy. With careful management, toxemia can be controlled with the help of drugs, regulation of weight gain and fluid intake, bed rest, and in some cases by early delivery of the baby. The fact that delivery of the child seems to resolve the problem of toxemia reinforces the theory of metabolic–physiologic relationships in the stresses of pregnancy in some women.

During pregnancy a number of complex changes take place in the mother's body—a different pattern of hormone activity, alterations in the glands secreting hormones, increased blood supply with greater demands on the heart, and a rapidly growing parasitic human in the uterus, which also grows and presses against other organs within the body. Each woman reacts somewhat differently to these changes, and toxemia is one of the reactions.

Backaches and Other Disorders

Some expectant mothers are concerned about whether the baby should be carried high or low. There is a belief among some women that a baby carried high will be a boy. The truth is that no single pregnancy is either high or low for the entire nine months. Some babies seem to be carried higher at certain stages of pregnancy while at other times they seem to be carried low. The position has nothing to do with the sex of the child.

Where the baby is carried also has nothing to do with a common complaint associated with pregnancy—backache. Backache in pregnant women is usually caused by changes in posture, and only rarely by abnormality of the organs within the pelvis. Usually it is due to bending, lifting, or walking without properly compensating for the added strain of the weight of the child, especially in the later stages of pregnancy. Generally, backache responds to rest, heat, and drugs, which relax the muscles—although the drugs should be used only on a physician's recommendation. The physician also may recommend that a lightweight maternity girdle be worn to help minimize the strain.

Improper posture in the final weeks may also be responsible for numbness and tingling or crawling sensations in the hands and arms. The hand-and-arm complaints frequently are related to what is called the *lordotic posture,* where shoulders are slumped, the spine curved forward, and the neck bent forward. The tingling sensations usually vanish when the posture is corrected. Exercises are used to help change the lordotic positioning of the spine and shoulders.

The mother-to-be must be careful about the use of seat belts when traveling by automobile or airplane. In the final months of pregnancy the belt should be fitted snugly around the lower third of the abdomen to protect the uterus from the steering wheel or dashboard in the event of an accident or sudden stop.

Pelvic X Ray

Occasionally, a physician will want to have X rays made of the pelvis of the mother to determine whether it is adequate to permit an uncomplicated childbirth. There is little hazard in a brief diagnostic X ray if modern equipment is used. Nevertheless, the mother should avoid exposure to unnecessary X rays, particularly during the first three months of pregnancy. Embryonic tissue is highly sensitive to radiation because the cells have not reached the degree of differentiation found in the fetus in the later months of pregnancy. In other words, the embryo's tissues are much more likely to be adversely affected by radiation.

Infection of the Urinary Tract

Urinary tract disturbances are not unusual during pregnancy, and may be recurrent in women who were treated for kidney or bladder infections before pregnancy. It is not unusual for women to void as frequently as once an hour or oftener and half a dozen times during the night. The disorder may be accompanied by fever and a burning sensation while voiding the urine. But most cases respond to the medications and special hygiene instructions prescribed by the physician.

Leg Cramps and Varicose Veins

Leg cramps and varicose veins affect a significant number of pregnant women. Leg cramps are the most common problem, and probably 85 percent of expectant mothers experience an occasional spasm of the calf muscles while carrying a child. The leg cramps may occur suddenly and be quite painful; at other times, the cramp may feel more like a simple kink in the muscles. The cramps occur more frequently in the last three months of pregnancy and are more likely to be experienced during a second or third pregnancy than during the first. Sluggish blood circulation and a dietary deficiency of calcium are thought to be the causes of leg cramps. The treatment consists of applying heat to the legs, massaging them, and sitting or lying down with the legs elevated. Drinking fortified milk will add calcium and vitamin D to the diet. In severe cases, muscle-relaxing drugs may be prescribed.

Varicose veins are more likely to appear during the second or third pregnancy, and tend to disappear after the birth of the baby. They are caused by a pooling of blood in the veins of the legs. Normally, the contraction of the leg muscles during walking has the effect of pumping blood from the legs back up toward the heart. But just the strain of standing can produce varicose veins even in normally active people who are on their feet for long periods. The strain of pregnancy also can upset the normal return flow of blood in the legs, so the veins become dilated. As with leg cramps, some relief can be had by sitting or lying with the feet raised. Additional relief can be obtained by wearing elastic stockings. If the varicosities remain after pregnancy, they can be treated by drugs or surgery.

Immunization

There are certain facts about immunization that a woman should know if she contemplates pregnancy. One is that the mother's reaction to smallpox vaccine can be transmitted through the placenta to the fetus. The disease can be fatal to an unborn child. Fortunately, smallpox has been eradicated from almost all areas in the world, and vaccination is no longer routinely required for travel abroad.

If the mother plans to be pregnant during the winter months, she should arrange to receive a series of influenza shots beginning in September and ending by mid-December. If she has been immunized against influenza within the past two years, a booster shot should be sufficient.

Rubella, or German measles, can be a serious threat to the normal development of a baby if contracted during the first 12 weeks of pregnancy. The rubella vaccine normally given to children should be given to women of childbearing age only with caution. Some medical scientists believe that the virus can be transmitted by the vaccine to the fetus if conception occurs within two months after the vaccine is given. If the virus infects the unborn child, particularly during the first trimester, the child may be afflicted with cataracts, deafness, or damage to the heart and nervous system.

Immunizations should also be obtained for diphtheria, malaria (if in an area where this is common), and mumps. If these diseases occur during pregnancy they result in spontaneous abortion in about one-third of the cases.

Tetanus is regarded as one of the most serious complications of pregnancy. The period of incubation for tenanus is shorter in pregnant than in nonpregnant women. It is particularly hazardous during the period immediately after abortion or childbirth. But the threat can be avoided by receiving proper tetanus immunization before pregnancy.

The Rh Factor

Blood incompatibilities between the mother and father can be another complication of pregnancy. The condition is caused by a blood protein known as the *Rh factor*. A person whose blood contains the protein is called *Rh-positive; Rh-negative* people lack the blood factor. Approximately 85 percent of the population is Rh-positive. The term *Rh* is derived from the first two letters of the name of the Rhesus monkey, a laboratory animal which was used for much of the basic research on the blood incompatibility problem.

About ten percent of all marriages in the United States involve an Rh conflict. If both husband and wife are either Rh-positive or Rh-negative, there is no problem. But if the wife has Rh-negative blood and her husband Rh-positive, the child of such a union may be threatened by death or mental retardation, particularly after the first pregnancy.

The Rh factor is inherited, and if the unborn offspring inherits the Rh-positive factor from its father while the mother has Rh-negative blood, the mother's blood may develop antibodies that destroy the baby's blood. The threat to the unborn child can be modified by a blood transfusion to the newborn infant or to the fetus before birth. The mother can also in effect be immunized against the development of antibodies by the injection of a gamma globulin blood fraction rich in passive Rh antibodies.

Usually, the first child is not affected by Rh blood conflicts. The red blood cells of the fetus can cross the placenta and trigger the reaction in the mother's blood system. But they do not reach their peak of entry into the mother's blood supply until the time of delivery. Thus, to prevent sensitization of the mother, physicians must eliminate the fetal red cells around the time of delivery—before the buildup of antibodies can begin. Once the antibodies have developed in the mother's blood, all future Rh-positive babies will be threatened unless preventive steps are taken.

If the husband of an Rh-negative woman has Rh-negative blood, or if he carries genes for both Rh-negative and Rh-positive, the baby will probably inherit the Rh-negative factor, and there will be no blood conflict. In nearly every case of Rh conflict today the baby can be saved and the production of antibodies suppressed in the mother. But the blood of both parents should be checked at the start of pregnancy plans, and arrangements made to protect the fetus if there is a threat of blood incompatibility.

Genetic Counseling

The genetic background of each marital partner has an influence on the fetus, since hereditary factors have a tendency to show up in the offspring. In addition to desirable hereditary traits, over 1,200 congenital defects have been catalogued. However, genetic factors do not always appear in a new generation, and environmental influences do not always affect mothers in the same manner. During the thalidomide episode of the 1960s, for example, only 20 percent of the pregnant women who used the drug had deformed babies; the other 80 percent had normal offspring.

While the expectant mother should take all normal precautions and follow her physician's orders faithfully with regard to diet, hygiene, and exercise, if she and her husband have normal family histories she should not be concerned with congenital birth defects. However, there are cases where there is cause for legitimate worry about the chances of an inherited disorder. If there are cases of cystic fibrosis, phenylketonuria (PKU), sickle-cell anemia, or other genetic diseases in the background of either prospective parent; if the prospective mother is over 40 (at which age there is an increased chance of giving birth to a child afflicted with *Down's syndrome* or Mongolism); or if the parents or others in the family have previously given birth to a mentally retarded child, then it is recommended that the couple seek the advice of a *genetic counselor.*

Genetic counseling is available through a network of genetic counseling and treatment centers which were set up to help couples who are planning a family but are troubled by the possibility that their children may be born with a genetic disorder. When the wife gets pregnant a prenatal diagnosis is made. This procedure, known as *amniocentesis,* involves obtaining a small sample of the amniotic fluid that surrounds the fetus by inserting a hypodermic needle through the abdominal wall. The sex of the fetus can also be determined by this method, and because many inherited disorders are sex-linked (for example, transmitted only from mother to son), this information can be critically important. If the fetus is found to be affected with the suspected disorder a therapeutic abortion is performed, if so desired by the parents. Those interested in consulting a genetic counselor should write to the National Genetics Foundation, 555 W. 57th St., New York, NY 10019.

Physicians can also use *chorionic villi sampling* (CVS) to determine the sex of a fetus before birth. Where amniocentesis cannot be performed before the fifteenth or seventeenth week of pregnancy, CVS can be done as early as the ninth week. The sampling process involves removal of genetic material for analysis. Like amniocentesis, CVS also indicates whether a fetus has any of the approximately 350 genetic abnormalities. As one advantage to parents

who want to avoid giving birth to a severely handicapped child, early CVS provides the option of a first trimester abortion.

Miscarriage

About ten percent of all pregnancies end in a *miscarriage,* often called a *spontaneous abortion.* A miscarriage can occur for a variety of reasons, many of which are related. Some of the reasons may be hormone malfunction or deficiency; a faulty sperm or ovum, which would, in the vast majority of cases, result in a cruelly malformed child or one incapable of staying alive if the pregnancy were carried to term; a poor *endometrium,* or lining of the uterus, in which the ovum is implanted; changes in the mother's body chemistry; or other factors that interfere with normal development of the child within the uterus.

Hormone Deficiency

Hormone malfunction is responsible for many spontaneous abortions. Once the placenta is established on the inner wall of the uterus, it ordinarily produces sufficient hormones to maintain the pregnancy. But the condition of the endometrium at the time the embryo becomes implanted in the uterine wall affects the later development of the placenta. That situation, in turn, may affect the secretion of the hormones needed to continue the pregnancy. The level of one hormone, called the human chorionic gonadotropic hormone, is frequently used as a barometer of the condition of the uterus. When the amount of that hormone excreted in the urine suddenly decreases, it is a warning signal that spontaneous abortion may be imminent.

Other physiological barometers are thyroid function and the rate of

excretion of a substance known as sodium pregnanediol. Normally, there is a rise in thyroid activity when a woman becomes pregnant. The level remains elevated as long as the pregnancy continues, declining when the pregnancy is terminated either by delivery of a child or abortion. The expectant mother who has an underactive or overactive thyroid gland needs special medical attention because the hormone secreted by the gland seems to influence both the ovaries and the pituitary gland. Thyroid dysfunction is associated with infertility and the tendency toward spontaneous abortions.

Hormone deficiencies can contribute to the failure of the ovaries to produce thriving ova. In younger girls, the ovaries may be too immature to yield ova that are capable of continuing life after they are fertilized. In older women, the egg cells may be faulty because of approaching menopause. Even if the egg cell is perfect, defective sperm from the husband may be responsible for failure of the egg cell to develop into a healthy embryo after fertilization.

Still another cause of spontaneous abortion related to unfavorable hormone levels is the infantile or underdeveloped uterus, which may not have the capacity to maintain the fetus as it grows toward normal size for delivery. The undersized uterus can be treated with a hormone, estrin, to make it large enough to sustain a full-term pregnancy.

Other Causes of Miscarriage

Fibroid tumors or polyps in the uterus can interfere with both conception and pregnancy. Congenital malformations, such as a divided uterus, may also result in miscarriage. These problems can usually be corrected by surgery. A retroverted, malpositioned or tipped uterus can also be corrected to make carrying to term possible if this situation has caused a spontaneous abortion. An abnormality of the uterus called incompetent cervix used to be the cause of many spontaneous abortions in the last half of pregnancy, but in recent years a simple operation has been devised to correct the defect. See Ch. 15, *Women's Health,* for further information on gynecological problems.

Symptoms of Miscarriage

Spontaneous abortions usually are classified as threatened or inevitable. Generally, an abortion is considered to be of the threatened type when there is bleeding or cramps or both. Even when bleeding and cramps seem to be severe, it is possible that they will stop, or can be stopped, and the pregnancy will continue. If the bleeding and cramps become progressive and there is dilation of the cervix with the passage of tissue, the abortion is considered inevitable. Physicians sometimes can estimate the length of time that a spontaneous abortion has been progressing by examining the blood. If the blood is dark brown rather than bright red, it suggests that bleeding may have started at some time in the past. The longer the bleeding continues, the less chance there is that the fetus will survive.

Ectopic Pregnancy

Bleeding and cramping are not always signs of spontaneous abortion. Bleeding may be caused by a polyp or a malignant growth on the cervix. Cramps or bleeding can also occur if there is an *ectopic pregnancy,* a pregnancy outside the uterus. For example, the fertilized egg may become implanted in a Fallopian tube or even in the abdominal cavity instead of in the uterus. Many cases of ectopic pregnancy go undiagnosed because the

symptoms are quite similar to those of a threatened abortion. Most ectopic pregnancies end in miscarriage when the pressure of the growing fetus causes the tube to rupture. In rare cases, the fetus may lodge in the abdominal cavity after rupture and continue to grow and develop. Such a fetus can be delivered by caesarian techniques, but is thought to be extremely dangerous for the mother. Most physicians prefer to perform a therapeutic abortion if this situation occurs.

Trophoblastic Disease

In about one of every 1,500 to 2,000 pregnancies in the United States, the placenta degenerates into a *hydatidiform mole,* a benign tumor consisting of a mass of grapelike cysts. This condition is known as *trophoblastic disease,* in reference to the *trophoblast,* a layer of cells that develops around the fertilized ovum and contributes to the formation of the placenta.

Signs and symptoms of a hydatidiform mole generally appear one to two months after conception. They include nausea and vomiting, persistent bleeding from the uterus, and an increase in uterine size more rapid than normal. X rays fail to show a developing skeleton and there is no fetal heartbeat perceptible at the usual stage of pregnancy. X-ray arteriograms and ultrasound scanning of the uterus also reveal signs of the mole. Spontaneous abortion commonly threatens and often occurs. Laboratory analysis of chorionic gonadotropic hormone levels in serum and vaginal smears are among other tests used to verify the presence of a hydatidiform mole.

The mole must be removed as soon as feasible after it has been identified, to decrease the chances of its invading the uterine wall and becoming cancerous. It is removed by sur-

gical methods, such as suction curettage, or occasionally surgical excision. In those few cases in which the mole invades the uterus, the uterus is removed. Following a molar pregnancy that is neither invasive nor cancerous, a woman should be examined regularly for a year or so. Subsequent pregnancies are permitted and have every prospect of being successful. If the mole is invasive or cancerous, antitumor chemotherapy is essential. Occasionally, radiation therapy also is used.

Habitual Abortion

Among some women, spontaneous abortion occurs repeatedly and is known as habitual abortion. Habitual abortion usually threatens at the same stage of each pregnancy, and the measures needed to prevent a repetition of the miscarriage should be started as soon as the expectant mother knows she is pregnant. The usual prenatal care should be followed conscientiously, including the rules about nutrition and exercise. Cigarette smoking should be curtailed or eliminated because, among other reasons, tobacco use seems to affect the carbohydrate metabolism of smokers, and pregnant women are particularly sensitive to changes in carbohydrate balance. The cells that form the placenta and fetal membranes require large amounts of carbohydrates that can be assimilated easily. Even before the fertilized egg cell becomes implanted in the lining of the uterus, the cells of the endometrium demand unusually large quantities of glycogen, or body starch, that has been converted to simple sugar molecules. Other nutrients are also needed, of course, but the demand for them is not as critical as that for carbohydrates.

Induced Abortion

Not all abortions are involuntary. The induced abortion is a deliberate interruption of the development of an embryo or fetus because of therapeutic or nonmedical reasons. Such an abortion, usually performed in a hospital or clinic, requires antiseptic conditions. Local anesthetics are used if needed. In the procedure called *dilation and curettage,* or *D and C,* the physician enlarges the opening of the uterus to permit entry of the surgical tools used to scrape the lining of the uterus. The tissue is removed from the lining with a *curette,* a surgical instrument resembling a scoop with sharpened edges. Another method often used, called *vacuum aspiration,* employs suction to pull the embryonic tissue from inside the uterus. These techniques—the D and C and vacuum aspiration—can be used only during the first trimester of pregnancy.

If the abortion is delayed beyond the first three months, more complicated surgery may be required. An alternative method called *salting out* (medically, *saline amniocentesis*) involves the injection of a saline solution into the amniotic fluid. The salt water kills the fetus and induces labor, and the fetus is delivered, thus terminating the pregnancy. This method involves somewhat greater risk of complications than the other methods.

If an induced abortion is performed by a physician in a hospital or clinic equipped with facilities to cope with possible complications the procedure is safe, with very low risk of complications. The notion that women are rendered sterile or more likely to have spontaneous abortions or premature deliveries of wanted children in later years can be true; but this is usually so only in those cases where women had the procedure performed under unsanitary conditions or by someone who was medically incompetent.

Approaching Delivery

When all is going well with a pregnancy—and it does in the vast majority of cases—a favorite guessing game becomes the prediction of delivery day. There are several ways in which to estimate the approximate birth date of the new addition to the family. One is to calculate 267 days from the date of conception. Another approach is to count 280 days from the first day of the last menstrual period. This method is easier, because women are more likely to know the date of the last menstrual period than the last time they ovulated. Still another method commonly used is to count back three months from the first day of the last menstrual period and add seven days. No matter what method is used it will probably be wrong, since surveys show that fewer than five percent of all babies arrive on the day they were expected. However, the majority of babies are born within five days of the anticipated date.

As delivery day approaches, the physician usually wants to make some last-minute studies of the position of the child and its general condition. He may also want to check the size of the bony area of the mother's pelvis in an effort to determine in advance whether there will be any complications in delivery. During the examination, the physician usually looks for varicose veins around the vulva and vagina; they are a common occurrence among pregnant women, and some women claim they can tell when they are pregnant—even before a period is missed—by the appearance of these varicose veins.

By pressing the abdomen with the palms of his hands and his fingers, the physician can determine the position of the unborn child in the uterus. He also can get a fair idea of the size of the fetus and can tell how low it is in the pelvic region. The physician listens to the heartbeat of the fetus and, if labor is near, he may mark the position of the fetus on the skin of the

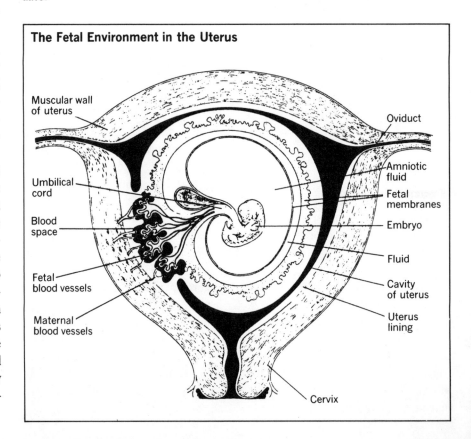

The Fetal Environment in the Uterus

Muscular wall of uterus

Umbilical cord

Blood space

Fetal blood vessels

Maternal blood vessels

Oviduct

Amniotic fluid

Fetal membranes

Embryo

Fluid

Cavity of uterus

Uterus lining

Cervix

mother's abdomen so that he can tell later if it has moved and in which direction.

In about half of all pregnant women, reddish streaks appear on the skin of the stretched abdomen. The streaks sometimes have the appearance of broken skin fibers because of stretching, but most physicians agree that the streaks are the result of hormone activity. It is another sign of a successful pregnancy.

In the final days before delivery, the physician usually makes an estimate of the space through which the baby must move to reach the outside world. He also must make a rough guess about the weight of the baby at birth. If the baby weighs less than five pounds at birth it is *premature* by definition and may require special care, which the physician would want to schedule.

Lightening

The phenomenon of *lightening* is a sign that pregnancy is approaching an end and that birth can be expected within about three weeks. When lightening occurs, the mother feels less pressure on the upper part of the abdomen and more discomfort in the pelvic region as the head of the fetus descends toward the birth canal. Lightening may be accompanied by strong contractions of the uterus, which may be mistaken for labor pains. If lightening does not occur during the final weeks, the physician may conduct further examinations to learn if the delay is due to a large fetus, twins (though a possible multiple birth is usually discovered earlier in the pregnancy), or another reason such as an unfavorable fetal position. When lightening does occur on schedule, the physician usually assumes that the head of the fetus is low in the pelvic region and can pass through the birth canal without difficulty, since it

Abnormal Presentations during Delivery

Breech

Buttocks presentation

Retroflexed uterus

Abnormal Shoulder-arm presentation

has already completed the first part of the obstacle course to the outside world.

Fetal Position

With X rays and fetal electrocardiograms, it can be determined whether the unborn baby is upside down or in some other position in the uterus. A fetal electrocardiogram is made by placing electrodes on the mother's abdomen while she is lying on an examination table. The electrical impulses of the fetal heart muscle will produce a pattern revealing the direction of the heart which, in turn, tells which way the head is positioned. If the pattern indicates the head is toward the top of the abdomen rather than the bottom, a *breech presentation* can be expected in the delivery room.

Although 95 percent of all babies are in the head-downward position

when labor begins, about three percent are in the more difficult breech presentation. Some physicians believe that a breech presentation is more likely if the fetus is delivered before term, since nearly 40 percent of the fetuses are in the breech presentation at the 20th week of pregnancy. However, this percentage declines as delivery day approaches, because the growing fetus finds it more comfortable to move its feet and bottom into the widest part of the pear-shaped uterus while the head fits into the narrow lower part.

Labor

The contractions of labor pains are something of a mystery. They are independent of the will of the mother. Women who are paralyzed or who feel no labor pains because of severed nerves can have a normal delivery. The uterus may even continue contractions automatically after it has been removed from the body.

First Stage of Labor

The first stage of labor is characterized by regular pains, which may occur at intervals of 5 to 15 minutes. During this stage the cervix becomes dilated and forms a passageway into the vagina. There is a rest period between the labor pains that lasts at least a minute and gives the mother a brief respite while permitting the flow of oxygen to the fetus by way of the placenta. (If the uterine contractions were continuous they would cut off the baby's oxygen supply.) During uterine contractions, the uterus rises in the abdomen; the change in shape can be observed at the start and end of each labor pain.

The so-called *bag of waters,* which actually is the *amniotic fluid* within the membrane, may be discharged at almost any time during labor. Sometimes the bag of waters ruptures before the labor pains begin, but this usually occurs during one of the strong contractions. The fluid generally comes out with a gush, but it may also be discharged in small amounts with each contraction. The term *dry labor* is used to describe contractions that begin after the bag of waters has ruptured. Ordinarily, the contractions become stronger and more frequent and the cervix dilates more rapidly after the amniotic fluid has been discharged.

Occasionally, the baby is delivered with the amniotic membrane still intact about its head. The membrane in such a case is known as a *caul.* At one time, a caul was regarded as a symbol of great superstitious value; midwives sold cauls to sailors who carried them for good luck on voyages.

Second Stage of Labor

Rupture of the bag of waters frequently climaxes the first stage of labor, which may last more than 12 hours if it is the first pregnancy. The second stage of labor is considerably shorter and can be expected to last around 2 hours in a first pregnancy, 30 minutes for a woman who has had children previously. The second stage may begin with rupture of the bag of waters if the amniotic fluid was not

Birth Sequence

Dilated cervix
During the first stage of labor the cervix dilates to form a passageway into the vagina, the birth canal. Contractions of the uterus may occur at intervals of approximately 5 to 15 minutes, with brief periods of rest in between, which permit oxygen to flow to the fetus.

Ruptured amniotic sac
Ruptured amniotic sac ordinarily signals the onset of the second and generally shorter stage of labor. Contractions during this stage occur in more frequent succession and are more intense. The so-called *bag of waters,* which contains the amniotic fluid, is ordinarily discharged during a strong contraction but may even rupture before labor begins.

Delivery
As the fetus moves into the lower pelvic region the mother naturally experiences a conscious impulse to bear down and help its entry into the world. She may feel a few moments of increased pressure or pain as the infant's head gradually appears and is followed by the rest of its body.

Placental stage
Placental stage is the third stage of labor and is characterized by the expulsion from the womb of the placenta, or *afterbirth,* to which the baby is connected by the umbilical cord. This cord is not cut until all the placental blood has pulsed into the baby's body.

released earlier. The contractions are more intense and frequent, occurring at intervals of 2 to 3 minutes rather than the 5- to 15-minute intervals of the first stage. There also is a conscious desire on the part of the mother to help expel the fetus. She may feel additional pains, pressures, or irritations because of the presence of the fetus in the lower pelvic area.

During this series of labor pains the baby gradually makes its appearance outside the mother's womb. At first a bit of the scalp shows, then recedes as the labor pain subsides. With the next labor pain more of the head appears. Finally, the entire head is outside the mother's body, followed by the shoulders, trunk, and lower extremities.

Anesthetics and Drugs

Although it is standard practice to refer to the uterine contractions as labor pains, the amount of actual pain varies, and there are numerous methods for reducing the pain. True painless labor is rare, and when it occurs it is sometimes attributed to an abnormality of the nervous system.

The physician is as concerned about the welfare of the mother and baby as the mother herself, and this concern is reflected in the approach taken to provide relief from labor pains. The drug or anesthetic the physician chooses to use will be one that gives optimum relief to the mother without creating an environment in the womb that would threaten the life of the baby. A number of rather common drugs that could be used to relieve pain without harm to the mother could very easily be fatal to the infant, who would share through the placenta substances injected into the mother's bloodstream.

The type of anesthetic or drug administered to the mother is usually one that affects only the part of the nervous system associated with pain. If the substance also affected the motor nerves, the delivery would become stalemated. On the other hand, it would be very simple to handle the childbirth in a satisfactory manner as far as the baby is concerned if the mother were given no relief from pain.

Drugs used as aids in childbirth include analgesics, tranquilizers, barbiturates, and the type of drugs used in so-called twilight sleep—scopolamine and morphine. They can be given orally or by injection. In nearly all cases the drugs are used with caution, and they are frequently administered in combination with a gas anesthetic.

The gases frequently used during delivery are nitrous oxide, which provides intermittent relief from pain during the second stage of labor, and cyclopropane, which may be administered for caesarian section or cases of delivery in which there are complications requiring unconsciousness or deep analgesia (incapacity to feel pain). Nitrous oxide sometimes is provided during labor pains on signal from the mother. When she wants relief for a few moments or when she feels a pain starting, the mother signals the anesthetist, who places the mask over her face so she can take a few deep whiffs. The procedure is repeated when the next labor pain begins. Nitrous oxide may also be used in conjunction with ether or one of the other standard anesthetic gases. When properly administered, ether is safe and reliable for producing deep anesthesia or relaxation.

Still another anesthetic commonly used during delivery is a drug injected either for local anesthesia or for putting the mother to sleep for the period of delivery. Sodium pentothal is injected intravenously in many cases, particularly when forceps are used to assist in delivery. However, the physician has to work fast in these cases, because this is one of the drugs that can be transmitted through the placenta in a short time.

A caudal anesthetic can be used to block pain in the entire pelvic area. In this case, a drug is injected into the area at the bottom of the spinal column. Most women who have had a caudal anesthesia like it as a means of obtaining relief from labor pains, but it requires the presence of specially trained personnel.

When delivery can be timed rather precisely, a spinal anesthetic, sometimes called a *saddle block,* is injected into the region of the spinal cord in the lumbar area while the mother is in a sitting position. After the injection, the mother lies on her back and, in most cases, is free of pain for the remainder of labor and delivery.

Natural Childbirth

Natural childbirth methods are preferred by some women who want to participate as consciously as possible in the act of bringing a child into the world. Others, by contrast, want to go into the delivery room completely anesthetized—to enter a pregnant woman and awaken as a mother. In natural childbirth, most women receive a local anesthetic for the *episiotomy* incision, to make the vaginal area large enough for passage of the baby, drugs to relieve tension when requested, and *oxytocin.* Oxytocin is a hormone naturally secreted by the pituitary gland to help the muscles of the uterus contract normally.

Lamaze Method

A woman who chooses the natural childbirth technique developed by Dr. Ferdinand Lamaze conditions herself for labor pains by substituting a different response. Instead of crying

Natural Childbirth

Pituitary
Naturally secreted by the pituitary gland, *oxytocin* helps the uterine muscles to contract normally during childbirth.

Muscle relaxants
Today many women choose natural childbirth to remain conscious during the birth of their babies. Muscle relaxants are still commonly used, however, to help some mothers feel more comfortable and relaxed during labor.

Episiotomy
An episiotomy incision is made by the physician to prevent tearing of the tissues and to make the vaginal opening large enough for the baby to pass through. In natural childbirth, most mothers will receive a local anesthetic before this procedure.

out, for example, her response is a pattern of rapid, shallow breathing which she begins at the first sign of a uterine contraction. The conditioning exercises take about 30 minutes a day and should be started two months before the expected delivery date. Although some women who start natural childbirth training lessons are not able to complete the course for various reasons, most agree that they were better prepared for labor because of what they learned about the control of muscles and breathing.

Fathers-to-be are encouraged to participate in preparations for natural childbirth by coaching their spouses in breathing exercises and timing their contractions. Many hospitals now permit husbands to be with their wives during the second stage of labor in the hospital and even to be present in the delivery room.

Hypnosis sometimes is used instead of drugs or anesthetics for childbirth. But only a minority of women are able to accept the long period of training for the effective deep trance required, some applicants are not susceptible to hypnosis, and few obstetricians are adequately trained to control the hypnotic situation during delivery. Many physicians feel that the type of woman who would be

a good subject for child delivery while hypnotized would get along just as well with the natural childbirth method.

LeBoyer Method

"The infant is like one possessed," writes Dr. Frederick LeBoyer of the moment preceding birth. "Mad with agony and misery, alone, abandoned, it fights with the strength of despair. The monster drives the baby lower still . . . The baby is now at the height of its travail. The effort required is too great. The end is surely near. Death seems certain. The monster bears down one more time, and it is then that . . .

"Then that everything explodes! The whole world bursts open. No more tunnel, no prison, no monster. The child is born."

In such terms Dr. LeBoyer focuses on the trauma that the child experiences at birth. The LeBoyer method seeks to train the mother to concentrate on that trauma while delivering her child. A form of natural childbirth, the technique also requires that silence or near-silence be maintained in the delivery room—to protect the newborn infant's ears and sensitivities.

"Relaxing, accepting the slow pace [of birth], letting it take command"— these responses on the mother's part lie at the heart of the LeBoyer method. When birth proceeds in this way, Dr. LeBoyer notes, the child enters the world relaxed and already adjusted. The painful aspects of birth have been eliminated; both mother and child enter on the new relationship outside the womb with calm acceptance.

Like other approaches to natural childbirth, the LeBoyer method requires the full understanding and cooperation of the mother-to-be. The benefits of natural methods are said to be shorter periods of labor and reduced birth trauma. Natural childbirth is also said to reduce morbidity and mortality rates among newborn babies.

Caesarian Section

A caesarian section may be performed in cases of diabetic mothers with rapidly growing fetuses, when delivery is complicated by breech or shoulder presentation, if the uterus is weak due to previous surgery or other reasons, or when the mother has a history of losing the child after carrying it to the time of delivery. There are several variations in caesarian techniques, some requiring a general anesthetic and others using local anesthetics and other medications. But all approaches are directed toward the same goal of saving the lives of both mother and baby. In nearly all instances, the uterus is closed after the baby and placental material are removed. Only in extremely rare cases is it necessary to remove the uterus. Most mothers who have caesarians can have more children in the future if they so desire.

Third Stage of Labor

After the baby is delivered through

the normal birth canal, the placenta is expelled by the same route. This is called the third, or placental, stage of labor. The placenta, also known as the *afterbirth,* is connected to the baby by the unbilical cord. The cord is not cut until the blood has drained from the placenta into the baby's body; to help the flow the placenta is held above the level of the baby to get an assist from gravity.

Before the infant leaves the delivery room, it is examined for a normal heartbeat, possible abdominal distention or evidence of fluid in the abdominal region, possible abnormalities of the ears, and possible deformities of the mouth area, such as cleft palate or lip. The health of newborn babies is scored by the *Apgar system* when the baby is 60 seconds old. Five items of physical condition are noted and scored on a scale of 0 to 2. They are heart rate, muscle tone, respiration, nerve reflexes, and skin color. Babies that score 8 to 10 points are considered in excellent condition and are given routine postnatal care. If they score 7 points or less, additional measures are taken to get the infants off to a normal start in life. Since the system was started, nearly three-fourths

of all newborn babies tested have passed with 8 points or more.

Breast and Bottle Feeding

Whether the infant is to be breast fed or bottle fed is usually a personal matter to be decided by the new mother. For the average healthy baby, there are no obstacles to breast feeding if the mother desires it and is able to produce and deliver milk. A few women are unable to produce a sufficient supply of milk and most supplement their output with bottle feedings. In a few cases, babies are allergic to mother's milk, but in such instances the allergen can be identified and removed from the mother's diet.

Feeding problems are sometimes fewer and less serious among breast-fed babies. The mother's milk contains most of the necessary nutrients and is available when needed at the proper temperature. It also is more likely to be fresh and free of infectious bacteria than bottled milk.

The mother's milk during the first few days after birth is yellowish in color and rich in proteins and miner-

als. It is called *colostrum,* and is replaced gradually by regular human milk by the fourth week. Mother's milk is low in iron and may lack vitamins C and D. However, the baby arrives in the world with enough stores of iron in its tissues to last through the first few months of life. Compared to cow's milk, human milk is richer in carbohydrates, but cow's milk has a greater proportion of proteins and minerals. The vitamin content of both mother's milk and cow's milk varies with the vitamin intake of each.

Mother's milk generally is more easily digestible in the baby's stomach than cow's milk, because the curd of mother's milk is fine and more rapidly metabolized. On the other hand, mothers who breast-feed sometime suffer from fissuring or cracking of the nipples, *mastitis* (breast inflammation) or diseases that require temporary or permanent discontinuance of breast feeding.

Surveys indicate that more than three-fourths of babies today are bottle fed. Many mothers avoid breast feeding because they feel it is socially unacceptable, that it interferes with employment or social life, that it will affect their physical attractiveness, or because of fear of failure. For mothers who select bottle feeding over breast feeding, the procedure is much simpler today than in previous years. Many of the differences in nutritional values of mother's milk and cow's milk have been reduced or eliminated by improved formula development. Equipment for preparing the bottled meals is superior to that used in previous generations. And there is less danger today of bacterial infection from cow's milk because of improved dairy sanitation methods. New mothers who choose not to breast-feed are usually given hormones, along with ice packs and analgesics, to relieve any breast discomfort that may appear during the first few days.

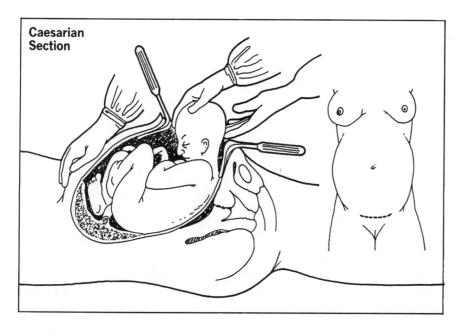

Caesarian Section

If the mother wants to breast-feed the baby, plans should be made in advance of delivery. The first feeding can be started as soon after delivery as is feasible for both mother and child, usually within hours after birth. Although the first breast feeding can be delayed for several days, because of the stimulation of milk secretion immediately after delivery, the first ten days to two weeks are crucial in the establishment of a breast feeding program. The sucking reflex of the baby at the mother's breast triggers release of the hormone oxytocin, which in turn influences the release of another substance of the pituitary gland, prolactin, needed for the production of milk in the mother's breast. See also "Feeding the Baby" in Ch. 2, *The First Dozen Years*.

Marriage and Parenthood

Early Marriage

Although young newlyweds are ready physically for marriage, and can prove it by having babies, they are not always ready for the responsibilities of marriage. Often, the parents of the newlyweds have to contribute to the support of the family in one way or another. If the older generation can afford it, they may help the young couple to purchase a home or help them finance an apartment that would not otherwise be available to them. Sometimes the newlyweds will move into the home of the parents of the bride or the groom.

In the view of some experts, a number of teenagers enter marriage as a kind of initiation into adulthood. These young couples marry not for

sexual reasons but to satisfy a desire to have the status of adulthood. Although the average age of marriage for men and women has been rising in recent years, a substantial number of young people are still marrying before the age of 21. About 50 percent of teenage marriages end in divorce within five years. The couples find that marriage and adult status do not offer the magic they had expected, and the bride and groom find themselves locked into a life that can be quite mundane and dull.

When the wife realizes that instead of a life of magic she faces a life of pots and pans and diapers, and the husband discovers that two cannot live as cheaply as one, arguments may evolve. Not all marriages of young couples are destined for failure, of course, and millions of unions that are threatened by divorce survive the rocky first years to develop into well-adjusted and realistic lifetime partnerships.

Marriage Counseling

At some point in the early years of marriage, the couple may decide to consult with someone outside their inner circle of friends and family when personal problems arise that defy an amicable solution. An outside point of view can be more objective, and the conflict may involve matters the couple would not want to discuss with family, friends, or a clergyman.

Rather than face separation or divorce, they can take their problems to someone professionally trained, such as a psychiatrist, psychologist, or a marriage counselor. However, they should be forewarned that solutions are not quick and easy. Several sessions, at least, may be needed. If the problems are serious enough to warrant professional help, the couple can expect that it will take time for a

stranger to separate facts from emotions and develop a future course acceptable to both parties.

Selecting the right counselor can be a problem in itself, because not all counselors are equally qualified. A family physician or a psychiatrist may be asked to give direct help or to make a referral. A counselor who uses systems or formulas, such as astrology charts or computer analysis, or who communicates by mail or telephone, should be avoided. Marital problems require a personal approach; it is unlikely that a marriage counselor could have simple solutions that might be applied to any couple who come to him with questions ranging from sexual incompatibility to the handling of family finances. The couple should also be suspicious of a counselor who offers a contract for his services or who suggests that a certain set number of sessions will be required.

Sexual Compatibility

Recent research suggests that sexual compatibility derives from many factors. Married couples who achieve compatibility generally enjoy one another's company as friends *and* as love partners. They share conversation, ideas, fears, hopes, and basic feelings. Their two-way relationships are characterized by mutual respect and an ability to deal with negative emotions and conflict. Mutual respect makes possible honesty; but it does not usually condone the kind of honesty that disregards the other person's feelings.

Couples achieving sexual compatibility have also, as a rule, committed themselves clearly and definitely to the relationship. A spirit of trust can then develop. Interests can be shared. As time passes, each partner learns to accept life and personality changes flexibly.

The research indicates, in effect, that sexual compatibility does not spring primarily from romantic notions of marriage and love but, much more directly, from mutual acceptance of one another, trust, and sincere regard. Compatibility emerges as a by-product of sharing and belief in the possibility of a permanent partnership. Where "like marries like," studies also show, the chance that such a relationship will develop is enhanced. Thus similarities in educational and age levels, religious convictions, and preferences regarding parenting all contribute to compatibility.

The Honeymoon

During the first weeks or months of marriage, the husband and wife have an opportunity to become better acquainted on an intimate basis. The honeymoon period usually provides ideal settings for intimate living, away from the daily pressures of earning a living and the social pressures of well-meaning friends and relatives. Even so, honeymoons frequently are disappointing, perhaps because of the disproportionate emotional investment in them. This does not, by any means, indicate that the marriage is doomed to fail.

Fatigue

After the honeymoon, both partners may suffer a bit from mental and physical fatigue in the evenings, particularly if both are employed; sexual intimacies might be less frequent than the couple had anticipated. The wife may be in the mood for sex play but the husband might be tired or distracted by financial worries. Or the husband may be in the mood, but the wife may be too tired physically or emotionally upset. However, if fatigue

serves as a frequent excuse for not having sexual relations, it may be rationalization, and the attitudes of both partners toward sex should be examined. One of the best ways to get the marriage off to a pleasant beginning is to make sure that the husband and wife can retire in the evening and leave the cares of the day for tomorrow.

Importance of Foreplay

Despite the seemingly open attitude toward sex among today's young people, many marital partners can be rather inept in the bedroom. If the sex act were a complicated procedure, the human race would not be around today. However, the many superstitions, fears, and restrictions superimposed upon a normal function almost from the time of birth until marriage can lead to emotional conflicts and frustrations when the young man and woman are face to face in a double bed.

If the husband does not take into account the importance of sexual foreplay and timing, the wife may not respond in the manner he expected, and he may reject her as frigid. Or the husband may experience premature ejaculation in his sexual excitement and complete the sex act before the wife has had time to respond. Premature ejaculation is one form of impotence. In another form, because of shyness or other psychological reasons, the man may not be able to sustain an erection.

The wife may not experience a true orgasm until after several months of marriage, and it may take the same amount of time for the husband to develop his techniques to the point where the wife is satisfied. The idea that practice makes perfect in *coitus,* or the sex act, may seem facetious, but it is nevertheless true. Patience and consideration for each oth-

er's preferences should result in a mutually pleasurable sexual adjustment.

Frigidity and Impotence

Only a small percentage of women fail to achieve orgasm eventually, and probably a smaller percentage of men remain impotent for an extended period of time. The most frequent cause of frigidity and impotency is psychological. For those who do feel frustrated in the sex act after many weeks or months of serious effort, advice should be sought from a psychotherapist, or the family physician may make a referral to a physician who specializes in this area of medicine. In some cases, impotence can be treated with drugs or medication. On the other hand, the wrong kinds of drugs or alcohol may interfere with normal sex functions.

Birth Control

Female frigidity can be caused by nothing more serious than fear of an unwanted pregnancy. If the couple has agreed to postpone starting a family or adding to it, the wife might feel insecure about her birth control method, especially if she depends upon a technique known to be less effective than the oral contraceptive.

Oral Contraceptives

Although "the pill," or *oral contraceptive,* has received a bad press in recent years, it probably ranks second only to sterilization as a birth control method. Oral contraceptives are composed of synthetic sex hormones; they are manufactured by pharmaceutical companies from substances found in plant materials such as Mexican yams. The hormones are chemical cousins of the hormones naturally secreted in the female body during a normal reproductive cycle. They work by "fooling" the woman's reproductive system with a simulated pregnancy.

How "The Pill" Works

Normally, an ovum is released from the ovaries once during each menstrual cycle. If the ovum becomes fertilized by male sperm and implanted in the uterus, the hormones send back chemical signals that tell the ovaries to suppress ovulation until further notice. If this natural defense did not occur, a woman could find herself carrying several embryos and fetuses of different ages at the same time.

In other words, when an ovum is fertilized, the mother's reproductive machinery is mobilized to protect and encourage the development of the newly created life, and the monthly release of ova is halted until the birth of the baby. The synthetic hormones in the pill are of the type that signal the body that a pregnancy has been started, even though it is not true. Ovulation is suppressed and menstruation is delayed as long as the pills are taken.

At the end of a series of approximately 20 pills, one per day, menstruation is allowed to occur. The periods of women using oral contraceptives usually are only of two to three days' duration, and the menstrual flow is considerably lighter than in women not taking the pill. Then the series of pills is resumed for another menstrual cycle, but the hormones again suppress ovulation with a false pregnancy message. Since no ovum is released, there is very little chance that pregnancy will result from intercourse while the pills are used. Oral contraceptives are almost 100 percent effective, but errors occur from time to time, usually human errors in which the woman forgets to take a pill each day.

Side Effects

Some women who use the pill have experienced undesirable side effects, which may range from break-through bleeding or cramps to hypertension, neurologic disorders, or *thromboembolism* (the blocking of a vein or artery by a blood clot). However, the most unpleasant side effects, such as blood clots and hypertension, usually occur when the woman taking the pill has high blood pressure. Therefore, women with this condition should not take the pill unless under strict medical supervision.

Although there is a danger of circulatory disorders and other side effects from the use of oral contraceptives, many physicians agree that the hazards of pregnancy are a greater threat to possibly millions of women. However, it is advisable for women using the pill to have periodic checkups. This is particularly important for women over 40 and from families with a tendency toward cancer. The Food and Drug Administration has recommended that all women over the age of 40 be made aware of the increased risk to their health of oral contraceptives and that physicians urge them to use other forms of contraception.

The IUD

Once a popular and effective method of contraception, the *intrauterine device*, or IUD, has greatly declined in popularity in the mid-1980s. In part the decline was associated with reports that one kind of IUD, the Dalkon Shield, led to a number of deaths from septic abortions—a massive infection during gestation—as well as to ectopic (tubal) pregnancies and thousands of cases of sterility. By 1986, only one pharmaceutical firm was manufacturing IUDs.

The IUD is a plastic or metal coil that a physician inserts through the cervix into the uterus. To make the insertion, the physician uses a syringelike device. The IUD typically is about an inch and one-half in length, and has an attached thread that hangs down through the cervix. Once the IUD is in place, the wearer checks after each menstrual period to make sure she can feel the thread. If she cannot feel it, the IUD may be out of place or has been expelled and the woman should call her physician.

How It Works

Once it has been inserted, the IUD can usually remain in the uterus indefinitely. It can be removed when the woman wants to become pregnant. The device apparently functions by interfering with the natural implantation of a fertilized egg in the wall of the uterus.

The effectiveness of IUDs has been estimated to be as high as 95 to 96 percent. If pregnancy should occur, or is suspected, while the woman is using an IUD she should see her physician because of the dangers of septic abortion or tubal pregnancy.

Side Effects

Women using the IUD have reported other side effects. Some users experience some cramping or dizziness at the time of insertion. With some women, bleeding, cramps, or backache may continue for a few days. Long-term, more serious side effects include occasional cases of pelvic inflammatory disease (PID), an infection marked by a vaginal discharge that is heavier than normal and by lower abdominal pain, with or without fever and headaches. If not treated, PID can cause sterility and, in rare cases, death.

Very rarely, use of the IUD has led to perforation of the uterus, a serious medical problem calling for immediate treatment. Perforations usually occur at the time of insertion or shortly afterward.

The Vaginal Sponge

The vaginal sponge, another kind of sperm barrier that also contains a spermicide, requires no visit to a physician or clinic. Made of a soft polyurethane that is permeated with nonoxynol-9, the spermicide used in many jellies, creams, gels, and foams, the sponge is inserted manually into the vagina. There it blocks the opening to the cervix and absorbs and traps semen.

How It Works

The sponge has to be dampened with water before insertion. A few tablespoons will do. When damp, it should feel slightly soapy. About the size of a collapsed golf ball, the sponge's sides are folded together, with the removal loop underneath. It is then inserted into the vagina as far as it will go—until it covers the cervix.

The sponge offers protection against conception for 24 hours. No additional spermicide, other than that already contained in the sponge, is necessary. But the sponge has to remain in place for at least six hours after the last act of coitus.

To remove the sponge, the woman hooks a finger into the removal loop or simply pulls the device out with two fingers. A new sponge can be inserted hours before intercourse. Each package of sponges contains detailed, printed instructions. Even though the sponge does not have to be fitted, as does the IUD, many women check with their physicians when first using the contraceptive to make sure they are inserting it properly. Many are also advised to avoid using the sponge during their periods.

Diaphragms and Cervical Caps

The oral contraceptive, the intrauterine contraceptive device, and two kinds of mechanical sperm barriers, the *cervical cap* and *diaphragm*, require a visit to the physician's office or birth control clinic. The diaphragm or cervical cap must be fitted to the size and shape of the female reproductive organs at the opening of the uterus.

How They Work

The main difference between the diaphragm and the cervical cap is that the diaphragm is placed at the back of the vagina in such a way that it serves as a barrier against spermatozoa that would be ejaculated during intercourse. The cervical cap, as the name suggests, is a cap that fits over the cervix to prevent the passage of spermatozoa.

The diaphragm must be coated on both surfaces as well as along the rim with a contraceptive jelly or cream. The soft rubber cup is placed at the back of the vagina and over the cervix before intercourse and should be left in place for at least 6 hours but not more than 16 hours after coitus. When removed, it should be cleaned according to directions and not used again for a period of 6 to 8 hours. Because of changes in weight and other factors, the diaphragm should be refitted at least once every two years. It should be replaced periodically, regardless of changes in size, because, being made of rubber, it does deteriorate with use, and the flaws are not always obvious to the naked eye.

A cervical cap may be made of rubber, plastic, or metal. It is carefully fitted over the cervix by a physician. During use, it is filled with contraceptive cream or jelly. The metal variety can be left in place from the end of one menstrual period to the beginning of the next, but other types should not remain in place for more than 24 hours. The cervical cap should be checked from time to time, because it can slip out of position during intercourse.

Condoms

Among birth control devices that do not require a visit to a physician is the *condom,* usually made of soft rubber and shaped to fit as a sheath over the penis. They are inexpensive and are the preferred method of contraception for many couples because they require the least advance preparation of all the methods except the oral contraceptive and the IUD.

Although condoms manufactured in the United States for the past 35 years have been subjected to quality control tests and are checked by federal inspectors, they are not immune to failure. For this reason, many women insert a spermicidal jelly or cream in the vagina when the man uses a condom.

The condom frequently is used by newlyweds as a birth control device while the wife waits to be fitted with a diaphragm after the first weeks of marriage. It also permits intercourse when one of the partners has an infectious disease affecting the genitals.

Because the condom dulls the sensation of intercourse somewhat, it is recommended for men who experience premature ejaculation. On the other hand, some men object to the lessened coital sensation associated with the wearing of a condom.

The Rhythm Method

In the *rhythm method,* the couple schedules intercourse before or after ovulation. In order for this method to be effective, a woman must keep extremely accurate charts of her basal temperature with a basal body thermometer in order to determine exactly when she ovulates. One problem with the rhythm method is that few women, especially newly married, have had experience keeping careful records of this kind and often misinterpret the results without a physician's counsel. About one in five women simply does not have regular menstrual cycles, which is the key to avoiding days of peak fertility.

Spermicides

Spermicides in the form of jellies, creams, foaming tablets, gels, aerosol foams, and suppositories are available in nearly any drugstore and can be obtained without prescription. The chemical substances are inserted with special applicators and form a film over the vaginal lining. The tablets and suppositories melt inside the vagina to spread a film over the lining.

The main objection to the use of chemical contraceptives is that coitus must take place within an hour after the substances are applied. When tablets are used, up to 15 minutes must elapse before coitus can begin. Generally, the chemicals should remain in the vagina for at least six hours after intercourse. If coitus is repeated during that period, another dose of chemicals must be inserted in advance.

Coitus Interruptus and Douching

Two of the least reliable birth control methods are *coitus interruptus* and *douching*. Coitus interruptus requires that the man withdraw his penis from the vagina before ejaculation. If carried out to its ideal conclusion, the technique requires a lot of self-control and split-second timing. Ejaculation is triggered by an automatic nerve reflex after the seminal vesicles are filled with semen; once the message gets through the nervous system,

there is little the man can do to prevent ejaculation. Needless to say, the coitus interruptus technique has a high rate of failure. Beyond that, it is psychologically bad because it places undue anxiety on both partners during coitus.

Douching with water or special solutions works on occasion, but it is rated only as better than no birth control method at all. The douching, or flushing, of the vagina seems to have some effect in that it reduces the number of spermatozoa in the female reproductive system. Water alone is sufficient to kill sperm, although special preparations are available. The important factor with a douche is timing. The douche must be used immediately after intercourse, because spermatozoa can be moving through the cervix within a couple of minutes after ejaculation and are normally able to reach the Fallopian tubes within 45 minutes.

Sterilization

About ten percent of the married couples in the United States have chosen to have one of the partners sterilized as a permanent form of contraception. A rather quick and simple operation called a *vasectomy,* performed on the male, has become increasingly common in recent years. A vasectomy consists of the removal of a portion of the *vas deferens,* or sperm ducts, thus preventing semen from reaching the seminal vesicles, where it would ordinarily be discharged during intercourse. A vasectomy can be performed in a physician's office with no more than a day or two lost from work.

The operation to sterilize a female is more involved; the abdomen is opened and the Fallopian tubes are cut or tied. A general anesthetic is employed and the operation is performed in a hospital. It is a safe and

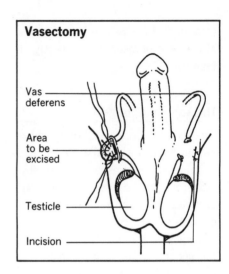

Vasectomy

Vas deferens

Area to be excised

Testicle

Incision

almost bloodless operation requiring hospitalization for only a few days. One variation of this procedure utilizes a *peritoneoscope* (or *laparoscope*) for viewing the Fallopian tubes through a small incision below the navel while the tubes are cut through a second incision. With this method the average hospital stay is reduced to one or two days.

The problem with sterilization is that it is generally not reversible. It does not interfere with sex activity once the patient has recovered, but if the couple decides later to have more children, or if the sterilized partner remarries and wants to have children, the odds are against success in patching together the Fallopian tubes or the sperm ducts so that normal reproductive function can be restored.

Research on Other Methods

There are other birth control methods in the research and testing stage, such as oral contraceptives for men, morning-after contraceptives, and once-a-month shots. Eventually, some scientists speculate, foods in the supermarket will be treated with harmless substances that prevent conception. They will be similar to the iodine in iodized salt or the vitamin D added to homogenized milk. When the wife wants a baby, she will merely change the menu for a few days to exclude birth control foods or switch to the foods in a special grocery store.

The Working Mother

A woman's place is in the home—and in the office, laboratory, factory, classroom, and almost any other place where she is qualified to fill a position. The woman must, of course, receive pay for her work and talents and have the right to fulfill her professional goals. Since World War II, when women took over assembly lines and women in uniform released military men from office tasks, the working mother has generally been an integral part of the modern social scene. Because they want to work, and find satisfaction and fulfillment in working part-time or full-time, women have, according to experts, found ways to function successfully in both the workplace and the home.

Agreement on Priorities

Managing a home and a job and trying to raise a family at the same time can be a frenzied routine beset with tension and emotional strain. The strain is frequently related to the priorities a working wife and mother assigns to her various responsibilities. If the family really cannot subsist adequately on the husband's income, most women can devote a considerable amount of time to an outside job without feeling they are neglecting other duties. Also, mothers who pursue a career for the sake of self-fulfillment have probably calculated the assorted risks and feel little or no anguish about the goals they have chosen.

The women most likely to suffer are the ones who believe that total, full-time devotion to home and family is necessary. These women may have intense guilt feelings if they take an outside job in order to improve the standard of living in the home.

The decision of a mother to take on a full- or part-time job should be based on mutual understanding and a thorough discussion between husband and wife. It is most important that both husband and wife realize each other's feelings and the changes a job can bring about. For example, the husband should realize that if his wife agrees to remain at home despite her desire to get a job, her frustrations will undoubtedly be transmitted to her children. He must also realize that if the couple cannot afford the services of a maid to help with the housework, he himself must help with the housework or care of the children.

On the other hand, the wife must realize that her husband's position may require him to work occasional evenings—at which time he cannot also help her with housework—and that she may have to entertain clients or other people for him, even on days when she has worked a full day and is tired. The important thing is to weigh all aspects of the problem and base the decision on whatever brings the most satisfaction to everyone concerned. When both husband and wife are satisfied with the home-and-job decision, the children will be in a more secure position, regardless of which choice was made.

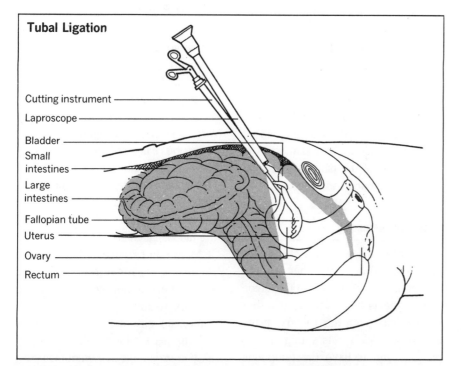

Tubal Ligation

Cutting instrument

Laproscope

Bladder

Small intestines

Large intestines

Fallopian tube

Uterus

Ovary

Rectum

Age of Children

The age of the children should also be considered. Although many experts feel that the mother should postpone working outside the home if possible until the children are about six years of age, others maintain that this is not necessary if the children are well cared for in her absence and are given ample love and attention by both parents. A child of six or younger is particularly vulnerable, and his emotional needs must be served just as completely as are his physical needs.

Parents' Division of Labor

The roles of both parents are often subjected to revisions and modifications in a family where both parents work. The father usually assumes more responsibility for the care of a child at the end of a workday, while the working mother gets dinner ready. This may actually enable father and child to know one another more intimately and may also result in the father's feeling more sympathy and understanding toward the problems involved in child care.

Limitations on the Mother's Time

One recent study revealed that working mothers spend an average of 34 hours a week at housework, compared to about 56 hours a week for mothers who stay at home. Because the 34 hours are in addition to the time spent on her job plus commuting time, the working mother obviously has little time for recreation or community activities.

However, many women drive themselves to exhaustion by trying to prove they can hold a job and be perfect housekeepers and community leaders. The working mother must be able to accept limitations and decide what is most important; otherwise, she may feel guilty and insecure as well as continually tired. At some point the couple might consider alternatives; perhaps the mother should give up all extracurricular activities in favor of a career, or she might drop out of the work force for a few years, resume community activities, and return to work when the children are old enough to be more self-sufficient.

She also might consider a part-time job until the children are older. Even when the children are in the early years of grammar school, the mother may want to find employment that allows her to be at home when they are dismissed from class in the afternoon.

Economic and Other Factors

If economic factors are the prime mo-

tive for the mother's outside job, her take-home pay should be considerably greater than the costs of a baby-sitter, maid, or housekeeper, nursery school or day-care center, clothing needed for the job, transportation, lunches, and so on. The economics of the situation may be complex. For example, the couple may decide that even though the wife's earnings are not that sizable to begin with, she will be a far better wage earner in the long run if she continues working now rather than tries to return to a career at some later date when her skills will be rusty or completely outdated. Besides, economic considerations are not the only criteria; the woman's emotional needs to be productive or challenged intellectually must also be considered.

Care of the Child

The baby-sitter must be a person responsible enough to assume the role of the parents in their absence, although the sitter does not have the authority to treat the child as she might her own. Because of the many gray areas, such as whether the sitter is authorized to punish the child, some firm ground rules should be established by the parents before the sitter begins work. Even if the sitter is a close relative, such as a grandmother or aunt of the child, there should be an understanding about what the child can and cannot do in the absence of the parents and what the sitter can and cannot do.

Teenage Sitters

If the sitter is a teenager, she should be instructed as to whether she can let her friends visit her at the home where she is baby-sitting, whether she can chat with her friends on the telephone while she is sitting, and so on. She should have the telephone

numbers where the parents can be reached if a problem arises, as well as the telephone numbers of doctors, friends, and neighbors who could assist in an emergency.

Usually, the main job of the baby-sitter is the safety and welfare of the child. But when a sitter is expected to spend as much as a full working day with a child, five days a week, parents should try to find a sitter who is emotionally compatible with the child and can provide warmth and companionship, particularly for the preschool-aged child.

If the sitter is a close relative, she probably will know all about changing diapers, bottle feeding, minor first aid for bumps and bruises, and so on. A teenager, however, may not be experienced in these areas. Just because she has never changed a diaper doesn't mean the girl is unqualified for the job of sitter. But the parents should learn in advance how experienced the sitter is. She may need only a brief lesson in formula preparation or diaper changing to make the grade.

Nursery Schools

There are good nursery schools and not-so-good nursery schools, as well as children who do and those who do not benefit from a nursery school experience. The facilities should supplement rather than substitute for home care of a child. Although the child may at first be reluctant to leave his home, he should be mature enough to spend part of each day away from home. The staff, physical setting, and equipment should be appropriate for the needs of the individual child.

Many states have strict licensing requirements for nursery schools, while others do not, so it is up to the parents to investigate thoroughly. Under no circumstances should a child be parked for the day in any facility in order to solve emotional conflicts of the child or the parents or because it is cheaper than others.

Nursery school can be a rewarding and enriching experience for the preschool youngster. Perhaps the most important purpose of nursery school is the opportunity it provides for children to experience peer relationships. This is particularly necessary if children lack frequent opportunities to play with other children. For most preschoolers, nursery school is the first time they experience a group situation, and what they learn in nursery school in terms of cooperation with others prepares them for the dynamics of the more formal learning situations to come.

The programs for nursery school children may include excursions, exposure to music, story books, creative work with clay and paints, and organized games. It is wise to investigate several schools in terms of staff, facilities, and professional standards before making a decision.

Parental Responsibilities

Parents who are separated from their children because of the demands of their jobs should not abdicate their responsibilities as mother and father either to baby-sitters or nursery school staff members.

Need for Strong Father

The father, particularly, must not avoid his responsibilities in the child-raising department. Too often in the past the father made himself unavailable for guidance by telling a child to "ask your mother," when what the youngster wanted was a decision from the father. The trend in recent years for the father to assume a greater share of the responsibility for the children is a wholesome one. Families need a male authority who can command the respect of the children, but the father cannot expect to have much of a voice in family affairs if he passes the responsibility to the mother.

Agreement on Discipline

Many children learn at an early age that they can play the parents against each other to gain their objectives. If the father continually tells a child to ask his mother for a decision, the youngster may learn to work the game into a "yes" from the mother whenever he wants his own way. This should not be interpreted to mean that the father should be harsh or stern, but rather that he be actively concerned and involved in all phases of his child's growth, particularly in guiding his behavior.

If parents cannot agree on a course of discipline, the effect on a child can be as bad as no direction at all. In such a home the growing child has difficulty in learning to discipline himself because of uncertainty as to whom to model himself after. Although the female influence in child raising may seem more immediate because it is the mother who nurtures the baby during his first few months, growing children need two loving and attentive parents to give them support and provide them with behavioral models.

For more information on child care and parental responsibilities, see the "Alphabetic Guide to Child Care" in Ch. 2, *The First Dozen Years*.

5

The Middle Years

Maintaining good health over the years is far simpler, less expensive, and more comfortable than restoring health that has become poor. Because some diseases cannot be cured after they are contracted, it is only logical to try to prevent all possible health problems. The techniques of modern preventive medicine are available to Americans of every age.

All people are not beautiful or handsome, but nearly everyone can have the kind of attractiveness and vitality that comes from good health. The health of an individual depends upon the kind of body he inherits and the care he gives it. Good health can be thought of as a state of social, physical, and mental well-being, a goal virtually everybody can attain—if the responsibility for maintaining one's own health, with occasional help from the health experts, is accepted.

Keeping Fit

Physical Changes

Physically, middle age should be a pleasant plateau—a time to look back on a vigorous youth, enjoy an active present, and prepare for a ripe old age.

Middle age should not be measured by chronological age but by biological age, the condition of various parts of the body. You might say that the middle-aged body is like a car that has been driven a certain number of miles. It should be well broken in and running smoothly, but with plenty of reserve power for emergencies, and lots of mileage left.

Biological age should be measured by the state of the heart, arteries, and other essential organs, the length of life and comparative health of parents and grandparents, temperament and outlook on life, and outward appearance. The way you have fed or treated yourself is important. Eating the wrong kinds of food, being overweight, smoking too much, or worrying too much can add years to biological age.

However, no one should be surprised if he is not in quite the shape he was when he was 25 or 30 years old. At age 40 to 50 it is perfectly normal to have only 80 percent of the maximum breathing capacity, 85 percent of the resting cardiac output, 95 percent of the total body water, and 96 percent of the basal metabolic rate. These factors, however, should not slow anyone down very much.

There is one difference, though, that can be anticipated in middle age. Reaction time and decision-making processes may be a bit slower. This is because the nervous system is one of the most vulnerable to aging. The cells of the central nervous system begin to die early in life and are not replaced, while other organs are still growing and producing new cells. Specific response to input is delayed because it takes a greater length of time for an impulse to travel across the connections linking nerve fibers.

Thus, though you may function as usual under normal conditions, you may find it a little harder to respond to physical or emotional stress. However, if you have followed a sound health maintenance program, including good nutrition, enough mental and physical exercise and rest, and moderate living habits, you should respond to unusual physiological or emotional stress quite adequately.

The Importance of Checkups

Physical disabilities associated with

chronic disease increase sharply with age, starting with the middle years. While more than half (54 percent) of the 86 million persons who have one or more chronic conditions are under age 45, the prevalence of disability from illness is greatest in the 45 and older age group. Of those under 45 who have chronic conditions, only 14 percent are limited in activity as compared with almost 30 percent of the 45 to 64 age group. And only 1 percent of those under 45 with chronic illness are completely disabled, as compared with 4 percent in the 45 to 64 age group.

These figures suggest that it is wise to have an annual checkup so that any disease process or condition can be nipped in the bud. Further evidence of the value of medical checkups comes from the Aetna Life Insurance Company, which compared two groups of policyholders over a five-year period. Those who did not have checkups and health counseling had a death rate 44 percent higher than the group who did. Regular checkups will not only help prolong life, they will also help you to live it more comfortably.

Here are some other good reasons for having a physical checkup:

- If an organ has been attacked by serious disease in youth, it may deteriorate at an early adult age.

- Heredity may play an important role in determining the speed at which various organs age. If your parents and grandparents had arteriosclerosis, there is a chance you might develop this condition in your middle years.

- Your environment (smog, poor climate, etc.) might affect the rate at which your body ages, particularly the skin.

- Individual stresses and strains or abuses or overuse (of alcohol, for example) may create a health problem in middle age.

- The endocrine glands (pituitary, thyroid, parathyroids, adrenals, ovaries, testicles) play important roles in aging. Serious disease of one or more of these glands may lead to premature aging of an organ dependent upon its secretions.

- At middle age you are more likely to be beset by emotional strains at work or at home that could make you an early candidate for heart disease, arteriosclerosis, and other degenerative disorders.

- The earlier a chronic disease is detected, the better the chance that it can be arrested before permanent damage is done. This is especially true in the case of glaucoma, diabetes, heart disease, cancer of the lung or breast or other cancers—all of which could have their onset in middle age.

To help detect disease and other debilitating conditions, many physicians utilize automated medical screening, which combines medical history with selected physiological measurements and laboratory tests to give the physician a complete health profile of the patient. This profile should indicate the probability of any chronic condition, which the physician could then pinpoint with more thorough tests.

Also, annual checkups enable the physician to observe changes taking place over a period of time. For example, he is able to observe gradually changing blood chemistry levels or a progressive increase in eye pressure that could signal the onset of disease.

Don't Try To Be Your Own Physician

A panel of medical specialists from the University of California at Los Angeles recently found that many men of 40 years and older were dosing themselves with unnecessary pills and "conserving" their energy by increasing bed rest to the point that it actually became enervating.

These physicians point out that increasing dependence on pills can be harmful as well as expensive. Laxatives are a good example of a popular commercial medicine taken unnecessarily by large numbers of people. Perhaps only one person in 100,000 may have an actual motor disability of the bowels, and most constipation can be easily corrected through proper foods and exercise, without resorting to laxatives. Also, taking vitamin pills or avoiding all high-cholesterol foods is unnecessary—unless recommended by a physician.

But, most important, "conserving" energy through prolonged bed rest or avoiding exercise can be fatal. The panel members pointed out that before age 40, a person exercises to improve his performance, but that after age 40 he exercises to improve his chances of survival.

Physical Fitness and Exercise

In middle age most of us stop performing most forms of exercise other than those that we enjoy doing. In other words, we find it easier to bend an elbow than lift weights. This is unfortunate, because in middle age most of us need regular exercise to maintain both mental and physical fitness and to increase endurance, strength, and agility.

As noted earlier, in middle age there is some decrease in breathing capacity, cardiac output, and metabolic rate; yet exercise can improve these functions. The more often the normal heart and circulatory system are required to move blood to active regions of the body through exercise or movement, the more efficient they become. Protracted exercise also improves the work of the lungs by increasing their ability to expand more fully, take in more air, and utilize a greater proportion of the oxygen in the inhaled air.

While exercise alone cannot eliminate obesity, it can help prevent it by improving digestion and bowel movements and by burning up excess calories. Exercise can also make you feel, look, and think better. Some traditional formal exercises, however, like touching the toes while keeping your knees stiff, or doing deep knee bends, are potentially harmful in middle age; they put too much stress on weak parts of the back and legs.

Despite protests about not having enough time, everyone has time to exercise, particularly if it is worked into the daily routine—for example, walking instead of riding to the train, office, store, or bus stop. You might find you'll get there faster, especially in traffic-clogged metropolitan areas, and you'll save money as well. More important, those minutes of "stolen" exercise accrue over the years in the form of improved health.

Sports and Games

If you don't like formal exercise, you can get exercise informally—through a favorite sport, whether it be golf, tennis, swimming, jogging, skiing, cycling, or whatever. Many sports and games are stop-and-go activities that do not provide helpful, rhythmic exercise, but here's how you can make them more beneficial.

Golf

Instead of riding in a golf cart between shots, walk—in fact, stride vigorously, lifting your head and chest. And don't make golf a cut-throat competition or business pursuit. Relax and enjoy it—count your blessings rather than your bogeys.

Tennis

Like golf, tennis can be a cut-throat competitive sport or a pleasant pursuit. If it's played with muscles tied in knots from nervous tension, it will not provide any fun or healthful exercise. Also, players over 30 are well-advised to play more doubles than singles and to avoid exhausting themselves in the heat of competition.

Swimming

Along with fast walking and jogging, swimming is one of the best all-around exercises. When swimming, most of the muscles are exercised and lung capacity and cardiac output are improved. The exercise potential can be increased by doing pull-ups with the diving board or ladder and by bobbing up and down in the water.

Jogging

This popular sport can be combined with walking, done in a group or alone, either outdoors or indoors, and alternated with other exercises. Moreover, it doesn't require any special equipment and has been recognized by fitness experts as one of the best exercises for the heart and circulation. However, it is wise to get your physician's advice and approval before embarking on a jogging program.

Skiing

Skiing is healthful as well as fun. You can get in shape for skiing and improve your ability by jogging and by practicing some of the techniques needed in skiing—such as the rhythmic left-right-left-right twist of foot, knee, and leg in short turns. To do this exercise, stand up straight with your feet quite close together and flex your knees forward so that the weight goes onto the balls of the feet. Now, arms apart for balance, twist your feet and knees to the left without twisting your upper body. As you do this, try the modified half-bends of the traversing position that all ski schools teach. Then reverse the position to the right, and keep repeating.

Other Sports

Other worthwhile sports for healthful exercise include badminton, bicycling, canoeing, rowing, table tennis, skating, and squash. However, they should be sustained for at least 30 minutes at a time, ideally four times a week, and should be combined with supplemental exercises.

A Word of Warning

Everyone should beware of becoming a weekend athlete and punishing himself with an overdose of exercise or sports only on weekends. It makes as much sense as stuffing yourself on weekends and starving the rest of the week. It's far more sensible—and healthful—to engage in sports activities for an hour or so at a time on a daily basis.

Exercises

Participating in sports activities is not the only way to keep fit. Special exercises can help reduce tension and build muscles. For instance, one way to relax is to do rhythmic exercises, particularly for the trunk, that help to improve circulation. You can also try exercises that will relieve tense muscles and improve breathing. The exercises described below were developed by Dr. Josephine L. Rathbone of Columbia University.

Breathing to Relax

Lie on your back on the floor with knees bent and feet resting on the floor. Take a deep breath, letting both the abdominal wall and chest rise. Hold the air for a few seconds, then expel it through your mouth with a gasp. Repeat four or five times at regular intervals.

For Tense Arms

Standing erectly, swing both arms forward, then to the side, letting them drop during the swings so that your hands brush your thighs with each motion. Keep your shoulders low. Repeat a few times. Then, sit on the edge of a chair and clench one hand tightly. Swing your arm vigorously in large circles, keeping your hand clenched. Then repeat with other arm.

For Tense Legs

Sit on the edge of a table with lower legs hanging free. Then, alternately, swing them backward and forward. Try to keep your legs moving in rhythm.

For Stomach Tension

Kneel with your feet under your hips and swing your trunk down to one side and around, sweeping your arms in a wide circle, coming up again on the opposite side. Or stand with your hips supported against the wall, feet apart and a few inches from the wall. Bend your body forward, arms drooping, and let your body sway from side to side, with your arms and head loose.

Relaxing at Work or Home

Relieve tension while sitting by holding the spine erect, shoulders low. Turn your head so that the chin touches first one collarbone, then the other. Move slowly and rhythmically.

Yoga

You can also relax and become revitalized through various Yoga exercises. Courses are taught at many recreational centers. Some of the exercises require only a minimum of time, and can be done not only before and after the workday but in the office during the lunch hour.

Isometrics

Isometric exercises—pitting one muscle against another without moving—can also be practiced at odd moments. These exercises should, however, be done only by healthy persons, and not by anyone with a cardiac problem. To strengthen arm and shoulder muscles through isometrics, put the fist of one hand against the palm of the other and push without moving. Or push up with your arms from a chair or the edge of a table. Strengthen arm and neck muscles by grasping the back of the neck with laced fingers and pulling forward—again, without movement.

All of the above exercises and sports can put you on the road to physical fitness. Just remember, whatever form of exercise or sport you choose, make it fun and do not strain yourself unduly.

Rest and Sleep

Rest and sleep adequate for one's personal needs are another vital component of good health and good appearance. They also influence human relationships and mental alertness. Scientists believe that during sleep the body replaces tissue cells and eliminates waste products created by fatigue at a faster rate than when awake.

Sleep also rests the heart and blood system, because heart muscle contractions and blood pressure are slower then. Excessive fatigue from lack of sleep increases susceptibility to a number of ailments, including the common cold. If an individual gets an adequate amount of sleep (usually seven to eight hours for an adult), he will feel ready to meet the day's activities. If not, his memory may not be sharp, and he may be irritable because his nervous system has had inadequate rest.

A quiet, dark, ventilated room, a fairly firm mattress, and performance of a moderate amount of exercise during the day will aid sleep. When worry, frustration, or anxiety make it difficult to sleep, a conscious attempt to relax will help. Sedatives or sleeping pills should not be taken unless they are prescribed or recommended by a physician.

Personal Hygiene

Disease germs can enter the body only in a limited number of ways. One of the major ways is through the skin. The skin is a protective covering which, when broken, can admit harmful bacteria or viruses easily.

Simple precautions are very effective. The hands come into contact with disease germs more than any other part of the body. Therefore, they should be washed whenever they are dirty, prior to preparing food or eating, and after using the lavatory.

The rest of the body must also be kept clean, because adequate bodily cleanliness will remove substances that, by irritating the skin, make it more susceptible to infection. Bathing also improves the muscle tone of the skin. Hair should also be washed frequently enough to prevent accumulation of dust and dead skin cells.

Openings in the body are also paths by which disease germs can enter the body. The nose and ears should be carefully cleaned only with something soft, for instance, a cotton swab. Genital orifices should be kept clean by frequent bathing. Any unusual discharge from a body opening should be promptly reported to a physician. The problem can then be treated at its earliest stage—the easiest time to solve the problem.

Personal hygiene includes care of the nails. They should always be kept clean and fairly short. Hangnails can be avoided by gently pushing back the cuticle with a towel after washing the hands.

Care of the Feet

"My feet are killing me!" is a complaint heard more frequently in middle age, especially from women. The devil in this case usually takes the shape of fashionable shoes, where the foot is frequently squeezed into shapes and positions it was never designed to tolerate. Particularly unhealthy for the foot was the formerly fashionable spike heel and pointed toe.

Any heel two inches or higher will force the full weight of the body onto the smaller bones in the front of the foot and squeeze the toes into the forepart of the shoes. This hurts the arch, causes calluses on the sole of the foot, and can lead to various bone deformities.

The major solution to this problem is to buy good shoes that really fit. The shoes should be moderately broad across the instep, have a straight inner border, and a moderately low heel. To fit properly, shoes should extend one-half inch to three-fourths inch beyond the longest toe.

Avoid wearing shoes that have no support; also, avoid wearing high heels for long periods of time. Extremely high heels worn constantly force the foot forward and upset body balance. Changing heel height several times a day will rest the feet and give the muscles in the back of the legs a chance to return to their normal position. It's highly desirable to wear different shoes each day, or at least alternate two pairs. This gives the shoes a chance to dry out completely. Dust shoes with a mild powder when removed.

Shoes should not be bought in the morning. They should be tried on near the end of the day, when the feet have broadened from standing and walking, and tightness or rubbing can be more easily detected.

As to hosiery, socks and stockings should extend a half-inch beyond the longest toe. Stretch socks are fine in many cases, but plain wool or cotton socks help if your feet perspire a lot.

Foot Exercises

Exercise your feet by trying these simple steps recommended by leading podiatrists:

- Extend the toes and flex rapidly for a minute or two. Rotate the feet in circles at the ankles. Try picking up a marble or pencil with your toes; this will give them agility and strength.

- Stand on a book with your toes extended over the edge. Then curl your toes down as far as possible, grasping the cover.

- After an unusually active day, refresh the feet with an alcohol rub. Follow this with a foot massage, squeezing the feet between your hands. When you are tired, rest with your feet up. Try lying down for about a half-hour with your feet higher than your head, using pillows to prop up your legs.

- Walk barefoot on uneven sandy beaches and thick grass. This limbers up the feet and makes the toes work. Walking anywhere is one of the best exercises for the feet if you learn to walk properly and cultivate good posture. Keep toes pointed ahead, and lift rather than push the foot, letting it come down flat on the ground, placing little weight on the heel. Your toes will come alive, and your feet will become more active.

Foot Ailments

Doing foot exercises is particularly important in middle age, because the foot is especially vulnerable to the following problems.

Bunions

A bunion is a thickening and swelling of the big joint of the big toe, forcing it toward the other toes. There is also a protuberance on the inner side of the foot. Unless treated, this condition usually gets progressively worse. Surgery is not always necessary or successful. Often, special shoes to fit the deformed foot must be worn.

Stiff Toe

People suffering from this problem find that the big joint of the big toe becomes painful and stiff, possibly due to a major accident or repeated minor trauma. This condition usually corrects itself if the joint is protected for a few weeks, usually by a small steel plate within the sole of the shoe.

Hammer Toe

This clawlike deformity is usually

caused by cramping the toes with too small shoes. The pressure can be eased with padding and, in some cases, the deformity can be corrected by surgery.

Ingrown Toenail

Cutting the nail short and wearing shoes that are too tight are major causes of ingrown toenails; the edge of the nail of the toe—usually the big toe—is forced into the soft outer tissues. In some cases the tissues can be peeled back after soaking the foot in hot water, and the offending part of the nail can be removed. To prevent ingrown toenails, the nails should be kept carefully trimmed and cut straight across the nail rather than trimmed into curves at the corners. For severe or chronic cases of ingrown toenails it is best to seek professional treatment.

Morton's Toe

This is the common name for a form of *metatarsalgia,* a painful inflammation of a sheath of small nerves that pass between the toes near the ball of the foot. The ailment is most likely to occur in an area between the third and fourth toe, counting from the large toe, and usually is due to irritation produced by pressure that makes the toes rub against each other. In most instances, the pressure results from wearing improperly fitted shoes, shoes with pointed toes, or high heel shoes, which restrict normal flexing of the metatarsals (the bones at the base of the toes) while walking.

Temporary relief usually is possible through removal of the shoes and massaging of the toes, or by application of moist, warm heat to the afflicted area. In cases of very severe pain, a doctor may inject a local an-esthetic into the foot. Additional relief sometimes can be obtained by wearing metatarsal arch supports in the shoes. However, continued irritation of the nerves can result in the growth of a tumor that may require surgical removal.

Care of the Teeth

An attractive smile is often the first thing that one notices about others. In addition to creating an attractive appearance, healthy teeth and gums are a basic requirement for good overall health. One cannot have a healthy body without a healthy mouth, and vice versa. The dentist should be visited at whatever intervals he recommends, usually every six months.

Neglect of oral hygiene and the forgoing of dental checkups are commonplace in the middle years. An often-heard excuse is that the eventual loss of teeth is inevitable. Years ago, loss of teeth really was unavoidable. Today, however, thanks to modern dental practices, it is possible for nearly everyone to enjoy the benefits of natural teeth for a lifetime.

Problems of Aging

When the human body reaches middle age, a number of problems and conditions that are the result of advancing years begin to make themselves felt. These include wrinkling of the skin, baldness, varicose veins, menopause and the male climacteric, and the body's decreased ability to deal with nicotine, caffeine, alcohol, and excess calories.

Skin

The skin usually starts to show its age in the mid to late 30s. At that time it starts to lose its elasticity and flexi-bility, and becomes somewhat thinner. Little lines—not yet wrinkles—start to show up, usually crow's feet around the eyes.

Wrinkling takes place at different times with different people, and sometimes in different areas of the skin. Heredity may play a part. For instance, one family may have the trait of wrinkling around the mouth rather than the eyes. In another family, wrinkling or crow's feet may start early and then stop.

Treatment for Wrinkles

While wrinkles do not hurt, many people want to do something about them. Experienced physicians and dermatologists have a number of techniques for removing or minimizing wrinkles. One accepted method is *dermabrasion,* or planing of the skin. The physician sprays on a local anesthetic, then scrapes the skin with a motor-driven wire brush or some other abrasive tool. The treatment usually takes one session, and no hospital stay is required. There will be some swelling and scab formation, but this should clear up in a week to ten days.

Another method is called *cryotherapy,* in which the physician freezes the skin with carbon dioxide. This induces peeling, which improves the appearance of flat acne scars and shallow wrinkles.

Still another procedure involves the application of chemicals, which are neutralized when they have obtained the desired action.

Skin Texture Change

Besides wrinkling, the skin has a tendency in some people to become thinner, leathery, and darkened as they move towards the 40s and 50s. This effect can be minimized if the skin is toned up with cold cream and other emollients that provide the moisture and oil the skin needs. Also, overexposure to the sun—one of the prime agers of the skin—should be avoided.

In fact, most physicians feel that the sun is a lethal agent, and that exposing the face to too much sun is like putting it in a hot oven. Many say that the sun destroys some inherent good qualities of facial skin, and ruins any chance of improving the appearance through cosmetic surgery.

Cosmetic Surgery

Cosmetic surgery for both men and women is becoming increasingly popular and sophisticated. Cosmetic surgery procedures include *rhinoplasty* (nose); *facial plasty* or *rhytidoplasty* (face lift); *blepharoplasty* (upper eyelids and bags under the eyes); breast augmentation and reduction; as well as the dermabrasion and other methods mentioned earlier. See "Plastic and Cosmetic Surgery" in Ch. 20, *Surgery.*

Baldness

The problem of baldness has its roots in ancient history. Men were worried about baldness 4,000 years ago. But until recently, medical opinion agreed largely with the statement by Dr. Eugene Van Scott, head of the Dermatology Service of the National Cancer Institute: "Baldness is caused by three factors: Sex, age, and heredity. And we can't do a thing about any of these."

Other causes of male baldness include infections, systemic diseases, drugs that have a toxic effect, mechanical stress, friction, and radiation. Diet does not usually affect baldness, but chronic starvation or vitamin deficiencies can contribute to dryness, lack of luster, and hair loss. Also, ex-

cessive intake of vitamin A can cause hair loss.

In women, loss of hair is quite common toward the end of pregnancy, after delivery, and during menopause. A hysterectomy, crash dieting, severe emotional stress, high fever, a major illness such as thyroid disease or diabetes, certain allergies, and the use of systemic drugs such as steroids and amphetamines—all can produce hair loss.

There are two common types of baldness in men: male pattern baldness (*alopecia*) and patchy baldness (*alopecia areata*). The latter is more common in women.

Male Baldness

Male pattern baldness may begin as early as the early 20s or 30s. Hair

falls out from the crown until a fringe of hair remains at the sides and along the back of the head. At the onset, a bald spot may appear on the crown of the head; balding spots in other areas may merge to form the fringe pattern.

In patchy baldness, hair may fall out suddenly in patches. In this case, hair usually returns after going through three growth periods. The new hair may be thinner than the original hair. Although patchy baldness is self-limiting and often self-curing, therapy is indicated for some patients. The therapy may consist of injections of soluble steroid suspensions directly into the scalp. Regrowth may begin in three to four weeks, but remains localized at the sites of injections.

Hair transplants remain the most dependable way to grow new hair—especially in men with male pattern baldness. The process involves cut-

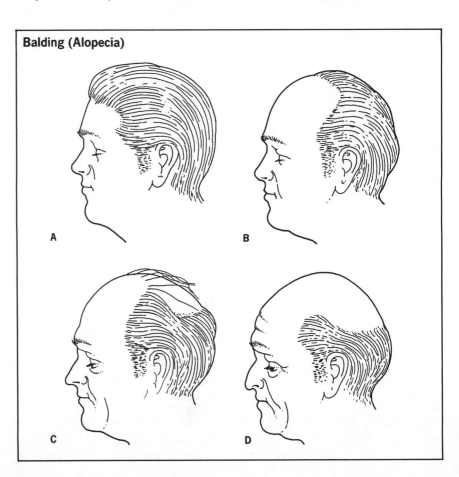

Balding (Alopecia)

A   B   C   D

ting out *punch grafts,* small patches or plugs of hair and follicle-bearing tissue, from the back or sides of the head. The grafts are immediately inserted into recipient incisions that are slightly smaller than the plugs. In a two- or three-hour session a physician can transplant 60 to 80 plugs of hair. Adequate coverage of a balding crown usually requires 200 to 400 plugs.

Female Baldness

The hair on the crown of a woman's head may thin out, but women seldom become bald as men do. Progesterone, administered in careful, dose-regulated treatments, has been used successfully by some dermatologists. The progesterone is applied to the scalp as a cream or ointment.

Drug Treatments

Other forms of therapy have come into experimental use for both men and women. Many of them involve the use of drugs. In one treatment carefully monitored doses of cortisone are injected into the scalp. In another, the drug psoralen may either be applied to the scalp directly or taken internally. A combination of drugs including 8-methoxypsoralen and inosiplex may be used in conjunction with ultraviolet irradiation.

Most acclaimed of all the new drug therapies is minoxidil, a derivative of the blood pressure-reducing drug Loniten. Physicians simply order Loniten reformulated as a topical solution. Thicker than water, the minoxidil has been used generally by prescription as a gel. Visible improvement is never guaranteed, and in most cases results can take from four months to a year.

Minoxidil must be prescribed by a physician and requires medical monitoring about every four months. It must be used indefinitely to maintain new hair growth. Early findings suggest that the drug works best on men who have not been bald for a long time. Some dermatologists believe that patients with minoxidil-generated growths of hair can gradually, over time, switch to low-dose, modified use patterns.

Excess Hair

For some middle-aged women, the problem is too much hair in the wrong place, instead of too little. Excess hair can grow on the face, chest, arms, and legs. In some instances, unwanted hair may be a sign of an endocrine disorder that can be detected by a physician. In other cases, it can be caused by chronic irritation, such as prolonged use of a cast, bandage, or hot-water bottle; it can also be due to excess exposure to the sun, iodine or mercury irritation, or localized rubbing.

Excess hair can be bleached, shaved, tweezed, waxed, or removed by chemical depilatories and electrolysis. Only electrolysis is permanent. See "Hair Removal" in Ch. 21, *Skin and Hair.*

Varicose Veins

Another complaint of middle-aged men and women is *varicose veins.* About half the women over 50 years of age have these enlarged veins with damaged valves in their thighs and calves.

Varicose veins are usually caused by years of downward pressure on the veins, causing the valves to break down. This often happens to people who must stand for many hours at a time. The large, bluish irregularities are plainly visible beneath the skin of the thighs and calves, and they cause a heavy dragging sensation in the legs and a general feeling of tiredness and lack of energy.

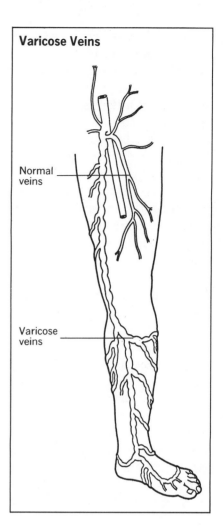

Varicose Veins

Normal veins

Varicose veins

Treatment

In most instances, the best treatment involves surgery to tie off the main veins and remove all superficial veins that lend themselves to this procedure (called *stripping*). In other cases, varicose veins can be relieved by wearing elastic stockings or compression bandages.

Varicose veins that remain untreated can cause *varicose ulcers,* which usually form on the inner side of the leg above the ankle. Treatment calls for prolonged bed rest, warm applications, and surgical ligation and stripping of the varicose veins responsible for the ulcers.

Menopause

At some point during middle age, women go through what is often called the *change of life,* when the capacity to bear children comes to an end. The start of the menopause usually comes between ages 40 and 50. However, about 12 percent of women reach the menopause between ages 36 and 40; 15 percent between ages 51 and 55; and another 6 percent earlier or later. As a general rule, it may be said that the later in a girl's life menstruation begins, the sooner menopause starts.

While menopause is sometimes abrupt, the onset is usually gradual, and the process normally lasts several years. The ovaries gradually reduce their ovulation and hormone secretion. Menstruation becomes irregular and finally ceases.

The periods between, during, and after the menopause are called *premenopausal, menopausal,* and *postmenopausal.* Premenopausal symptoms include skipped menstrual periods and scanty or lessened menstrual flow. During the menopausal period, menstruation ceases, and there are sometimes various systemic disturbances. The postmenopausal period is characterized by the return of bodily equilibrium and a renewed feeling of good health.

Symptoms of Menopause

Physical symptoms of the menopause are believed to be caused by an estrogen deficiency that upsets the hypothalamic control of the autonomic nervous system. While many women go through menopause with little or no distress, about one out of five may feel hot flashes and chills, nervousness, insomnia, heart palpitation, dizzy spells, or increased or diminished appetite. Generally, most women suffer from only a few of these symptoms, sudden hot flashes and dizziness being the most common.

Surgical Menopause

Many women develop benign uterine tumors called *fibroids,* and these tumors may cause irregular bleeding, prolonged menstrual periods, massive hemorrhages, or pain and discomfort because of pressure on other organs. In these cases a *hysterectomy,* or surgical removal of the uterus, may be performed. In cases where the cervix is also removed, the procedure is called total hysterectomy. It is only when the complete removal of the ovaries and tubes, called radical hysterectomy, is also necessary that the production of ova and the normal menstrual cycle are stopped abruptly and surgical menopause occurs. See "Benign Tumors" in Ch. 25, *Women's Health,* for further information about fibroids.

Though more abrupt and severe than menopause that occurs naturally, surgical menopause is treated in much the same manner as natural menopause. Tranquilizers or sedatives may be prescribed. In some cases, the physician may prescribe hormone replacement therapy to supplement the body's reduced supply of estrogen. This can be especially beneficial in the relief of hot flashes.

Emotional Aspects of Menopause

In addition to physical symptoms, a woman often has a pronounced psychological reaction to menopause. Though there is no medical basis for believing that menopause adversely affects her sex life or appearance, a woman may feel this is true. Common emotional problems may include the following: the feeling that she has lost her beauty, sex appeal, or sexual desire; a fear of cancer; the idea that the onset of menopause means the loss of her husband's love; fears that her job may be lost because of illness, bad nerves, or general debility; or a feeling that menopause means that

she has lost youthful energy and spirit and is becoming old.

It is only normal to feel sad occasionally about growing older, but there is no need to identify the menopause with loss of attractiveness, an end to sexual desire, or a so-called nervous breakdown. For anyone who is emotionally unstable, this transition may be especially hard to weather, but for such a personality, any time of change—such as marriage or motherhood—might also be accompanied by emotional turbulence.

Probably those women who see their total identity in terms of motherhood are the ones hardest hit when faced with the loss of their child-bearing functions. A woman who has a more complete sense of herself can accept the menopause with equanimity and can also face the tapering off of her child-rearing activities without feeling useless and discarded.

The most satisfying way to continue to express a strong maternal instinct after the menopause is in the role of grandmother, and if there are no grandchildren, in the role of occasional baby-sitter. Volunteer work in the children's ward of a local hospital or as a helper in a day-care nursery has also brought satisfaction to women who miss mothering as their own children leave them.

A Healthy Attitude toward Change

"Change of life," the old-fashioned term for the menopause, really isn't accurate, because change is a rule of life at all times. It is the ability to adjust to different circumstances and to find contentment in new outlets that marks the happy woman of any age.

Instead of feeling frustrated, or wallowing in self-pity, or hunting for sexual adventures, a woman whose emotions are disturbed during the menopause should set herself the goal of finding better ways to cope with them.

If depression and anxiety are deep enough to result in a loss of interest in daily affairs, the wisest thing to do is to have an honest conversation with the family physician or gynecologist. He may be able to alleviate these symptoms by such temporary measures as prescribing hormones or tranquilizers. Or he may feel that a few sessions with a psychiatrist would be helpful. It is no sign of personal failure or weakness of will to need professional guidance, and no woman should feel guilty if she seeks it out.

Advice to the Husband

A husband can help his wife through this difficult period if he makes an effort to be especially considerate. For example, he can take special care to show her that she is appreciated and still physically attractive. When she is in a bad humor or moody and depressed, he can sympathize with her moods and remain tolerant. He can pamper her and show his interest by remembering anniversaries and birthdays and by taking her out more often. Instead of hiding behind a newspaper or watching television in the evening, he can talk to his wife and show an interest in what she is doing.

By taking a realistic view of menopause as a natural process of life, and with the aid of an understanding husband, friends, and family, most women can get through the menopause without frequent visits to a family physician. However, if a woman experiences any unusual symptoms—abnormal vaginal discharge, spotting between periods, too frequent periods, periods that last too long, or unusual irritation of the genitals—she should by all means see a physician.

Pap Test

Cancer may be a major fear during the menopause, especially cancer of the cervix. Such fears can easily be allayed by having a simple diagnostic test called the *Papanicolaou* (or *Pap*) *smear.* This is a painless process in which the cervix is exposed by an instrument that dilates the cavity to make it more visible. The physician can then take samples of the cells, which are examined for the possible presence of cancer. All women should have a pelvic examination and Pap test at least once a year.

A number of other forms of cancer, including cancer of the lining of the uterus, cancer of the ovaries, cancer of the breast, and cancer of the vulva and other sexual organs, appear more frequently in women over 50. However, these conditions can be detected before they do much, if any, damage by having regular examinations during and after the menopause. If such cancers are caught in an early stage, they are much easier to treat and cure. See also Ch. 25, *Women's Health.*

Male Climacteric

Many men go through a psychological equivalent of the menopause, which may be called the "foolish forties," the "frenzied fifties," or the *male climacteric.*

According to Dr. Charles Wahl, a psychiatrist at the University of California (Los Angeles), some men tend to blame all sorts of symptoms—forgetfulness, self-doubt, worry, depression, and a declining sexual interest—on this mythical male menopause. "These symptoms are of psychic origin," says Dr. Wahl, "when found in a middle-aged man who is not afflicted by a specific disease. The body undergoes no organic or functional changes that might account for

such complaints."

This may be of small comfort to the man who—for whatever emotional reasons—goes through this period of psychological upset. But there is some help in this remark from Dr. John F. Briggs, Associate Professor of Clinical Medicine at the University of Minnesota: "The best way to steer a successful course through the hazards of the frenzied fifties is to assay your assets and liabilities dispassionately, and adapt to the circumstances and changes they dictate."

Advice to the Wife

Just as a husband can help his wife through her menopause, so can a wife help her husband. The thoughtful wife can bolster her husband's ego by being aware of what deflates him and what builds him up. Concentrate on building up his self-confidence and avoid nagging criticisms and arguments. Show your husband how much you need him and depend on him; sustain his sense of self-importance. Be affectionate and give him tender loving care, especially if you feel that he is worried or tense. He may want more company than usual, or he may prefer not to go out socially. Whatever the case, give in to him. He will assume his normal pace after a while.

Physiological Problems

There can be a physical reason for the male change of life, called primary testicular failure. In such cases, the testes fade out earlier in life than might be expected. Because it is an illness, like diabetes or kidney trouble, testicular failure can happen at any age. When it does occur, the physical discomforts may be surprisingly similar to a woman's symptoms in menopause.

Any man who suspects he may be

really ill should see a physician who can make a thorough examination. This is necessary because any treatment with hormones (androgen) could hurt as much as it could help if the case is not a true testicular failure. Androgen could also be harmful in the case of prostate trouble, which becomes more prevalent after the age of 40. See Ch. 6, *The Later Years,* for a fuller discussion of prostate trouble.

Other than testicular failure, which is rare, there is no physical reason why a man should be impotent in middle age. As the late Dr. Kinsey reported: "Only a slight portion of the male population ever becomes impotent before death."

If a man thinks that he needs "one last fling" before his virility is curtailed by glandular deterioration, he will not find support for this idea from Dr. Josiah Brown, an endocrinologist with the University of California (Los Angeles). Says Dr. Brown: "There is no significant change in the endocrine function between the ages of 40 and 55."

Also, if a man looks for a sex stimulator for flagging interests, he need look no farther than this statement by the late Dr. Kinsey: ". . . good health, sufficient exercise, and plenty of sleep still remain the most effective of the aphrodisiacs known to man."

Nicotine

Used in moderation, nicotine is not harmful, and according to some researchers may be helpful, improving memory and learning ability, perhaps by stimulating the flow of adrenaline. Nicotine also stimulates the adrenal glands, causing blood vessels to constrict and skin temperatures to drop.

Interestingly enough, nicotine is thought to get into the system through the membranes of the mouth and related areas. Thus, a person who holds an unlighted cigar in his mouth may absorb nicotine.

While a little nicotine is not harmful, most steady smokers absorb too much nicotine for their own good. Lung cancer kills over 85,000 persons a year, about 80 percent of whom are cigarette smokers. Also, cigarette smoking is believed to be a primary cause of *emphysema* (a disease that decreases efficiency of the lungs) which kills over 15,000 persons a year. Approximately 100,000 cigarette smokers die from heart attacks each year.

In their book *Vigor for Men Over 30,* the authors, Drs. Warren R. Guild, Stuart Cowan, and Samm Baker, suggest these tips on giving up smoking:

- *Try a program of enjoyable physical activity.* They suggest that if the urge to smoke becomes overpowering, the smoker should take a brisk walk, do a set of invigorating exercises at home or in the office, or engage in an enjoyable sport.

- *Don't use antismoking drugs or other nostrums without a physician's advice.* Such devices may do more harm than good. Your physician is the one who can advise you on the best way to cut down on smoking, and he can help you cope with any withdrawal symptoms such as nervousness, dizziness, or insomnia.

- *Don't try to cut down on too many things at the same time.* Concentrate on cutting down on your smoking, and relax about cutting down on diet and drinking, too. One reduction at a time is best.

- *You've got to quit completely.* Like the alcoholic, you've got to say, "This is my *last* cigarette"—and mean it.

- *Quit when there's a major break in your routine.* The recovery from an operation or illness is a good time to stop. After you have established the habit of *not* smoking, make that habit a part of your daily life.

- *Try something different to throw desire off the track.* Take a shower—you can't light a match under water. Also, you can't hold a cigarette if you're playing table tennis or practicing your golf swing.

Caffeine

Like nicotine, *caffeine* can be a pleasant stimulant if used in moderation. Laboratory studies show that caffeine appears to work on the central nervous system: fatigue and drowsiness fade while mental activities quicken. But too much caffeine can produce headaches, irritability, and confusion.

Although tea leaves contain almost twice as much caffeine as an equal weight of coffee, smaller amounts of tea are used to make a cup of tea, thus lessening the per-cup intake rate. Cola and chocolate also contain caffeine. Although these drinks are not addictive, abstaining from them is no easy matter, as anyone who has tried to give up coffee drinking can attest.

Ordinarily, drinking a few cups of coffee or other caffeine beverage is not harmful—unless your physician tells you to cut down for some reason. But if you find that you need a caffeine beverage to keep going, you might be better off taking a rest instead.

Alcohol

Many physicians feel that a person's capacity to handle liquor diminishes after age 40, and that alcohol intake should be cut down after this age. Also, some people seem to develop an allergic reaction to alcohol—an allergy that can be fatal. One physician described the extra dry martini as "the quick blow to the back of the neck."

Drinking too much and too fast can jar the whole system. It tends to make the drinker nervous and on edge instead of providing calming relief from tensions. The hard-pressed executive is especially vulnerable to the quick, fast drink he takes to provide instant relaxation when he is fatigued.

"The key to the real value of alcohol is intelligent drinking," says Dr. Harry J. Johnson, of the Life Extension Institute. Dr. Johnson says that he sometimes recommends a drink or two before dinner, which he says is the best time to indulge. However, Dr. Johnson suggests a tall, well-diluted highball taken in a peaceful, quiet setting.

How to Avoid Drinking

If you find that drinking is a problem at business luncheons, conventions, and cocktail parties, Dr. Warren R. Guild recommends the following commonsense ways to pass up drinks:

- Say "no thanks" if you do not like the taste or effect of alcohol. Order a juice or nonalcoholic beverage just to have something to sip. Actually, many more jobs and clients have been lost through drinking too much than by not drinking at all.

- Wait for others to order drinks. If someone else refuses a drink, you can decline too. Or, you could say, "I'm not having one but you go ahead." This usually sets the pace for drinking.

- Instead of a powerhouse martini, try vermouth on the rocks, beer, wine, or a well-diluted highball.

- Use dieting as a reason to cut down or out on drinking. You have a good excuse—a drink has 100 or more calories.

- Make arrangements with your favorite restaurant or bar to serve you "your usual." You could make this a nonalcoholic drink.

Remember that alcohol definitely decreases your ability to concentrate, absorb, or produce thoughts or ideas. After drinking you will not be as efficient at writing, drawing, handling objects, or driving. If the level of alcohol in your blood exceeds 0.05 percent—which, depending on weight, is approximately the equivalent of two ounces of hard liquor or two bottles of beer at one session—*you are not a safe driver.*

Treating a Hangover

What if you do drink too much and have a hangover? Is there anything you can do about it? Dr. Harold T. Hyman, formerly of the Columbia University College of Physicians and Surgeons, recommends calling a physician if the case is particularly bad. He will probably prescribe a large dose of paraldehyde or a tranquilizer such as Librium or Thorazine, and put the patient to bed.

Less acute sufferers should, on awakening after a binge, take warmed fluids (tea, consommé, clam broth). As soon as your stomach feels in shape, eat warm, soft foods at frequent intervals—poached egg, milk toast, pureed soup, mashed potatoes. Despite your craving for cold, carbonated fluids, avoid them; they may cause stomach cramps.

To prevent a hangover as you drink, Dr. Guild recommends taking *fructose*. Fructose, or *levulose*, is a crystalline sugar, the sweetest of the sugars. It increases the rate at which the body metabolizes and eliminates alcohol. It seems to work best when the alcohol is combined with something naturally high in fructose, as the tomato juice in a Bloody Mary, for example. Or just sip tomato juice between drinks.

Looking for quick panaceas in the medicine cabinet to cure a hangover or any other condition seems to become increasingly popular after age 40. Panaceas are all right up to a point, but indiscriminate self-treatment can do a great deal of harm, because it may mask a more serious illness or may prevent a condition from clearing up if left alone. In drinking, as in eating, the key is moderation.

Proper diet

Proper diet is an important contribution an individual can make to his good health, because foods build body tissues and provide energy for the body to work. Adequate diet planning is not difficult. The basic rules of good nutrition must be learned. See Ch. 27, *Nutrition and Weight Control,* for a full treatment of diet and nutrition. Applying these rules to a daily diet will take only a few minutes of planning when the menu is decided upon, and will reap enormous rewards in good health and appearance. The hardest part of planning a balanced diet is to avoid selecting food solely on the basis of taste or convenience and ignoring nutritional value.

Vitamins

Eating a proper, balanced diet generally fulfills vitamin and other nutritional requirements. Nutritious diet habits are important to the maintenance of good health. In instances of vitamin and mineral deficiencies brought about by health problems, and in instances of poor diet habits, vitamins and other food supplements have proven very beneficial. It is important, however, not to attempt to treat a physical or health problem of any kind without the advice and help of a physician.

Breakfast

Many Americans neglect breakfast, an important contribution to good diet. Studies prove that men, women, and children need an adequate breakfast. A good breakfast can provide a start in obtaining the day's vitamin and mineral requirements. It is also a help to dieters and those trying to maintain a stable weight, since those who have eaten a good breakfast are able to avoid mid-morning snacks such as sweet rolls, cakes, and the like, which are usually high in carbohydrates and calories.

Weight and Health

Overweight is one of the biggest deterrents to successful middle age, and is also one of the greatest threats to health and longevity. As one physician said, "Consider how few really obese persons you see over 60 years of age." Unfortunately, in middle age most of us maintain the eating habits of our youth while we cut down on our exercise. The result: added weight that acts as a deterrent to our physical well-being.

The overweight person is more likely to develop arthritis, diabetes, heart disease, high blood pressure, kidney trouble, and many other disabling or fatal disorders. As the American Heart Association said recently: "Pity the fat man; the statisticians number his days."

As reported in *Nation's Business,* "If you are overweight by 10 percent,

your chances of surviving the next 20 years are 15 percent less than if you had ideal weight; if you are 20 percent overweight, your chances are 25 percent less; if you are 30 percent overweight, 45 percent less." In other words, the odds are against the overweight.

If you do not know what your ideal weight should be, a physician can tell you. To check yourself, try the "pinch" test. Take a pinch of skin on your upper arm just below the shoulder. If more than a half-inch separates your fingers, you are too fat. Try the same test on your stomach when you're standing erect. And, of course, your mirror can reveal the tell-tale signs of middle-age fat—the double chin, sagging belly, flabby arms and legs.

Good Eating Habits

Is there any magic way to reduce? The only sure way is to *eat less,* and to continue this practice all the time. It will not help if you go on a crash diet and then resume your normal eating habits. And while exercise will help control weight and burn up excess calories, probably the best exercise is to push yourself away from the table before you've overeaten.

Calories do count, and usually the caloric intake of a person in the 40- to 55-year age bracket should be about one-third less than that of a person between ages 25 and 40. Again, your physician or a good calorie-counter can help you determine what to eat and how much.

Here are some additional tips from nutritionists to help you lose weight:

- *Cut down on quantity.* Eat just enough to satisfy your appetite— not as much as you can. Even low-calorie foods will add weight if you eat enough of them.

- *Eat less more often.* Spread your food intake over several meals or snacks. Some hospitals have been experimenting with five meals a day, spreading the recommended total food intake over two full meals a day (brunch and dinner) and three snacks (continental breakfast, afternoon snack, and before-bedtime). They find that the stomach handles small amounts of food better, that metabolism keeps working at a good pace all day, and that blood sugar levels (your energy reserve) do not drop between meals. Also, the process of digestion burns up calories.

- *Avoid high-calorie foods.* Cut out breads, rolls, jellies, jams, sauces, gravies, dressings, creams, and rich desserts. These are the villains that add calories and are not as rich in nutrients.

- *Look for natural flavors.* Cultivate an interest in the natural flavor of what you eat. Try vegetables without butter, coffee and tea without cream and sugar. You might want to substitute a pinch of salt or a squeeze of lemon on your vegetables or noncaloric sweeteners in your beverages, but chances are you will find the natural flavors new and interesting.

- *Serve only just enough.* Keep portions small and put serving dishes with leftovers out of sight. Taking seconds is often just a habit. Cultivate the idea of just one serving, and you will find it satisfies the appetite. Another idea: serve meals on smaller plates. the portion will look big if only in relationship to the size of the plate.

In order to maintain a healthy body and a youthful appearance while dieting, you must make sure you eat the necessary proteins and nutrients.

This can be done by selecting foods from the four basic food groups. See Ch. 27, *Nutrition and Weight Control.*

As a panel of experts on middle age said in a recent interview: "Two factors are vital to successful middle age: physical activity and a variety of interests. Move around but don't rush around. Keep an open mind and a closed refrigerator. Remember that variety is more than the spice of life— it's the wellspring of life. The person who pursues a variety of activities will usually stay fit long after middle age."

Living Life to the Fullest

No wise man ever wished to be younger.   —JONATHAN SWIFT

Staying young is looked on by most of the rest of the world as a peculiarly American obsession. This obsession is certainly fostered and exploited by the advertising industry, but its causes have to be looked for elsewhere.

In many countries, it is the old who are venerated for their wisdom and authority. This point of view is likely to prevail in societies that stay the same or that enjoyed their greatest glories in the past.

America is another matter. Because of its history, it is literally a young country. It is also a nation built on the idea of progress and hope in the future. And to whom does the future belong if not to youth?

Keeping up with change is unfortunately identified by too many people with how they look rather than how they think or feel. To be young in heart and spirit has very little to do with wearing the latest style in clothes—no matter how unbecom-

ing—or learning the latest dances. Maintaining an open mind receptive to new ideas, keeping the capacity for pleasure in the details of daily living, refusing to be overwhelmed by essentially unimportant irritations can make the middle years more joyful for any family.

A Critical Time

Nowadays, the average American can expect to reach the age of 70. Thus, for most people, the middle years begin during the late 30s. Ideally, these are the years of personal fulfillment accompanied by a feeling of pride in accomplishment, a deeper knowledge of one's strengths and limitations, and a growing understanding and tolerance of other people's ideas and behavior.

Emotional Pressures

In many families, however, the pleasures of maturity often go hand in hand with increased pressures. It's no simple matter for the typical husband and wife in their 40s to maintain emotional health while handling worries about money, aging parents, anxiety about willful teenagers, tensions caused by marital friction, and feelings of depression about getting older. To some people, the problems of the middle years are so burdensome that instead of dealing with them realistically—by eliminating some, by compromising in the solution of others—they escape into excessive drinking or into sexual infidelity. It doesn't take much thought to realize that those escapes do nothing except introduce new problems.

Physical Symptoms of Emotional Problems

For others, deep-seated conflicts that come to a head during the middle

years may be expressed in chronic physical symptoms. Many physicians in the past intuitively understood the relationship between emotional and physical health, but it is only in recent years that medical science has proved that feelings of tension, anxiety, suppressed anger, and frustration are often the direct cause of ulcers, sexual impotence, high blood pressure, and heart attacks, not to mention sleeplessness and headaches.

Of course, there are no magic formulas that guarantee the achievement of emotional well-being at any time of life. Nor does any sensible person expect to find a perfect solution to any human problem. However, it is possible to come to grips with specific difficulties and deal with them in ways that can reduce stress and safeguard emotional health.

Sexuality during the Middle Years

In spite of the so-called sexual revolution and all its accompanying publicity, it is still very difficult for most people to sort out their attitudes towards sexual activity. It is a subject that continues to be clouded by feelings of guilt and anxiety, surrounded by taboos, and saddled with misinformation. For each individual, the subject is additionally complicated by personal concepts of love and morality.

Many people were shocked when the Kinsey reports on male and female sexual behavior appeared. More recently, militant efforts have been made in various communities to prevent the schools from including sex education in their courses of study. Yet marriage counselors, family physicians, ministers, and all other specialists in human relations can attest to the amount of human misery caused by ignorance about sex—all the way from the ignorance that results in a 15-year-old's unwanted pregnancy to the ignorance of a 50-year-old man about his wife's sexual needs.

Pioneering Work in Sexual Response

According to the research of Dr. William H. Masters and Mrs. Virginia E. Johnson, directors of the Reproductive Biology Research Foundation in St. Louis and authors of *Human Sexual Response* and *Human Sexual Inadequacy,* 50 percent of all married couples can be considered sexually inadequate. These authorities define sexual inadequacy as the inability to achieve sexual communication in marriage or insecurity about whatever sexual communication does exist.

In the intensive sexual therapy they offer to married couples professionally referred to the Foundation, Dr. Masters and Mrs. Johnson concentrate on the relationship between husband and wife. They stress the concept of sexual activity as communication between two human beings, each with unique needs and desires that must be fulfilled by the other. The basic attitude they hope to instill in those who come to them for help is that pleasure in sex is natural and can be achieved through an understanding of giving and receiving it.

Emotional Causes of Sexual Inadequacy

It is not unusual for a couple whose marriage began with a satisfactory sexual adjustment to find the relationship deteriorating as they approach their 40s. From the point of view of how the body itself functions during the middle years, there is rarely a physical reason for a decline in the ability to perform sexually. Almost always, male impotence or lack of female responsiveness is caused by

psychological factors, some deeply buried, others superficial.

The Impotent Husband

Because of particular circumstances and differing personalities, many middle-aged men spend their days in a state of impotent anger. They may have suppressed feelings of hostility against an unreasonable boss; they may feel put down by a successful neighbor; they may be unable to deal effectively with a rebellious son. With such men, a chain of cause and effect sometimes develops that cannot be broken without professional help.

The tensions generated by impotent anger may result in impotence during the sex act. Because the underlying causes for sexual impotence are probably unknown to him, a middle-aged husband may develop deep anxieties about his waning sexuality. These anxieties in turn cause the sexual incompetence to continue.

There is also the husband who unconsciously builds up resentments against his wife because he thinks she is paying too much attention to the house and the children or to her career and too little to him. Their surface relationship may not be affected, but his body will express his feelings by withholding itself from her as a form of punishment.

Another typical cause of temporary impotence is a feeling of guilt about an adventure in sexual infidelity. Impotence with the marital partner under these circumstances is usually the husband's way of punishing himself for behavior that he considers wrong.

The Unresponsive Wife

Many men complain about their wives' waning interest in sex during the middle years. It is true that women sometimes give or withhold

themselves from their husbands as a reward or a punishment, but more commonly, wives who are unresponsive are likely to be expressing resentment about the fact that the only time they get any attention is in bed, and even there, the attention is apt to be perfunctory rather than personally gratifying and meaningful.

When this is the case, the breach in a marriage is likely to widen unless there is a willingness on the part of both partners to confront the problem openly, if necessary with a marriage counselor, minister, or physician, so that a satisfactory solution can be found. Otherwise, the wife's resentment of neglect expressed in sexual coldness may lead her husband to look elsewhere for gratification.

Sometimes a woman seems unresponsive only because she feels she is being used as a sex object instead of having her needs satisfied. This unconscious feeling may express itself in the lack of responsiveness that is mistakenly called frigidity. As a result of their experience in helping many couples achieve good sexual relationships, Dr. Masters and Mrs. Johnson assert that the word *frigidity* has little meaning. There are very few women incapable of being physically aroused and satisfied by an understanding sexual partner.

Being Honest

In most cases of sexual inadequacy, insight and honesty about feelings are usually a more effective treatment than hormones, sex manuals, and so-called aphrodisiacs.

Any married couple whose sexual problems have become acute during the middle years should look for the causes in their own emotions about themselves and each other. They should also examine any persistent feelings of tension and anxiety that might be the result of practical matters in their daily lives, such as worry about money or children.

New Treatments

Where other approaches fail, the impotent male can either undergo a test for erectability or try one of the new treatments currently available. Conducted during sleep, the tests provide evidence indicating that impotence in any given case has physical or psychological causes. Physical causes may include such diseases as diabetes; some drugs or medication, including those used to treat high blood pressure; and alcohol abuse, hardening of the arteries, or testosterone or thyroid hormone deficiencies.

These tests have shown that physical causes underlie impotence in nearly half of all cases. As a result much research has been conducted into physical "cures." All of the tests operate on the accepted medical principle that "normal" men have approximately five erections during every sleep period. In what is called the *stamp test,* a strip of stamps is wrapped around the penis before the subject retires for the night. Fitted snugly around the shaft of the penis, the strip tears along one of the perforated edges if the subject experiences an erection while sleeping.

Two other tests are more reliable. In one, a *snap gauge band* made of elastic fabric and Velcro is wrapped around the penis; the band has three snaps designed to open at various stages of penile rigidity. A third test utilizes a *Nocturnal Penile Tumescence Monitor* to tell exactly when erections occur, with what rigidity, and for how long. Two circular elastic silicone bands are attached to the penis; sensor wires connect the bands to an apparatus like an electrocardiograph machine.

Of the prosthetic devices used to "cure" impotence, three can be im-

planted in the penis in operations that take one to three hours under local anesthetic. The simplest utilizes two semirigid rods that keep the penis permanently erect. A second implanted type, made of flexible, plastic-covered metal wire, also maintains the penis in a constantly erect state but can be bent into an erect or downward position. A third type works hydraulically to pump the penis into a naturally erect state. Two expandable metal tubes implanted in the penis function with an attached tiny pump in the scrotum and a water reservoir placed behind the muscles of the lower abdomen. Pressure on the pump causes the penis to erect; valves make possible penile relaxation.

Beyond Motherhood: New Goals

There are many women casting about to find ways of spending their newly found spare time, women who are bored by bridge and gossip, who enjoy being a wife and mother and grandmother but also want an outlet that is their very own, disengaged from their role in the family. Such women might do some thinking about unfulfilled aspirations and the interests of their younger years, abandoned because of practical pressures.

Each one must find a way of spending leisure time in a way that is personally meaningful. Never mind that the children think it's funny for their mother to be going back to school for a college degree; or that the husband doesn't understand why his wife isn't taking it easy instead of taking a part-time job in a department store; or that the neighbors make remarks about the easel and paints that have suddenly appeared on the back porch.

Returning to Work or School

More middle-aged, middle-class women are taking jobs after years of housekeeping than ever before. Many companies are eager to hire them—on a part-time basis if necessary—because they are usually serious, competent, and reliable. Colleges make special provisions for women who want to complete their education after a long absence from studies. Even in small towns, there are many fruitful avenues for earning money or engaging in a productive hobby.

A feeling of pride in accomplishment at a time when household chores and child-raising no longer require much daily attention is usually the best medicine for depressed spirits. Personally meaningful activities outside the home are also an excellent way to keep in touch with what's happening in the world. Nowadays there is no reason for a woman in her 40s or 50s to feel restless, bored, or useless. The opportunities for self-expression and personal fulfillment are sufficiently varied to satisfy anyone's individual needs. All it takes is the genuine desire to find them.

More Than a Breadwinner: Vocation and Avocation

Everybody knows that it takes money to maintain a household and raise a family, and there is no doubt that during the middle years financial pressures reach their highest point, what with sending children through school, helping to support aging parents, and meeting increased medical and dental expenses. At this time, even those men who truly enjoy their work often feel they scarcely have the time or peace of mind to enjoy anything else.

Need for Other Outlets

Just as most women need personal

outlets for their individuality away from home and family, so most men can achieve better emotional health if they find avenues of self-expression unrelated to their job or their role as husband and father. This does not mean becoming so passionately involved in playing golf or going fishing that the family is constantly neglected. Nor does it mean spending excessive amounts of money on rare stamps at the expense of the family budget.

On the other hand, if a man chooses a hobby that doesn't include the family, such as singing in a choir or studying a foreign language, rather than choosing one that does—such as going on camping trips or taking pictures—there is no reason for the rest of the household to be resentful. Togetherness is a good thing to strive for, but it isn't a hard and fast principle to be applied to all activities.

It's healthier for a man to take an occasional fishing trip with his cronies, enjoy every minute of it, and come home relaxed and refreshed, than to take along a wife who will be bored and children who will be restless. In such far-too-frequent cases, no one has a good time. Nor should a father insist on teaching his son how to play chess so that they can share a hobby when his son would rather spend his time otherwise.

A Satisfying Hobby

The choice of a satisfying leisure-time activity is an entirely individual matter. Some men prefer a hobby that is sedentary, such as model-building. Others who have to sit in an office all day find the vigorous play of the hand-ball court physically and emotionally exhilarating.

Some men, oppressed by constant association with other people, enjoy solitary hobbies such as long nature walks; others, whose jobs involve working alone, like to get together with a group for bowling or bridge playing. There are those who like competitive hobbies and those who want to escape the competitiveness of their work by puttering around in the basement or studying the fine points of the Civil War or experimenting in haute cuisine.

Many men as well as women find the idea of community service appealing as a productive way of using free time. The opportunities are endless: going into poorer neighborhoods and training athletic teams; starting a tutoring group as part of a church activity; getting involved in grass-roots politics and pressing for local reforms; organizing a block association for property maintenance and improvement.

Building a collection can be a gratifying hobby, and the collection need not involve much money. The pleasures usually come from finding a rare specimen—whether it's a matchbook cover or an old comic book—from satisfying a need to own something unique, and from learning in the process of looking for items of interest.

Flexing Mental Muscles

Healthy human beings, regardless of age, need a certain amount of intellectual stimulation to keep their spirits refreshed. The arteries of the body may harden slowly with age, but there are people whose minds remain young and limber in spite of their increasing years.

Housewives commonly complain that they do not get enough stimulation from their daily chores. Men talk about getting into a rut on their jobs—going stale. Yet stimulation for the mind is no farther away than the nearest library, if the mind is hungry for food for thought. There's plenty of mental exercise available for those in the middle years who are willing to review their old ideas and to examine some new ones.

Family Discussions

Having relaxed discussions with teenage children can be a fine source of intellectual refreshment if both generations can listen to each other with tolerance and mutual respect. Some parents get huffy and defensive if their views are challenged. This defensiveness—in some cases, downright hostility—results in closing the channels of communication.

This is not to suggest that every idea espoused by the young should be adopted by their elders. But opinions can be exchanged and challenges involving facts and figures can be met in the spirit of civilized discussion. There are areas in which parents can be educated by their children, and the areas can range all the way from trying out new recipes suggested by a venturesome daughter to getting a book on drugs from the library in order to answer a son who cheerfully calls his father a drug addict because he has to have three drinks when he comes home from work.

Community Resources

Some families find they need go no farther than their own home for intellectual activity. For those who want broader opportunities to use their heads, there are community resources that can be explored. Church organizations, parent-teacher associations, or social clubs can be used as forums. These might include public discussions, film presentations, and meetings on problems of current interest, such as drug addiction and slum clearance.

For those looking for enlightenment of a specific kind, the facilities of schools in the area should be investigated. Many colleges and universities offer adult education programs that cover a wide range of subjects—from real estate evaluation to philosophy. It's also possible to set up a study group composed of friends and associates who want to find out more about American history or the history of art, to study anthropology or the behavior of social insects, and to hire a lecturer to meet with the group once or twice a week.

Travel

Travel is a wonderful way of broadening interests, even if the trip means going to a nearby city or dairy farm. When children are in their later teens and can safely be left on their own for a few days—with some neighborly supervision—a husband and wife can enjoy going places of special interest to them rather than having to take younger tastes into account.

The destination needn't be another continent to provide fascinating new sights and information. People who live in Chicago will find the small seacoast villages of New England a totally new world; Bostonians will find a way of life strange to them if they drive through the Smoky Mountains; people who live in a small town or a farm can get a big lift out of wandering about in a big city.

In traveling abroad, the more advance planning that is invested in the trip, the greater the rewards. Every effort should be made to learn at least a little of the language of the country to be visited, and instead of settling for a group tour in which each moment is planned, there's much pleasure to be gained from exploring a particular enthusiasm, whether it be food, architecture, history, or a return to the village of one's foreign-born ancestors.

Separation and Divorce

Marriage in this country is based on the highly personal concept of love rather than on such traditional foundations as a property merger between two families or an arrangement determined by the friendship of the young people's parents. It is often assumed, therefore, that if mutual love is the basis for embarking on a marriage, its absence is a valid reason for dissolving it, either by legal separation or divorce.

The idea of divorce is not particularly modern; in practically every time and place where a form of marriage has existed, so has some form of divorce, with reasons ranging from excessive wife-beating to failure to deliver a piece of land mentioned in the marriage contract.

The High Rate of Divorce

What is new is the high rate of divorce. Figures now indicate that in the United States as a whole, approximately one in every four marriages is terminated by legal arrangement. However, these figures by no means indicate that the family as an institution is on the way out, because a constantly increasing number of people who get divorced get married again.

There are many reasons for the growing rate of separation and divorce:

- Over the last 50 years, a continually increasing percentage of the population has been getting married.

- Although the trend toward earlier marriages has leveled off in recent years, a significant number of people still marry at earlier ages than was common in the past. (The number of divorces is highest among the poorly educated group who marry under the age of 21.)

- The legal requirements for separation and divorce are less rigid than formerly.

- With increasing independence and earning capacity, women are less frightened of the prospect of heading a family.

- The poorer groups in the population, in which desertion was a common practice, are more often obtaining divorces.

Contrary to popular belief, there are more divorces among the poor than among the rich, and more among the less well-educated than among the educated. Also, most divorces occur before the fifth year of marriage.

Telling the Truth to Children

Most people with children who are contemplating a breakup of their marriage generally make every effort to seek professional guidance that might help them iron out their differences. When these efforts fail and steps are taken to arrange for a separation or divorce, it is far healthier for parents to be honest with each other and with their children than to construct elaborate explanations based on lies.

A teenager who is given the real reason for a divorce is less likely to have something to brood about than one who is told lies that he can see through. If the real reason for a divorce is that the parents have tried their best to get along with each other but find it impossible, the child who is in his teens or older can certainly understand this. If the marriage is coming to an end because the husband or wife wants to marry someone else, the explanation to the child should avoid assigning blame. When the rejected parent tries to enlist the child's sympathy by blackening the character of the parent who is supposedly the cause of the divorce, results are almost always unpleasant. Under no circumstances and no matter what his age should a child be called on to take the side of either parent or to act as a judge.

Nor should children be told any more about the circumstances of the breakup of a marriage than they really want to know. Young people have a healthy way of protecting themselves from information they would find hurtful, and if they ask few questions, they need be told only the facts they are prepared to cope with. Of course, as they grow older and live through their own problems, they will form their own view of what really happened between their parents.

After the Separation

Traditionally, in separation and divorce proceedings, the children have remained in the custody of the mother, with financial support arrangements and visiting rights spelled out for the father. Although an increasing number of fathers have been awarded custody of their children in recent years, it is still commonly the mother who must face the problems of single parenthood after divorce. Although teenage children may need some extra attention for a while, there is no need for a mother to make a martyr of herself, nor should she feel guilty when she begins to consider remarrying.

The father should be completely reliable in his visiting arrangements, and if he has remarried, should try to establish good relationships between the offspring of his former marriage and his new family.

Stepchildren

People who remarry during the middle years frequently find themselves in the role of stepparent. This is a role with many problems and many rewards; the chief requirements are patience and tact.

The stepchild has to deal with many complicated feelings: his sense of loss, either through death or divorce, of his own parent; his resentment against the parent who has remarried, and his hostility to the stranger who has become his new parent.

A stepparent should proceed affectionately but cautiously, and should not try to be accepted by the child as a replacement for the parent who has gone. If the child and stepparent have achieved a friendly rapport before the remarriage, they should build on the friendship rather than trying to transform it into a parent–child relationship immediately. When the child's trust has been gained, the stepparent can gradually assume some of the authority of a true parent, always waiting for the child to indicate a desire and need for it first.

A Death in the Family

When a husband or wife dies during the middle years, there is a general feeling that the death is unnatural because it is in all ways premature: the normal life expectancy has been cut short, the one who remains is prematurely bereaved, and the children are deprived of a parent too soon.

There are a few consolations in the presence of death: some people are sustained by their religious beliefs, others by the rallying of relatives and friends, and still others by happy memories of the years spent together in a fulfilled relationship.

The bereft parent should share his grief with the children, but they should not be thought unfeeling if they seem to be going about their business almost in the usual way. They may be dealing with a tangle of feelings that will take some time to come to the surface—feelings of guilt about past thoughtlessness, of confusion about

wishing that the parent who remains had died instead, and of fear connected with the thought of their own death.

When the time seems right, young people can be encouraged to talk about the parent who died. Remembering funny incidents and times of anger, reliving shared experiences—these can act as a restorative to the living and make family ties closer.

As for remarrying, although the children and the deceased's relatives may consider such a step a disloyalty to the memory of the dead, it is actually a tribute, because it implies that the state of marriage was a happy one.

The Single Parent

When the job of being a single parent has to be faced, either because of death or divorce, the problems may seem overwhelming. Although they differ considerably depending on whether the parent is the father or mother, they are nonetheless difficult to sort out, particularly at a time when morale may be at a low ebb.

The Single Father

The single father with growing children often feels helpless in dealing with household tasks and gains some insight into the number of tasks involved in keeping things running smoothly at home. If he has a teenage daughter or son, he can depend on him or her to do part of the job, but young people should not be burdened with all the responsibilities of housekeeping if some other arrangement can possibly be made. Perhaps a relative can be called on to help out part-time, or a professional housekeeper can be engaged for a few hours a day. Outside help is particularly important if the care of younger children is involved.

A motherless girl in adolescence may seek out the companionship and occasional guidance of an older woman who was a friend of her mother's, or she may spend more and more time at the home of a friend whose mother she likes and respects. Such a transfer of affection should not be considered as disloyalty.

The Single Mother

The mother who is a single parent usually has to cope with problems of earning and managing money. Fortunately, the job opportunities for middle-aged women are varied, and if the family finances can be worked out on the basis of a part-time job, this is a good transitional solution for making the adjustment of handling a job and running the household. A widow or divorcee may need to call on a friend or relative to help her with such practical matters as income tax, mortgages, loans, or investments. If these matters can be handled by a family lawyer without the fees being prohibitive, so much the better.

A widow or divorced woman should avoid concentrating too much on her children, nor should she give a son in his tccns the understanding that he is now the head of the family. He is and must remain her son and nothing more. If an authority figure is needed as partial replacement for the departed husband, he should be sought among neighbors or relatives for whom the children feel respect.

In many communities, single parents have formed groups for discussion and mutual help. Such groups can usually be located through local social work agencies. Parents Without Partners, 7910 Woodmont Ave., Ste. 1000, Bethesda, MD 20814, specializes in the problems of single parents and publishes literature of interest to them.

6

The Later Years

Aging
and What To Do About It

Growing older could mean growing healthier. In many ways you are as old as you think and feel. Consider these points:

- No disease results just from the passage of years.

- We age piecemeal—each organ separately rather than uniformly.

- In retirement you have less daily stress and strain, and you have more time to take care of yourself.

What, then, makes a person think and feel old?

The Aging Process

Physically, we mature at about 25 to 30, when the body reaches maximum size and strength. Then, body tissues and cells are constantly being rebuilt and renewed. Nutrition, rest, exercise, and stress influence the length of time that the body can maintain a balance between the wearing down and rebuilding of body tissues. When more cells die than can be reproduced, they are replaced by a fibrous, inert substance called *colagen*. The living process slows down to compensate, and we begin aging; strength and ability start to decline.

But this happens at various intervals. For instance, vision is sharpest at age 25; the eye loses its ability to make rapid adjustments in focus after age 40. Hearing is sharpest at about age 10, then diminishes as you grow older. Sensitivity to taste and smell lessens after age 60.

The decline in strength and muscle ability is long and gradual; there are even gratifying plateaus. At age 50, a man still has about four-fifths of the muscle strength he had when he was 25.

Although physical abilities may decline, mental abilities may actually improve during the middle years, and memory and the ability to learn can remain keen. Dr. Alfred Schwartz, dean of education at Drake University, was asked: "Can a 70-year-old man in reasonably good health learn as rapidly as a 17- year-old boy?" Dr. Schwartz answered:

Indeed he can—provided he's in the habit of learning. The fact that some older people today are not active intellectually is no reflection on their ability to learn. There is ample proof that learning ability does not automatically decline with age.

Regardless of what you may have heard, organic brain damage affects less than one percent of those over age 65.

But in thinking about physical change, remember that this is just one aspect of aging. Age is determined by emotional and intellectual maturity as well as by chronological years.

Can a person do anything to retard aging?

Most *gerontologists* feel that the reason more people don't live longer is that they are not willing to follow a regimen of diet, exercise, rest, recreation—coupled with the exclusion of various excesses. And while there isn't anything you can do to set back the clock, you can keep in good health by making sure to have regular physical examinations, sufficient exercise, adequate rest, nutritious food, and a positive mental attitude.

A Positive Mental Attitude

Mark Twain once said: "Whatever a

man's age he can reduce it several years by putting a bright-colored flower in his buttonhole." A lively, fresh outlook is essential for enjoyable living at any age. Most physicians believe there is a direct connection between one's state of mind and physical health. This is especially true when you are faced with the challenges of retirement. Plato said: "He who is of a calm and happy nature will hardly feel the pressure of age, but to him who is of an opposite disposition, youth and age are equally a burden."

Experts in the field of aging have found that most older people can relieve transitory depression by a deliberate shift of thought or by physical activity. If you look upon retirement as an opportunity to take better care of yourself and to pursue old and new interests, you'll go a long way toward better health.

The Annual Checkup

For peace of mind and to maintain and improve your health, make it a habit to see your physician at least once a year. To remind themselves, many people make an appointment on their birthday. An annual checkup is especially important in later years and should not be put off or neglected.

During a routine checkup, the physician pays special attention to enlarged lymph nodes of the neck, armpits, and groin, and the front of the neck. He also checks the condition of veins and arteries and looks at your knees and arches—which are of particular importance to older people.

He makes tests for arteriosclerosis, high blood pressure, diabetes, brain tumors, and other diseases. He can feel and tap your body to check your lungs, liver, and spleen, and he can take electrocardiographs to detect changes in your heart. Simple tests can note bladder and kidney conditions.

In addition, the physician usually asks about personal habits—smoking, drinking, eating. He also wants to know about any unusual symptoms you might have. Be completely frank with your physician, answer his questions as directly as possible, and give all information that might be helpful.

When explaining the nature of your ailment or symptom, tell him what part of the body is involved, what changes are associated with the symptoms, and whether symptoms occurred after a change of diet or medicine. Tell him about any previous experiences with this condition and what treatments you might have had.

It is extremely important to tell your physician about any pills you are taking—including aspirin, tranquilizers, and sleeping tablets. Even the most common drug can affect the potency of medication he might prescribe.

After he has taken your case history and after he has all the reports from your tests, the physician will want to talk with you, explain his findings, and perhaps make some recommendations. Take his advice; don't try to be your own physician.

If you have questions, don't be afraid to ask them. Have him explain the nature of your ailment, how long it may take for relief or cure, how the therapy or medication is expected to work, and the possible impact on your everyday activities.

Hopefully, by following his advice you'll stay healthy and well. However, if you are at home and feel ill, call your physician if:

- Your symptoms are so severe you can't endure them.

- Apparent minor symptoms persist without explainable cause.

- You are in doubt.

For more information, see "The Physical Examination" in Ch. 26, *Physicians and Diagnostic Procedures.*

Oral Health

It is especially important in later years to have regular dental checkups. After age 50, over half of the American people have some form of *periodontal disease*, and at age 65 nearly all persons have this disease.

Brushing teeth and gums regularly is a defense against periodontal disease. Use dental floss to remove all food particles and plaque from areas between the teeth, especially after each meal. See "Periodontal Disease" in Ch. 22, *The Teeth and Gums*, for more information on this subject.

Dentures

If you do lose some teeth, they should be replaced with bridges or partial or full dentures, because the cheeks and lips will otherwise sag and wrinkle and make you look older than you really are. Chewing ability and the clarity of speech are also impaired if missing teeth are not replaced. See "Dentures" in Ch. 22, *The Teeth and Gums.*

Diet and Health

Just what are your food requirements as you grow older? Basically you need the same essential nutrients that you have always needed, except that you face special problems. You need to:

- Select food more carefully to eat adequate proteins, vitamins, and minerals—while cutting down on calories.

- Get the most nutritious food for the least money and make the most of what you buy.

- Avoid bad eating habits—make mealtime a pleasure rather than a chore.

- Learn new techniques to stretch meals, use leftovers, and substitute lower-priced items with the same nutritional value for higher-priced foods. In other words, learn how to shop well.

Basic Requirements

How can you get the essential nutrients every day? A good rule is first to eat recommended servings from the Basic Four Food Groups (see below) established by the National Research Council. Then, eat other foods that you like, as long as they do not go over the recommended daily caloric intake. The average man in the 55-to-75-year age group should consume 2,200 calories a day; the average woman in the same age group, 1,600 calories a day. This is a drop of between 500 and 600 calories a day from what was needed at age 25. As you grow older, your physical activity decreases and your metabolism slows, causing body fats to build up at a much higher rate and making you more prone to hardening of the arteries and certain heart conditions.

Here are the Basic Four Food Groups:

Meat Group

Two or more servings from this group of foods are recommended daily. A serving is two to three ounces of cooked meat, fish, or poultry; two eggs; occasionally one cup of cooked dry beans or peas; one-half cup peanut butter; or one cup cottage cheese.

Dairy Foods

Dairy food requirements may be satisfied by two cups of milk or its equivalent in cheese, ice cream, etc. A one and one-third ounce slice of cheddar-type cheese or one scant pint of ice cream is equivalent to one cup of milk. Imitation ice cream or ice milk where vegetable fat has been substituted for butterfat has just as much protein.

Vegetables and Fruit

The daily vegetable and fruit requirement consists of four or more servings. A serving is one-half cup. Include one serving of citrus fruit each day and dark green or deep yellow vegetables every other day.

Bread and Cereal Group

Each day have four or more servings of whole grain, enriched, or restored products such as breads, cereals, rice, hominy grits, noodles, or macaroni. One serving is a slice of bread; one-half to three-fourths cup cooked cereal, pasta, or rice; one medium potato.

Use other foods such as sweets, baked goods, or desserts to complete meals and treat the sweet tooth. But remember to count calories. Nutritionists have found that skinny animals live longer than fat ones, and this seems to be true of people, too.

Beware of food fads and so-called health foods unless these are recommended by your physician. Also, do not buy vitamins and mineral tablets unless prescribed. When you obtain vitamins from food, your body uses the amount necessary to maintain proper health, appetite, and resistance to infection. Your body promptly eliminates excesses of vitamin C and the B complex, and stores an excess of vitamins A and D in your liver and other body organs. It may take up to seven years of practically complete deprivation for a previously healthy adult to show signs of a vitamin deficiency.

Some older people may go on low-fat diets because of fear of cholesterol caused by talk and advertisements for unsaturated fats. Get a physician's recommendation before curtailing your fat intake—too little fat and dairy products can be as harmful as too much.

Also, unless prescribed, do not take iron tonics or pills. Usually you'll get adequate iron intake if you eat meat, eggs, vegetables, and enriched cereals regularly. Adding more iron to a normal diet may even be harmful.

Eating Habits

If you find that mealtime is a chore rather than a pleasure, try these tips to enhance your meals:

- Try a two-meal-a-day schedule. Have a late breakfast and early dinner when you are really hungry. But be sure to get your Basic Four requirements in these two meals.

- Drink a glass of water as soon as you wake up to promote good digestion, weight control, and bowel movements.

- Try a walk or light exercise to stimulate appetite and to regulate body processes. Moderate exercise also will help regulate weight because it burns up calories.

- You might sip glass of wine before dinner. Recent research shows wine is very useful to older people in improving appetite and digestion. Port, a light sherry, and vermouth with a dash of soda are good appetite stimulators.

- Make meals interesting by including some food of distinctive flavor to contrast with a mild-flavored food; something crisp for contrast with softer foods, even if it is only a pickle or a lettuce leaf; some brightly colored food for eye appeal.

- Pep up your food with a judicious use of herbs and spices or flavor-enhancers like wine, bottled sauces, fruit juices, and peels.

- If some food causes you distress, eliminate it and substitute something else of equal nutritive value. Green salad may include too much roughage for the intestinal tract; ham or bacon may be supplying your body with too much salt, which increases water retention. Or you may be drinking too much coffee, tea, or soft drinks.

- Be realistic about your chewing ability. Food swallowed whole may be causing digestive problems. If your teeth are not as good as they were or if you are wearing dentures, try cubing, chopping, or grinding foods that are difficult to chew. Let your knife or meat grinder do part of the work.

- Try a different atmosphere or different setting for your meals. Use candlelight, music, and your best linen on occasion. Move outdoors when the weather is good; eat your lunch in the park and dinner on the patio.

- Occasionally invite a friend or relative to dine with you. It's surprising what stimulating conversation and an exchange of ideas can do to boost your mood and appetite.

- Try a new recipe or a new food. Thanks to modern transportation, foods are available in larger cities from many areas and other countries. Eat eggplant or okra, avocado or artichoke, gooseberry jam, or garbanzo beans in a salad. And why not have a papaya with lemon juice for breakfast?

Cooking Hints

Try these ideas for preparing food more easily; they are especially useful if you have only a single gas or electric burner:

- Combine your vegetables and meat—or some other protein food—in a single pot or pan. You can cook many hot, nourishing meals of this kind: Irish stew, braised liver or pot roast with vegetables, ham-and-vegetable chowder or fish chowder, a New England boiled dinner.

- Combine leftovers to make a one-dish meal. Leftover meat combines beautifully with vegetables, macaroni, or rice. Add a cheese or tomato sauce or a simple white sauce and heat in a baking dish. Chopped tomatoes or green onions or chives will give extra flavor and color to the dish.

- Round out one-dish meals with a crisp salad topped with cut strips of leftover cooked meat or poultry or another raw food, bread, a beverage, and perhaps a dessert.

- Mix leftover cooked vegetables with raw fresh ones, such as chopped celery, cucumber slices, tomatoes, green pepper, shredded cabbage, to make an interesting salad.

- Cream vegetables, meat, fish, or chicken. Or serve them with a tasty sauce. Use canned tomato or mushroom soup for a quick and easy sauce. If the dish is a bit skimpy, a hard-boiled egg may stretch it to serving size.

- Add a bit of relish, snappy cheese, or diced cucumber to a cooked dressing for meat or vegetable salad.

- If you cook a potato, an ear of corn, or some other vegetable in the bottom of a double boiler, you can use the top to warm rolls, heat leftover meat in gravy, or heat such foods as creamed eggs or fish.

The Value of Exercise

As you grow older, exercise can help you look, feel, and work better. Various organs and systems of the body, particularly the digestive process, are stimulated through activity, and, as a result, work more effectively.

You can improve your posture through exercise that tones supporting muscles. This not only improves appearance but can decrease the frequency of lower-back pain and disability.

Here are some other benefits of exercise: it can increase your ability to relax and tolerate fatigue; it improves muscle tone; reduces fat deposits; increases working capacity of the lungs; improves kidney and liver functions; increases volume of blood, hemoglobin, and red blood cells, leading to improved utilization of oxygen and iron.

Also, physically active people are less likely to experience a heart attack or other forms of cardiovascular disease than sedentary people. Moreover, an active person who does suffer a coronary attack will probably have a less severe form. The Public Health Service studied 5,000 adults in Framingham, Mass., for more than a decade. When any member of the group suffered a heart attack, his physical activity was reviewed. It was found that more inactive people suffered more fatal heart attacks than active members.

Walking for Exercise

Exercise need not be something you *must* do but rather something you *enjoy* doing. One of the most practical and enjoyable exercises is walking. Charles Dickens said:

Walk and be happy, walk and be healthy. The best of all ways to lengthen our days is to walk, steadily and with a purpose. The wandering man knows of certain ancients, far gone in years, who have staved off infirmities and dissolution by earnest walking—hale fellows close upon eighty and ninety, but brisk as boys.

The benefits of walking were revealed in a recent Health Insurance Plan study of 110,000 people in New York City. Those who had heart attacks were divided into two groups—walkers and nonwalkers. The first four weeks of illness were reviewed for both groups. At the end of the time 41 percent of the nonwalkers were dead, while only 23 percent of the walkers were. When all physical activity was considered, 57 percent of the inactive had died compared to only 16 percent of those who had some form of exercise.

Walking is as natural to the human body as breathing. It is a muscular symphony; all the foot, leg, and hip muscles and much of the back musculature are involved. The abdominal muscles tend to contract and support their share of the weight, and the diaphragm and rib muscles increase their action. There is automatic action of the arm and shoulder muscles; the shoulder and neck muscles get play as the head is held erect; the eye muscles are exercised as you look about you.

Other Types of Exercise

Swimming and bicycling exercise most of the muscles, and gardening is highly recommended. The fresh air is beneficial, the bending, squatting, and countless other movements exercise most parts of the body.

Surprisingly, most games do not provide good exercise. According to a physical fitness research laboratory at the University of Illinois, the trouble with most games is that the action is intermittent—starting and stopping—a burst of energy and then a wait. The bowler swings a ball for two and one-half seconds and gets about one minute of actual muscular work per game. Golf is a succession of pause, swing, walk—or, more often, a ride to the next pause, swing, and so on. Also, you spend a lot of time standing and waiting for the party ahead and for your partners. Tennis gives one more exercise but it too involves a great deal of starting and stopping, as does handball. No game has the essential, tension-releasing pattern of continuous, vigorous, rhythmic motion found in such activities as walking, running, or jogging.

For formal exercises, you could join a gym, but you might find your enthusiasm waning after a few weeks. You could also exercise at home; there are many excellent books on exercise that provide programs for you to follow at home on a daily basis.

But everyone's exercise capacity varies. It is best to discuss any new exercise program with your physician, especially if you have some illness or are out of practice. Then select an exercise which is pleasant for you and suitable to your condition.

It is most important always to warm up before any strenuous exercise. The U.S. Administration on Aging's booklet, *The Fitness Challenge in the Later Years*, states:

> The enthusiast who tackles a keep-fit program too fast and too strenuously soon gives up in discomfort, if not in injury. A warm-up period should be performed by starting lightly with a continuous rhythmical activity such as walking and gradually increasing the intensity until your pulse rate, breathing, and body temperature are elevated. It's also desirable to do some easy stretching, pulling, and rotating exercises during the warm-up period.

The booklet outlines an excellent program—*red* (easiest), *white* (next), and *blue* (the most sustained and difficult). Each program is "designed to give a balanced workout utilizing all major muscle groups."

A Word of Caution

You may be exercising too strenuously if the following happens:

- Your heart does not stop pounding within 10 minutes after the exercise.

- You cannot catch your breath 10 minutes after the exercise.

- You are shaky for more than 30 minutes afterwards.

- You can't sleep well afterwards.

- Your fatigue (not muscle soreness) continues into the next day.

Sensible, moderate exercise geared to your own physical capacity can help to give you a sense of all-around well-being. As Dr. Ernest Simonson, associate professor of physiological hygiene at the University of Minnesota Medical School, has said:

> Those who exercise regularly never fail to mention that it makes them feel better in every way. It's common logic if one feels better, his attitude towards others will be more congenial. When one is in a cordial, happy frame of mind, he will likely make wiser decisions, and his world in general will look better.

Weight Control

Importantly, both diet and exercise affect the individual's ability to control his weight (see Ch. 27, *Nutrition and Weight Control*; "Weight Problems" in Ch. 23, *Aches, Pains, Nuisances, Worries*; and Ch. 37, *Physical Fitness*). Healthy habits in both areas provide a complete answer for many older persons. For others, some additional effort is required.

The same diet rules that help the older person feel well and function adequately will make weight control simpler. But persons beyond middle age who have weight problems should make extra efforts to bring their weight down. Extra pounds of fat only make it harder for the vital organs to function; excess poundage also forces the heart to work harder. A variety of diets may be used to bring your weight back to where it should be. But the calorie-counter program may suffice for most persons.

Exercise provides the second key to weight control. Many physicians feel that older persons of both sexes should walk at least a mile daily. Other exercises acclaimed by physicians include golf, gardening, working on or around the house, and similar activities. Some other basic rules regarding exercise and diet should be noted:

- Avoid junk, or high carbohydrate, food where possible.

- Make certain you are eating foods that provide enough protein.

- Eat to assuage hunger, not to drive away boredom.

- Remember that appetite usually decreases with age, and act accordingly.

- Avoid vitamins unless they are prescribed by your physician, and use them accordingly.

- Try every day to eat foods in the four basic groups.

- Keep moving; walk daily—to the store, post office, church, around the block.

- If you exercise already, do it regularly; a little exercise daily is better than a lot on weekends.

- If you don't exercise but are thinking of starting a program of workouts of some kind, start slowly and build up—following your physician's recommendations.

- If stress gives you problems, find ways to relax without eating or drinking; consider light exercises, yoga, meditation, breathing exercises, or some other method.

Skin Problems

As a person grows older, his skin begins to wrinkle; oil and sweat glands slow down, causing the skin to become dry. Also, the skin may lack the elasticity and tone of normal skin, and this might cause changes in facial contours.

However, the skin, like other parts of the body, tends to age according to various factors. Among prime agers of the skin are exposure to sunlight and weather; the sailor and chronic sunbather may have older-looking skin than their years. Also, hereditary and racial factors influence skin age.

Itching

The skin often itches as one grows older. Itching usually stems from external irritations or internal diseases. External irritations may be more severe in winter because of lack of humidity and because the skin oil does not spread properly. Too many baths or wearing wool garments could also cause itching. You can correct this by cutting down on bathing, maintaining correct temperature and humidity, and applying skin creams.

If itching does not clear up in about two weeks, the trouble may be due to any of a number of internal diseases, some of them serious. Thus, it is wise to see your physician if itching persists.

Skin Cancer

Skin cancer can be easily diagnosed and treated. The two most common types are *basal cell* and *squamous cell*.

The basal cell type begins with a small fleshy *nodule*, usually on the face. It may take several months to reach one-half to one inch in diameter. In about a year it begins to ulcerate and bleed. Then it forms a crust, which it sheds at intervals, leaving another ulcer. If you notice anything like this, see your physician. He can usually remove the ulcer by a local operation.

Squamous cell cancer is often aided by smoking and exposure to the sun. The lesions may appear on the lips, mouth, and genitalia, and they tend to spread and increase in size. Horny growths in exposed areas—face, ears, neck, and scalp—may be forerunners of squamous cell cancer. Again, your physician can treat or operate effectively. See also Ch. 18, *Cancer*.

Vitiligo

Vitiligo, loss of pigment, is not caused by a disease, but it could be a hereditary problem. The affected area of skin has patches of whiteness throughout, but these can be masked by cosmetics.

Senile Purpura

Sometimes the skin develops *senile purpura* as one grows older. The characteristic hemorrhages of this condition usually appear on the extremities, and the purple color gradually fades and leaves mottled areas of yellow-brown. Generally, the skin is thin, fragile, and transparent in appearance.

Stasis Dermatitis

Sometimes in association with such conditions as varicose veins, the skin may develop *stasis dermatitis*, an acute, chronic condition of the leg, associated with swelling, scaling of the skin, and in some cases, ulcer formation. It may exist for years with or without ulceration.

If any of the above conditions develop, it is wise to consult your physician rather than try to treat yourself.

Other Skin Conditions

Other skin conditions that may develop in the later years may include an increase in coarse hairs on exposed places such as the upper lip or chin. The downy hairs in the ears and nose become become thicker and more apparent, and the eyebrows may become bushy. Graying hair is popularly associated with aging, but its onset often depends upon genetic factors and varies so much that it cannot be used as a reliable measure of age.

The earlobes may elongate as you grow older and the nails may become coarse and thickened or thinner and brittle.

Relieving Skin Conditions

As mentioned earlier, you can use some creams to relieve dryness and scaliness in older skin. The best of such creams are the water-in-oil emulsions (cold creams) such as Petrolatum Rose Water Ointment USP XVI, or oil-in-water emulsions such as Hydrophilic Ointment USP XVI. Wrinkle creams will not help much, but some conditions may be masked by regular cosmetic items such as powder, rouge, mascara, hair dyes, etc.

Sunscreens may aid in preventing acute and chronic overexposure to the sun's rays.

Various types of surgery may be performed to correct older skin conditions, but they won't work for everyone. Among some of the more common types of surgery are plastic surgery, dermabrasion (skin planning), chemosurgery (chemical cautery), cryosurgery (freezing of the skin), and electrosurgery (employing electricity). See "Plastic and Cosmetic Surgery" in Ch. 20, *Surgery*.

Hearing Loss

About three out of ten persons over age 65 have some hearing loss; at age 70 to 80 this percentage increases greatly.

Causes

While some hearing loss can be blamed on bad listening habits (tuning out people and conversation a person does not want to hear), the two major causes are conduction loss and nerve defects. A person with conduction loss hears high-pitched sounds best; a person with nerve impairment hears low sounds best. A combination of the two is called mixed deafness.

Conduction loss can be caused by wax, diseases of the ear, disturbances of the eardrum, or abnormalities inside the ear. It can also be caused by *otosclerosis*, a bony growth over the window to the inner ear. Most of these conditions can be treated by an ear doctor (*otologist*). He can remove wax from the ear, repair or replace eardrums, remove bony growths, and loosen or remove fixed ear bones.

Nerve defects may be another story. They are caused by wear and tear on the ear, disease, certain drugs, and blows and skull fractures, and usually cause permanent damage that cannot be helped by surgery or medical treatment.

Some persons complain about ringing in the ears (*tinnitus*) that may start without warning and vary in intensity and quality. What causes tinnitus in one person may not cause it in another, but often it is caused by wax in the ear, middle ear infection, arteriosclerosis, or certain drugs.

Hearing Aids

In most cases a hearing loss can be helped with a hearing aid or surgery. But if you think you have a hearing problem your first task is to see your physician. If your problem is not medically treatable, and if your physician believes a hearing aid will help you, you should see a dispensing audiologist. The American Speech-Language-Hearing Association, 10801 Rockville Pike, Rockville, MD 20852, will supply a directory of certified practitioners on request. If you have trouble finding an audiologist, an experienced hearing-aid dealer may be able to advise you on the device best suited to your needs. The National Hearing Aid Help Line (800/521-5247), a service of the National Hearing Aid Society, provides lists of dealers certified as dispensing audiologists.

A hearing test at a hearing aid clinic may be your next stop. Here trained audiologists will scientifically measure your hearing and assist you in trying on different kinds of aids. The audiologists do not sell hearing aids, but can tell you what kind is best for you. Basically, there are five kinds of aids:

- Body types that operate with a cord running to the receiver mold in the ear from a miniature microphone carried in a pocket, pinned to the clothing, or worn in a special carrier. These devices are about one to one and one-half inches long and weigh about two ounces.

- Behind-the-ear types that weigh only about one-half ounce and fit behind the ear. A plastic tube leads from the microphone to the receiver that fits in the ear.

- Hearing aids that fit inside the ear canal and weigh about one-sixth of an ounce. This model has become the most popular among hearing aid wearers.

- A type that fits in the outer ear.

- A "bionic ear" that requires surgery to make possible a *cochlear implant*. In the surgery a strip of 22 platinum electrodes is inserted into the inner ear, or cochlea (see "The Ear," in Ch. 1, *The Body*). A tiny cable connects the electrodes to a microchip planted under the skin behind one ear and to a microphone and transmitter attached to a headset.

A sixth kind of hearing aid, one that was built into eyeglasses, has virtually disappeared from use.

Buying a Hearing Aid

No single hearing aid is ideal for every hard-of-hearing person. Thus testing is essential if you are to find the right aid. You may want to bring a friend or relative when you are being fitted. A familiar voice serves as a yardstick to help you judge which aid is best.

It takes time to get used to a hearing aid. An aid amplifies all sounds— wanted and unwanted. It also changes most sounds, giving them an "electronic" character. Voices may sound unnatural and tinny. Normal noises may be harsh and grating. But special circuiting in many of today's aids limits the sound level reaching the eardrum. These *automatic gain controls* prevent discomfort but may distort speech. A still newer approach is to use filters to screen out background noises.

In addition to greatly reducing the sizes of many hearing aids, technological advances are expanding the usefulness of hearing aids continually. Noise blockers filter out sounds that do not fit with speech patterns. Tiny microphones reduce the buzzing noises picked up by some older hearing aid models. Treble and bass dials give the wearer a way to adjust sound quality to background noises. With the dials the wearer can also make adjustments to the hearing fluctuations resulting from bodily changes.

If you do not want to wear a hearing aid, or cannot adjust to one, you can try lip reading or speech reading. Each involves watching the lips and vocal chords to determine what another person is saying.

Talking to the Hard-of-Hearing

If you are talking to someone who has some hearing difficulty, he'll understand you better if you speak slowly and distinctly and use the lower range of your voice. Face him when you speak; let him see the movements of your lips. It also helps to point to visible objects.

Above all, don't shout. In fact, raising your voice sometimes pitches it into a higher frequency which a hard-of-hearing person may find difficult to understand.

Other Health Problems

The following health problems might also confront an older person. (Many of these conditions are discussed at greater length elsewhere in the book; in such cases, cross-references are supplied for your convenience at the end of the section.)

Heart Disease

The heart is the strongest, toughest muscle in the body. It is like an engine that could run 70 years or more without an overhaul. The heart has a complete maintenance and repair system, enabling many heart disease victims to continue long and useful lives.

While heart disease is not necessarily a product of aging, some heart and blood vessel problems become more acute as one grows older.

The following symptoms do not necessarily indicate heart disease, but it is wise to see a physician if you notice any of them:

- Shortness of breath

- A feeling of tightness in the chest or pain directly related to exertion or excitement

- Swelling of the feet and ankles

- Unusual fatigue

There is much that physicians can do to prevent heart conditions or to relieve them once present. But there is much that you can do to help yourself.

Weight

Extra pounds of fat mean more work for the heart.

Diet

The rules of sound nutrition apply to proper heart care.

Smoking

Heavy cigarette smokers suffer three times as many heart attacks as do pipe or cigar smokers. Nonsmokers are safest.

Exercise

Exercise improves the pumping action of the heart as well as circulation, digestion, and general health.

Worry

Worry increases tension and elevates blood pressure. Try to cultivate a philosophical approach to the daily ups and downs. See Ch. 10, *Heart Disease*.

Strokes

Strokes are not hopeless; even severely paralyzed patients may make remarkable progress. A *stroke* occurs when the blood supply to a part of the brain tissue is cut off and, as a result, the nerve cells in that part of the brain can't function. When this happens, the part of the body controlled by these nerve cells can't function either.

Whenever the blood supply is cut off from an area, small neighboring arteries get larger and take over part of the work of the damaged artery. In this way nerve cells that have been temporarily put out of order may recover, and that part of the body affected by the stroke may eventually improve or even return to normal.

Once a stroke has occurred, a sound rehabilitation program can help the patient resume as many normal activities as possible. This program can be worked out in cooperation with the physician, patient, family, and local organizations. See Ch. 9, *Diseases of the Circulatory System*.

Arthritis

There are two main types of arthritis: *rheumatoid arthritis* and *osteoarthritis*.

Rheumatoid arthritis—which can cause pain and swelling in joints, nerves, muscles, tendons, blood vessels, and connective tissue in the whole body—can strike at any age, but it occurs mainly in the 25-to-40-year age group. The exact cause of rheumatoid arthritis is unknown.

Osteoarthritis is a degenerative joint disease that affects almost everyone who lives long enough; it is a product of normal wear and tear on the joints over the years. Poor posture and obesity are contributing causes, as are heredity and trauma.

Osteoarthritis is usually mild, and it seldom cripples. Pain is generally moderate. Unlike rheumatoid arthritis, which is inflammatory, spreads from joint to joint, and affects the whole body, osteoarthritis confines its attack locally to individual joints. Rarely is inflammation a problem.

Osteoarthritis is likely to develop in any joint that has been required to take a lot of punishment or abuse: the knee or hip joints of someone who is overweight; joints injured in an accident; joints injured or overused in sports; joints subjected to unusual stresses and strains in work or play; joints with hidden defects that were present at birth.

There is no specific cure for arthritis, but the pain and swelling can be controlled. In other than acute cases, common aspirin has proved the safest and most popular medication.

Adequate rest for both the body and the affected joint is a fundamental treatment. Heat, controlled exercise, hydrotherapy, and massage are all effective if done under a physician's supervision. See "Arthritis and Other Joint Diseases" in Ch. 7, *Diseases of the Skeletal System*.

Cancer

Cancer strikes at any age, but it does strike more frequently in the later years. Many factors are believed to contribute to cancer; frictional and chemical irritations like cigarette smoking, irritation of the skin and mouth (such as poor dentures), exposure to the sun, X rays, or radioactive elements. Common sites are the lips, mouth, stomach, intestines, rectum, liver, pancreas, lungs, breast, kidney, bladder, skin, uterus, and prostate.

Early detection and prompt treatment are the best protection against cancer. If any of the following seven danger signals lasts longer than two weeks, be sure to get a checkup.

- Unusual bleeding or discharge

- A lump or thickening in the breast or elsewhere

- A sore that does not heal

- Change in bowel or bladder habits

- Hoarseness or cough

- Indigestion or difficulty in swallowing

- Change in wart or mole

Great strides have been made in treating cancer through surgery, radiotherapy, and chemotherapy. See Ch. 18, *Cancer*. For cancers affecting women only, see "Cancers of the Reproductive System" and "Cancer of the Breast" in Ch. 25, *Women's Health*.

The Eyes

The eye does age. After age 40, failing vision is usually caused by natural hardening of the lens, making it difficult to see close objects. However, failing vision may also be the first symptom of a serious bodily disorder, or of glaucoma or of a cataract, which requires a physician's immediate attention.

Both glaucoma and cataract can be treated effectively. About 90 percent of glaucoma cases can be checked with eye drops and about 95 percent of cataracts can be removed by a painless operation.

Other diseases that may develop in later years affect the blood vessels of the eye. A common condition is *senile macula degeneration* which causes a blind spot to appear when the victim looks directly at something. The exact cause of senile macula degeneration is not known. See under Ch. 16, *Diseases of the Eye and Ear.*

Diabetes

Most likely candidates for diabetes are overweight persons past 40, particularly those who have a hereditary history of diabetes, and especially older women.

The exact cause of diabetes is not known, but it is a functional disorder in which the body cannot handle certain foods—mainly sugars and starches. Symptoms include increased thirst, constant hunger, frequent urination, loss of weight, itching, easy tiring, changes in vision, and slow healing of cuts and scratches.

Treatment and control consist of planned diet, exercise, and, in many cases, insulin shots or oral medication. Well-controlled diabetics can lead active lives. See Ch. 15, *Diabetes Mellitus.*

Constipation

There is no truth in the notion that a daily bowel movement is necessary for good health. A movement every day or twice a day may be all right for one person; for another every three or four days may be enough.

The two most common causes of chronic constipation are physical inactivity and poor food and water habits. Ironically, constipation may be caused by swallowing a cathartic nightly to induce a bowel movement. The habit eventually leads to chronic constipation because normal bowel movement ceases and bowel evacuation depends on using a cathartic.

To maintain proper bowel movement, try the following:

- Drink eight to ten glasses of water a day. Take two glasses of water on an empty stomach as soon as you get up.

- Drink more fruit juices and eat more dried and fresh fruits.

- Get at least one-half hour of moderate exercise daily. Walking, for example, is excellent, particularly if you relax while you walk.

- Give yourself enough time for normal bowel movement and set up a regular time for evacuation.

- If you are constipated, consult your physician to make sure it is simple and functional. See under Ch. 23, *Aches, Pains, Nuisances, Worries.*

Back Problems

As we grow older, the back muscles—weakened by inactivity, poor posture, and almost unavoidable wear and tear—start to complain.

Other causes of back problems are muscle and joint strain, changes in the spine, psychological tension, and internal diseases. Here are some tips to help avoid backache:

- Learn to lift correctly. Use your leg muscles, which are stronger than back muscles, by placing your feet closer to the base of the object, bending your knees outward, and pushing up with your legs.

- Avoid subjecting your back to any sudden, erratic motion.

- Try to improve your posture when sitting and walking.

- Sleep on a firm bed; a bed board may be helpful.

- Get regular exercise of a type that stimulates all your muscles rather than just a few.

- If you sit for a long period, get up and stretch occasionally.

- Beware of excess weight. Extra weight on the abdomen pulls on the vertebrae at the small of the back, increasing the spine's normal curve and causing pain.

- Try never to become overfatigued or exhausted, either physically or mentally. Emotional pressure, from work or personal problems, causes muscle tension. See "Backaches" in Ch. 23, *Aches, Pains, Nuisances, Worries.*

Because the feet are farthest away from the heart's blood supply, they are often the first areas affected by circulatory diseases. Also, arthritis and diabetes might first show up in the feet.

Warning signs include continued cramping of the calf muscles, pain in the arch and toes, and unusually cold feet—especially if accompanied by a bluish skin. Brittle or thickened toenails or burning, tingling, and numbness may also signal a circulatory disease.

Foot ulcers may be one of the first signs of diabetes. Some *bunions*—swollen, tender, red joints—are caused by arthritis. Swelling around the feet and ankles suggests a possible kidney disorder.

If you have these symptoms, go to a *podiatrist* (a foot doctor) or to your own physician. They are trained to recognize these symptoms.

Most older people, however, suffer from minor aches and pains in the feet that are caused by poor foot care or abuse. See "The Vulnerable Extremeties" in Ch. 23, *Aches, Pains, Nuisances, Worries.*

Care of the Feet

To prevent these problems, treat yourself to daily foot care. Dry your feet thoroughly and gently after bathing and inspect the skin for abrasion, rough spots, or cracks. Dry carefully between the toes. If the skin is dry or scaly, lubricate it with lanolin or olive oil. Next, apply a medicated foot powder recommended by your podiatrist or physician over the entire foot, especially between the toes, as a preventive measure against athlete's foot.

When you cut your nails, do it with a strong light and be careful to cut straight across the nail to prevent ingrown toenails. Avoid the use of strong medications containing salicylate and strong antiseptics like iodine, carbolic acid, lysol, or bleach. Harsh chemicals that attack toughened skin can irritate normal tissue and cause infection. Avoid using hot water bottles, electric pads, or any form of extreme heat or cold. Diabetics should visit a podiatrist regularly.

The Prostate

Men over 50 may have an enlarged *prostate*. (This is not caused by sexual excesses or venereal disease.) The exact cause is not known, but it's estimated that some type of enlarged prostate is present in about 10 percent of 40-year-olds and 80 percent of 80-year-olds.

The prostate is a rubbery mass of glands and muscle tissue about the size and shape of a horse chestnut. It is wrapped around the urethra and base of the bladder at the point where they join. The prostate functions as part of a man's sexual apparatus, providing a fluid that transports and nourishes the spermatozoa.

Symptoms of an enlarged prostate include difficulty in urination. There might be an initial blocking of the urine, or the stream may lack force. You may feel that you can't empty the bladder, and you may have urgent needs to urinate. You may have pain or blood in the urine from straining.

If you have any of these symptoms, your physician can easily check for enlarged prostate by a simple rec-

tal examination. If he discovers an enlargement, he can usually treat it in early stages with simple massage. But if it has progressed too far, he may have to operate.

An operation is usually performed through the urethra or by an incision in the lower abdomen. The choice depends upon the individual problems of the patient and the judgment of the surgeon. In either case, the patient usually recovers completely in a short time.

A rectal examination can also discover early stages of cancer of the prostate, which is not uncommon in men over 40. Some 20 percent of men over 60 have this condition, and it is most common in men over 70.

Unfortunately, this disease does not manifest itself early, so it is important that men over 40 have the diagnostic rectal examination. If the disease is detected early and treated—usually by surgery, hormonal therapy, and possibly radiation—the cure rate is very high. If found late, the cure rate is low.

When treatment is by surgery, the entire prostate and upper urethra may be removed. In some cases, the disease may be retarded or relieved by treatment with female hormones. (The male hormone is known to hasten prostate cancer.)

In both enlargement and cancer of the prostate, early detection is vital to a successful cure. That is why it is important to have a rectal examination. See also "Cancer of the Prostate" in Ch. 18, *Cancer.*

Alzheimer's Disease

Alzheimer's disease is a group of brain disorders marked by progressive deterioration and affects both memory and reasoning abilities. Victims of Alzheimer's, which is a form of dementia, or mental deterioration (see "Dementia" in Ch. 8, *Diseases of*

the Muscles and Nervous System), undergo various behavioral changes. These include an inability to concentrate, anxiety, irritability, agitation, withdrawal, and petulance. Persons suffering from Alzheimer's may wander about and lose their way. They may have temper tantrums and engage in obsessional behavior, such as repeatedly washing dishes. Time and place disorientation may be accompanied by delusions and depression. In the later stages of the disease, sufferers often lose bladder and bowel control.

Diagnosing Alzheimer's in its early stages is difficult despite its numerous symptoms. Laboratory tests that could identify the disorder do not exist. Adding to the problems of diagnosis, various other disorders have similar symptoms. The best medical alternative, a complete physical examination, generally includes a review of any drugs or medications the patient has been taking as well as standard laboratory tests. The latter help to rule out other diseases or disorders that may be treatable. A clinical evaluation can include a CT (computed tomography) scan, an EEG (electroencephalogram), and assessment of evidence from family members and the patient regarding the latter's (or patient's) mental state.

Even when diagnosed with relative certainty, Alzheimer's disease cannot be cured. But some symptoms, including depression and delusions, can be treated. The effect is to slow the progress of the disorder. Where Parkinson's disease or heart problems accompany Alzheimer's, treatment can focus on alleviation of those conditions.

Theories regarding the causes of Alzheimer's abound. Because it is known that the disease leads to severe atrophy and distortion of the cerebral cortex, researchers have explored both genetic and physiological theories. On the genetic side, studies have indicated that persons with relatives who had or have Alzheimer's face three or four times the normal risks of becoming victims. On the physiological side, Alzheimer's patients have been shown to lack adequate supplies of *choline acetyltransferase* (CAT), a neurotransmitter, or chemical, that enables brain signals to travel from one cell to another. Such findings, it is hoped, will lead eventually to cures.

Meeting the Challenge of Leisure

Leisure Activities

In ten years of retirement, you will have the leisure time equivalent of working 40 hours a week for 21 years. You cannot fish this time away and you cannot rest it away. Whatever you do for long must have meaning—must satisfy some basic need and want. Certain needs remain constant throughout life:

- Security—good health, income, and a recognized role in society

- Recognition—as an individual with your own abilities and personality

- Belonging—as a member of a family, social group, and community

- Self-expression—by developing abilities and talents in new areas and at new levels

- Adventure—new experiences, new sights, and new knowledge

There are many activities that can satisfy these basic needs and wants to keep you mentally and physically in top shape.

Travel

Travel satisfies your need for adventure in many ways. If you travel off-season at bargain rates, you'll find that time truly is money. Most travel problems stem from rushing to meet a schedule. Making every minute count on a fast-paced European tour can be expensive and exhausting. For the· same transatlantic fare, you can spend a full year in Europe at one-third the daily cost of a three-week vacation.

Wherever you travel, it isn't enough just to sightsee. Try to center your travel around an interest or a hobby. You can take art or music tours—tours that stress education, night life, culture, or special interests. You can travel on your own or with a group. But whatever you do, participate; don't just observe.

Doing things instead of just observing adds new dimensions to the pleasure of going places. For people who participate, travel means the adventure of enjoying exciting new places, people, and experiences. To help plan your trip, write to the government tourist offices of foreign countries (ask your library for addresses); to the National Park Service, Washington, DC; and to state or local chambers of commerce (no street addresses necessary).

Gardening

Gardening satisfies one's need for self-expression in many ways. Being outside in the fresh air and planting living things can bring satisfaction and peace of mind.

Gardening is a many-faceted hobby that offers many challenges. You can go into plant breeding, growing for resale, introducing new plants, collecting the rare and unusual, plant selecting, or simply cultivating what you find personally appealing and satisfying.

Your local library or bookstore has many books on the subject. There are local and national garden clubs that you can join to learn about your hobby and to meet other people who are interested in gardening. Write the Government Printing Office, Washington, DC 20401, for help and advice. In addition, state extension directors at state colleges and universities, county agricultural agents, and local plant nurseries can give expert advice and information.

Reading

Reading offers excitement, adventure, pursuit of knowledge, and an introduction to new people and places. Your local library is the best place to launch a reading program—and you may be surprised to find that it offers more than books. Most libraries have art and music departments, audiovisual services (films and microfilm copies), foreign language departments, periodical rooms (newspapers and magazines), writing classes, genealogy workshops, and special courses of general interest.

Hobbies

A hobby can be any physical or mental activity that gives you happiness, relaxation, and satisfaction. It should not be just a time killer—it should offer some tangible reward. Also, it should have continuity, not be too expensive, and not make undue demands on time and energy. Perhaps you would prefer a series of hobbies, some serious and some just for fun. They can be related to your work or completely unrelated. In any event, a hobby should be something you've always wanted to do.

Before selecting a hobby, consider these points:

- Do you like to do things alone? Consider arts, crafts, reading, sewing, fishing—activities that are not dependent on others, although you can enjoy them with others.

- Do you like groups? Seek hobbies that include other people—organizational, sport, game, or craft activities.

- Do you like to play to win? Try your luck in competitive or team games that stress winning.

- Do you have to be an expert? Too many of us are afraid to try new activities because we hate to fail or look clumsy. But be fair; judge your efforts in light of your past experience and present progress; do not compare yourself to someone who's been at it longer than you.

- Do you put a price tag on everything? Many people will not engage in an activity if it costs too much. Yet, many hobbies fail because they're tried on a shoestring without adequate equipment. Also, some people do not want to do anything unless it brings in money. If so, perhaps you should look for something that's an offshoot of the work or business you know best.

Creative Crafts

Creative crafts are difficult for most of us because we are conservative, afraid to make mistakes, sensitive because of buried and almost forgotten blunders. Yet creativity is essential to life. Without it we don't live fully; through creative skills we refurbish old interests and develop new ones.

Most of us are happiest with creative crafts that do not require intri-

cate work or fine detail and that are not too demanding physically. Some crafts best suited to retirement years include weaving, rug making, sewing, ceramic work, knitting, plastic molding, woodwork, leathercraft, and lapidary.

You can learn these and other crafts and also market your products through senior centers, adult education classes, and senior craft centers.

Volunteer Work

Through community service and volunteer work, thousands are not only helping others but are serving themselves. Such activities keep time from hanging heavy, give purpose to retirement, and in some cases may lead to paying jobs and a second career.

Participating in community activities is not difficult. In some communities a call to the city clerk is enough to get started. In others, a letter to the mayor will bring faster results. In larger cities, call the Volunteer Bureau in your area; this is a United Fund agency that acts as a clearing house for volunteer jobs.

If you wish to have the type of volunteer job that leads to a second career, you might consider doing work for one of the government programs utilizing the skills of older people. All of these programs have been assembled under the umbrella of one organization called ACTION. For additional information about any of the following programs, write to ACTION, Washington, DC 20525.

- The Foster Grandparent Program hires low-income men and women over 60 to give love and attention to institutionalized and other needy children.

- The Peace Corps is seeking the skills of retirees. However, you must be skilled in some trade or

profession, pass a tough physical examination, and complete a rigorous orientation and training program. For information, write to ACTION, Washington, DC 20525, and request a copy of *Older Volunteers in the Peace Corps*. It lists specific skills needed in the Peace Corps.

- Other programs within ACTION include the Retired Senior Volunteer Program, the Service Corps of Retired Executives, the Active Corps of Executives, and VISTA (Volunteer in Service to America). Many of the workers in these programs are paid.

There are other volunteer jobs that may not pay a salary, but do fill a basic need by allowing you to pass along your skills and ideals to younger people. You can do this through the Boy Scouts, Girl Scouts, Boys Clubs of America, YMCAs and YWCAs, hospitals, schools for the handicapped and mentally retarded, and many other organizations.

Continuing Social and Intellectual Activities

The one organ we can depend upon in old age is the brain. At 80, a person can learn at approximately the same speed he could when he was 12 years old. But like any organ, the brain must be kept active and alert by constant use.

One of the best ways to exercise the brain is through some process of continuing education. This does not have to mean going back to school or taking formal classes. Continuing education can take the form of participating in discussions in senior centers, "Y's," town meetings, or study courses. You can find out about educational opportunities and possibilities by contacting local, state, or national offices of education; state employment offices; the information service of your Community Council or Health and Welfare Federation; the Adult Education section of the U.S. Office of Education, Washington, DC 20202; the National Education Association, 1201 Sixteenth Street, NW, Washington, DC 20036; the State Commission on Aging (write to your state capital).

Your local library may have some suggestions (and perhaps offers some classes), and your local "Y" is probably offering some programs.

The federal government continues to be a prime source of educational literature. Each year the government prints about 50 million books, pamphlets, brochures, reports, and guidebooks on everything from astrology to zoology. For a free price list of specified subjects, write to the Superintendent of Documents, Government Printing Office, Washington, DC 20401.

Formal and informal learning situations can help you keep pace with change and the future. Continuing education prepares you to live contentedly with a free, independent spirit and mind—while providing you with the means for improved social integration, participation, and satisfaction.

Sexual Attitude and Activity in the Aged

We have come far since the Victorian era when talk about sex was taboo. Now science is taking a candid look at sex in the later years and is exploding old myths as well as exploring new truths. Such enlightenment can help reduce any remaining guilt in this area.

After Age 60

In one study to determine the pattern of sexual behavior after 60, researchers at Duke University quizzed 250 people aged 60 to 93 about their sexual activities. Of the 149 who were married, 81 reported they were still sexually active; even in the single group, 7 of the 101 questioned reported "some sexual activity."

Dr. Gustave Newman, who conducted the study, reported 10 percent of the couples over 60 as having sexual relations more than once a week, though couples over 75 unanimously reported less activity.

"No age is an automatic cut-off point for sex," claims the late Dr. Isadore Rubin in his study, *Sexual Life After Sixty*. "But," he continues,

> sexuality cannot flourish in a climate where rejection of aging as a worthwhile stage of life leads inevitably to self-rejection by many older persons . . . the men and women who "act old" in their sexual activity before their bodies have really called a halt become sexually old long before their time.

Sexual Interest after Menopause

Actually, many women take a renewed interest in sex after menopause. Dr. William H. Masters and Mrs. Virginia E. Johnson in their study *Human Sexual Response* credit the tendency of many women to experience a second honeymoon in the early 50s to the fact that they no longer have to worry about pregnancy and usually have resolved most of the problems of raising a family.

On the other hand, they tell us:

> Deprived of normal sexual outlets, women exhaust themselves physically in conscious or unconscious efforts to dissipate their accumulated and frequently unrecognized sexual tensions. Many demonstrate their basic insecurities by · casting themselves unreservedly into their religion, the business world, volunteer social work, or overzealous mothering of their mature children or grandchildren.

Lessened Response of Men

While some women become more responsive as they grow older, Masters and Johnson point out, "There is no question that the human male's responsiveness wanes as he ages." They attribute this to attitudes arising from:

- Boredom—being taken for granted by his wife

- Economic pursuits—occupational competition becomes a demanding, all-consuming activity

- Fatigue from unusual or excessive physical strain, such as that induced by sports; or mental fatigue induced by such factors as a "bad day at the office"

- Overindulgence in food and drink, usually alcohol

- Physical and mental infirmities

- Fear of failure

Myths about Sex

One common reason for an older person's termination of sex life is the often mistaken idea that continued sexual activity in middle and old age may adversely affect health. Although the old myths that sex is weakening or speeds the aging process have been largely dismissed by physicians today, some people still cling to them; what sexual activity they do have is troubled by fear.

Heart Patients

Cardiac patients are no longer admonished to lead sexless lives except in extreme cases. After a heart attack most are able to resume sexual activity within a few months, although patients with angina pectoris may be advised to proceed cautiously.

According to Dr. Philip Reichert, former executive secretary of the American College of Cardiology:

> We must get rid of the notion that every heart patient lives under an overhanging sword and that he faces the constant threat of sudden death. The congenial married couple, accustomed to each other and whose technique is habituated through many years of companionship, can achieve sexual satisfaction without too great an expenditure of body energy or too severe a strain upon the heart. . . .

Hypertension sufferers may sometimes indulge in a restricted form of sexual activity with medical supervision. And modern therapy and surgical methods can often prevent or delay impotence caused by prostate disease or diabetes.

Other Health Problems

But where any health problem is involved, it is best to analyze your sex needs and those of your partner; consult with your physician and partner as to how you can both attain satisfaction without harm to your health; see your physician regularly and report accurately distress symptoms and the conditions causing them.

Recent research has dispelled other long-held ideas about sex, too—among them the myth that masturbation is childish and harmful to health. Moreover, Rubin points out: "All studies of older persons have shown that autoerotic activity, while not as common as in the younger years, is far more prevalent in later years than most of us have imagined." He quotes a survey by *Sexology* magazine that showed that of 279 married men studied, 1 out of every 4 masturbated after age 60.

Dr. Lester W. Dearborn, marriage consultant, in pointing out the role masturbation plays in the lives of the single or widowed, comments:

It is to be hoped that those interested in the field of geriatrics will . . . encourage the aging to accept masturbation as a perfectly valid outlet when there is a need and other means of gratification are not available.

The "dirty old man" myth has run its course, too. Although society tends to picture both the child molester and the exhibitionist as older men, experts point out that both typically belong to much younger age groups. Donald Mulcock, child welfare specialist, in studying men who assaulted children sexually in England and Wales, found most offenses against boys were committed by men between the ages of 39 and 50, those against girls by men between 33 and 44. Only six percent of the men he studied were 63, and none was older.

Cellular Therapy and Hormone Treatment

To keep older people vigorous and active, some researchers have experimented with *cellular therapy* as a means of retarding aging. Dr. Paul Niehans, a Swiss physician, introduced the idea of cellular therapy in the 1930s with his theory that organs begin to deteriorate in old age when the body fails to replace the cells that compose it. He prescribed a treatment whereby a person is injected with cells from healthy embryonic animal organs. (He used sheep, pigs, and calves.) He believed that the animal cells from a particular organ would migrate to the same organ in the aging body and reactivate it. Thus, kidney troubles could be cured with cells from an embryonic animal kidney. Although such notables as Sir Winston Churchill, Pope Pius XII, Somerset Maugham, and Dr. Konrad Adenauer submitted to it, cellular therapy is not widely accepted in the United States today as an effective agent against aging.

More to the point, most researchers feel, are the current experiments with hormones. Hormones help women through the tension of menopause and are used to treat impotence and loss of sexual desire. However, some studies have linked estrogen hormone therapy statistically with uterine cancer. For this reason and because of side effects, hormones face many years of testing before they will be used extensively to retard aging.

Mental Outlook

Good health plus a romantic outlook promote sex appeal at any age. Being romantic and showing affection, whether sexually or not, keep you sparkling and lively no matter what your age.

A good wholesome attitude toward life, a hearty sense of humor, a sympathetic interest in other people—all help make up the indefinable something that makes us appealing to the opposite sex. Good grooming plays an important role, too. Cleanliness, neat suitable apparel, and good posture all add to the image we create of ourselves in other people's minds. So do the manners we reflect in the courtesies we show the people around us—the thoughtful little things we do for them, our reactions to the things they do for us.

If you're a woman over 65 who is looking for companionship, you'll probably find a good personality uplift will get you farther than a face or bust lift. If you're a man who is hoping to find feminine companionship, you will probably find a good spiritual overhaul more image-enhancing than dyeing your hair. Also, a good night's sleep is the best aphrodisiac.

The Right Housing

Selecting retirement housing is like

selecting a spouse; there are many possibilities, but few that are right.

Ideally, the right housing should take care of you rather than requiring you to take care of it. It should give you shelter, security, and privacy; allow you freedom; and keep you near friends, relatives, and a grocer who delivers.

To Move or Not to Move

What is the right housing for you—the one that you are in or some other place? The answer to this question depends upon the state of your pocketbook and the state of your health.

Advantages of Moving

Right now you might be in good health, but this could change. Would stairs become a problem? Could you keep up the house and garden? Would you want more adequate heat? Older people are more comfortable when the temperature is over 75° F. You might also need better lighting in several rooms.

If you are retired, you might find that you cannot keep up expenses on the old house. You might find that your larger, older house does not suit the reduced size of your family or your need for work or recreation. You could probably save money by living in a smaller place that requires less upkeep. You could also arrange to move nearer children and grandchildren, or into an area where you could find new opportunities for work and recreational activities.

Advantages of Staying Put

But by staying in your home you would remain in familiar surroundings and near old friends. You could maintain your comfortable routine and remain independent as long as possible. If you have unused space, you could move into the first floor and shut off the second floor to save on heat and maintenance. Or you could convert part of the house into apartments.

Where to Live?

Many older persons fulfill ambitions of long standing by moving to warmer climates after retirement. The question whether such a move should be undertaken should be considered with other questions relating to housing.

Moving to a different climate makes sense for many reasons. Many elderly persons feel threatened or restricted by cold winters and their usual accompaniments—snow, sleet, and high winds. Having more leisure time, older persons feel that warmer temperatures will make it possible to take part in more activities for more hours of the day than if they "stay put." Some persons move so that they can live closer to friends who have already moved—or to children or other relatives. Some move to play golf or tennis outdoors the year around.

An individual or couple considering a move to a warmer climate should look at a number of basic considerations. A key one relates to the cost of living in the new area or state. Living on incomes that may have been substantially reduced by retirement, older persons without special preferences may select that state that offers the cheapest living. Studies indicated in 1979 that the "10 best states to retire to" from a personal-financial point of view were, in order:

1. Utah, because of lower energy costs, growing job opportunities, moderate living costs. A drawback: Utah may have extremely cold winters.

2. Louisiana, because of cheap living costs—about 10 percent lower than other states—and low real estate taxes.

3. South Carolina, for the same reasons. A drawback: physician shortages in some communities.

4. Nevada, because of new housing, jobs, no state income or inheritance taxes, and average living costs.

5. Texas, with moderate housing costs away from major cities, and normal, if rising, living costs.

6. New Mexico, where energy costs are low, jobs are increasing in number, and cheap housing is plentiful.

7. Alabama, the cheapest and lowest as regards costs of living. Drawbacks: few new jobs, medical care lacking in some areas.

8. Arizona, because of good, relatively inexpensive housing, warm climate, good medical care. Drawbacks: rising living costs, high taxes.

9. Florida, with a warm climate, no income tax, good medical services. Drawbacks: living costs high in coastal areas; property taxes rising.

10. Georgia, because of mild climate, low living costs. Drawbacks: slow growth in jobs, locally poor medical services.

"Retirement to the sun" entails many other decisions. States like New Mexico offer a wide range of sites, from urban to desert, from high mountains to empty plains. Some of the states with favorable tax laws and cheap living costs have little to offer in the way of cultural attractions. Other states may lack recreational activities.

Psychological Trauma

Moving 100 or 1,000 or 2,000 miles to live in a warmer climate obviously involves some pain of separation and loss. The psychological trauma occasioned by a departure from old friends and familiar surroundings has caused major problems for some older persons. For that reason, the psychological challenge should be given deep consideration *before* any move is made.

How to alleviate the trauma of leaving the familiar for the unfamiliar? Some persons spend a year in the new locale, return home, and *then* make up their minds to move or not to move. Others, including those who cannot afford such trial living, at least visit the target region to "get a feel" for it and its way of life. Whatever your situation, the wisdom of considering at least five factors cannot be disputed:

● In the new home under the sun, will you be able to entertain family, including children and grandchildren, and in that way to minimize the pain of separation?

● Are friends or relatives already located in the new area—and can you live near them (not *with* them, if possible)?

● Will you be able to swing into enough new activities to eliminate any possibility that you might feel useless, wasted, or frustrated?

● Can you maintain your old, or a decent, standard of living once you have moved?

● Can you stand the first 9 to 12 months in the new home without climbing the walls? Studies have shown that those who can last out a year or more will very likely adjust and continue to enjoy life.

Requirements of Retirement Housing

Whatever you plan to do, your retire-ment housing should be located near or be easily accessible to shops and recreation centers by public transportation. To make living arrangements more pleasant, individual housing units should contain at least 400 square feet, and there should be two or more rooms.

The new dwelling unit should be equal to or better than the housing you have been used to in the past. It should be suitable for comfortable living in both health and sickness—easily adaptable to convalescent needs with either two bedrooms or a bedroom and sleeping alcove.

In addition, retirement housing should incorporate the following:

● All rooms on one floor, and that floor reached by few, if any, steps

● No thresholds or tripping hazards

● Nonslip surfaces in hallways, bedrooms, and kitchens

● Handrails by all steps and inclines

● Adequate illumination in halls, near steps, and in other potentially hazardous areas

● Fully automatic central heating

● Doors and halls wide enough to accommodate a wheelchair

Public Housing

If you decide to move and to rent instead of buying, consider public housing projects. These projects are available to single men and women 62 or older, as well as to families whose head is 62 or older or has a spouse at least 62. Local housing authorities build, purchase, or lease the units and set entrance requirements and maximum income limits. Rents are comparatively low.

The Housing and Urban Development Agency also makes loans for nonprofit (and profit) sponsors that will build housing for senior citizens with moderate or higher incomes.

Retirement Hotels and Communities

You might also consider retirement hotels, which are especially numerous in Florida, California, and Texas. These hotels are usually refurbished former resorts that provide room and board at a fixed monthly rent.

Retirement communities offer housing of various types, usually apartments, cooperatives, and individual units. It usually costs about $450 a month or more to cover mortgage payments, living, and maintenance expenses.

Would you like retirement community living? It's usually the life for people who like people and who enjoy being active. For those who don't, it can be a bit tiring. Some couples do not like the closeness and activity found in a retirement community and prefer living in a less social environment.

Lifetime Care Facilities

In contrast to the emphasis on independent living in retirement communities, many projects sponsored by church, union, and fraternal organizations stress lifetime care (room, board, and medical care for life), with fees based on actuarial tables of life expectancy at age of entry. Housing alone costs from $10,000 to $30,000, depending upon age and type of living accommodation, *plus* a monthly charge of around $250 per person to cover meals, medical care (exclusive of Medicare), maintenance, and other expenses. In many cases, lifetime care for a couple could cost around $90,000.

Cooperatives and Condominiums

In addition to lifetime care facilities,

many church, fraternal, and union groups offer other types of housing. In the case of church-sponsored housing, residence usually is not restricted to members of the sponsoring faith.

Some of these units are operated as *cooperatives;* others as *condominiums.* The major difference in the two is that condominium owners have titles to their units, while cooperative residents are stockholders in the cooperative association with occupancy rights to specific units. Condominium owners pay their own taxes; cooperative residents pay taxes in their monthly charges.

Mobile Homes

You might also want to consider a mobile home. A suitable one must be at least 10 feet wide and 50 feet long.

What is it like to live in a mobile-home park? Certainly, there is a closeness in these parks that you would not have in a normal neighborhood. Typically, the mobile home is placed on a lot 25 to 30 feet wide and 75 feet deep. This means that you could have 12 families within a radius of 100 feet.

Residents visit back and forth and hold frequent picnics, barbecues, and other social activities. This would not be the way of life for someone who did not enjoy group activities.

Be Realistic

To find out what type of housing is best for you, look around the area to see where you want to live. Each community is different, shaped by the people who live there. Talk to the residents and do some serious thinking before you move, not forgetting to carefully consider your financial position in regard to the new locale. Try to be realistic; don't expect to find the perfect climate for health and happiness. The nearest thing to it would be

a place that encourages outdoor life, is neither too hot nor too cold, has a relative humidity of around 55 percent, and enough variety in weather, with frequent but moderate weather changes, to be interesting and not too monotonous.

If you have any doubts about the location as far as health is concerned, check with your physician.

When Faced with Ill Health

How can you help yourself or others when faced with a serious or terminal illness?

Alvin I. Goldfarb, M.D., former consultant on Services for the Aged, New York State Department of Mental Hygiene, notes the importance of self-esteem, self-confidence, sense of purpose, and well-being to a person who is seriously ill or dying. Supported by the idea, "I've led a good and full life," older people can face a serious or terminal illness with dignity. Sometimes this acceptance may be almost an unspoken and tacit understanding between the aging and society to help the separation process along.

When a person is terminally ill, the chances are that he is not in severe pain. With the increasing supply of pain-relieving drugs and the possibility of sedation, very few elderly patients suffer greatly with pain. While a fear of death probably exists in most people, when death is actually encountered the fear is seldom overwhelming, even though it may deeply affect others directly involved with the dying patient.

Most patients are at least aware of the possibility of dying soon; those with lingering conditions are particularly adept at self-diagnosis. But more often, they notice a change in social relationships with friends, family, and medical personnel.

Patient–physician relationships can be vital in helping the seriously ill patient retain peace of mind. It is the physician's responsibility to give compassion and recognize fear, even when it is hidden. Likewise, he should respond to a patient's hidden wish to discuss his illness. Of course, there is no set formula for communicating with seriously ill patients. Each individual needs a different approach, and most physicians are sensitive to this.

Many physicians report that death, except in unusual cases, is not accompanied by physical pain. Rather, there is often a sense of well-being and spiritual exaltation. Physicians think this feeling is caused by the anesthetic action of carbon dioxide on the central nervous system and by the effect of toxic substances. Ernest Hemingway wrote, "The pang of death, a famous doctor once told me, is often less than that of a toothache."

Stages of Death

According to physicians, people die in stages—rapidly or slowly, depending on circumstances. First comes *clinical death*, when respiration and heartbeat cease. The brain dies as it is deprived of oxygen and circulating blood, and *biological death* occurs.

Life can be restored in the moments between clinical death and brain death if circulation and respiration are continued through the use of medical devices that stimulate the heart and lungs.

After the brain ceases to function, cellular death begins. Life is not considered to be completely lost until the brain stops functioning. It is possible for surgeons to remove viable organs after biological death for transplant or other use.

Many clergymen and physicians insist that we need more honest communication about death, as such communication is probably the single most useful measure to avoid unnecessary suffering. Sound knowledge never made anyone afraid. And although death will probably always remain essentially a mystery, scientists will continue to search for a better understanding of its nature. By such means they may learn a great deal more about life.

The Autopsy

Family members adjusting to the death of a loved one may face the question of whether or not an autopsy should be performed. More and more, medical experts are underscoring the need for an autopsy as a means of confirming the cause of death. The postmortem examination may also "provide a reasonable context for accepting death," according to Daniel W. McKeel, director of autopsy pathology at Washington University School of Medicine. From a family and genetic point of view, the autopsy may reveal information about specific conditions or medical problems in the deceased that survivors can use to guide their own health practices and concerns.

Contrary to some reports, the autopsy need not delay funeral arrangements or disfigure the body so as to require a closed casket. Autopsies are generally mandatory in homicide, suicide, burn deaths, deaths resulting from on-the-job injuries, operating room deaths, and questionable or unwitnessed deaths.

7

Diseases of the Skeletal System

The bones and joints of the human body, although designed to withstand a great deal of stress, are subject to a variety of disorders that can affect people of all ages. Some skeletal deformities are the result of congenital defects, and can be treated by physical therapy or surgery with varying degrees of success. Arthritis and related joint diseases, caused by wear and tear over the years, probably affect more people than any other skeletal disorder.

Man's erect posture makes the spine especially vulnerable to problems of alignment, often causing considerable pain. Bone tissue can also be invaded by tumors and by infections of the bone marrow. Also, stress to bones and joints can cause fractures or dislocations, which require prompt medical treatment to prevent deformity or loss of mobility.

Congenital Defects

As the fetus develops in the womb, its bony skeleton first appears as soft cartilage, which hardens into bone before birth. The calcium content of the mother's diet aids the fetus in bone formation and in the development of the normal human skeleton. Thus the basic skeletal structure of an individual is formed before his birth. In some instances, the bones of the fetus develop abnormally, and such defects are usually noticeable soon after delivery.

The causes of skeletal birth defects are not always known. Some may result from hereditary factors; others have been traced to the mother's exposure to X rays, radiation, chemicals, drugs, or to disease during pregnancy. Among the more common birth defects are extra fingers, toes, or ribs, or missing fingers, hands, toes, feet, or limbs. Sections of the spine may be fused together, often without causing serious problems later in life, although some fused joints can hinder the motion of limbs. The sections of the skull may unite prematurely, retarding the growth of the brain.

Defects of the Skull, Face, and Jaw

Various malformations of the skull, face, and jaw can appear at birth or soon after. They include *macrocephaly* (enlarged head) and *microcephaly* (very small head). Microcephaly is caused by the premature fusion of the cranial sutures in early childhood. If brain growth increases very rapidly during the first six months of life in infants whose skulls have fused prematurely, the brain cannot expand sufficiently within the rigid skull, and mental retardation results. Surgery is used to widen the sutures to permit normal brain development.

Cleft lip and *cleft palate* are common facial deformities and are visible at birth. These are longitudinal openings in the upper lip and palate. They result from failure of the area to unite in the normal manner during embryonic stages of pregnancy. They should be corrected at an early age. If surgery is performed in infancy there is a good chance that the child will mature with little or no physical evidence of the affliction and with no psychological damage as a result of it. See "Cleft Palate and Cleft Lip" in Ch. 2, *The First Dozen Years*, for further information.

The Human Skeleton

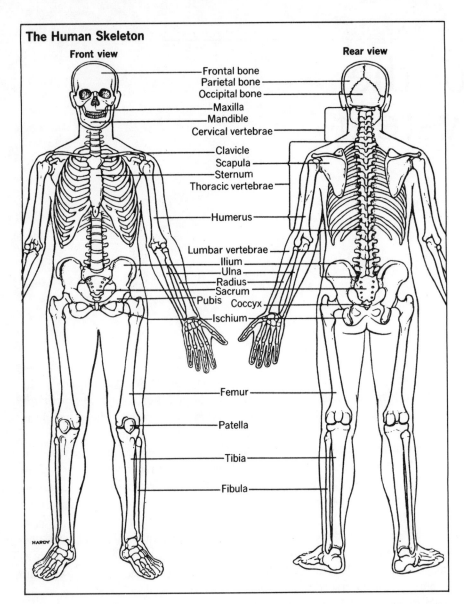

Front view

- Frontal bone
- Parietal bone
- Occipital bone
- Maxilla
- Mandible
- Cervical vertebrae
- Clavicle
- Scapula
- Sternum
- Thoracic vertebrae
- Humerus
- Lumbar vertebrae
- Ilium
- Ulna
- Radius
- Sacrum
- Pubis
- Coccyx
- Ischium
- Femur
- Patella
- Tibia
- Fibula

Rear view

HARDY

Defects of the Rib Cage

Every normal human being has 12 pairs of ribs attached to the spine, but some people are born with extra ribs on one or both sides.

Although such extra ribs are usually harmless, one that projects into the neck can damage nerves and the artery located in that area. In adults extra neck ribs may cause shooting pains down the arms, general periodic numbness in the arms and hands, weak wrist pulse, and possible diminished blood supply to the forearm. Surgery may be required to remove the rib and thereby relieve the pressure on the nerves or artery. Minor symptoms are treated by physiotherapy.

Congenital absence of one or more ribs is not uncommon. An individual may be born with some ribs fused together. Neither condition creates any serious threat to health.

Congenital Dislocation of the Hip

Dislocation of the hip is the most common congenital problem of the pelvic area. It is found more often in girls than in boys in a five to one ratio. Babies born from a breech presentation, buttocks first, are more likely to develop this abnormality than those delivered head first. The condition may be the result of inherited characteristics.

Clinical examination of infants, especially breech-born girls, may reveal early signs of congenital hip dislocation, with the affected hip appearing shorter than the normal side. If the condition is not diagnosed before the infant is ready to walk, the child may begin walking later than is normal. The child may develop a limp and an unsteady gait, with one leg shorter than the other.

Early diagnosis of this condition is important, followed by immediate reduction and immobilization by means of a plaster cast or by applying traction. Permanent deformity, dislocation, uneven pelvis, retarded walking, limping, and unsteady gait are possible complications if this condition remains untreated. Surgery is sometimes required.

Arthritis and Other Joint Diseases

Arthritis is probably the most common of all disabling diseases, at least in the temperate areas of the world. It has been estimated that 10 percent of the population suffers from one of the many forms of arthritis. In the United States alone, more than 13 million persons each year seek professional medical care for arthritis. Of this number, some three million must restrict their daily activities, and about 750,000 are so disabled by arthritis that they are unable to attend school, work, or even handle common household tasks.

Arthritis apparently is not associated with any stage of civilization; it has been diagnosed in the skeletons of prehistoric humans. There is even evidence that arthritic diseases afflict a variety of animals, including the dinosaurs that inhabited the earth more than 100 million years ago. Arthritis caused pain and suffering to such famous personages as Goethe, Henry VI, Charlemagne, and Alexander the Great.

Arthritis and *rheumatism* are terms sometimes used interchangeably by the layman to describe any abnormal condition of the joints, muscles, or related tissues. Many rheumatic or arthritic diseases have popular names, such as "housemaid's knee," "baseball finger," or "weaver's bottom." Physicians usually prefer to apply the term *arthritis* to disorders of the joints, especially joint disorders accompanied by inflammation. More than 75 different diseases of the joints have been identified; they are classified according to their specific signs, symptoms, and probable causes. The list includes bursitis, gout, and tendinitis in addition to the major disorders, rheumatoid arthritis and osteoarthritis.

Rheumatoid arthritis and osteoarthritis are examples of two types of arthritic ailment that are quite different diseases. Rheumatoid arthritis usually develops from unknown causes before the age of 45 and is marked by a nonspecific inflammation of the joints of the extremities; the inflammation is accompanied by changes in substances found in the blood. A victim of rheumatoid arthritis may develop limb deformities within a short period of time. Osteoarthritis, on the other hand, is most likely to produce symptoms after the age of 45. Here the cause is simply wear and tear on the cartilage cushions of the joints, mainly weight-bearing ones such as the hips and knees. Both kinds of joint disorders afflict millions of persons with painful and disabling symptoms.

Osteoarthritis

The most common form of arthritis is *osteoarthritis*, which is also known by the terms *hypertrophic arthritis* and *degenerative joint disease*. It can be said quite accurately that if you live long enough you will experience osteoarthritis. In fact, osteoarthritis is most common in areas of the world where people have the greatest longevity. The first signs of osteoarthritis may appear on X-ray pictures of persons in their 30s and 40s, even though they have not yet felt pain in the weight-bearing joints, the hips and knees, where discomfort usually appears first. Studies show that nearly everybody has at least the beginning signs or symptoms of osteoarthritis after they reach their 50s. It affects both men and women, although women may not experience symptoms until after they have reached the menopause.

Causes

A somewhat simplified explanation of the cause of osteoarthritis is this: the joints between the bones of a young person are cushioned and lubricated by cartilage pads and smooth lining membranes; normal wear and tear on

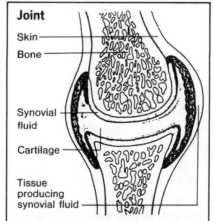

Joint

Skin

Bone

Synovial fluid

Cartilage

Tissue producing synovial fluid

All of the body's joints allow movement of the bones through this combination of ball and socket contours. Cartilage allows the bones to move without scraping or catching. Synovial fluid helps reduce friction in the movement.

the joints during a lifetime of activity gradually erodes the protective layers between the bones. In addition, the bones may develop small growths at the joints, a factor that aggravates the situation. There is evidence that heredity plays a role in the development of these bone growths, which are ten times more likely to occur in women than in men.

While hips and knees are among the most likely targets of osteoarthritis, the disease also can involve the hands, the shoulders, or back. Weight-bearing joints are commonly involved when the patient is overweight and spends a great deal of time standing or walking.

Symptoms

Except for the descriptions of aches and pains by victims of osteoarthritis and X-ray examination of the joints, a physician frequently has little information to go on in making a diagnosis of this disease. In some cases, there may be enlargement of the joint and some tenderness. But few cases are marked by the excessive warmth, for example, associated with rheumatoid arthritis. There are no laboratory tests that can distinguish the disorder from other rheumatic or arthritic diseases.

Osteoarthritis seldom causes the degree of discomfort experienced by patients afflicted by rheumatoid arthritis; the disease is not as disabling for most patients, and even the stiffness associated with osteoarthritis is milder, usually lasting only a few minutes when activity is attempted, while the stiffness of rheumatoid arthritis may continue for hours.

Arthritis of the Hip

Although most cases of osteoarthritis are not seriously disabling, arthritis of

Hip Disorders

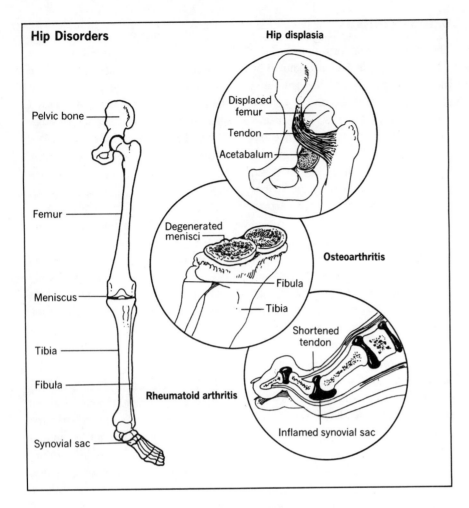

the hip is a prominent cause of disability in older persons. It produces pain in the hips, the inner thigh, the groin, and very often in the knee. Walking, climbing steps, sitting, and bending become very painful, because the joint is destroyed by degeneration of bone and cartilage. Stress and strain on the hip joint further aggravate the condition, which becomes worse with advancing age.

Surgery to replace the head of the femur or the entire hip joint with metal or plastic parts has brought relief from pain and restored mobility to some patients suffering from severe arthritis of the hip.

Small children sometimes suffer from transient arthritis of the hip, of unknown cause, manifested by pain, limitation of hip movement, and impeded walking. Because the condition usually disappears within six weeks, the only treatment is bed rest. Transient arthritis must not be mistaken for the more serious pyrogenic hip arthritis of children and adults, marked by high fever.

Spinal Arthritis

The aging process is the prinicipal cause of spinal arthritis. Other contributing factors are disk lesions and injury. Spinal arthritis causes pronounced bone degeneration and disability. The sufferer experiences severe back pain radiating to the thighs as a result of interference of the nerve roots from *osteophytes*, or spurs, formed in the joints. In mild cases, physical therapy may be the only treatment required.

Treatment of Osteoarthritis

For most patients, osteoarthritis is not likely to be crippling or disabling. The effects generally are not more serious than stiffness of the involved joints, with occasional discomfort and some pain. When weight-bearing joints are involved, the basic remedies are weight control and adequate rest for the areas affected. In some instances, the patient may have to learn new postural adjustments; symptoms often appear in another joint after the first has been affected because the patient tends to favor the joint that first caused pain and shifts weight or muscle stress to the second joint.

Physical therapy and corrective exercises are helpful. A physician may recommend the use of aspirin or another analgesic for the pain. Steroid drugs may be injected into an injured joint, but usually only for temporary relief. Surgery is sometimes recommended for removal of troublesome bone spurs or to correct a serious problem in a weight-bearing joint, where a metal cup or other device may be inserted as part of an artificial joint.

Rheumatoid Arthritis

Rheumatoid arthritis occurs at a much earlier age than osteoarthritis, appearing at any time from infancy to old age, but most commonly afflicting persons between the ages of 20 and 35. Women are three times as likely to be victims of rheumatoid arthritis as are men, although men seem to lose that advantage after the age of 50. All races seem to be equally vulnerable. Recent studies also suggest that two common beliefs about rheumatoid arthritis probably are untrue. The facts show that the disease is not hereditary and that it is not more prevalent in cold, damp climates.

Symptoms

Rheumatoid arthritis can begin as part of an acute illness, with high fever and intense inflammation of the joints, or it can develop insidiously with little or no discomfort except for fatigue, loss of appetite, weight loss, and perhaps a mild fever. Sometime later the victim becomes aware of aches and pains in the joints and muscles and seeks medical attention. Frequently, deformities develop before the patient realizes that rheumatoid arthritis may be the cause of swollen joints, pain, redness, or excessive warmth about the affected area.

The inflammation of a joint caused by rheumatoid arthritis may continue for weeks or it may last for a period of years. During inflammation, tendons become shortened and muscles lose their normal balance. The result is the deformity of joints commonly associated with rheumatoid arthritis, such as a swan-neck shape in the fingers. Muscular weakness develops and there is a loss of grip strength in the hands when that area is affected. Patients may be unable to make a tight fist.

A common symptom of rheumatoid arthritis is a stiffness that develops during periods of rest but gradually disappears when activity resumes. After a night's sleep, the stiffness may persist for a half hour or much longer. The stiffness may result, at least in part, from the muscular weakness that accompanies the disease.

Although the effects of rheumatoid arthritis are most commonly observed in the hands or feet of patients, other body joints such as the elbows, shoulders, knees, hips, ankles, spine, and even the jawbones may be involved. It is possible for all of a patient's joints to be involved, and the involvement often is symmetrical; that is, both hands will develop the symptoms at the same time and in the same pattern.

Probable Causes

The exact cause of rheumatoid arthritis is unknown, although a variety of factors have been associated with the onset of the disease. Emotional upsets, tuberculosis, venereal disease, psoriasis, and rheumatic fever are among conditions associated with the beginnings of the disease. Various viruses and other microorganisms have been isolated from the inflamed tissues of patients, but medical researchers have been unable to prove that any of the infectious agents is the cause. Efforts have also been made to transmit rheumatoid arthritis from a known victim to a normal volunteer by transfusions and injections of substances found in the victim's tissues, but without success in tracing the causative factor.

Treatment

The symptoms of rheumatoid arthritis intensify or abate spontaneously and unpredictably. Available methods of treatment do not cure the disease but relieve the symptoms so that the pain is reduced and some normal movement is facilitated. Proper nutrition, heat, rest, and exercise are also helpful. A number of drugs can reduce the inflammation of the joints, but they may have undesirable toxic side effects. Accordingly, before any drug therapy is embarked upon, the patient should seek the advice of a physician specializing in arthritic disorders.

Aspirin

The most common drug used to treat all kinds of arthritis is aspirin; it is also the most economical. Occasional side effects, such as irritation of ulcers or other gastrointestinal upsets, as well as buzzing in the ears, can result from aspirin use, especially in massive doses; such complications can some-times be avoided by the use of specially coated aspirin tablets. The size of the dose usually is started at a minimum level and gradually increased until the physician finds a level that is most helpful to the patient but does not result in serious side effects.

Several other types of medication have been tried as alternatives to aspirin. One of the newer drugs, *indomethacin*, is about as effective as aspirin, but when taken in large doses it also seems to cause side effects, including nausea, heartburn, and headache.

Sulindac, a nonsteroidal antiinflammatory drug (NSAI), made its appearance on the U.S. market in the late 1970s. Under the trade name Clinoril, sulindac came into wide use in the treatment of a variety of arthritic disorders. These included osteoarthritis, rheumatoid arthritis, gouty arthritis, and painful shoulder.

Sulindac both relieves pain and reduces fever while attacking inflammations. In those respects it resembles other antiarthritis drugs such as fenoprofen (trade name: Nalfon), naproxen (trade name: Naprosyn), and tolmetin (trade name: Tolectin). Sulindac can be ingested on a twice-daily basis; but in use it was found to have adverse side effects, some of them serious. For example, some patients reported abdominal pains, nausea, and constipation. Diarrhea can also occur. Some side effects involved the central nervous system, and included dizziness, drowsiness, and headache.

Among other drugs used to treat arthritis, DMSO (dimethylsulfoxide) attracted widespread attention in the early 1980s. Research indicated that DMSO might have value as an antiarthritic agent. The Arthritis Foundation of the United States indicated, however, that DMSO might serve as "a short-term analgesic for pain due to limited conditions." A liquid that arthritis sufferers rubbed on their skin,

DMSO was reported to have such negative side effects as skin rashes and halitosis.

Many other drugs promising relief for victims of arthritis have made their appearance in recent years. For example, penicillamine (trade name: Cuprimine) was found to help patients with rheumatoid arthritis. Experiments with many other drugs—including aclofenac, flurbiprofen, and proquazone—are under way.

Steroids

The cortisone-type (steroid) drugs have proven effective in controlling severe cases of rheumatoid arthritis. They can be given orally or injected directly into the affected joints. However, these drugs generate a number of undesirable side effects, and withdrawal often results in a severe recurrence of the original symptoms. Thus, steroid drug therapy is a long-term process that can make the patient totally dependent on the medication. Some physicians are reluctant to inject steroid drugs into the joints because the effect is temporary and there is a danger of introducing infection by repeated use of the needle. In addition, some patients do not seem to respond to the steroid drugs and X-ray studies of the joints may show progressive destruction of the tissues despite the medications.

Rest

Bed rest is recommended for acute cases and up to 10 hours of sleep per day is advised for mild cases of rheumatoid arthritis. The patient also should take rest periods during the day whenever possible, reducing fatigue and stress on the affected joints. As in severe cases of osteoarthritis, the patient should try to adjust his daily work habits to avoid strain on weight-bearing joints.

Exercise

Patients tend to avoid moving arthritic joints because of pain and stiffness. Exercise of an arthritic joint, however, helps prevent the adjoining muscles from shrinking and weakening. A program of physiotherapy—including hot packs and exercise—can be extremely helpful.

The exercise program should carry the joints through their normal range of movement. Exercises should be performed every day but not carried to the point of fatigue. In addition to exercises intended to prevent limitation of normal joint movement, isometric-type exercises should be used to maintain or increase muscle power in other parts of the body that might otherwise be neglected because of limited activity by the patient.

Posture

The patient should be encouraged to maintain proper posture as much as possible, through correct positioning of the body when standing, sitting, or reclining in bed. A sheet of thick plywood may be used under a mattress to prevent it from sagging. Chairs should be firm with straight backs. Pillows should be avoided whenever possible.

Crutches, canes, leg braces, and other devices may be needed by the patient in advanced stages of rheumatoid arthritis. In some cases, orthopedic surgery is recommended to help reconstruct the limbs and joints as a part of rehabilitation.

Heat

Massages or vibrating equipment are not recommended as part of the therapy for rheumatoid arthritis patients. Heat in the form of hot baths, hot compresses, or heating pads, however, may be helpful. Paraffin baths are particularly helpful in treating hands or wrists.

Diet

While osteoarthritis patients are advised to lose as much weight as possible, rheumatoid arthritis patients tend to suffer from weight loss and nutritional deficiencies. Part of the cause may be a loss of appetite that is a characteristic of the disease and part may be the gastrointestinal problems that frequently accompany the disorder and that may be aggravated by the medications prescribed. Some physicians advise that rheumatoid arthritis patients include adequate amounts of protein and calcium in their diets as a preventive measure against a loss of bone tissue.

Juvenile Rheumatoid Arthritis

A form of arthritis quite similar to adult rheumatoid arthritis afflicts some children before the age of 16. Called *juvenile rheumatoid arthritis* or *Still's disease*, it includes a set of symptoms that nevertheless differentiate it from adult rheumatoid arthritis. In addition to the rheumatoid joint symptoms, the patient may have a high fever, rash, pleurisy, and enlargement of the spleen. The onset of the disease may appear in the form of an unexplained childhood rash and fever, with arthritic symptoms developing as much as several weeks later. A possible complication is an eye inflammation that can lead to blindness if untreated.

Treatment

Juvenile rheumatoid arthritis is treated with aspirin or steroid drugs, or both, along with other kinds of therapy used for the adult version of rheumatoid arthritis. Steroid therapy is often more effective against rheumatoid arthritis in children than in adults. There may be a complete remission of the disease or the patient may experience rheumatoid symptoms into adult life.

Ankylosing Spondylitis

A kind of arthritis that affects the spine, causing a fusion of the joints, is known as *ankylosing spondylitis*. About 90 percent of the patients are young adult males. There is some evidence that it may be a hereditary disease.

Like other forms of arthritis, ankylosing spondylitis is insidious in its start. The patient may complain of a backache, usually in the lumbar area of the back. Some victims of the disease have claimed they were without pain but felt muscle spasms and perhaps tenderness along the lower part of the spine. Then stiffness and loss of motion spread rapidly over the back.

Along with fusion of the spine, the ligament along the spine calcifies like a bone. X-ray photographs of the spinal column may show the backbone to resemble a length of bamboo. A complication is that the spine is bent and chest expansion is limited by the fusion so that normal breathing is impaired.

Treatment of the disease consists of physical therapy and exercises to prevent or limit deformity and the use of aspirin or other drugs to reduce pain.

Gout

Gout is an arthritic disease associated with an abnormality of body chemistry. There is an excessive accumulation of uric acid in the blood resulting from the chemical abnormality, and the uric acid, in the form of sharp urate crystals, may accumulate in the joints, where they cause an inflammation with symptoms like those of arthritis. A frequent target of the u-rate crystals is the great toe, which is why gout patients occasionally are pictured as sitting in a chair with one foot propped upon a pillow.

Primary Gout

There are two forms of gout, primary gout and secondary gout. Primary gout is presumed to be linked to a hereditary defect in metabolism and afflicts mostly men, although women may experience the disease after menopause. The painful inflammation may develop overnight following an injury or illness or after a change in eating habits. The patient may suddenly feel feverish and unable to move because of the tenderness of the affected joint, which becomes painfully swollen and red.

Although the great toe is a common site for the appearance of gout, it also may develop in the ankle, knee, wrist, hand, elbow, or another joint. Only one joint may be affected, or several joints might be involved at the same time or in sequence. The painful attack usually subsides within a week or so but it may return to the same joint or another joint after an absence of a few years. The inflammation subsides even if it is not treated, but untreated gout may eventually result in deformity or loss of use of the affected joint. During periods between attacks the patient may show no signs of the disease except for high blood serum levels of uric acid and the appearance of *tophi*, or *urate* (a salt or uric acid) deposits, visible in X-ray photographs of the joints.

Secondary Gout

Secondary gout is related to a failure of the kidneys to excrete uric acid products or a variety of diseases that are characterized by overproduction of certain types of body cells. Failure of the kidneys to filter out urates can, in turn, be caused by various drugs, including aspirin and diuretics. Gout symptoms can also be caused by efforts to lose weight rapidly through a starvation diet, because this speeds up the breakdown of stored body fats. Among diseases that may precipitate an attack of secondary gout are Hodgkin's disease, psoriasis, and some forms of leukemia.

Chronic Gouty Arthritis

A form of arthritis called *chronic gouty arthritis* is associated with patients who have abnormal levels of uric acid in their blood. While they may or may not be plagued by attacks of acute joint pain, the urate deposits apparently cause a certain amount of stiffness and soreness in various joints, especially during periods of stormy weather or falling barometric pressure. The tophi or urate crystals may spread to soft tissues of the body, such as bursae, the cartilage of the ear, and tendon sheaths. More than ten percent of gout patients eventually develop kidney stones formed from urate deposits in the kidney.

Treatment of Gout

Because gout was traditionally associated with certain meats that are rich in chemicals called *purines*, special diets were once a routine part of the treatment. In recent years, there has been less emphasis placed on maintaining a low-purine diet for gout patients. This change in therapy is mainly the result of the relatively good success in maintaining proper uric-acid levels in gout patients with medications. However, adequate fluid intake is still recommended to prevent development of urate kidney stones.

Infectious Arthritic Agents

There are at least 12 types of arthritis

and rheumatism that are associated with infections involving bacteria, viruses, fungi, or other organisms. One of these diseases is known as *pyrogenic arthritis*. The arthritis-causing organisms infect a joint and induce pain and fever and limitation of joint movement by muscle spasm and swelling. Treatment includes bed rest and antibiotics. If untreated, destruction of the joints is possible.

Gonococcal Arthritis

This disease is transmitted by the gonococcal bacteria associated with venereal disease. As in the venereal disease itself, the arthritic effects are more likely to be treated at an early stage in men than in women because men are more likely to develop obvious infections of the urethra and thus seek medication from a physician. In females, the initial infection is likely to go unrecognized and untreated by antibiotics. The infection, meanwhile, may spread to body joints and produce acute attacks of arthritis. The symptoms tend to appear first in the wrists and finger joints; there may also be skin lesions that occur temporarily in areas near the joints.

Tuberculous Arthritis

As the name suggests, this disease is associated with tuberculosis and can be serious, leading to the destruction of involved joints. The infection spreads to the joints from other areas of the body. The early symptoms include pain, tenderness, or muscle spasm. In children and young adults the infection tends to settle in the spinal joints. If there is an absence of pain, the disease may go unnoticed until changes in posture or gait are observed. If untreated, the disease may progress toward spinal deformity. When detected early in the course of the disease, treatment with anti-

tuberculosis drugs and physical therapy may control the disorder. In some cases, surgery may be required.

Rubella Arthritis

This form of arthritis derives from an infection involving the rubella virus. The arthritis symptoms may appear shortly after a rash appears, or they may be delayed until after the rash has faded. The onset of the arthritis effects may be accompanied by fever and a general feeling of illness; pain and swelling are most likely to occur in the small joints of the wrists, knees, or ankles. The physician usually advises aspirin for the pain while it lasts, usually about a week. Eventually all signs and symptoms may subside without joint destruction.

Bacteria That Cause Arthritis

A type of bacteria that causes spinal meningitis also may cause symptoms of arthritis. The pain usually is not severe and may be limited to a few body joints. Antibiotics are administered to control the infection, although this form of the disease does not respond as rapidly to the medication as some of the other versions of arthritis caused by infection.

Several other kinds of bacteria may invade the joints and precipitate or aggravate arthritic symptoms. They include the increasingly common strains of bacteria that have become resistant to control by antibiotics. Patients who are being treated with steroid drugs or those whose resistance to infection has been lowered by disease are among the most vulnerable victims.

Fungal Arthritis

While fungal infections are relatively rare causes of arthritis, there are at least four kinds of fungus that have been identified as the responsible or-

ganisms in joint inflammations. The fungus seems to be carried by the bloodstream to the area of the joint where it causes an inflammation in the tissues surrounding the bony structures. The infection usually can be treated with special antibiotic remedies that destroy fungal organisms, but surgery is occasionally necessary to ensure eradication of the source of the inflammation.

Psoriatic Arthropathy

Arthritis also may be associated with psoriasis (a chronic skin condition marked by bright red patches and scaling) in a disease known as *psoriatic arthropathy*. This variation of the disease is marked by a deep pitting of the nails along with a chronic arthritic condition. The disease may be mild or very destructive and the sacroiliac region of the spine may be involved. The uric acid levels associated with gout frequently are elevated in patients with psoriasis, so gout symptoms also can appear. Unfortunately, one of the medications commonly used in the treatment of rheumatoid arthritis and gout, chloroquine, cannot be used as therapy for psoriatic arthropathy symptoms because the drug aggravates the psoriasis. Otherwise, the treatment is quite similar to that used for rheumatoid arthritis—analgesics such as aspirin and steroid drugs. In severe cases, methotrexate may be administered to control both the joint and skin symptoms.

Other Arthritic Diseases

Two kinds of arthritis once associated with venereal diseases are no longer considered a hazard of intimate contact. One is syphilis-caused arthritis, which is a possible problem but actually quite rare because of improved control of syphilis. The second is *Rei-*

ter's syndrome, a form of arthritis in which there is also involvement of urethritis, or inflammation of the urethra, and conjunctivitis, an inflammation of the eye. The disease also may be accompanied by skin lesions and a fever, pain in the heels, and a urethral discharge. Perhaps because Reiter's syndrome seems to affect young men and symptoms may be similar to those of gonococcal arthritis, it was once assumed that this form of arthritis was a kind of venereal disease. However, there is a lack of evidence that the disease is transmitted by sexual contact.

Rheumatic Fever

This generalized inflammatory disease, which affects the entire body with pain and swelling of the joints, sometimes is classified as a form of arthritis. Rheumatic fever usually follows a sore throat or tonsillitis caused by streptococcus bacteria; however, the disease is not regarded as a streptococcal infection by itself. A common effect of rheumatic fever is a scarring of the heart valves due to inflammation of that tissue. The heart valve damage is permanent. The streptococcal infection itself can be controlled by antibiotic medications. For further information, see "Rheumatic Fever and Rheumatic Heart Disease" in Ch. 10, *Heart Disease.*

Bursitis

The *bursa* is a fluid-filled sac located in the muscle near most joints. The fluid lubricates the joint, thereby providing smooth joint movement. Infection or injury may cause inflammation of the bursa. This condition is known as *bursitis* and can be very painful. The most commonly affected joints are the shoulder, knee, and hip.

Calcium deposits in the shoulder

tendon or calcification of the bursa (*calcific bursitis*) leads to more painful shoulder problems. This may be similar to *interstitial calcinosis*, a condition in which calcium deposits are found in the skin and subcutaneous tissues of children. Recovery from calcific bursitis is achieved by medical care, minor surgery, and resting the inflamed joint. Radiation treatments can sometimes speed the recovery process.

Living with Joint Diseases

The control of arthritis requires skilled medical supervision over extended periods of time. The causes of the major forms of arthritis are still unknown, although various theories have been formulated to explain it based on metabolic, biochemical, and microscopic tissue studies. Despite years of intensive research, it has not been possible to isolate a microorganism that is generally agreed to be a cause of rheumatoid arthritis. Viruses have been implicated in a number of arthritic diseases and may be a cause of rheumatoid arthritis; the evidence remains elusive, however, and the vi-

rus theory will remain a theory until the specific causative organism has been isolated and tested.

Whatever the mystery surrounding the causes of osteoarthritis and rheumatoid arthritis, severe crippling can be prevented in 70 percent of the cases if the patient seeks medical care early in the disease and receives proper medical treatment. The course of the disease varies from patient to patient and in many cases is confined to a few joints, causing little or no impairment of function. Commonly, however, there is a tendency toward relapse or continued inflammation.

The arthritis patient needs to develop a sense of coexistence with the disease, a tolerant attitude toward the problems of possible pain or disability without surrendering to arthritis. Millions of people have learned to live with arthritis and have found that it is possible to work, travel, raise families, and enjoy many of the recreational activities pursued by people not afflicted by the disease.

Joint Replacement

Over the years, various methods of

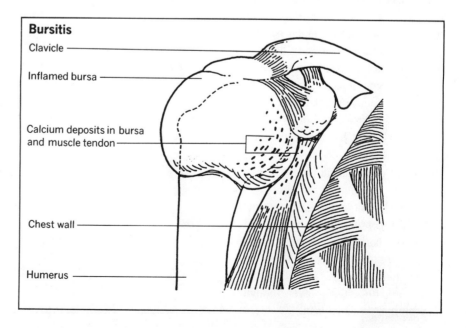

Bursitis

Clavicle

Inflamed bursa

Calcium deposits in bursa and muscle tendon

Chest wall

Humerus

Joint Replacement (Hip)

Fracture   Fracture

Nail   Nail with side plate   Plastic (acrylic) prosthesis

replacing joints have evolved. Like artificial hips, artificial knee, elbow, ankle, shoulder, toe, and finger joints are becoming more and more common. Technically known as arthroplasty, joint replacement both relieves pain, including the pain of arthritis, and improves function.

Materials used in joint replacement operations include metal, plastic, and ceramic components. Because of the tasks they perform in bodily movement, hip, knee, and ankle arthroplasties are undertaken much more often than those involving other parts. Developments in knee replacement surgery include a "cementless knee" that has a porous surface of chrome cobalt beads; aided by the beads, the patient's bone cells grow right into the knee replacement.

In each type of operation, the surgeon faces special problems. The elbow, for example, is not a simple hinge or joint but has three sections. Each involves one of the three arm bones that meet at that point: the humerus, the radius, and the ulna.

Surgical joint replacement techniques are continually evolving. In all cases, the patient faces some risks. Patients are also told usually that joint replacements do not really cure arthritis or osteoarthritis even though they normally relieve pain.

Defects and Diseases of the Spine

Spine Curve Deformities

When looked at from the side, the normal human spine follows a shallow S-shaped curve. If there is an exaggerated forward curvature of the spine, that condition is described as a *lordosis*. This type of spinal curvature is uncommon except in late pregnancy, and is caused by hip deformity or a defect in posture.

Kyphosis

Kyphosis is an exaggerated backward spinal curvature characterized by a humpback appearance. A person with this disorder develops an abnormal-looking thorax (or chest) due to the hump in the back and may sometimes find it difficult to lie on his back. The condition is brought on by untreated fractures of a vertebral body, a spinal tumor, osteoporosis, or spinal tuberculosis. If the principal cause is diagnosed and treated, recovery is possible.

Scoliosis

Scoliosis is a lateral curvature of the central part of the spine and appears mostly in children from birth and young adults up to age 15. Early diagnosis and proper orthopedic care are important. If scoliosis appears in early adulthood, the prognosis is better than if the disease starts in infancy. Growth of the curvature ends

Vertebral Column

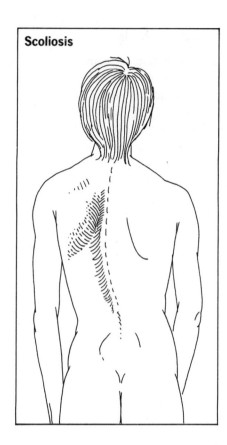

Scoliosis

when the individual's skeletal development ceases.

Scoliosis creates an ugly spinal deformity, and this is usually the only symptom. Sometimes there may be an acute attack of sciatica. Treatment of scoliotic children requires hospitalization. In simple cases, a cast is applied from the chest to the waist to reduce the curvature. Fusion of the vertebral bodies with bone grafting to maintain the fusion may be necessary.

Spinal Tuberculosis

Chronic pulmonary tuberculosis can spread to the skeletal system, including the vertebral column. Spinal tuberculosis, also known as *Pott's disease*, affects one or more vertebrae in children and young adults. It is currently a relatively rare disease.

The diseased vertebrae may col-

lapse because of the pressure from the vertebrae above, resulting in a humpback deformity and possible paralysis of the lower limbs. The usual symptoms are back pain, stiffness, and limited movement. Antibiotics are administered to combat and cure the infection.

Spinal Infections

Fever-inducing microorganisms may reach the spine via the blood and lymph channels, resulting in spinal osteomyelitis or a general inflammation of the vertebrae. This results in bone destruction, pressure on the spinal cord, and paralysis of the legs. Successful treatment includes bed rest, drug therapy, and sometimes a body jacket (for immobilization) made from plaster of Paris.

Tumors

The spinal column is affected by both malignant and benign tumors. They can either destroy the bony makeup of the affected vertebra, apply pressure to the spinal cord with resultant paralysis, or interfere with the nerve roots.

Spinal tumors are generally destructive. Some, like *meningiomas* and *neurofibromas*, result in lack of control over bowel and bladder function in addition to the loss of functioning of the lower extremities. Malignant tumors of the spinal column may originate from cancer of the prostate, uterus, bladder, lungs, or breast.

The symptoms of spinal tumors are pain, deformity, weakness, and lower limb paralysis. Diagnosis requires careful study of the subjective symptoms, as well as special tests and radiological examinations. Treatment may involve radiation therapy and chemotherapy; some tumors can be surgically removed. In many instances, the patient may be given analgesics to relieve the pain.

Back Pain and Its Causes

Most adults have experienced some form of back pain. Back pain is a serious physical impairment in persons of all ages, but it occurs more frequently in older persons.

Lumbago and Sciatica

Lumbago refers to general pain in the lower back. Technically, it is not a disease but a symptom that is accentuated by bending, lifting, turning, coughing, or stooping. Pain from neu-

Sciatica

Fifth lumbar root

Sciatic nerve

ritis of the sciatic nerve adds to one's misery, with pain shooting down the legs. This form of back pain is commonly known as *sciatica*, and, like lumbago, can be considered a symptom of some other condition. Treatment depends on the underlying cause of both.

Slipped and Herniating Disks

Between each two vertebrae is a fibro-cartilaginous disk that acts as a cushion. These disks are subjected to strain with every movement of the body, especially in the erect position. Increased pressure may cause a disk to protrude or herniate into the vertebral canal, causing what is referred to as a *slipped disk*. This condition can also be brought on by injury, degeneration caused by aging, unaccustomed physical activity, or heavy lifting.

The herniating disk presses against nerves in the area, resulting in low back pain, sciatica, and in some instances, disabling muscle spasm. Back rest and a surgical corset may help milder forms of slipped disk by allowing natural healing to take place. Treatment may also include bed rest with intermittent traction to the legs for several weeks. Spinal fusion may be required in severe cases.

A severely herniated disk can be surgically removed to relieve pain and other symptoms. Disk removal is followed by fusion of the vertebral bodies on both sides of the removed disk. Fusion is accomplished by bridging the vertebral space with a bone graft. For a fuller description of surgical repair of a slipped disk, see under "Orthopedic Surgery" in Ch. 20, *Surgery*.

Spondylolisthesis

A forward displacement of one vertebral body over another results in a painful condition known as *spondylolisthesis*. In mild cases there may be no symptoms at all. But in more advanced forms, there is severe low back pain when in the erect position and on bending, with the pain radiating to the legs. The displaced vertebra interferes with nerve roots in that area.

Mild cases require no treatment. Severe cases may require fusion of the vertebral segments with bone grafting; less severe symptoms can be relieved by a specially fitted corset.

Muscle Spasms and Strained Ligaments

Lack of physical exercise and unaccustomed bending can cause acute backache from undue muscle strain. Backache from strain on the ligaments is not uncommon in women following childbirth. The symptoms are similar to general low back pain. Physiotherapy with moist heat and massage helps restore muscular tone and relieve the pain. Muscle-relaxing drugs are sometimes prescribed.

Sacroiliac Pain

The *sacroiliac* joints in the lower back, where the *iliac* (hipbone) joins the sacrum, are a common location for osteoarthritic changes, rheumatoid arthritis, tuberculosis, and ankylosing spondylitis. The most common site of pain is in the lower lumbar region, radiating to the thighs and legs. X-ray diagnosis helps to pinpoint the cause of this particular form of back pain.

Herniated Disk

Spinal cord

Spinal column (vertebra)

Herniated disk pressing against cord

Intervertebral disk

Lumbar region

Other Disorders of the Skeletal System

Because bone consists of living cells, it is constantly changing as old cells die and new cells take their places. Any systemic disease during the growing period may temporarily halt the growth of long bones. As the aging process continues, dead bone cells are not replaced as consistently as in earlier life. The bony skeleton thus loses some of its calcium content, a process known as *decalcification* or *bone atrophy*, and the bones become fragile.

Pelvis and Hip Disorders

The hip joint presents most of the problems in the pelvic area. Symptoms may appear in early infancy in the form of congenital hip dislocation, in older children as tuberculous and transient arthritis, as slipped epiphysis in young adults (discussed below), and as osteoarthritis in adults and the aged. Early diagnosis of these conditions is very important in reducing the possibility of permanent deformity.

Diagnosis is achieved by physical examinations for signs of abnormal joint stability and mobility, postural changes, unstable and painful hip movement, fixed joint deformity, and pain in the lower back. Measurement of both lower limbs may indicate the presence of abnormal hip structure. X-ray examination of the pelvic area and both hips aids in diagnosis, as does blood analysis, which may yield evidence of early signs of gouty or arthritic conditions.

Slipped Epiphysis

This condition occurs in late child-

hood, between the ages of 9 and 18. The head of the *femur*, or thighbone, slips from its normal position, affecting one or both hips. The individual feels pain in the hip and knee, has limitation in joint movement, and walks with a limp. Usually there is evidence of endocrine disturbances.

Legg-Perthes' Disease

This is an inflammatory condition of unknown origin involving the bone and cartilage of the femoral head. It is found mostly in children between 4 and 12 years old and usually affects one hip. The symptoms are thigh and groin pain, joint movement limitation, and a walking impediment.

Successful treatment requires extended hospitalization with weight traction applied to the diseased hip and limitation of body weight on the affected side. Untreated Legg-Perthes' disease leads to permanent hip joint deformity and possible osteoarthritis around middle age.

Coxa Vara

This hip deformity is caused by a misshapen femur and causes shortening of the leg on the affected side; as a result, the person walks with a limp. The condition may be related to bone softening brought on by rickets, poorly joined fractures of the hip, or congenital malformation of the hip joint. Some cases may require surgical correction.

Any attack of persistent unexplained hip pains, limitation of movement, and walking impediments should be referred to the family physician for further investigation. Early diagnosis is crucial in controlling and eradicating many of the crippling diseases of the pelvic area.

Other Bone Disorders

Osteoporosis

This metabolic disorder is marked by porousness and fragility of the bones. When the condition is associated with old age, it is called *senile osteoporosis*. While the exact cause of the disorder is unknown, most physicians believe that calcium deficiencies—or inadequate calcium intake—may be a primary cause. Other contributing causes may be protein deficiency and a lack of the sex hormones androgen and estrogen. Postmenopausal women experience a dramatic decrease in the production of estrogen, which maintains bone strength. Because of its link with estrogen, osteoporosis is quite common among postmenopausal women.

Researchers stress the need for

Osteoporosis

Demineralization

both good diet and exercise as means of arresting or preventing osteoporosis. Calcium, estrogen, and vitamin D supplements may also help. A calcium-rich diet should include low-fat milk and cheeses; yogurt and ice cream; red kidney, lima, and soybeans; fish; watermelon, oranges, raisins, and strawberries; Brazil and other nuts; and green, leafy vegetables.

New methods of diagnosis have made possible earlier detection of osteoporosis. Three noninvasive methods include *absorptiometry*, measuring bone loss in the wrist and foot; *dual-photon absorptiometry*, a similar technique that indicates degrees of bone loss in the spine and hip; and an application of the CT scan that also measures loss of spinal bone. Blood tests, today the subject of research, may provide a means of very early detection. Once bone loss has been found to be too rapid, physicians can suggest ways to slow the rate of loss before fractures occur.

Osteogenesis Imperfecta

During the formation and development of bones, a process called *osteogenesis*, the bones may grow long and thin but not to the required width, becoming brittle so that they fracture easily. This condition is known as *osteogenesis imperfecta*. The individual may grow out of the condition in the middle twenties after suffering numerous fractures while growing up. A child thus afflicted cannot participate in games or other strenuous activities.

Paget's Disease

Paget's disease is characterized by a softening of the bones followed by an abnormal thickening of the bones. Its cause is unknown, and it manifests itself after the age of 30. It may cause pain in the thighs, knees, or legs, as well as backache, headache, and general fatigue. Symptoms include deafness, deformity of the pelvis, spine, and skull, and bowed legs. Although there is no known cure, Paget's disease is not usually fatal, but is eventually disabling.

Osteomyelitis

Osteomyelitis is an inflammation of the bone caused by fever-inducing bacteria or mold organisms. The invading microorganisms usually reach the bone through the bloodstream after entering the body through a wound or ulcer; the infection also can begin through a compound fracture or during surgery. The staphylococcus germ is most frequently the causative agent, and the most frequent site is the shaft of a long bone of a child. In adults, osteomyelitis usually occurs in the pelvis or spinal column.

Symptoms

Symptoms are fever, chills, and pain, with nausea and vomiting, especially in younger patients. There also may be muscle spasms around the affected bone. The infected bone usually is sensitive to the touch but X rays may reveal no abnormality during the early stages. Redness and swelling sometimes appear in tissues above the inflamed bone, and as the disease progresses the patient may find that simply moving the affected limb is painful. The infection can involve a joint, producing misleading symptoms of arthritis.

Causes

Examination by a physician usually reveals signs of a recent wound, ulceration, or similar lesion that may have been accompanied by pus from the invading bacteria. Laboratory tests of the blood usually will show an abnormal number of white cells and the presence of the infectious microorganism. Signs of anemia also may be found.

Treatment

Treatment may include the use of antibiotics for a period of several weeks. In difficult cases, surgery may be required to drain abscesses or to remove dead bone tissue. Before the advent of antibiotic drugs, osteomyelitis could be a fatal disease; early and proper treatment with modern medications has virtually eliminated that risk.

Diet and Bone Disorders

A proper diet is necessary to maintain the health of the skeletal system. The body's retention of the bone-building minerals, phosphorus and calcium, depends on vitamin D, which is manufactured in the human skin through the action of the sun's ultraviolet radiation.

Rickets

An insufficient supply of vitamin D and a lack of exposure to sunlight leads to a vitamin deficiency disease known as *rickets*. It can occur in infants and small children who live in northern latitudes and thus are not exposed to sufficient sunlight to permit their body to manufacture vitamin D. Rickets slows growth and causes bent and distorted bones and bandy legs. Symptoms first appear between the age of six months and the end of the first year. If rickets is recognized in time, it can be cured by a diet containing adequate vitamin D and by exposure to sunlight. If the disease is unchecked, the bones may develop permanent curves.

Bone Tumors

Benign and malignant tumors can occur in bone and bone marrow, although these growths are far less common than tumors of the body's soft tissues. Children and adolescents are more susceptible to bone tumors than adults. Since X rays cannot show whether a bone tumor is benign or malignant, surgical biopsy of the affected tissue is necessary in all cases.

Benign Tumors

These tumors usually take the form of an overgrowth of bone tissue, often near a joint, with many cysts or hollow spaces in the affected tissue. These growths often cause pathological fractures, in which a bone breaks for no apparent reason. Swelling, pain, and limited mobility in the joint nearest the tumor are the most common symptoms. Treatment consists of surgical removal of the tumor, after which the surrounding bone gradually repairs itself as it does after a fracture.

Malignant Tumors

Bone cancers may be primary (originating in the bone tissue itself) or caused by metastasis of cancer cells from a site elsewhere in the body. The most common types of primary bone cancer are *osteogenic sarcoma*, a rapidly growing form of cancer that often spreads into nearby muscles; *chondrosarcoma*, which begins in cartilage at the end of a bone; and *Ewing's sarcoma*, a highly malignant cancer of the shafts of the long bones in children.

Bone cancer of the extremities is treated by amputation of the affected limb, followed by radiation therapy. If treatment is begun early enough and all the cancerous tissue is removed, the prognosis for survival is favorable.

Injury to Bones and Joints: Fractures and Dislocations

Bones can be broken or displaced when the body is subjected to a violent impact or when a limb is suddenly wrenched out of its normal position. Auto and bicycle accidents and accidents in and around the home account for many such injuries. See Ch. 31, *Medical Emergencies*, for information on accidents and how to provide treatment.

A *fracture* is a break in a bone as a result of injury or pathological weakness. Tumors, for example, can destroy bones to such an extent that a spontaneous fracture occurs due to pathological weakness. Osteoporosis can also cause such fractures.

A *dislocation* is a displacement of any part, especially a bone. During this process the joint-capsule ligaments and muscle may be torn. The displaced bones must be reset by a bone specialist in their original position and immobilized until healing is complete. If this is not done, there is every possibility that the unhealed muscles will not provide the necessary support, thereby causing chronic spontaneous dislocation.

Injury (*trauma*) to bones and joints should not be dismissed lightly, especially if pain persists. If untreated, fractures and dislocations may heal with the bones out of alignment. Permanent deformity and joint degeneration are two possible complications.

Crush injuries, such as those occurring in some industrial and automobile accidents, may result in the clogging or blockage of blood vessels that supply blood to an extremity. When this happens, tissues below the blockage may die, and wounds do not heal because of lack of oxygenated blood and nutrition. If the fractures and wounds are not properly treated, *gangrene*, or the death of soft tissues, can sometimes result, requiring amputation just above the site of blockage and at a location that will make the healing process possible.

Kinds of Fractures

Incomplete fractures are those that do

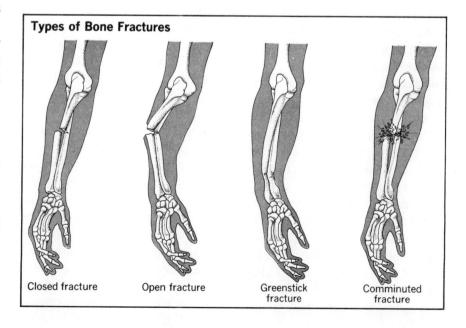

Types of Bone Fractures

Closed fracture   Open fracture   Greenstick fracture   Comminuted fracture not destroy the continuity of the bone. In a *complete fracture*, the bone is completely broken across. A *simple* or *closed fracture* is one in which the fragments are held together under the surface of the skin by the muscles and soft tissues. In a *compound* or *open fracture* one or both fragments pierce the skin, resulting in an open wound. In some cases the bony fragments can be seen protruding through the skin.

Comminuted fractures are the result of crushed bones. Several fragments appear at the trauma site. *Greenstick fractures* occur when one side of the bone is broken and the other bent. This type of fracture is more common in long bones, especially the forearms, clavicle, and legs of young children. *Stress fractures*, tiny cracks in the bone, can occur in the bones of the foot or leg of athletes who put these bones under repeated stress, such as ballet dancers and long-distance runners.

Healing of Fractures

When a bone breaks, new bone cells called *callus* are laid down at the ends of the fracture to unite the fragments. This is the beginning of the healing process, the speed of which is dependent on the nature of the fracture.

Simple, incomplete, and greenstick fractures heal readily. Rest is usually sufficient to heal stress fractures. However, compound fractures have wounds and fragments to complicate the healing process. Cleaning and suturing the wound and administering antibiotics reduce the chance of infection and promote healing.

Comminuted fractures may have to be disimpacted and all fragments reset, usually by an orthopedic or general surgeon. Some very serious fractures of the extremities may require surgical insertion of metallic pins, nails, plates, wires, or screws to hold the fragments in proper position, thereby promoting rapid healing with minimal deformity. Such devices must be made from corrosion-free and rustproof metals because they may remain in the body for a few months or throughout the person's lifetime.

Age and the Healing Process

The age of the fracture victim determines the speed of healing. In healthy, normal children, broken bones mend quickly because a rapid bone-cell manufacturing process is constantly in progress during the growth of the child. This is further advanced by proper diet, including daily intake of milk and milk products to provide the calcium required to build healthy bones.

In young adults, new bone cells do not develop as rapidly as in the growing child, but under normal circumstances, this will not present problems with the healing of fractures. Fractures in the aged heal slowly or not at all, depending on the age and health of the individual.

Treatment of Fractures

Correction of a fracture or dislocation is called *reduction* and is usually performed by an orthopedic surgeon. Bones that are merely cracked do not require reduction; they heal with the aid of immobilization. More serious fractures require manipulation, pressure, and sometimes, as mentioned above, wires, pins, nails, and screws, to bring the fragments together so that they can unite.

Healing of fractures and dislocations following reduction requires proper immobilization, which also reduces pain by preventing movement of the fragments. Immobilization is usually accomplished by the use of splints or plaster casts or by applying

(Top) A metal plate is fastened with screws to secure a fractured bone in the arm (the radius). The enlarged portion shown in cross section is also shown as it appears in the patient's arm. *(Bottom)* A steel rod has been driven through the center of the femur of the leg to hold the jagged ends of the fractured bone in proper alignment. Such appliances are sometimes left in place indefinitely when there are no adverse reactions.

traction. Traction subjects the fractured member to a pulling force by means of a special apparatus, such as a system of weights and pulleys.

After a fracture or dislocation is reduced and immobilized in a cast, the injury is X-rayed to ensure that the immobilized reduction will heal without deformity. If the reduction is not satisfactory, the cast is removed, the fragments are remanipulated to provide better reduction, and a new cast or bandage is applied. Periodic X-ray rechecks help the physician ascertain the degree of new bone formation as the healing continues. Casts are also checked to make sure there is not excess swelling of tissues and compression of blood vessels in the area.

How long a cast must remain depends on the extent of the injury and the rapidity of healing. A broken wrist may heal in four to six weeks while a fractured tibia may require four months of immobilization in a plaster cast.

Fracture of the Pelvis

Pelvic injuries are most often caused by falls in the home or on slippery streets and by industrial or automobile accidents.

The pelvis bears the entire weight of the body from the waist up and must bear the stress of general body motion during daily activity. The bony architecture of the pelvis does not readily permit the use of a plaster cast to immobilize a fracture. Consequently, fractures of the pelvis require bed rest for at least three weeks, depending on the nature of the injury and the age of the patient.

Simple fractures in children and young adults heal readily with complete bed rest and proper home care. Among the aged, the creation of new bone cells occurs more slowly, and this complicates the management of serious pelvic fractures in people over 65. Prolonged inactivity from extensive bed rest presents other health hazards for the aged, such as sluggish digestion and respiratory or vascular complications.

Fracture of the Hip

Falls are a major cause of hip fractures—the most common type of pelvic injury. Intense pain with limitation of hip movement and external rotation of the lower leg are indications of a hip fracture. When this occurs, a physician should be contacted immediately. The patient should be placed flat in bed until medical advice has been obtained. Proper diagnosis requires X-ray examinations.

Patients with hip fractures must be hospitalized. Although a hip fracture may be treated with traction, this method requires months of bed rest and is rarely used. The best method for treating such fractures is to nail the hip together with a metallic pin. The operation is performed by a surgeon, usually an orthopedist, who uses X-ray examinations during surgery to ascertain that the pin is in the correct position. Some hip fractures may also require a metallic plate screwed to the bone to help immobilize the fracture.

After plates and pins have been inserted, the patient can be out of bed within a day. This speeds recovery and prevents the complications of prolonged bed rest. Hip nails are usually left in the patient, depending on the nature of the fracture and the patient's age. Recuperation includes periodic medical checkups and X-ray examinations.

Hip Replacement

In recent years the technique of total hip replacement has become well advanced. The technique can be used where the hip joint has been injured or severely weakened by disease.

Called *total prosthetic replacement of the hip*, the operation involves removal of the upper portion of the large leg bone, the femur, and of the ball-like joint that holds it in the hip socket. A substitute piece shaped like the removed section of bone is attached to the femur. Care has to be taken during the operation to make certain the new part is firmly attached—by embedding the replacement part in the shaft of the bone. In addition, the surgeon tries not to destroy or damage the muscles and other tissues surrounding the hip. The replacement part is usually made of metal; a commonly used material is a durable cobalt-chromium alloy that produces no painful reactions in surrounding bones and tissues.

With modern techniques, hip replacement surgery can restore most patients to virtually normal levels of functioning. The implanted parts can carry weight and stand the strains of everyday use. Metal screws and a grouting agent (mortar of plastic cement or other material) help to join the metal implant to the leg bone. Patients may begin to walk one to three days after surgery. While they can later play golf or other nonstrenuous games, they are usually told to avoid more demanding activities, such as tennis or handball, because of the danger that they might fall and injure the replacement hip.

Some patients have had successful hip replacement surgery on both their right and left sides. Later they were able to function with good mobility and without pain.

Pubic Fracture

Pubic fractures can cause ruptures of the bladder with urine leaking into the pelvic cavity. Routine urinalysis for the presence of blood cells is always necessary in cases of pelvic fractures. Surgical repair of the bladder may be required.

Skull Injury

Although the skull is very thick, it is not invulnerable. Head injuries can result from sports or playground accidents, falls, automobile or industrial accidents, or sharp blows to the head. Head injuries can cause linear or hairline skull fractures, depressed skull fractures (dents), brain injury due to fracture fragments or foreign bodies piercing the brain (as in the case of a bullet wound), or *concussion* with or without bone damage. The effects of concussion can show up as dizziness, nausea, irritability, the tendency to sleep deeply or lose consciousness, a weak pulse, and slowed respiration.

Any of these injuries can cause blood vessels to rupture and bleed. The resulting blood clots form what is known as a *subdural hematoma*, which may cause increased pressure on the brain. Patients with a subdural hematoma feel dizzy, slip slowly into unconsciousness, and may die unless immediate hospital care is available. Usually half of the body on the opposite side of the clot becomes paralyzed.

A depressed fracture can also apply pressure on the brain at the area of the depression. Surgery is required to relieve the pressure.

No skull injury should be treated lightly. A child may hit his head in a playground or in the backyard and conceal this from his parents, or a baby-sitter may be afraid of losing her job if she reports such a fall. An alcoholic may slip on the street and strike his head on the sidewalk. Anyone who suffers a blow to the head or who falls on his head should be observed carefully for possible later complications. If such incidents are followed by vomiting, drowsiness, and headaches, immediate medical attention should be sought.

Facial Injury

A blow to the eye may fracture the upper or lower borders of the eye socket. It can also cause what is commonly known as a black eye, the blue-black appearance of which results from bleeding under the skin. The swelling can be reduced by applying an ice pack to the area.

Fractures of the facial bones, jaw, and nose result from a direct blow to these areas. The impact may rupture blood vessels and cause facial deformity. Dislocation of the jaw is a common problem caused by trauma. It may also occur spontaneously in certain individuals by an unusually wide-mouthed yawn or laugh. It is an uncomfortable rather than painful experience.

Serious facial injury requires hospitalization and surgical restoration.

Skin lacerations may have to be sutured and the scars removed by plastic surgery; fractures of the jaw and mouth may require surgical wiring for stabilization and immobilization before healing can take place. In some instances both jaws may be wired together until healing takes place.

Injury to the Rib Cage

Accidents, athletic injuries, and fights account for most injuries to the rib cage. Any blow to the chest can cause rib fractures, which hurt when one coughs or inhales. Hairline and incomplete fractures are less serious than complete fractures, where the fragments are usually sharp and pointed. Such fractured ribs can tear the lungs, causing air to leak into the pleural space, with possibly serious results. The lung can collapse as a result of being punctured. Punctured blood vessels can hemorrhage into the pleural space. The accumulated blood may have to be withdrawn before it reduces the capacity of the lungs to carry out their normal function.

Severe chest injuries—crush injuries with multiple fractures—require hospitalization. The patient must be confined to bed and kept under constant medical observation and treatment. If the lung has collapsed, it has to be reinflated. In simple rib fractures the chest may be strapped to immobilize the fragments and promote rapid healing. Generally, analgesics alone are enough to relieve pain.

Fractures of the sternum are caused by direct blows to the sternal area, as is usually the case with automobile accidents when the steering wheel hits the driver's chest. This injury can be avoided if the driver wears a shoulder-restraining belt, and if his car is equipped with a collapsible steering column.

Chest pains following a blow to the area of the sternum should be medically investigated by means of X-ray diagnosis for possible fracture. The fracture fragments may have to be wired together and remain in place until the injury has healed. For simple fractures, rest may be the only treatment required. The serious complication of a fractured sternum in a steering-wheel accident is contusion of the heart; it should be evaluated by means of an electrocardiogram.

Spinal Injury

Most spinal injuries originate from automobile accidents, industrial mishaps, falls, athletics, or from fights and beatings. Spinal injuries can create fractures that compress or sever the spinal cord, with resultant paralysis. A diving accident or headlong fall may cause a concussion and possible fractures of the cervical spine. Head-on collisions in the sports arena and automobile accidents are the chief causes of cervical spine fractures.

An individual who jumps from a considerable height and lands on his feet, especially on his heels, may easily fracture his spine. Sudden pain in the thoracic spine following a jump should receive immediate medical attention and investigation.

Whiplash

These injuries, the most common form of injury to the spine, occur most often during head-on and rear-end automobile accidents that suddenly jerk the neck and injure the cervical vertebrae. Accident victims thus injured may undergo months of agonizing headaches and pain in the neck. Immobilization of the neck by a surgical collar will reduce some of the pain and aid the healing process.

First Aid for Spinal Injuries

Victims of spinal injuries should be moved as little as possible. While waiting for professional help, the patient should be placed on his back and made as comfortable as possible. If an accident or explosion victim is wedged between debris, attempts should be made to free him, but his body should be kept flat with as little movement as possible. No attempt should be made to have the person sit up or stand before he has been examined by a physician. Unnecessary movement of victims of spinal injury can damage the spinal cord and cause permanent paralysis.

Decompression of Fractures

Anyone with a spinal injury should be taken to the emergency ward of the nearest hospital for X-ray examinations that will reveal possible fractures. If the fracture compresses against the spinal cord, the extremities may be paralyzed. In such cases, a neurosurgeon or an orthopedist may perform a delicate operation, lifting the fracture fragments away from the spinal cord, thereby relieving the pressure and reestablishing control and movement of the paralyzed extremities.

Fractures of the cervical spine can be decompressed by applying traction to the neck. Frequent X-ray rechecks are required to assess the degree of healing and new bone formation. Patients with fractured vertebrae undergo a lengthy rehabilitation with frequent medical rechecks and physical therapy. In some severe cases of spinal fractures that result in paralysis, the individual is never able to walk again.

8

Diseases of the Muscles and Nervous System

We have the capacity to perceive our environment by receiving sensory messages—such as hearing, sight, touch, pain, and awareness of our posture—to associate all the incoming messages, store the information, and then call it back to our consciousness as needed. Another function of the nervous system is the control of the body by sending signals to the muscles to perform movements ranging from the broadest to the most delicate—from wielding a pickax to playing the flute. Further, many aspects of our behavior are not at all mysterious and can be explained in terms of a series of neuroelectrochemical events. In short, our day-to-day existence is a reflection of the state of our nervous system, the normal function of which can be disturbed in many ways.

Diseases of the Nervous System

If any part of the brain has developed abnormally, the usual function of that structure would be expected to be altered. Abnormalities present at birth are called *congenital* defects. If the nervous system does not receive a normal blood supply because of the obstruction of a blood vessel, or if there is a tear in the vessel with subsequent hemorrhage, the cells are deprived of blood and will die. These lesions are *vascular* or *cerebrovascular* accidents. Cerebral injury, or *trauma,* can destroy brain tissue, with consequent loss of normal function; infections of the nervous system may also permanently injure tissue. Finally, brain function can be altered by *metabolic, toxic,* or *degenerative* changes in normal body chemistry. It is not surprising, then, that such a beautifully organized nervous system is vulnerable to the hazards of living.

Diagnostic Tests

A patient who has been referred to a *neurologist,* a physician who specializes in diseases of the nervous system, will be asked to tell the history of the problem in great detail, for that history will describe the nature of the disorder; the neurological examination will help to localize the problem.

After the neurological examination is completed, the physician may order radiographs (X-ray pictures) of the skull and spinal column and an electroencephalogram. The *electroencephalogram* (EEG), or brain wave recording, assists in localizing a brain abnormality or describing the nature of a convulsive disorder. A specific diagnosis is not based upon the EEG alone, but the EEG is used to corroborate the physician's clinical impression of the disease process.

It may also be necessary to perform a *lumbar puncture (spinal tap)* in order to obtain a specimen of the *cerebrospinal fluid (CSF),* the fluid that bathes the brain and spinal cord. This laboratory test is a benign, relatively painless procedure when performed by a skilled physician and is extremely useful in making a diagnosis. It entails a needle puncture under sterile conditions in the midline of the lower spine as the patient lies on his side or sits upright.

Occasionally, other more specialized diagnostic tests are used to better enable the physician to visualize the structure of the brain and the spinal cord. In a process called *ventriculography,* the cerebrospinal fluid is replaced by air introduced directly into the cavities (*ventricles*) of the brain. In *pneumoencephalography,* the air or other gas is inserted by means of a needle similar to that used in a lumbar puncture. In either case the outlines of the brain structure are photographed by X ray.

Another specialized neuroradiological test is the *angiogram.* A material that is opaque to X rays is injected into the blood vessels that supply the brain. Because the vessels can be plainly seen on the X-ray film, any displacement of those vessels from the normal position is evident.

A more recent diagnostic tool is the *brain scanner* or *CT scanner* (for *computed tomography*). CT scanning may in many cases make angiography, which can be painful and is not without risk, unnecessary. The scanner takes a series of computer-generated X-ray pictures of "slices" of the brain as it rotates about the patient. It can thus provide better pictures of parts of the brain (and of other internal areas of the body) than any older process.

A later version of the CT scanner takes stop-action photos of the beating heart. Called the *cine CT,* the imaging procedure enables cardiologists to measure blood flow through grafted coronary arteries. Only by using a catheter could physicians take such measurements earlier. With the cine CT it is also possible to measure the weights of different parts of the heart with almost 100 percent accuracy and to detect minute holes in the hearts of children suffering from congenital heart defects. Surgeons use these pictures to become familiar with a defective heart before surgery.

More advanced than either the CT scanner or radiography, *nuclear magnetic resonance* (NMR) uses neither X radiation, as does the CT scanner, nor needle-injected contrast fluids. Instead, NMR uses magnetic forces 3,000 to 25,000 times as strong as

Nervous System
Cranial Nerves

Optic nerve (vision)
Olfactory nerve (smell)
Oculomotor nerve (eye muscles)
Trigeminal nerve (face)
Trochlear nerve (eye muscles)
Facial nerve (facemuscles)
Acoustic nerve (hearing and balance)
Glossopharyngeal nerve (taste)
Vagus nerve (heart, lungs, abdomen)

Central Nervous System
Cerebrum
Cerebellum
Brachial plexus
Spinal cord

Autonomic Nervous System
Peripheral Nervous System
Thoracic nerves
Radial nerve
Ulnar nerve
Femoral nerve
Sciatic nerve

the earth's magnetic field. Taking three-dimensional "pictures" of various parts of the body, NMR "sees" through bones. It can differentiate between the brain's gray and white matter. NMR can also show blood moving through an artery or the reaction of a malignant tumor to therapy.

Another type of contrast study is called a *myelogram.* A radiopaque liquid similar to that used in angiography is introduced through a spinal needle into the sac-enclosed space around the spinal cord. Any obstructive or compressive lesion of the spinal cord is thus seen on the radiograph and

helps to confirm the diagnosis.

Each of these contrast studies helps the physician better understand the structures of the brain or spinal cord and may be essential for him to make a correct diagnosis.

Cerebral Palsy

The term *cerebral palsy* is not a diagnosis but a label for a problem in locomotion exhibited by some children. Definitions of cerebral palsy are many and varied, but in general refer to nonprogressive abnormalities of the brain that have occurred early in life from many causes. The label implies that there is no active disease process but rather a static or nonprogressive lesion that may affect the growth and development of the child.

Symptoms

Included in the category of cerebral palsy are such problems as limpness (flaccidity), *spasticity* of one or all limbs, incoordination, or some other disorder of movement. In some patients, quick jerks affect different parts of the body at different times (*chorea*); in others, slow, writhing, incoordinated movements (*athetosis*) are most pronounced in the hands and arms. Incoordination of movement may also occur in muscles used for speaking and eating, so that speech becomes slurred, interrupted, or jerky; the patient may drool because incoordinated muscle action prevents efficient swallowing of saliva. This does little to improve the physical appearance of the child and, unfortunately, he may look mentally subnormal.

The fact that a patient has an abnormality that is responsible for difficulty in locomotion or speech does not mean that the child is mentally retarded. There is some likelihood that he will be mentally slow, but patients in this group of disease states range from slow to superior in intelligence, a fact that emphasizes that each child must be assessed individually.

A complete examination must be completed, and to determine the patient's functional status complete psychological testing should be performed by a skilled psychologist.

Treatment

Treatment for cerebral palsy is a continuing process involving a careful surveillance of the patient's physical and psychological status. A physical therapist, under the physician's guidance, will help to mobilize and maintain the function of the neuromuscular system. Occasionally, an orthopedic surgeon may surgically lengthen a tendon or in some way make a limb more functional. A speech therapist can provide additional speech training, and a vocational therapist can help the patient to find appropriate work. The key professional is the primary physician, usually the pediatrician, who with care and understanding guides the patient through the years.

Bell's Palsy

Bell's palsy is a paralysis of the facial nerve that was first described by Sir Charles Bell, a Scottish surgeon of the early nineteenth century. It may affect men and women at any age, though it occurs most commonly between the ages of 30 and 50. The onset of the facial paralysis may be abrupt: the patient may awaken one morning unable to move one side of his face. He can't wrinkle one side of his forehead or raise the eyebrow; the eye will not close on the affected side, and when attempting to smile, the face is pulled to the opposite side. Occasionally the patient may experience discomfort about the ear on the involved side. There is no difficulty in swallowing, but because the muscles about the corner of the mouth are weak, drooling is not uncommon, and food may accumulate in the gutter between gum and lip.

Bell's palsy may affect the branch of the facial nerve that supplies taste sensation to the anterior part of the tongue and the branch that supplies a small muscle in the middle ear (the *stapedius*) whose function it is to dampen loud sounds. Depending on the extent to which the facial nerve is affected, the patient may be unable to perceive taste on the side of the paralysis and may be unusually sensitive to sounds, a condition known as *hyperacusis*.

The most probable causes of Bell's palsy are inflammation of the facial nerve as it passes through a bony canal within the skull or inflammation of that bony canal with subsequent swelling and compression of the nerve. It is not uncommon that the patient has a history of exposure to a cold breeze, such as sleeping in a draft or riding in an open car. Any patient who has a facial weakness should be carefully evaluated by a physician, preferably a neurologist, to be quite certain that there is no other neurologic abnormality. When the diagnosis of Bell's palsy is certain, some therapeutic measures can be taken.

Treatment

There is no specific treatment for Bell's palsy, but many physicians recommend massage, application of heat, and exercise of the weak muscles, either passive (by external manipulation) or active (by use). These therapeutic measures do not specifically influence the course of the facial nerve paralysis, but they are thought to be useful in maintaining tone of the facial muscles and preventing permanent deformity. Occasionally a V-shaped adhesive tape splint can be applied to the affected side of the face, from the corner of the mouth to the temple. Some physicians treat the condition with steroids such as cortisone, which may hasten recovery if begun at the onset of the illness.

In treating Bell's palsy, it is important to remember that when the eyelid does not close normally, the conjunctiva and cornea are not fully lubricated, and corneal lesions may develop from excessive dryness or exposure to the air. For this reason, some ophthalmic lubrication may be recommended by the physician.

About 80 percent of the patients with Bell's palsy recover completely in a few days or weeks, and about 10 to 15 percent recover more slowly, over a period of three to six months. The remaining 5 to 10 percent will have some residual facial deformity.

Parkinson's Disease

Patients with *Parkinson's disease,* or *parkinsonism,* are easily recognized because of the characteristic symptoms of tremor, rigidity, and a decrease of movement. This group of symptoms had another name, *shaking palsy,* long before it was scientifically described nearly a century and a half ago by an English physician, James Parkinson. It is associated with degeneration of nerve cells deep within the brain (*basal ganglia*) and the brain surface (*cerebral cortex*). It may follow encephalitis, a brain injury, or exposure to toxic substances, but in most cases, especially when the symptoms appear in a patient who is middle-aged or older, there is no known cause.

The tremor, or shaking, usually involves the fingers and the wrist, but sometimes the arms, legs, or head are involved to the extent that the entire body shakes. Characteristically, the tremor occurs when the patient is at rest. It stops or is much less marked during a voluntary muscle movement, only to start once again when that movement has been stopped. There is no tremor when the patient is asleep.

Early in the disease, the patient is aware that one leg seems a bit stiff; later, the arm does not swing normally at his side when he is walking. He moves about more slowly with stooped-over head and shoulders. Often he has difficulty in starting to walk, but once started he cannot stop unless he grabs at the wall or some

other object. The face appears expressionless, the speech is slurred, and handwriting is small and uneven (*micrographia*) because of the rigidity and the tremor. Mental faculties are usually not impaired but, as might be expected in such a chronic disease in which the patient cannot move or communicate normally, mood disturbances are common.

Treatment

For many years parkinsonism was treated with drugs derived from belladonna. Many other remedies were tried, among them such toxic compounds as strychnine and cigarettes made from jimsonweed. In nearly all cases the results were less than gratifying. Neurosurgical procedures were then devised to produce very small destructive lesions in the brain, with subsequent lessening of the symptoms. The most gratifying improvements following surgery are usually seen in patients under 60 whose symptoms are confined primarily to one side of the body.

Today, three basic categories of drugs are used to relieve the symptoms of parkinsonism: anticholinergics, levodopa-containing compounds, and a single dopamine agonist.

The anticholinergic drugs include trihexyphenidyl hydrochloride (trade name: Artane), benztropine mesylate (trade name: Cogentin), diphenhydramine hydrochloride (trade name: Benadryl), biperiden (trade name: Akineton), and procyclidine hydrochloride (trade name: Kemadrin). All of these drugs reduce tremors and rigidity to a modest degree, but none affects bradykinesia, or slow movement. Patients using the drugs may experience such side effects as gingivitis or inflammation of the gums, constipation, mild dizziness, nausea, nervousness, and slightly blurred vision. More serious side effects could

include urinary retention, confusion, and psychosis.

The levodopa-containing compounds reduce all the main symptoms of parkinsonism. One such compound combines levodopa, also known as L-dopa, with carbidopa (trade name: Sinemet). Levodopa is also sold alone under the trade names Larodopa and Dopar. Because L-dopa's effectiveness may dwindle after several years, physicians sometimes delay treatment until a patient shows more severe symptoms.

Side effects associated with L-dopa include nausea, involuntary movements, some mental changes, cardiac irregularities, and urinary retention. "End-of-dose" akinesia, the return of symptoms a few hours after taking medication, can be relieved in some cases by taking the patient off drugs entirely for three to seven days. The patient is usually hospitalized. During the "drug holiday" some patients take part in physical, occupational, and speech therapy programs.

The one drug in the dopamine agonist class, bromocriptine (trade name: Parlodel), stimulates the brain's dopamine receptors. Used in combination with L-dopa, bromocriptine reduces the end-of-dose response. But clinical studies have not established the drug's safety in long-term use (more than two years). Patients with histories of coronary or peripheral vascular disease should not take bromocriptine. Side effects may include confusion, nasal congestion, liver problems, and swelling of the feet.

One other drug used to treat Parkinson's disease, amantadine hydrochloride (trade name: Symmetrel), has brought rapid improvement when given along with L-dopa. But the drug may also produce such side effects as hypotension, urinary retention, depression, and congestive heart failure.

Epilepsy

Epilepsy is a common disorder of the human nervous system. In the United States, about five persons of every 1,000, or more than one million people, suffer from epilepsy.

Epilepsy affects all kinds of people, regardless of sex, intelligence, or standard of living. Among the more famous epileptics of history were Julius Caesar, Napoleon, Lord Byron, Dostoyevsky, Handel, Mendelssohn, and Mozart. The I.Q. range for epileptics is the same as that of the general population.

Unfortunately, epilepsy has been one of the most misunderstood diseases throughout its long history. Because of the involvement of the brain, epilepsy has commonly been associated with psychiatric disorders. Epilepsy differs strikingly from psychiatric disorders in being manifested in relatively brief episodes that begin and end abruptly.

Causes and Precipitating Factors

A single epileptic seizure usually occurs spontaneously. In some cases, seizures are triggered by visual stimuli, such as a flickering image on a television screen, a sudden change from dark to very bright illumination, or vice versa. Other patients may react to auditory stimuli such as a loud noise, a monotonous sound, or even to certain musical notes. A seizure is accompanied by a discharge of nerve impulses, which can be detected by electroencephalography. The effect is something like that of a telephone switchboard in which a defect in the circuits accidentally causes wrong number calls. The forms that seizures take depend upon the location of the nervous system disturbances within the brain and the spread of the nerve impulses. Physicians have found that certain kinds of epilepsy cases can be traced to specific areas of the brain

where the lesion has occurred.

Epilepsy can develop at any age, although nearly 85 percent of all cases appear before the age of 20 years. Hence, it is commonly seen as an affliction of children. There is no indication that epilepsy itself can be inherited, but some evidence exists that certain individuals inherit a greater tendency to develop the condition from precipitating causes than is true for the general population. According to the Epilepsy Foundation, studies show that if neither parent has epilepsy, the chances are one in 100 that they will have an epileptic child, but the chances rise to one in 40 if one parent is epileptic.

About 70 percent of epilepsy cases are *idiopathic*—that is, they are not attributable to any known cause. In the remaining 30 percent, the recurrent seizures are *symptomatic*—they are symptoms of some definite brain lesion, either congenital or resulting from subsequent injury. Because it can reasonably be assumed that some of the idiopathic cases are a result of lesions that have not been identified, epilepsy is perhaps best regarded not as a specific disease but as a symptom of a brain abnormality due to any of various causes.

Aura Preceding a Seizure

Unusual sensory experiences have been reported to occur before a seizure by about half the victims of epilepsy. The sensation, which is called an *aura,* may appear in the form of an unpleasant odor, a tingling numbness, a sinking or gripping feeling, strangulation, palpitations, or a gastrointestinal sensation. Some patients say the sensation cannot be described. Others report feeling strange or confused for hours or even days before a seizure. Such an early warning is known as a *prodrome.*

The various types of epilepsy can

be broadly grouped under four general categories: grand mal, petit mal, focal, and psychomotor. Only one feature is common to all types of epilepsy—the sudden, disorderly discharge of nerve impulses within the brain.

Grand Mal Seizure

The *grand mal* is a generalized convulsion during which the patient may initially look strange or bewildered, suddenly groan or scream, lose consciousness and become stiff (*tonic phase*), hold the breath, fall to the ground unless supported, and then begin to jerk the arms and legs (*clonic phase*). There may be loss of bowel and bladder control. The tongue may be bitten by coming between clenched jaws. The duration of the entire seizure, both the tonic and clonic phases, is less than two minutes—frequently less than one minute—followed by postconvulsive confusion or deep sleep that may last for minutes or hours.

Following a Seizure

The patient may be able to resume normal activities shortly after the spell has ended. But after recovering from a long postconvulsive sleep, the patient may show a variety of signs or symptoms known as postconvulsive phenomena, which may include headache, mental confusion, and drowsiness.

Variations in the Pattern

The sequence of events in grand mal seizures is not invariable. The tongue-biting and urinary and fecal incontinence do not occur as frequently in children as in adult patients. Children may also demonstrate a type of grand mal seizure in which the patient suddenly becomes limp and falls to the floor unconscious; there is no apparent tonic or clonic phase and the muscles do not become stiff. Other cases may manifest only the tonic phase, with unconsciousness and the muscles remaining in a stiffened, tonic state throughout the seizure. There also is a clonic type of seizure, which begins with rapid jerking movements that continue during the entire attack. In one very serious form of convulsive seizure known as *status epilepticus,* repeated grand mal seizures occur without the victim's becoming conscious between them.

Petit Mal Seizure

Petit mal seizures are characterized by momentary staring spells, as if the patient were suspended in the middle of his activity. He may have a blank stare or undergo rapid blinking, sometimes accompanied by small twitching movements in one part of the body or another—hands, legs, or facial muscles. He does not fall down. These spells, called *absence* or *lapse attacks,* usually begin in childhood before puberty. The attacks are typically very brief, lasting half a minute or less, and occur many times throughout the day. They may go unnoticed for weeks or months because the patient appears to be daydreaming.

Focal Seizure

Focal seizures proceed from neural discharges in one part of the brain, resulting in twitching movements in a corresponding part of the body. Usually, one side of the face, the thumb and fingers of one hand, or one entire side of the body is involved. The patient does not lose consciousness and may in fact remain aware of his surroundings and the circumstances during the entire focal convulsion. Focal

convulsions in adults commonly indicate some focal abnormality, but this is less true in a child who may have a focal seizure without evidence of a related brain lesion.

With their knowledge of the nerve links between brain centers and body muscles, physicians are able to determine quite accurately the site of a brain lesion that is involved with a focal seizure.

Jacksonian Epilepsy

One type of focal seizure has a distinctive pattern and is sometimes called a *Jacksonian seizure,* and the condition itself *Jacksonian epilepsy.* The attack begins with rhythmic twitching of muscles in one hand or one foot or one side of the face. The spasmodic movement or twitching then spreads from the body area first affected to other muscles on the same side of the body. The course of the twitching may, for example, begin on the left side of the face, then spread to the neck, down the arm, then along the trunk to the foot. Or the onset of the attack may begin at the foot and gradually spread upward along the trunk to the facial muscles. There may be a tingling or burning sensation and perspiration, and the hair may stand up on the skin of the areas affected.

Psychomotor Seizures

Psychomotor seizures, or *temporal lobe seizures,* often take the form of movements that appear purposeful but are irrelevant to the situation. Instead of losing control of his thoughts and actions, the patient behaves as if he is in a trancelike state. He may smack his lips and make chewing motions. He may suddenly rise from a chair and walk about while removing his clothes. He may attempt to speak or speak incoherently, repeating certain

words or phrases, or he may go through the motions of some mechanical procedure, like driving a car, for example.

The patient in a psychomotor seizure usually does not respond to questions or commands. If physically restrained during a psychomotor episode, the patient may appear belligerent and obstreperous, or he may resist with great energy and violence. Usually, the entire episode lasts only a few minutes. When the seizure ends, the patient is confused and unable to recall clearly what has happened.

The aura experienced by victims of psychomotor seizures may differ from that of other forms of the disorder. The psychomotor epileptic may have sensations of taste or smell, but more likely will experience a complex illusion or hallucination that may have the quality of a vivid dream. The hallucination may be based on actual experiences or things the patient has seen, or it may deal with objects or experiences that only seem familiar though they are in fact unfamiliar. This distortion of memory, in which a strange experience seems to be a part of one's past life, is known as *déjà vu,* which in French means literally "already seen."

Other visual associations involved in various forms of epilepsy include those in which the patient experiences sensations of color, moving lights, or darkness. Red is the most common color observed in visual seizures, although blue, yellow, and green also are reported. The darkness illusion may occur as a temporary blindness, lasting only a few minutes. Stars or moving lights may appear as if visible to only one eye, indicating that the source of the disturbance is a lesion in the brain area on the opposite side of the head. Visual illusions before an epileptic attack may have a distorted quality, or consist of objects arranged in an unnatural pattern or of an unnatural size.

Auditory illusions, on the other hand, are comparatively rare. Occasionally a patient will report hearing buzzing or roaring noises as part of a seizure, or human voices repeating certain recognizable words.

Treatment of the Epileptic Patient

Usually the physician does not see the patient during a seizure and must rely on the description of others to make a proper diagnosis. Because the patient has no clear recollection of what happens during any of the epileptic convulsions, it is wise to have someone who has seen an attack accompany him to a physician. First, the physician begins the detective work to find the cause of the seizure. He will examine the patient thoroughly, obtain blood tests, an electroencephalogram, and a lumbar puncture, if indicated. Even after all these studies, however, the physician often can find no specific cause that can be eradicated. Efforts are then made to control the symptoms.

The treatment of epilepsy consists primarily of medication for the prevention of seizures. It is usually highly effective. About half of all patients are completely controlled and another quarter have a significant reduction in the frequency and severity of attacks. The medication, usually in tablet or capsule form, must be taken regularly according to the instructions of the physician. It may be necessary to try several drugs over a period of time to determine which drug or combination of drugs best controls the seizures. Phenobarbital and diphenylhydantoin (Dilantin) may be prescribed for the control of grand mal seizures and focal epilepsy, and the physician may find that a combination of these drugs or others offers the best anticonvulsant control. Trimethadione frequently is administered to petit mal patients; primidone or phenobarbital may be prescribed for psychomotor attacks.

Surgery may be recommended when drugs fail to control the seizures. But this approach usually is used only as a last resort and is not always effective.

However, medicine and surgery are not the only treatments for epilepsy patients. Emotional factors are known to influence convulsive disorders. Lessening a patient's anger, anxiety, and fear can help to control the condition. An understanding family and friends are important, as are adequate rest, good nutrition, and proper exercise. The exercise program should not include vigorous contact sports, and some activities such as swimming should not be performed by the patient unless he is accompanied by another person who understands the condition and is capable of helping the epileptic during a seizure.

There is nothing permanent about epilepsy, although some patients may endure the symptoms for much of their lives. It is a disorder that changes appreciably and constantly in form and manifestations. Some experts claim that petit mal and psychomotor cases if untreated may progress to more serious cases of grand mal seizures. On the other hand, epilepsy that is given proper medical attention may eventually subside in frequency and severity of attacks. In many cases, seizures disappear or subside within a short time and treatment can be discontinued gradually.

While some effort has been made by medical scientists to determine if there is an "epileptic personality," evidence indicates there is no typical personality pattern involved. Whatever behavior patterns and emotional reactions are observed are the result of individual personality makeup rather than being directly related to epilepsy. Most epilepsy patients are capable of performing satisfactory work at various jobs; one study showed that only nine percent were partially dependent and four percent were incapable of holding a job. In some areas there may be restrictions on issuing driver's licenses to epileptics or other legal regulations that limit normal activities for epilepsy patients. As a result, some epileptics may conceal their condition or avoid medical treatment that might be reported to government agencies.

Because of ignorance and misinformation, some people regard epilepsy as frightening or mysterious, and patients may suffer unnecessarily and unjustly. In fact, behavioral abnormalities in patients with seizures are commonly the reflection of how they are viewed by others. The patient should be carefully observed by an understanding physician who watches not only for medical but for psychological problems.

When epilepsy has been diagnosed in a child, the parents must be instructed about the condition and the need for continuous careful medical supervision. If the child is old enough to understand, he also should learn more about the nature of the condition. Misbeliefs should be corrected. Both parents and child should understand that seizures are not likely to be fatal and that a brain lesion does not lead to mental deterioration. Parents and child should learn what actions should be taken in the event of a seizure, such as loosening clothing and taking steps to prevent injury. Natural concern should be balanced with an understanding that overprotection may itself become a handicap. The child should be encouraged to participate in social and physical activities at school and in the neighborhood as long as they do not strain his capabilities. Finally, parents should not feel guilty about the child's condition and think that some action of theirs contributed to the child's condition. See "Epileptic Seizures" in Ch. 31, *Medical Emergencies,* for a description of what to do when a seizure occurs.

Further information about epilepsy, including causes, effects, treatment, rehabilitation, and laws regulating employment and driver permits, can be obtained from the Epilepsy Foundation of America, 4351 Garden City Dr., Landover, MD 20785, and from the U.S. Department of Health, Education and Welfare, Public Health Service, National Institutes of Health, Bethesda, MD 20014.

Multiple Sclerosis

Multiple sclerosis is a disease involving the progressive destruction of myelin, the fatty material that covers the nerves of the body. The disease affects mainly the brain and spinal cord. It is termed *multiple* because there are distinct and separate areas of the nervous system involved, seemingly distributed in a random pattern.

Incidence

The incidence of multiple sclerosis is puzzling. It occurs most frequently in the temperate geographic areas of the world; the high-risk regions generally are between 40 and 60 degrees of latitude on either side of the equator, where the incidence is about 40 cases per 100,000 population. Within the high-risk latitudes, however, there are countries in Asia where the disease is relatively rare, and in the Shetland and Orkney Islands to the north of Scotland the incidence of the disease is approximately five times that in the United States, Canada, and Northern Europe. Multiple sclerosis has never been found in certain black populations in Africa, but black persons living in the United States develop the disorder at about the same rate as white persons.

Multiple sclerosis rarely appears before the age of 15 or after 55. A person aged 30 years is statistically at peak risk of developing the disease. The typical patient, statistically speaking, is a woman of 45 who was born and raised in a temperate climate. Women are more susceptible to the disease than men by a ratio of 1.7 to 1, and women are more likely than men to experience the onset of symptoms before the age of 30.

Symptoms and Diagnosis

There are no laboratory tests that are specific for multiple sclerosis, although there are certain tests that may suggest the presence of the disease. Diagnosing the disorder depends to a large extent upon tests that rule out other diseases with similar signs and symptoms. The first symptom may be a transitory blurring of vision or a disturbance in one or more of the limbs, such as numbness, a tingling sensation, clumsiness, or weakness. There may be a partial or total loss of vision in one eye for a period of several days, sometimes with pain in moving the eye, or the patient may experience double vision or dizziness. In some cases, the patient may develop either a lack of sensation over an area of the face or, paradoxically, a severe twitching pain of the face muscles. In more advanced cases, because of involvement of the spinal cord, the patient may have symptoms of bladder or bowel dysfunction and male patients may experience impotence.

When brain tissues become invaded by multiple sclerosis, the patient may suffer loss of memory and show signs of personality changes, displaying euphoria, cheerfulness, irritability, or depression for no apparent reason.

Multiple sclerosis is marked by periods of remission and recurrence of symptoms. Complete recovery can occur. About 20 percent of the patients may have to spend time confined to bed or wheelchair. In severe cases, there can be complications such as infections of the urinary tract and respiratory system.

Treatment

There is no known cure for multiple sclerosis, and treatment techniques generally are aimed at relieving symptoms, shortening the periods of exacerbation, and preventing complications that can be crippling or life-threatening. Most patients experience recurrences of symptoms that last for limited periods of days or weeks followed in cycles by periods of remission that may last for months or years, making it difficult to determine whether the therapy applied is actually effective or if the disease is merely following its natural fluctuating course. Because multiple sclerosis appears to be a disease that affects only humans, medical scientists are unable to use animals in experiments to develop effective remedies.

Among several types of medications now used are anti-inflammatory drugs such as adrenocorticotrophin (ACTH), a hormone that seems to reduce the severity and duration of recurrences. Cortisone and prednisone, two steroid hormones, also can be used and have an advantage over ACTH in that they can be taken by mouth rather than intramuscular injection. But not all patients react favorably to steroid drugs and serious side effects may be experienced. Several immunosuppressive drugs ordinarily used in the treatment of cancer and after organ transplants have been employed but they can be administered only in small doses for limited periods of time without undesirable side effects. Other therapies tested with varying effectiveness include vitamins and special diets.

Physical therapy and antispasmodic medications may be employed for patients suffering weakness or paralysis of the limbs. Bed rest during periods of exacerbation is important; continued activity seems to worsen the severity and duration of symptoms during those periods. Muscle relaxants and tranquilizers may be prescribed in some serious cases and braces could be required for patients who lose some limb functions.

Because of the lower incidence of multiple sclerosis in warmer climates, patients may be led to believe that moving to a "sunshine" state can have curative effects. But experience indicates that once the disease becomes established a change of climate does not change the course of the disorder. Living in a warmer winter climate, however, can lessen the impact of the physical handicaps faced by a multiple sclerosis patient.

Causes

The cause of multiple sclerosis has not been established. Multiple cases of the disease have been reported in only a small percentage of families but they occur often enough to suggest that the risk in brothers and sisters of patients is several times greater than the risk among the population at large. It is possible that patients with multiple sclerosis have inherited a specific susceptibility to the disease, a factor that could explain the vulnerability of members of the same family to acquire the disorder through one of several environmental causes, such as a virus or other infectious organism. Speculation about causes has covered dietary deficiencies, ingestion or inhalation of toxic substances,

and occupation.

A theory that researchers consider promising suggests that a virus similar but not identical to HTLV-I (human T-cell leukemia virus-I) may cause multiple sclerosis. HTLV-I causes an unusual form of leukemia. Some T-cells, a type of white blood cell, have been found to contain genetic material from this virus. These T-cells were taken from the cerebrospinal fluid of multiple sclerosis victims, establishing a possible link between the cells and the virus.

Infections of the Nervous System

Like any other organ system, the brain and its associated structures may be host to infection. These infections are usually serious because of the significantly high death rate and incidence of residual defects. If the brain is involved in the inflammation, it is known as *encephalitis;* inflammation of the brain coverings, or *meninges,* is called *meningitis.*

Encephalitis

Encephalitis is usually caused by a virus, and, because the symptoms are not specific, the diagnosis is usually made by special viral immunologic tests. Both sexes and all age groups can be afflicted. Most patients complain of fever, headache, nausea or vomiting, and a general feeling of malaise. The mental state varies from one of mild irritability to lethargy or coma, and some patients may have convulsions. The physician may suspect encephalitis after completing the history and the physical examination, but the diagnosis is usually established by laboratory tests that include examination of the cerebrospinal fluid (CSF), the EEG, and viral studies of the blood, CSF, and stool. Because there is no specific treatment for viral

encephalitis at the present time, particular attention is paid to general supportive care.

Meningitis

Meningitis can occur in either sex at any time of life. The patient often has a preceding mild respiratory infection and later complains of headache, nausea, and vomiting. Fever and neck stiffness are usually present early in the course of the disease, at which time the patient is commonly brought to the physician for examination. If there is any question of meningitis, a lumbar puncture is performed and the CSF examined. It is not possible to make a specific diagnosis of meningitis without examination of the cerebrospinal fluid.

Meningitis is usually caused by bacteria or a virus. It is important to learn what the infectious agent is in order to begin appropriate therapy. Bacterial infections can be treated by antibiotics, but there is no known specific treatment for viral (*aseptic*) meningitis. Meningitis is a life-threatening disease and, despite modern antibiotic therapy, the mortality rate varies from 10 to 20 percent.

Poliomyelitis

Poliomyelitis is an acute viral illness affecting males and females at any time of life, though most commonly before the age of ten. It is also called *polio, infantile paralysis,* or *Heine-Medin disease.*

Polio is caused by a virus that probably moves from the gastrointestinal tract via nerve trunks to the central nervous system, where it may affect any part of the nervous system. The disease, however, most often involves the larger motor neurons (*anterior horn cells*) in the brain stem and spinal cord, with subsequent loss of nerve supply to the muscle. The neuron may be partially or completely damaged; clinical recovery is, therefore, dependent on whether those partially damaged nerves can regain normal function.

There are two categories of polio victims: asymptomatic and symptomatic. Those persons who have had no observed symptoms of the disease, but in whom antibodies to polio can be demonstrated, belong in the *asymptomatic* group. The *symptomatic* group, on the other hand, comprises patients who have the clinical disease, either with residual paralysis (paralytic polio) or without paralysis (nonparalytic polio).

Symptoms

The symptoms of poliomyelitis are similar to those of other acute infectious processes. The patient may complain of headache, fever, or *coryza* (head cold or runny nose), or he may have loose stools and malaise. One-fourth to one-third of patients improve for several days only to have a recurrence of fever with neck stiffness. Most patients, however, do not improve, but rather have a progression of their symptoms, marked by neck stiffness and aching muscles. They are often irritable and apprehensive, and some are rather lethargic.

Whether or not the patient will have muscle paralysis should be evident in the first few weeks. Some have muscle paralysis with the onset of symptoms; others become aware of loss of muscle function several weeks after the onset. About half of the patients first notice paralysis during the second to the fifth day of the disease. Patients experience a muscle spasm or stiffness, and may complain of muscle pain, particularly if the muscle is stretched.

The extent of the muscle paralysis is variable, ranging from mild localized weakness to inability to move most of the skeletal muscles. Proximal muscles (those close to the trunk, like the shoulder-arm or hip-thigh) are involved more often than distal muscles (of the extremeties), and the legs are affected more often than the arms. When the neurons of the lower brain stem and the spinal cord at the thoracic level and above are affected, the patient may have a paralysis of the muscles used in swallowing and breathing. This circumstance, obviously, is life-threatening, and particular attention must be paid to the patient's ability to handle saliva and to breathe. If independent, spontaneous respiration is not possible, patients must be given respiratory assistance with mechanical respirators.

Treatment

There is no specific treatment for acute poliomyelitis. The patient should be kept at complete bed rest and given general supportive care, assuring adequate nutrition and fluid intake. Muscle spasm has been treated with hot as well as cold compresses, and no one method has been universally beneficial. Careful positioning of the patient with the musculature supported in a position midway between relaxation and contraction is probably of benefit, and skilled physical therapy is of great importance.

Immunization

Since the early 1900s, attempts had been made to produce an effective vaccine against poliomyelitis, with success crowning the efforts of Dr. Jonas Salk in 1953. Today, vaccination is accomplished with either the Salk vaccine (killed virus), which is given intramuscularly, or the Sabin (live attenuated virus), given orally. There is little question that immunization with poliomyelitis vaccine has proven to be highly effective in eradicating the clinical disease within the community, and it is now a part of routine immunization for all children.

Dementia

Dementia is a term for mental deterioration, with particular regard to memory and thought processes. Such deterioration can be brought about in various ways: infection, brain injury, such toxic states as alcoholism, brain tumors, cerebral arteriosclerosis, and so forth.

The presenile dementias (*Alzheimer's disease*) represent a group of degenerative diseases of the brain in which mental deterioration first becomes apparent in middle age. Commonly, the first clue may be demonstrations of unusual unreasonableness and impairment of judgment. The patient can no longer grasp the content of a situation at hand and reacts inappropriately. Memory gradually fades and recent events are no longer remembered, but events that occurred early in life can be recalled. The patient may wander aimlessly or get lost in his own house. There is progressive deterioration of physical appearance and personal hygiene, and, finally, the command of language deteriorates. Unfortunately, there is a relentless progression of the process, and the patient becomes confined to bed and quite helpless.

Whether the mental deterioration seen in some aged patients, senile dementia, is a specific brain degeneration or is secondary to cerebral arteriosclerosis is not yet settled. It does appear, however, that senile dementia is probably secondary to a degenerative process similar to that of Alzheimer's disease but occurring late in life.

Whether or not dementia can be halted depends upon its cause. If, for example, the dementia is secondary to brain infection or exposure to toxic material, eradication of the infectious agent or removal of the toxin may be of distinct benefit in arresting the dementing process. Unfortunately, there is no specific treatment for the brain degenerative processes.

Muscle Diseases

When one hears the words "muscle disease," one may think of only muscular dystrophy and picture a small child confined to a wheelchair. But there are many diseases other than muscular dystrophy in which muscle is either primarily or secondarily involved, and many of these diseases do not have a particularly bad prognosis. Muscle diseases may make their presence known at any time, from early infancy to old age; no age group or sex is exempt.

Any disease of muscle is called a *myopathy*. The hallmark of muscle disease is weakness, or loss of muscle power. This may be recognized in the infant who seems unusually limp or *hypotonic*. Often the first clue to the presence of muscle weakness is a child's failure to achieve the developmental milestones within a normal range of time. He may be unusually clumsy or have difficulty in running, climbing stairs, or even walking. Occasionally a teacher is the first one to be aware that the child cannot keep up with classmates and reports this fact to the parents. The onset of the muscle weakness can be so insidious that it may go unnoticed or be misinterpreted as laziness until there is an obvious and striking loss of muscle power.

This is true in the adult as well who at first may feel tired or worn out and then realize that he cannot keep up

his previous pace. Often his feet and legs are involved in the beginning. He may wear out the toes of his shoes and may then recognize that he must flex his ankles more to avoid tripping or dragging the toes. Or he finds that he must make a conscious effort to raise the legs in climbing stairs; he may even have to climb one step at a time. Getting out of bed in the morning may be a chore, and rising from a seated position in a low chair or from the floor may be difficult or impossible. Those with arm involvement may recognize that the hands are weak; if the shoulder muscles are involved, there is often difficulty in raising the arms over the head. The patient may

take a long time in recognizing the loss of muscle power because the human body can so well compensate or use other muscles to perform the same motor tasks. If the weakness is present for a considerable length of time, there may be a wasting, or a loss of muscle bulk.

Diagnostic Evaluation of Muscle Disease

In evaluating patients with motor weakness, the physician must have a complete history of the present complaints, past history of the patient, and details of the family history. A general physical and neurological examination is required, with particular

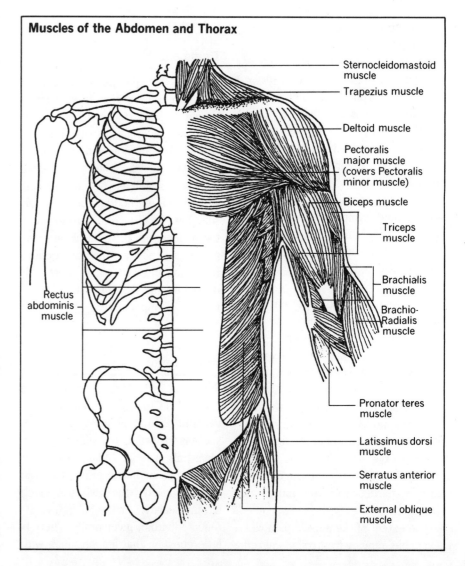

Muscles of the Abdomen and Thorax

Sternocleidomastoid muscle

Trapezius muscle

Deltoid muscle

Pectoralis major muscle (covers Pectoralis minor muscle)

Biceps muscle

Triceps muscle

Brachialis muscle

Brachio-Radialis muscle

Pronator teres muscle

Latissimus dorsi muscle

Serratus anterior muscle

External oblique muscle

Rectus abdominis muscle

reference to the motor, or musculo-skeletal system. In most cases, the physician will be able to make a clinical diagnosis of the disease process, but occasionally the examination does not reveal whether the nerve, the muscle, or both are involved. In order to clarify the diagnosis, some additional examinations may be required, mainly determination of serum enzymes (a good indicator of loss of muscle substance), a muscle biopsy, and an electromyogram.

Serum Enzymes

Enzymes are essential for the maintenance of normal body chemistry.

Because the normal concentration in the blood serum of some enzymes specifically related to muscle chemistry is known, the determination of concentrations of these enzymes can provide additional evidence that muscle chemistry is either normal or abnormal.

Muscle Biopsy

The first step is the surgical removal of a small segment of muscle, which is then prepared for examination under the microscope. The examination enables the physician to see any abnormality in the muscle fibers, supporting tissue, small nerve twigs, and

blood vessels. The muscle biopsy can be of great value in making a correct diagnosis, but occasionally, even in good hands, there is not sufficient visible change from the normal state to identify the disease process.

Electromyograph (EMG)

This is a technique for studying electrical activity of muscle. Fine needles attached to electronic equipment are inserted into the muscle to measure the electrical activity, which is displayed on an *oscilloscope,* a device something like a television screen. It is not a particularly painful process when performed by a skilled physician, and the information gained may be important in establishing a diagnosis.

Muscular Dystrophy

Muscular dystrophy (MD) is defined as an inborn degenerative disease of the muscles. Several varieties of MD have been described and classified according to the muscles involved and the pattern of inheritance. There is no specific treatment for any form of MD, but the patient's life can be made more pleasant and probably prolonged if careful attention is paid to good nutrition, activity without overfatigue, and avoidance of infection. Physical therapists can be helpful in instructing the patient or the parents in an exercise program that relieves joint and muscle stiffness. Sound, prudent psychological support and guidance cannot be overemphasized.

Duchenne's Muscular Dystrophy

In 1886, Dr. Guillaume Duchenne described a muscle disease characterized by weakness and an increase in the size of the muscles and the supporting connective tissue of those

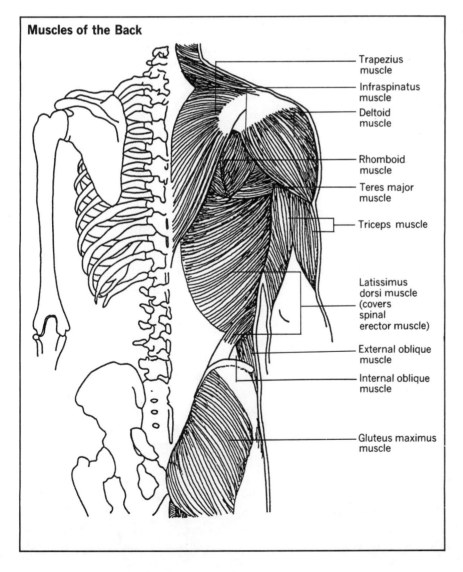

Muscles of the Back

- Trapezius muscle
- Infraspinatus muscle
- Deltoid muscle
- Rhomboid muscle
- Teres major muscle
- Triceps muscle
- Latissimus dorsi muscle (covers spinal erector muscle)
- External oblique muscle
- Internal oblique muscle
- Gluteus maximus muscle

muscles. He named the disease *pseudohypertrophic* (false enlargement) *muscular paralysis,* but it is now known as *Duchenne's muscular dystrophy.*

Duchenne's MD is observed almost entirely in males. It is inherited, however, like many other sex-linked anomalies, through the maternal side of the family. The mother can pass the clinical disease to her son; her daughters will not demonstrate the disease but are potential carriers to their sons. More than one-quarter of the cases of Duchenne's MD are sporadic, that is, without any known family history of the disease. There are rare cases of Duchenne's MD in females who have *ovarian dysgenesis,* a condition in which normal female chromosomal makeup is lacking.

The disease process in Duchenne's MD may be apparent during the first few years of life when the child has difficulty in walking or appears clumsy. The muscles of the pelvis and legs are usually affected first, but the shoulders and the arms soon become involved. About 90 percent of the patients have some enlargement of a muscle or group of muscles and appear to be rather muscular and strong; however, as the disease progresses, the muscular enlargement disappears. Most patients progressively deteriorate and at the age of about 10 to 15 are unable to walk. Once the child is confined to a wheelchair or bed, there is a progressive deformity with muscle contracture, with death usually occurring toward the end of the second decade. A small percentage of patients appear to have a remission of the disease process and survive until the fourth or fifth decade. Despite herculean attempts to unravel the riddle of muscular dystrophy, the problem is yet unsolved.

A benign variety of MD, *Becker type,* begins at 5 to 25 years of age and progresses slowly. Most of the reported patients with Becker type are still able to walk 20 to 30 years after the onset of the disease.

Facio-Scapulo-Humoral Muscular Dystrophy

This type of muscular dystrophy affects males and females equally and is thought to be inherited as a dominant trait. The onset may be at any age from childhood to adult life, but is commonly first seen in adolescence. There is not false enlargement of the muscles. The muscles affected, as indicated by the name of the disease, are those of the face and shoulders, usually with abnormal winging of the *scapula* (either of the large, flat bones at the backs of the shoulders). There is also a characteristic appearance of lip prominence, as if the patient were pouting. Occasionally there is an involvement of the anterior leg muscles and weakness in raising the foot. The disease progresses more slowly than Duchenne's type, and some patients can remain active for a normal life span.

Limb-Girdle Muscular Dystrophy

This type of muscular dystrophy is less clearly delineated than the others. Males and females are equally affected and the onset is usually in the second or third decade, but the process may start later. It is probably inherited as a recessive trait, but many cases are sporadic. It may first affect the muscles of the pelvis or the shoulder, but in 10 to 15 years both pelvis and shoulder girdles are usually involved. The disease varies considerably from patient to patient; sometimes the disease process appears to be arrested after involvement of either the pelvis or the shoulder, and the course thereafter may be a benign one. Most, however, have significant difficulty in walking by middle age.

Other Varieties of Muscular Dystrophy

These include ocular, oculopharyngeal, and a distal form (involving the muscles of the hands or feet).

Ocular MD

This type involves the muscles that move the eye as well as the eyelids; occasionally, the small muscles of the face and the shoulder girdle are affected.

Oculopharyngeal MD

This type involves not only the muscles that move the eye and the eyelids but may also affect the throat muscles, so that patients have difficulty in swallowing food (*dysphagia*).

Distal MD

This type is rare in the United States but has been reported in Scandinavia. Both sexes can be affected. Usually after the fifth decade, the patient recognizes weakness of the small muscles of the hands and anterior leg muscles that assist in raising the toes. The disease is relatively benign and progresses slowly.

The Myotonias

This is a group of muscle diseases characterized by *myotonia,* a continuation of muscle contraction after the patient has voluntarily tried to relax that contraction. It is best observed in the patient who holds an object firmly in his hand and then tries to release his grasp suddenly, only to realize that he cannot let go quickly. There are two major members of this group of diseases and several other less common variants.

Treatment

As in the case of muscular dystrophy, there is no specific treatment for myotonia. Some drugs, such as quinine, have limited value in decreasing the abnormally prolonged muscular contractions, but as yet no treatment has been completely effective.

Myotonia Congenita

This condition is usually present at birth, but is recognized later in the first or second decade of life when the child complains of stiffness or when clumsiness is noted. A child with this condition appears very muscular and has been called the "infant Hercules." The unusual muscular development persists throughout life, but the myotonia tends to improve with age.

Myotonic Dystrophy

The other major variety of myotonia, *myotonic dystrophy,* is a disease in which many organ systems in addition to muscle are involved. Both males and females are affected equally, and the onset may occur at any time from birth to the fifth decade. It is not unusual for a patient to recognize some clumsiness, but he may not be aware that he has a muscle disease. The myotonia may range from mild to severe. There is a striking similarity in the physical appearance of patients with myotonic dystrophy, the features of which include frontal baldness in the male, wasting and weakness of the temporal muscles (that control closing the jaws), muscles of the forearm, hands, and anterior leg muscles. Other physical abnormalities include cataracts in about 90 percent of the patients, small testicles, and abnormality of the heart muscle. Thickening and other bony abnormalities have been seen in the skull radiogram and, with time, many patients become demented.

Polymyositis

Polymyositis is a disorder of muscular and connective tissues affecting both sexes, males more commonly than females. It can occur at any age, although usually after the fourth decade. It is characterized by muscle weakness with associated muscle wasting; about half of the patients complain of muscle pain or tenderness. The disease may begin suddenly, but often follows an earlier mild, febrile illness. Changes in the skin are common, including a faint red-violet discoloration, particularly about the eyelids, and these changes are often associated with mild swelling. There may be a scaly rash. Some patients have ulcerations over the bony prominences. About one-quarter of the patients with polymyositis complain of joint stiffness and tenderness and an unusual phenomenon in which the nail beds become blue (*cyanotic*) after minor exposure to cold.

Treatment

The treatment involves the administration of cortisone preparations, which may be required for many years. General supportive care, including appropriate physical therapy, is recommended.

Myasthenia Gravis

Myasthenia gravis is characterized by muscle weakness and an abnormal muscle fatigability (pathologic fatigue); patients are abnormally weak after exercise or at the end of the day. The disease affects males and females at any period, from infancy to old age, but it is most common during the second to the fourth decades. There is no complete explanation for myasthenia gravis, but it is believed that there is some defect in the transmission of a nerve impulse to the muscle (*myoneural junction defect*). The disease may occur spontaneously, during pregnancy, or following an acute infection, and there appears to be a curious association with diseases in which there is an immunologic abnormality, such as tumors of the thymus gland, increased or decreased activity of the thyroid gland, and rheumatoid arthritis.

Usually there is an insidious onset of generalized weakness or weakness confined to small groups of muscles. Normal muscle power may be present early in the day, but as the hours pass the patient notices that one or both eyelids droop (*ptosis*) or he may see double images (*diplopia*). If he rests and closes his eyes for a short time, the ptosis and the diplopia clear up, only to return after further muscle activity. The weakness can also be seen in the trunk or the limbs, and some patients have involvement of the muscles used in speaking, chewing, or swallowing (*bulbar* muscles). Some are weak all the time and have an increase in that weakness the longer they use their muscles. The muscles used in breathing may be affected in patients with severe myasthenia, and these patients must be maintained on a respirator for varying periods of time.

Treatment

Myasthenia gravis is treated with drugs that assist in the transmission of the nerve impulse to the muscle. Medication is very effective, but the patient should be carefully observed by the physician to determine that the drug dose and the time of administration are adjusted so that the patient may have the benefit of maximal muscle power. Surgical removal of the thymus gland, *thymectomy,* may prove of benefit to some patients in lessening the symptoms of muscle weakness; however, not all patients have clinical improvement of the disease after thymectomy, and patients must be selected very carefully by the physician. Myasthenia gravis is another chronic disease in which long-term careful observation by the physician is most important in obtaining an optimal medical and psychological outcome.

9

Diseases of the Circulatory System

It's called the river of life, the five or six quarts of blood that stream through the 60,000 tortuous miles of arteries, veins, and capillaries.

Blood contains many elements with specific functions—red cells to transport oxygen from the lungs to body tissues, white cells to fight off disease, and tiny elements called *platelets* to help form clots and repair tears in the blood vessel wall. All float freely in an intricate complex of liquid proteins and metals known as *plasma*.

Because of the blood's extreme importance to life, any injury to it— or to the grand network of channels through which it flows—may have the most serious consequences. The troubles that beset the circulation may be grouped conveniently into two categories: diseases of the blood and diseases of the blood vessels.

Diseases of the Blood

Diseases of the blood include disorders that affect the blood elements directly (as in the case of *hemophilia*, where a deficiency in clotting proteins

is at fault) as well as abnormalities in the various organs involved in maintaining proper blood balance (i.e., spleen, liver and bone marrow). The various ills designated and described below are arranged according to the blood component most affected (i.e., clotting proteins, red blood cells, and white blood cells).

Hemorrhagic or Clotting-Deficiency Diseases

The blood has the ability to change from a fluid to a solid and back to a fluid again. The change to a solid is called *clotting*. There are mechanisms not only for sealing off breaks in the circulatory system when serious blood loss is threatened, but also for breaking down the seals, or clots, once the damage has been repaired and the danger of blood loss is eliminated. Both mechanisms are in continuous, dynamic equilibrium, a delicate balance between tissue repair and clot dissolution to keep us from bleeding or literally clogging to death.

Clotting involves a very complex chain of chemical events. The key is the conversion of an inactive blood protein, *fibrinogen,* into a threadlike

sealant known as *fibrin*. Stimulus for this conversion is an enzyme called *thrombin,* which normally also circulates in an inactive state as *prothrombin* (formed from vitamin K in the daily diet).

For a clot to form, however, inactive prothrombin must undergo a chemical transformation into thrombin, a step requiring still another chemical—*thromboplastin*. This agent comes into play only when a tissue or vessel has been injured so as to require clot protection. There are two ways for thromboplastin to enter the bloodstream to spark the chain of events. One involves the release by the injured tissue of a substance that reacts with plasma proteins to produce thromboplastin. The other requires the presence of blood platelets (small particles that travel in the blood) and several plasma proteins, including the so-called antihemophilic factor. Platelets tend to clump at the site of vessel injury, where they disintegrate and ultimately release thromboplastin, which, in the presence of blood calcium, triggers the prothrombin-thrombin conversion.

The clot-destroying sequence is very similar to that involved in clot formation, with the key enzyme, *fi-*

brinolysin, existing normally in an inactive state (*profibrinolysin*). There are also other agents (e.g., *heparin*) in the blood ready to retard or prevent the clotting sequence, so that it does not spread to other parts of the body.

Naturally, grave dangers arise should these complex mechanisms fail. For the moment, we shall concern ourselves with hemorrhagic disorders arising from a failure of the blood to clot properly. Disorders stemming from excessive clotting are discussed below under "Diseases of the Blood Vessels" because they are likely to happen as a consequence of preexisting problems in the vessel walls.

Hemophilia

Hemophilia is probably the best known (although relatively rare) of the hemorrhagic disorders, because of its prevalence among the royal families of Europe. In hemophilia the blood does not clot properly and bleeding persists. Those who have this condition are called *hemophiliacs* or bleeders. The disease is inherited, and is transmitted by the mother, but except in very rare cases only the male offspring are affected. Hemophilia stems from a lack of one of the plasma proteins associated with clotting, *antihemophilic factor* (*AHF*).

The presence of hemophilia is generally discovered during early childhood. It is readily recognized by the fact that even small wounds bleed profusely and can trigger an emergency. Laboratory tests for clotting speed are used to confirm the diagnosis. Further investigation may occasionally turn up the condition in other members of the family.

In advanced stages, hemophilia may lead to anemia as a result of excessive and continuous blood loss. Bleeding in the joints causes painful

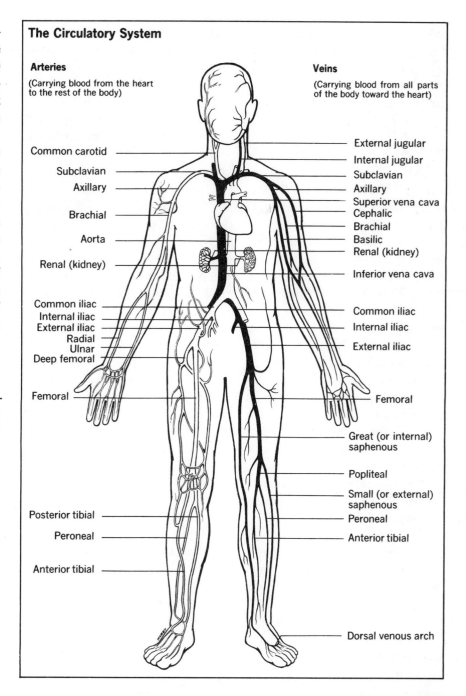

The Circulatory System

Arteries
(Carrying blood from the heart to the rest of the body)

Common carotid
Subclavian
Axillary
Brachial
Aorta
Renal (kidney)
Common iliac
Internal iliac
External iliac
Radial
Ulnar
Deep femoral
Femoral
Posterior tibial
Peroneal
Anterior tibial

Veins
(Carrying blood from all parts of the body toward the heart)

External jugular
Internal jugular
Subclavian
Axillary
Superior vena cava
Cephalic
Brachial
Basilic
Renal (kidney)
Inferior vena cava
Common iliac
Internal iliac
External iliac
Femoral
Great (or internal) saphenous
Popliteal
Small (or external) saphenous
Peroneal
Anterior tibial
Dorsal venous arch

swelling, which over a long period of time can lead to permanent deformity and hemophilic arthritis. Hemophiliacs must be under constant medical care in order to receive quick treatment in case of emergencies.

Treating bleeding episodes may involve the administration of AHF alone so as to speed up the clotting sequence. If too much blood is lost a complete transfusion may be necessary. Thanks to modern blood bank techniques, large quantities of whole blood can be made readily available. Bed rest and hospitalization may also be required. For bleeding in the joints, an ice pack is usually applied.

Proper dental hygiene is a must for all hemophiliacs. Every effort should be made to prevent tooth decay. Parents of children with the disease should inform the dentist so that all necessary precautions can be taken. Even the most common procedures, such as an extraction, can pose a serious hazard. Only absolutely essential surgery should be performed on hemophiliacs, with the assurance that large amounts of plasma are on hand.

Purpura

Purpura refers to spontaneous hemorrhaging over large areas of the skin and in mucous membranes. It results from a deficiency in blood platelets, elements essential to clotting. Purpura is usually triggered by other conditions: certain anemias, leukemia, sensitivity to drugs, or exposure to ionizing radiation. In newborns it may be linked to the prenatal transfer from the maternal circulation of substances that depress platelet levels. Symptoms of purpura include the presence of blood in the urine, bleeding from the mucous membranes of the mouth, nose, intestines, and uterus. Some forms of the disease cause arthritic changes in joints, abdominal pains, diarrhea and vomiting—and even gangrene of the skin, when certain infectious organisms become involved.

To treat purpura in newborns, physicians may exchange the infant's blood with platelet-packed blood. Sometimes drug therapy with *steroids* (i.e., cortisone) is prescribed. In adults with chronic purpura it may be necessary to remove the spleen, which plays an important role in eliminating worn-out blood components, including platelets, from the circulation. Most physicians prescribe large doses of steroids coupled with blood transfusions. Purpura associated with infection and gangrene also requires appropriate antibiotic therapy.

Red Cell Diseases

Half the blood is plasma; the other half is made up of many tiny blood cells. The biggest group in number is the red blood cells. These cells contain a complicated chemical called *hemoglobin*, which brings oxygen from the lungs to body cells and picks up waste carbon dioxide for expiration. Hemoglobin is rich in iron, which is what imparts the characteristic red color to blood.

Red blood cells are manufactured by bones all over the body—in the sternum, ribs, skull, arms, spine and pelvis. The actual factory is the red bone marrow, located at bone ends. As red cells mature and are ready to enter the bloodstream, they lose their nuclei to become what are called *red corpuscles* or *erythrocytes*. With no nucleus, a red corpuscle is relatively short-lived (120 days). Thus, the red cell supply must be constantly replenished by bone marrow. And a busy factory it is because 20 to 25 trillion red corpuscles normally travel in the circulation. The spleen is responsible for ridding the body of the aged corpuscles, but it is not an indiscriminate sanitizer; it salvages the hemoglobin for reuse by the body.

To measure levels of red cells, physicians make a blood count by taking a smidgen of blood from a patient's fingertip. The average number of red cells in healthy blood is about five million per cubic millimeter for men, and four and one-half million for women.

Anemia

Anemia exists when the red cell count stays persistently below four million. Abnormalities in the size, shape, or hemoglobin content of the erythrocytes may also account for anemic states. Any such irregularity interferes with the red cell's ability to carry its full share of oxygen to body tissues. It also tends to weaken the red cells so that they are more likely to be destroyed under the stresses of the circulation.

Anemia may result from:

- nutritional deficiencies that deprive the body of elements vital to the production of healthy cells

- diseases or injuries to organs associated with either blood cell formation (bone marrow) or blood cell destruction (spleen and liver)

- excessive loss of blood, the consequences of surgery, hemorrhage, or a bleeding ulcer and

- Heredity, as in the case of *sickle cell anemia* (where the red cells are misshapen)

Hemolytic Anemia

There are also several kinds of disorders known as *hemolytic anemias* that are linked to the direct destruction of red cells. Poisons such as snake venom, arsenic, and lead can cause hemolytic anemia. So can toxins produced by certain bacteria as well as by other organisms, such as the parasites that cause malaria, hookworm, and tapeworm. Destruction of red cells may also stem from allergic reactions to certain drugs or transfusions with incompatible blood.

The various anemias range from ailments mild enough to go undetected to disorders that prove inevitably fatal. Many are rare; following are the more common.

Pernicious Anemia

Pernicious anemia, or *Addison's anemia,* is associated with a lack of hydrochloric acid in the gastric juices, a defect which interferes with the body's ability to absorb vitamin B_{12} from the intestine. Because the vitamin acts as an essential stimulus to the production of mature red blood cells by the bone marrow, its lack leads to a reduced output. Moreover, the cells tend to be larger than normal, with only half the lifespan of the normal erythrocyte.

The symptoms are characteristic of most anemias: pale complexion, numbness or a feeling of "pins and needles" in the arms and legs, shortness of breath (from a lack of oxygen), loss of appetite, nausea, and diarrhea (often accompanied by significant weight loss). One specific feature is a sore mouth with a smooth, glazed tongue. Advanced stages of the disease may be marked by an unsteady gait and other nervous disorders, owing to degeneration of the spinal cord. Red cell count may drop to as low as 1,000,000. Several kinds of tests may be necessary to differentiate pernicious anemia from other blood diseases—a test for hydrochloric acid levels, for example.

Pernicious anemia, however, is no longer so pernicious, or deadly, as it once was—not since its cause was identified. Large, injected doses of vitamin B_{12} usually restore normal blood cell production.

Sickle-Cell Anemia

Sickle-cell anemia, an inherited abnormality, occurs almost exclusively among black people. Widespread in tropical Africa and Asia, sickle-cell anemia is also found in this country, affecting perhaps 1 in 500 American blacks. The blood cells are sickle-shaped rather than round, a structural aberration arising from a defect in the manufacture of hemoglobin, the oxygen-carrying component. Such misshapen cells have a tendency to clog very small capillaries and cause the complications discussed below.

A differentiation should be made between sickle-cell anemia, the full-blown disease, and sickle-cell trait. Anemia occurs when the offspring inherits the sickle-cell gene from both

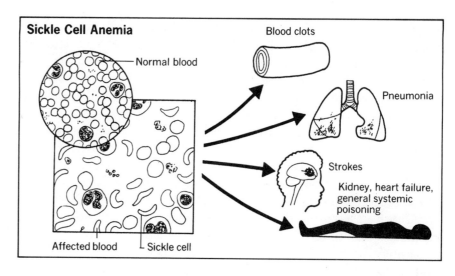

Sickle Cell Anemia

Normal blood

Affected blood — Sickle cell

Blood clots

Pneumonia

Strokes

Kidney, heart failure, general systemic poisoning

parents. For these people life stretches out in endless bouts of fatigue punctuated by a series of crises of excruciating pain lasting days or even weeks. In some cases there is permanent paralysis. The crises often require long-term hospitalization. The misshapen cells increase the patient's susceptibility to blood clots, pneumonia, kidney and heart failure, strokes, general systemic poisoning because of bacterial invasions, and, in the case of pregnant women, spontaneous abortion. Ninety percent of the patients die before age 40, with most dead by age 30. Half are dead by age 20, with a number also suffering from poor physical and mental development.

Those with only one gene for the disease have *sickle-cell trait*. They are not likely to have too much trouble except in circumstances where they are exposed to low oxygen levels (the result, say, of poor oxygenation in a high-altitude plane). Administration of anesthesia or too much physical activity may also bring on some feverish attacks. Those with the trait are also carriers of the disease because they can pass it on to the next generation. Two out of every 25 black Americans are said to be carrying the trait.

Iron-Deficiency Anemia

Iron-deficiency anemia is a common complication of pregnancy, during which time the fetus may rob the maternal blood of much of its iron content. Iron is essential to the formation of hemoglobin. The deficiency can be further aggravated by digestive disturbances (e.g., a lack of hydrochloric acid) that may hinder the absorption of dietary iron from the intestines. Some women may not observe proper dietary habits, thereby aggravating the anemic state. Successful treatment involves increasing iron intake, with iron supplements and an emphasis on iron-rich foods, including eggs, cereals, green vegetables, and meat, especially liver.

Polycythemia

Polycythemia is the opposite of anemia; the blood has too many red corpuscles. The most common form of the disease is *polycythemia vera* (or *erythremia*). In addition to the rise in corpuscle count, there is a corresponding rise—as much as threefold—in blood volume to accommodate the high cell count, and increased blood viscosity. Symptoms include an enlarged spleen, bloodshot eyes, red mouth, and red mucous membranes—all resulting from excess red cells. Other common characteristics are weakness, fatigue, irritability, dizziness, swelling in the ankles, choking sensations, vise-like chest pains (angina pectoris), rapid heartbeat, and sometimes severe headaches. There is also an increased tendency toward both clotting and hemorrhaging.

The disease occurs primarily in the middle and late years and is twice as prevalent in males as in females. The cause is unknown, but polycythemia is characterized by stepped-up bone marrow production activity.

Radioactive phosphorus therapy is one method for controlling this hyperactivity. Low iron diets and several forms of drug therapy have been tried with varying degrees of effectiveness. A one-time panacea, bloodletting—to drain off excess blood—appears to be of considerable value. Many patients survive for years with the disease. Premature death is usually the result of vascular thrombosis (clotting), massive hemorrhage, or leukemia.

The Rh Factor

Rh disease might also be considered a form of anemia—in newborns. The disorder involves destruction of the red blood cells of an as-yet unborn or newborn infant. It is brought about by an incompatibility between the maternal blood and fetal blood of one specific factor—the so-called Rh factor. (Rh stands for rhesus monkey, the species in which it was first identified.) Most of us are Rh positive, which is to say that we have the Rh protein substance on the surface of our red cells. The Rh factor is, in fact, present in 83 percent of the white population and 93 percent of the black. Those lacking it are classified as Rh negative.

A potentially dangerous situation exists when an Rh negative mother is carrying an Rh positive baby in her uterus. Although the mother and unborn baby have separate circulatory systems, some leakage does occur.

When Rh positive cells from the fetus leak across the placenta into the mother's blood, her system recognizes them as foreign and makes antibodies against them. If these antibodies then slip across into the fetal circulation, damage is inevitable.

The first baby, however, is rarely affected because it takes time for the mother's body to become sensitized to the Rh positive cells. But should she become pregnant with another child, the now-sensitized mother's blood produces a large quantity of destructive antibodies that could result in stillbirth, death of the infant shortly after birth or, if the child survives, jaundice and anemia.

Modern medicine has reduced the fatality rate and considerably improved the prognosis. Severely affected newborns are being treated by complete blood transfusion—even while still in the womb—to draw off all the Rh positive cells. After birth and as it grows older, the child will once again produce Rh positive cells in its bone marrow—but by that time the danger from the mother's antibodies is past. Recently an Rh vaccine to prevent the problem from ever occurring was developed. After Rh negative women give birth to their first Rh positive baby, they are immunized with the anti-Rh serum to prevent them from manufacturing these dangerous antibodies.

White Blood Cell Diseases

For every 600 to 700 or more red corpuscles, there is one white blood cell, or *leukocyte*. White cells, unlike red corpuscles, have nuclei; they are also larger and rounder. About 70 percent of the white cell population have irregularly-shaped centers, and these are called *polymorphonuclear leukocytes* or *neutrophils*. The other 30 percent are made up of a variety

of cells with round nuclei called *lymphocytes*. A cubic millimeter of blood normally contains anywhere from 5,000 to 9,000 white cells (as compared with the four to five million red cells).

White cells defend against disease, which explains why their number increases in the bloodstream when the body is under infectious assault. There are some diseases of the blood and blood-forming organs themselves that can increase the white count. Disorders of the spleen, for example, can produce white cell abnormalities, because this organ is a major source of lymphocytes (cells responsible for making protective antibodies). Diseases of the bone marrow are likely to affect neutrophil production.

Leukemia

Leukemia, characterized by an abnormal increase in the number of white cells, is one of the most dangerous of blood disorders. The cancerlike disease results from a severe disturbance in the functioning of the bone marrow. Chronic leukemia, which strikes mainly in middle age, produces an enormous increase in neutrophils, which tend to rush into the bloodstream at every stage of their development, whether mature or not. Patients with the chronic disease may survive for several years, with appropriate treatment.

In acute leukemia, more common among children than adults, the marrow produces monster-sized, cancerous-looking white cells. These cells not only crowd out other blood components from the circulation, they also leave little space for the marrow to produce the other elements, especially the red cells and platelets. Acute leukemias run their fatal course in a matter of weeks or months—although there have been dramatic instances of sudden remission. The cause is unknown, but recent evidence strongly suggests that a virus may be responsible for at least some forms of the disease.

Modern treatment—radiation and drugs—is aimed at wiping out all of the malignant cells. A critical stage follows treatment, however. For with the disappearance of these abnormal cells and the temporary disruption of marrow function, the patient is left with his defenses against infection down. He also runs a great risk of hemorrhage. Therefore, he is usually kept in isolation to ward off infections. In addition he may be given white cell and platelet transfusions along with antibiotic therapy. Eventually—and hopefully—the marrow will revert to normal function, freed of leukemic cell production. For additional information on leukemia, see Ch. 18, *Cancer.*

Other White Cell Diseases

Agranulocytosis

Agranulocytosis is a disease brought on by the direct destruction of neutrophils (also called *granulocytes*). Taken over a long period of time, certain types of drugs may bring about large-scale destruction of the neutrophil supply. Symptoms include general debilitation, fatigue, sleeplessness, restlessness, headache, chills, high fever (often up to 105° F.), sore mouth and throat, along with psychologically aberrant behavior and mental confusion. White cell count may fall as low as 500 to 2,000. Sometimes agranulocytosis is confused with leukemia.

Treatment involves antibiotic therapy to ward off bacterial invasion, a likelihood that is increased owing to the lowered body resistance. In advanced cases, hospitalization and transfusions with fresh blood are necessary. Injections of fresh bone marrow may also be prescribed.

Leukopenia

Leukopenia is less severe than agranulocytosis. It too involves a reduction of circulating white cells to counts of less than 5,000. It is usually the result of allergic reactions to some chemical or drug.

Infectious Mononucleosis

Infectious mononucleosis, also known as *glandular fever* or *kissing disease,* is characterized by the presence in the bloodstream of a large number of lymphocytes, many of which are abnormally formed. The disease is mildly contagious—kissing is thought to be one popular source of transmission—and occurs chiefly among children and adolescents. The transmitting agent, however, has yet to be discovered, though some as yet unidentified organism is strongly suspected.

The disease is not always easy to diagnose. It can incubate anywhere from four days to four weeks, at which point the patient may experience fever, headache, sore throat, swollen lymph nodes, loss of appetite, and a general feeling of weakness.

The disease runs its course in a matter of a week or two, although complete recovery may take a while longer. Bed rest and conservative medical management is often enough for complete patient recovery. A few severe cases may require hospitalization because of occasional complications, such as rupture of the spleen, skin lesions, some minor liver malfunctions, and occasionally hemolytic anemia or purpura.

Diseases of the Blood Vessels

Diseases of the blood vessels are the result primarily of adverse changes in the vessel walls, such as hardening of the arteries, stroke, and varicose veins.

A healthy circulation depends to a large extent not only on the condition of the blood-forming organs but on the pipelines through which this life-sustaining fluid flows. The arteries, which carry blood away from the heart, and the veins, which bring it back, are subject to a wide range of maladies. They may become inflamed, as in the case of arteritis, phlebitis, and varicose veins; or they may become clogged—especially the arteries—as a result of atherosclerosis (hardening of the arteries) or blood clots (thrombosis and embolism), which can prevent the blood from reaching a vital organ.

The Inflammatory Disorders

Arteritis

Arteritis, or inflammation of the arterial wall, usually results from infections (e.g., syphilis) or allergic reactions in which the body's protective agents against invading organisms, the antibodies, attack the vessel walls themselves. In these instances, the prime source of inflammation must be treated before the arterial condition can heal.

Phlebitis

Phlebitis is an inflammation of the veins, a condition that may stem from an injury or may be associated with such conditions as varicose veins, malignancies, and infection. The extremities, especially the legs, are vulnerable to the disorder. The symptoms are stiffness and hot and painful swelling of the involved region. Phlebitis brings with it the tendency of blood to form blood clots (*thrombophlebitis*)

Phlebitis

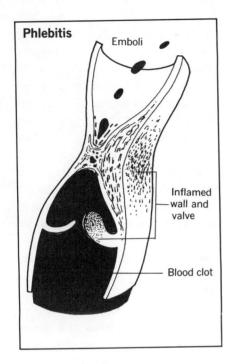

Emboli

Inflamed wall and valve

Blood clot

at the site of inflammation. The danger is that one of these clots may break away and enter the bloodstream. Such a clot, on the move, called an *embolus*, may catch and become lodged in a smaller vessel serving a vital organ, causing a serious blockage in the blood supply.

Physicians are likely to prescribe various drugs for phlebitis—agents to deal with the suspected cause of the disorder as well as *anticoagulants* (anticlotting compounds) to ward off possible thromboembolic complications.

Varicose Veins

Varicose veins, which are veins that are enlarged and distorted, primarily affect the leg vessels, and are often troublesome to people who are on their feet for hours at a time. Varicose veins develop because either the walls or the valves of veins are weakened. Some people may be born with weakened veins or valves. In others, the damage may develop from injury or disease, such as phlebitis. More women than men seem to have this condition, but it is common among both sexes. In women, the enlarged

veins sometimes occur during pregnancy, but these may well diminish and disappear after delivery. Some elderly people are prone to this condition because the blood vessels lose their elasticity with aging, with the muscles that support the vein growing less sturdy.

In most instances, the surface veins lying just beneath the skin are involved. If there are no other complications, these cases are seldom serious, although they may be disturbing because of unsightliness. Physicians have remedies, including surgery, for making varicose veins less prominent.

When varicose veins become severe, it is usually because the vessels deeper in the leg are weak. Unchecked, this situation can lead to serious complications, including swelling (*edema*) around the ankles and lower legs. The skin in the lower leg may beome thin and fragile and easily irritated. Tiny hemorrhages may discolor the skin. In advanced stages, hard-to-treat leg ulcers and sores may erupt.

Most of the complicating problems can be averted with early care and treatment. Physicians generally prescribe elastic stockings even in the mildest of cases and sometimes elastic bandages to lend support to the veins. They may recommend some newer techniques for injecting certain solutions that close off the affected portion of the vein. On the other hand, surgery may be indicated, especially for the surface veins, in which the varicose section is either tied off or stripped, with the blood being rerouted to the deeper vein channels. See under "Vascular Surgery" in Ch. 20, *Surgery,* for more information about surgical treatment of varicose veins.

While long periods of standing may be hard on varicose veins, so are uninterrupted stretches of sitting, which

may cause blood to collect in the lower leg and further distend the veins. Patients are advised to get up and walk about every half hour or so during any extended period of sitting. A good idea, too, is to sit with the feet raised, whenever possible, to keep blood from collecting in the lower legs.

The Vessel-Clogging Disorders

Atherosclerosis

Atherosclerosis (hardening of the arteries) is the nation's most serious health problem, the underlying cause of a million or more deaths each year from heart attack and stroke. It is the process whereby fats carried in the

Varicose Veins

Normal veins

Varicose veins

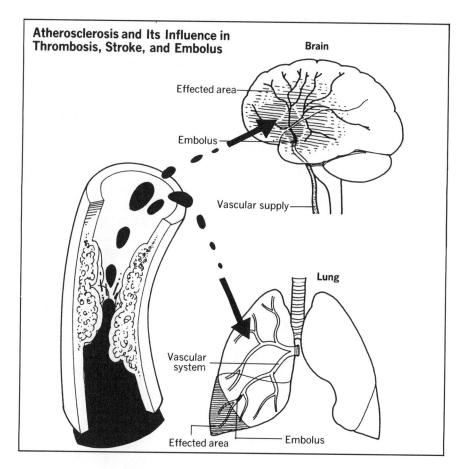

Atherosclerosis and Its Influence in Thrombosis, Stroke, and Embolus

Brain

Effected area

Embolus

Vascular supply

Lung

Vascular system

Effected area — Embolus

roughened wall surfaces, forming clots. If the clot blocks the coronary arteries, it may produce a heart attack—damage to that part of the heart deprived by vessel obstruction. For a detailed account of atherosclerosis and heart attack, see under Ch. 10 *Heart Disease.*

Stroke

Stroke, like heart attack, is a disorder usually resulting from blockage brought on by the atherosclerotic process in vessels supplying the brain. This sets the stage for a *thrombus,* or blood clot fixed within a vessel, which would not be likely to occur in arteries clear of these fatty deposits. A stroke may be a result of an interruption of blood flow through arteries in the brain or in the neck vessels leading to the brain.

Sometimes the shutoff of blood flow, or *embolism,* may be triggered by a wandering blood clot that has become wedged in cerebral vessels. This kind of clot, known as an *embolus,* is a thrombus that has broken free into the circulation.

A stroke may also stem from hemorrhaging, where a diseased artery in the brain bursts. A cerebral hemor-

bloodstream gradually pile up on the walls of arteries, like rust in a pipe. The vessels become brittle and roughened; the channel through which blood flows grows narrower. Eventually the organs and tissues supplied by the diseased arteries may be sufficiently deprived of their normal oxygen delivery so as to interfere with proper function. Such a cutback in the pipeline supply is called *ischemia.* This fat deposit poses its greatest hazard when it occurs in the vessels serving the heart, brain and, sometimes, the lower extremities.

A reduced supply of blood to the lower extremities may cause irreversible damage and ultimately lead to death of the leg tissues unless proper circulation is restored. Bacterial invasion may follow; the area may swell, blacken, and emit the distinctly offensive smell of the deadly infection. Such a condition is known as *gangrene,* a severe disorder that may

require amputation above the site of blockage if other measures, including antibiotic therapy, fail. Diabetics more commonly than others may develop atherosclerotic obstructions in leg arteries. Such persons must take care to avoid leg injuries, because even minimal damage in an already poorly served tissue area can bring on what is termed *diabetic gangrene.*

When the coronary arteries nourishing the heart are involved, even a moderate reduction in blood delivery to the heart muscle may be enough to cause angina pectoris, with its intense, suffocating chest pains.

Thrombosis

Thrombosis, a blood clot that forms within the vessels, is a great ever-present threat that accompanies atherosclerosis. The narrowed arteries seem to make it easier for normal blood substances to adhere to the

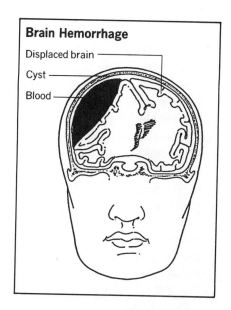

Brain Hemorrhage

Displaced brain

Cyst

Blood

rhage is most likely to occur when a patient has atherosclerosis in combination with hypertension (high blood pressure). (For a discussion of hypertension, see "Hypertensive Heart Disease" in Ch. 10, *Heart Disease*.) Hemorrhage is also a danger when an aneurysm forms in a blood vessel. An *aneurysm* is a blood-filled pouch that balloons out from a weak spot in the artery wall. Sometimes, too, pressure from a mass of tissue—a tumor, for example—can produce a stroke by squeezing a nearby brain vessel shut.

When the blood supply is cut off, injury to certain brain cells follows. Cells thus damaged cannot function; neither, then, can the parts of the body controlled by these nerve centers. The damage to the brain cells may produce paralysis of a leg or arm; it may interfere with the ability to speak or with a person's memory. The affected function and the extent of disability depend on which brain region has been struck, how widespread the damage is, how effectively the body can repair its supply system to this damaged area, and how rapidly other areas of brain tissue can take over the work of the out-of-commission nerve cells.

Symptoms

Frequently there are symptoms of impending stroke: headaches, numbness in the limbs, faintness, momentary lapses in memory, slurring of speech, or sudden clumsiness. The presence of these symptoms does not always mean a stroke is brewing; sometimes they are quite harmless. But should they be stroke warning signals, the physician can take some preventive action. He may recommend anticoagulant therapy as well as drugs to bring down elevated blood pressure. In some cases, he might decide to call for surgical replacement of diseased or weakened sections of arteries leading to the brain.

Treatment

Following a stroke, medical personnel may use *single photon emission computed tomography* (SPECT) to assess quickly the effects of a stroke. A refinement of nuclear scanning (See Chapter 26, Physicians and Diagnostic Procedures), SPECT shows the nature and extent of brain damage. The next critical step is intensive rehabilitation. Not everyone needs a rehabilitation regimen; some strokes have little effect. Some persons recover quickly from what appears to be a severe stroke. Others may suffer serious damage, and may take a long time to recover even partially. Treatment can usually help—especially those who are partially paralyzed and those with *aphasia*, the inability to speak properly because of damage to the brain's speech center.

Embolism

An embolus, or thrombus that has broken away into the bloodstream, is, as we have seen, sometimes the direct cause of a stroke. A heart attack may also cause a stroke. Bacterial action may soften a thrombus so that it separates into fragments and breaks free from its wall anchorage. Thrombi are not the only source of emboli; any free-floating mass in the bloodstream, be it an air bubble, clumps of fat, knots of cancer cells, or bacteria, can prove dangerous.

Usually, however, emboli originate as thrombi in the veins, especially the leg veins. Breaking free, the clump of clot material wanders into the bloodstream to be carried towards the right chamber of the heart and then onward into the lungs, unless dissolved before that. Once in the pulmonary arteries there is a growing threat that the moving mass will catch in one of the smaller branches of the lung circulation. This life-threatening blockage is called a *pulmonary embolism*.

This disorder takes at least 50,000 lives a year; most occur during or following prolonged periods of hospitalization and bed rest. The lack of activity slows the blood flow and increases the danger of thrombi—and ultimately emboli. Prevention requires getting the patient out of bed as soon and as often as possible to stimulate leg circulation. The nonambulatory patient, meanwhile, is encouraged to move his legs by raising them, or changing positions so as to step up blood flow.

The detection of a large embolus—symptoms include shortness of breath and chest pains—may require emergency surgery for removal. In most instances, however, treatment means administering anticoagulants to prevent new clots from emerging while allowing the body to rid itself of the embolus.

10

Heart Disease

Heart disease is the commonly used, catch-all phrase for a number of disorders affecting both the heart and blood vessels. A more apt term is cardiovascular disease, which represents America's worst health scourge. More than 27 million Americans of all ages are afflicted with some kind of cardiovascular ailment. When considered together, heart and circulatory system diseases, including stroke, account for more than one-half of all deaths each year in the United States, a total of more than one million people.

The most frequent cause of death from cardiovascular disease is *coronary artery disease,* brought on by obstructions that develop in the coronary vessels nourishing the heart muscle. These fatty blockages impair adequate delivery of oxygen-laden blood to the heart muscle cells. The result may be *angina pectoris:* short episodes of viselike chest pains that strike when the heart fails to get enough blood; or it may be a full-blown attack, where blood-starved heart tissue dies.

One out of every five American males will have a heart attack before the age of 60. Heart attacks strike about 1.6 million annually, killing more than 600,000. Overall, more than six million adults either definitely have or are suspected of having some degree of coronary disease; for this reason it has been labeled the "twentieth-century epidemic," or the "black plague of affluence."

Hypertensive heart disease is an impairment of heart-pumping function stemming from persistent *hypertension* (high blood pressure). Untreated, elevated pressure makes the heart work harder, causing it to enlarge and sometimes to fail. It can also

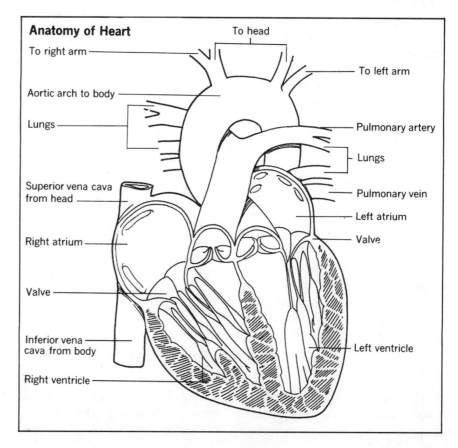

Anatomy of Heart

To right arm

To head

To left arm

Aortic arch to body

Lungs

Pulmonary artery

Lungs

Superior vena cava from head

Pulmonary vein

Left atrium

Right atrium

Valve

Valve

Inferior vena cava from body

Left ventricle

Right ventricle

lead to serious damage to the kidneys and acceleration of the vessel-clogging process responsible for most heart attacks and strokes. Hypertension is the most common of the cardiovascular diseases, affecting about 22 million Americans, with more than half having some degree of heart involvement. A little more than 60,000 deaths are directly attributable to hypertension and hypertensive heart disease.

Rheumatic heart disease, the leftover scars of a rheumatic fever attack, claims the lives of 13,000 annually. It generally strikes children between the ages of 5 and 15. All told, 1.6 million persons are suffering from rheumatic heart disease, with about 100,000 new cases reported each year.

Congenital heart disease includes that collection of heart and major blood vessel deformities that exist at birth in 8 out of every 1,000 live births, or 25,000 cases yearly. Nine thousand deaths annually are attributable to these inborn heart abnormalities.

This grim portrait of death and disability is improving rapidly, however, because of research uncovering new knowledge for protecting the heart and its pipelines. For example:

- Rheumatic fever, once a major menace of childhood, has been subdued effectively through the use of antibiotics, which can eradicate streptococcal infections, the precursor of rheumatic disease; theoretically, the disease has been made wholly preventable. In the last two decades the death rate from rheumatic heart disease has dropped more than 85 percent within the 5- to 24-year-old age group.

- Bold new surgery makes it possible to cure or alleviate most congenital heart defects, to replace

defective heart valves with plastic substitutes, and to open new sources of blood to a heart with diseased coronary arteries.

- A broad arsenal of drugs that makes almost all cases of hypertension—whether it is mild or severe—controllable, helps explain the 63 percent drop in the death rate as compared with that recorded in 1950.

- Advances in coronary care are lowering the heart attack death rate. Physicians, having learned to recognize the coronary-prone individual, are able to prescribe life-styles to forestall heart attack.

- Out-of-kilter heart rhythms are being restored to normal with permanently implanted pacemakers.

Coronary Artery Disease

To keep itself going, the heart relies on two pencil-thick main arteries. Branching from the aorta, these vessels deliver freshly oxygenated blood to the right and left sides of the heart. The left artery is usually somewhat larger and divides into two sizable vessels, the circumflex and anterior branches. The latter is sometimes called the artery of sudden death, since a clot near its mouth is common and leads to a serious and often fatal heart attack. These arteries wind around the heart and send out still smaller branches into the heart muscle to supply the needs of all cells. The network of vessels arches down over the heart like a crown—in Latin, *corona*—hence the word *coronary.*

Atherosclerosis

Coronary artery disease exists when flow of blood is impaired because of narrowed and obstructed coronary arteries. In virtually all cases, this

blockade is the result of atherosclerosis, a form of *arteriosclerosis,* the thickening and hardening of the arteries. *Atherosclerosis,* from the Greek for porridge or mush, refers to the process by which fat carried in the bloodstream piles up on the inner wall of the arteries like rust in a pipe. As more and more fatty substances, including cholesterol, accumulate, the once smooth wall gets thicker, rougher, and harder, and the blood passageway becomes narrower.

This fatty clogging goes on imperceptibly, a process that often begins early in life. Eventually, blood flow may be obstructed sufficiently to cause the heart muscle cells to send out distress signals. The brief, episodic chest pains of angina pectoris announce that these cells are starving and suffering for lack of blood and oxygen. Flow may be so severely diminished or totally plugged up that a region of the heart muscle dies. The heart has been damaged; the person has had a heart attack.

Angina

Angina pectoris means chest pain. Usually the pain is distinctive and feels like a vest being drawn too tightly across the chest. Sometimes it eludes easy identification. As a rule, however, the discomfort is felt behind the breastbone, occasionally spreading to the arms, shoulders, neck, and jaw. Not all chest pain indicates angina; in most cases it may simply be gas in the stomach.

Symptoms

Angina attacks are likely to appear when sudden strenuous demands are placed on the heart. They may come from physical exertion—walking uphill, running, sexual activity, or the effort involved in eating and digesting

Angina Pectoralis

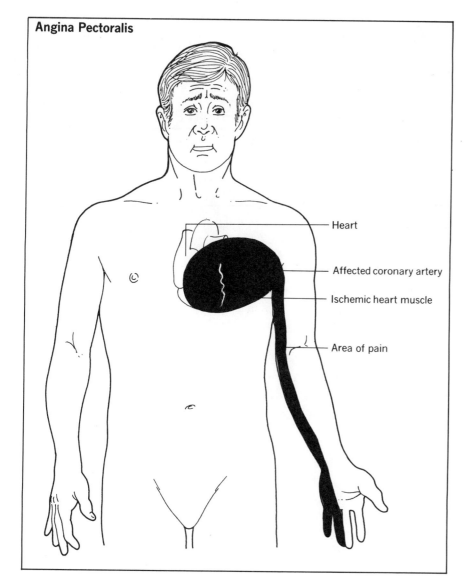

Heart

Affected coronary artery

Ischemic heart muscle

Area of pain

a heavy meal. Watching an exciting movie or sporting event can trigger it; so might cold weather. An attack can occur even when the individual is lying still or asleep—perhaps the result of tension or dreams.

Whatever the trigger, the heart is called upon to pump more blood to meet the body's stepped-up needs. To do so means working harder and faster. If one or more of the heart's supply lines is narrowed by disease, the extra blood and oxygen required to fuel the pump cannot get through to a region of the heart muscle. Anginal pain is a signal that muscle cells are being strained by an insufficiency of oxygen; they are, as it were, gasp-

ing for air.

The attacks usually are brief, lasting only a matter of minutes. Attacks stop when the person rests. Some people, apparently, can walk through an attack, as if the heart has gotten a second wind, and the pain subsides.

Treatment

Treatment may involve merely rearranging activity to avoid overly taxing physical labors or emotional situations likely to induce discomfort. A major medication used for angina is *nitroglycerine*. It dilates small coronary blood vessels, allowing more blood to get through. Nitroglycerine pellets are

not swallowed but are placed under the tongue, where they are quickly absorbed by blood vessels there and sped to the heart; discomfort passes in minutes. Often anginal attacks can be headed off by taking the tablets before activities likely to bring on an attack.

Still other drugs have been found to relieve angina pains. One group, called the beta-blockers, slows down the heart's action and thus its need for oxygen. Widely used to treat high blood pressure as well as heart disease, the beta-blockers may cause shortness of breath. For that reason, physicians usually prescribe other medications for persons with asthma.

The first of the beta-blockers to come into use was *propranolol*. But at least five chemically related drugs may be prescribed: atenolol, timolol, metoprolol, nadolol, and pindalol. Physicians generally try to fit one of these drugs to the problems of the individual patient. There is some evidence that propranolol and nitroglycerin taken together may increase the effectiveness of therapy.

A second group of drugs for angina is known as the calcium slow channel blockers, or simply calcium channel blockers. These drugs prevent coronary spasms, one cause of angina chest pains, by blocking the flow of calcium ions to the heart. Unblocked, the calcium ions enter the muscle cells of coronary arteries, in some cases causing the muscles to contract suddenly. Three chemically different calcium channel blockers in use are verapamil, nifedipine, and diltiazem.

Angina does not mean a heart attack is inevitable. Many angina patients never have one, probably because their hearts have developed collateral circulation. Fortunately, an auxiliary system of very tiny pipelines lacing the heart exists in a dormant state as a potential escape hatch for the diseased heart. As the coronary arteries narrow, the collateral vessels gradually grow larger and wider, switched on, presumably, by the oxygen shortage. Thus, they may provide an alternate route for blood to the afflicted area of the heart muscle. As the collateral system continues to develop, it may cause anginal symptoms to lessen. Although this may not prevent a heart attack, these newly activated pathways might make the attack less severe.

Coronary Artery Surgery

In general, surgery for angina is reserved for the severely restricted, incapacitated patient for whom medical treatment has been a failure. A procedure devised in Canada for bringing new sources of blood to the heart with clogged arteries may be of value in some cases. It involves implanting into the wall of the left ventricle an artery that normally supplies blood to the chest. One drawback is the time it takes—often a matter of months—for the implanted artery to develop the necessary collateral linkages to be of help to the heart.

Ideally, surgeons would like to operate directly on the coronary arteries, especially when the obstructing atherosclerotic deposits are confined to short, accessible vessel segments. Early attempts to do this, however, have brought high mortality and a low percentage of cures.

Endarterectomy, which means reaming out the trouble-making blockage, is still in the experimental stage. Carbon dioxide, forced in under high pressure to blow the deposits loose, has been used as a reaming tool in experiments. The diseased core is then cut free and pulled out through an incision in the coronary artery. Still another direct technique involves bypassing the diseased portion of the artery with a synthetic blood vessel graft taken from the patient's leg artery.

Heart Surgery

Direct surgery on the heart is possible because of the development of the heart-lung machine, which takes over the job of oxygenating and pumping blood into circulation, thus giving surgeons time to work directly on a relatively bloodless heart.

To choose patients appropriate for surgery, physicians use a reviewing system called *arteriography,* which allows them to watch blood flowing through the coronary artery system and to evaluate with accuracy the degree and location of obstruction. A substance opaque to X rays is injected into the coronary arteries and then followed by X ray as it runs its course through the vessels supplying the heart muscle.

Newer diagnostic methods dispense with injections of the opaque fluid and with X-ray technology. Nuclear magnetic resonance (NMR), for example, uses magnetic forces to scan the interior of the body for abnormalities. In heart disease diagnoses, NMR can identify specific problems in specific areas of the heart and its arteries.

Despite the newspaper headlines and dramatic history-making operations of recent years, heart transplants must still be considered experimental. One reason is the logistics problem: getting and storing enough donor hearts to meet the demand. More important, however, is the immunological barrier. The body's defense against disease regards the new heart as foreign and attacks it, just as it would bacteria and viruses. Until scientists have learned how to thwart rejection consistently, heart transplants will have to be performed only on a limited, highly selective basis. For more information see "Heart Surgery" in Ch. 20, *Surgery.* See also "Organ Transplants" in Ch. 20, *Surgery.*

Heart Attack

Physicians have other names for heart attack: coronary occlusion, coronary thrombosis, myocardial infarction. *Coronary occlusion* means total closure of the coronary artery. This may be caused by fatty deposits that have piled up high enough to dam the flow channel.

Or it may be that a blood clot, or *thrombus,* forming in the coronary artery, has suddenly caught on the roughened, fat-clogged area and plugged up the vessel. In this case the occlusion is called a *coronary thrombosis. Myocardial infarction* refers to the actual damage or death of heart muscle (*myocardium*) resulting from the occlusion.

Heart attacks hit males hardest. The frequency of heart attacks begins to build rapidly among men between the ages of 30 and 40 but is almost unknown in women of the same age group. The odds begin evening out as women approach and pass menopause. Despite this, during the same 40- to 44-age period, the ratio of male to female heart attacks may be as high as 24 to one.

The incidence of heart attacks increases with age. The peak years for male heart attacks are in the 55- to 59-age bracket. The percentage of deaths from first heart attacks, however, is higher among men in their forties than those in their sixties, presumably because the younger men do not have as well-developed collateral circulation to protect them.

Symptoms

Sometimes heart attacks are so vague or indistinct that the victim may not

Myocardial Infarct

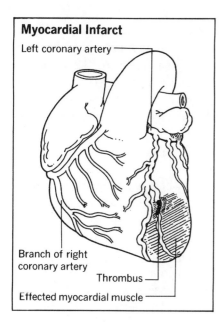

Left coronary artery

Branch of right
coronary artery

Thrombus

Effected myocardial muscle

know he has had one. Often a routine electrocardiogram—the squiggly-lined record of the heart's activity—turns up an abnormality indicative of an *infarct,* or injured area. This is another instance of the importance of periodic checkups. Special blood tests can also detect substances that may leak out into the circulation when heart muscle cells are injured.

Most heart attacks, however, do not sneak by. There are well-recognized symptoms. The most common are:

- A feeling of strangulation

- A prolonged, oppressive pain or unusual discomfort in the center of the chest that may radiate to the left shoulder and down the left arm

- Abnormal perspiring

- Sudden, intense shortness of breath

- Nausea or vomiting (because of these symptoms, an attack is sometimes taken for indigestion; usually, coronary pains are more severe)

- Occasionally, loss of consciousness

Treatment

Knowing these warning signals and taking proper steps may make the difference between life and death. Call a physician or get to a hospital as soon as possible. Time is crucial. Most deaths occur in the initial hours after attack. About 25 percent, for example, die within three hours after onset of their first heart attack.

Often, death is not due to any widespread damage to the heart muscle, but rather to a disruption in the electric spark initiating heart muscle contraction—the same spark measured by the electrocardiogram. These out-of-kilter rhythms, including complete heart stoppage or cardiac arrest, are often reversible with prompt treatment.

Nonsurgical methods of treating heart disease have multiplied in recent years. In balloon angioplasty, a catheter is pushed through blood channels into a coronary artery that has been narrowed by fatty deposits, which cut off the flow of blood. Inflated, a balloon attached to the catheter forces open the affected artery. The catheter and balloon are then removed. In another new technique, the Multiwire Gamma Camera assesses heart damage, working six times faster than conventional cameras, which emit 150,000 X rays a second. The Gamma camera can reportedly detect small areas of the heart that are receiving inadequate oxygen because of reduced blood flow.

Pharmaceutical firms have developed many products that aid in cardiographic imaging. The products may be used with X rays, nuclear imaging, or ultrasound to provide pictures of the heart. Once a diagnosis of heart attack is reached, any of six types of therapeutic drugs may be used. The classes include thrombolytics like TPA (tissue plasminogen activator), Streptokinase, and others that dissolve blood clots; antiarrhythmics,

which restore a regular beat to an irregularly beating heart; and vasopressors or inotropic agents that stimulate the heart and enhance heart function. Among the many cardiostimulants, or inotropic drugs, is a large group called partial beta 1 agonists that accelerate the rehabilitation process and increase exercise tolerance.

Of two other classes of therapeutic drugs, calcium and beta channel blockers are used to slow the heart rate while angiotensin converting enzyme (ACE) inhibitors increase blood flow to the kidneys. The ACE inhibitors also block an enzyme that raises blood pressure. Among the diuretics are Dyazide and furosemide, marketed as Lasix. Both help to prevent fluid accumulation in the lungs.

Coronary Care Units

Special hospital centers called coronary care units (CCUs) have been created to provide for heart attack victims. Here, around-the-clock electronic devices keep watch over each patient's vital functions, particularly the heart's electrical activity. The critical period is the first 72 hours, when up to 90 percent of heart attack patients experience some type of electrical disturbance or *arrhythmia* (irregular heartbeat).

In planning the CCU, each hospital assesses the number of heart attack victims reaching the hospital annually. It estimates how many patients would have to be kept in the CCU at any given time. The CCU is always integrated into the hospital system so that it can work with other departments.

Patient rooms in the CCU are designed to ensure privacy and a tranquil, cheerful environment. Rooms may be separated from one another by curtains or partial or full walls. Beds usually stand in a space adequate for movement of heavy equipment such as the portable X-ray apparatus.

Very importantly, the CCU provides for heart monitoring at each bed. Using a "slave" monitor, nurses can check on a patient's condition without leaving the nurse's station. There is one slave for each bedside monitor. Both types of monitor have pulse rate meters and readout triggers that enable a nurse or physician to take a recorded electrocardiogram (EKG) simply by pressing a button. An alarm system on the slave monitor notifies the nurse when a major change is taking place in the patient's condition.

Where possible, CCUs have two defibrillators for treatment of the condition called ventricular fibrillation, with one kept for standby use. Other emergency equipment includes intravenous pacemakers and a crash cart stocked with such items as the drugs needed for emergency cardiac care (ECC) and endotracheal tubes.

Fibrillation

The most dangerous rhythmic disorder is ventricular *fibrillation,* in which the lower chambers of the heart contract in an uncoordinated manner, causing blood-pumping to cease completely. Treated within one minute, the patient has a 90 percent or better chance of surviving. A delay of three minutes means a survival rate of less than 10 percent because of extensive and irreversible brain and heart damage.

Treatment involves the use of an instrument called a *defibrillator.* Through plates applied to the chest, the device sends a massive jolt of electricity into the heart muscle to get the heart back on the right tempo.

More significantly, it is now also possible to head off ventricular fibrillation, so that the already compro-

mised heart will not have to tolerate even brief episodes of the arrhythmia. Ventricular fibrillation is invariably heralded by an earlier, identifiable disturbance in the heartbeat. Most frequently, the warning signal is a skipped or premature ventricular beat. Picked up by the coronary care monitoring equipment, the signal alerts the unit staff to administer heart-calming medicaments that can ward off the danger. One such drug is *lidocaine,* a long-used dental anesthetic found to have the power to restore an irritated heart to electrical tranquillity.

The advent of coronary care has produced striking results. Where in use, these units have reduced heart attack deaths among hospitalized patients up to 30 percent. If all heart victims surviving at least a few hours received such care, more than 50,000 lives could be saved annually.

Failure of Heart Muscle

Most deaths in coronary care units, however, result not from electrical failure but power failure—the result of massive injury to the heart muscle. So large an area of the muscle is put out of commission, at least temporarily, that the still healthy portion is unable to cope with the body's ceaseless blood needs.

Success in treating failures of the heart muscle has not been great. Various devices for assisting the weakened heart with its pumping burden are still in the experimental stage. The problem is to create a device that will do most, if not all, of the work for the struggling left ventricle over a period of days or weeks to give the heart muscle a chance to rest and recover.

Emergency Care

Most heart attack victims never reach the hospital. About 400,000 die be-

fore getting there, as many as 60 percent in the first hour. Evidence suggests that many of these sudden deaths result from ventricular fibrillation or cardiac arrest—reversible disturbances when treated immediately.

These considerations led to the concept of mobile coronary care units—of bringing the advanced techniques of heart resuscitation to the victims. Originated in 1966 in Belfast, Northern Ireland, the practice of having a flying squad of specially equipped ambulances ready to race with on-the-spot aid to heart attack patients has been spreading to more U.S. communities, successfully reducing mortality.

An emergency technique called *external cardiopulmonary resuscitation* (ECPR), more popularly known as *cardiac massage* or *closed-chest massage,* has also reduced out-of-hospital heart attack mortality figures. Used in conjunction with mouth-to-mouth breathing, ECPR is an emergency procedure for treating cardiac arrest. The lower part of the breastbone is compressed rhythmically to keep oxygenated blood flowing to the brain until appropriate medical treatment until appropriate medical treatment can be applied to restore normal heart action; often ECPR alone is enough to restart the heart. The technique should be performed only by trained personnel, however, because it involves risks, such as the danger of fracturing a rib or rupturing a weakened heart muscle if too much pressure is applied.

Recuperation

Beyond the 72-hour crisis period, the patient will still require hospitalization for three to six weeks to give the heart time to heal. During the first two weeks or so, the patient is made to remain completely at rest. In this period, the dead muscle cells are being cleared away and gradually replaced by scar tissue. Until this happens, the damaged area represents a dangerous weak spot. By the end of the second week, the patient may be allowed to sit in a chair and then to walk about the room. Recently, some plysicians have been experimenting with getting patients up and about earlier, sometimes within a few days after their attack. Although most patients are well enough to be discharged after three or four weeks, not everyone mends at the same rate, which is why physicians hesitate to predict exactly when the patient will be released or when he will be well enough to resume normal activity.

About 15 percent of in-hospital heart attack deaths come in the post-acute phase owing to an *aneurysm,* or ballooning-out, of the area where the left ventricle is healing. This is most likely to develop before the scar has toughened enough to withstand blood pressures generated by the heart's contractions. The aneurysm may kill either by rupturing the artery or by so impairing pumping efficiency that the heart fails and the circulation deteriorates.

Most heart attack patients are able to return to their precoronary jobs eventually. Some, left with anginal pain, may have to make adjustments in their jobs and living habits. What kind of activity the patient can ultimately resume is an individual matter to be worked out by the patient with his physician. The prescription usually involves keeping weight down and avoiding undue emotional stress or physical exertion; moderate exercise along with plenty of rest is encouraged.

The Holter Monitor

Before or after a heart attack victim returns to work and more normal life habits, physicians may want to know how he or she will react to stresses, medicines, and other factors and conditions. A "Holter monitor," named after the physicist Dr. Norman J. Holter, makes such measurements possible. The portable monitor delivers electrocardiographic readings for 6 to 24 hours or longer while the patient goes about his normal activities.

Called "ambulatory electrocardiographic monitoring," the process of recording heart signals is relatively simple. Electrodes are attached to the patient's chest over the heart. The electrodes connect with a tape recorder that makes electrocardiograms. Completely portable because of its weight—less than two pounds—the tape recorder/monitor is carried on a strap hung over the patient's shoulder or is attached to the wearer's belt.

The monitor's recordings tell physicians a number of things that may be crucial to the patient's survival. Where a patient has experienced heart palpitations or irregularities, the physician can adjust treatment to the recorded findings. Medication designed to prevent rhythm disorders may be adjusted as regards dosage and timing. These readings would typically be taken before the patient returns to work, either in the hospital or at home.

Where a patient has dizzy spells, the monitor can often detect the specific problems affecting heart functioning. Those problems, mainly slow or rapid nonrhythmic beats or heart blockage, may be found to be causing the dizziness. The possibility of pacemaker failure may also be indicated. The pacemaker provides a regular electrical impulse to keep heart action regular.

Patients using the ambulatory monitor are generally asked to supplement the cardiographic record by keeping notes on their activities. These notes show the physician the activities in which the patient was engaged from hour to hour during the day. The notes may be matched up with the EKG to show what stresses accompanied particular activities. Some monitors have a special band on which the patient can record oral reports of his activities. With the monitor's tape record and the patient's written or dictated notes, the physician can often:

- Give the patient specific instructions on when and to what extent he or she can resume normal home activities

- Provide an accurate schedule for resuming work tasks

- Guide the patient on the need for future evaluations and therapy

Prevention

Scientists do not have all the answers to atherosclerosis as yet. What is apparent, though, is that not one but a mosaic of factors is involved.

Long-term population studies have helped to point up individual characteristics and living habits that raise heart attack risk. These include such factors as sex, heredity, overweight, high blood pressure, lack of exercise, cigarette smoking, high blood levels of cholesterol and other fatty substances, and the presence of diabetes.

Identification of these risk factors has given the physician an important new weapon: a way to spot coronary-prone individuals years before any overt symptoms appear and a practical program for reducing this risk.

The program:

- Eat less saturated fat and cholesterol. Egg yolks are rich in cholesterol. Saturated animal fats, as in butter, cheese, cream, and whole milk, help to raise cholesterol levels. Use skimmed (fat-free) milk. Substitute polyunsaturated vegetable fats for saturated fats whenever possible—and use monounsaturated fats, found in such foods as olive oil, avocados, and nuts, in moderate quantities. Eat more poultry and fish.

- If recommended by your physician, bring your cholesterol levels under control with drugs as well as diet. One new drug, Gemfibrozil, helps by reducing low-density lipoproteins (LDLs, or "bad" cholesterol) while increasing high-density lipoproteins (HDLs, or "good" cholesterol) in the blood.

- Undergo periodic—at least annual—tests of your total cholesterol level. A total cholesterol reading under 200 is desirable; a reading from 200 to 239 ranks as "borderline high"; and levels above 240 indicate a need to consult a physician and possibly to make dietary changes.

- Control high blood pressure. Hypertension sharply increases the chances of a heart attack. A man whose blood pressure at *systole* (the moment the heart contracts) is higher than 160 runs four times the risk of an individual with a systolic blood pressure under 120.

- Don't smoke. The heart attack death rate is 50 to 200 percent higher, depending on age and number of cigarettes consumed, among men who smoke as compared with nonsmokers. Giving up the habit can decrease the coronary risk to that of the nonsmoker; the danger from smoking is reversible.

- Count calories. Get down to your proper weight and stay there. Excess weight taxes the heart, making it work harder. Middle-aged men who are 20 percent overweight run as much as two to three times the risk of a fatal heart attack as their trimmer counterparts.

- Exercise regularly. Your physician can tell you what the best exercise program is for your age and physical condition.

- Take one aspirin every other day if you're a man at risk of a heart attack. A six-year study showed that men who took aspirin on the every-other-day schedule had approximately half as many heart attacks as those who did not. Women should consult their doctors before starting an aspirin regimen. The aspirin keeps the blood platelets from sticking together.

Hypertensive Heart Disease

Hypertension, or elevated blood pressure, results from a persistent tightening of the body's very small arterial branches, the *arterioles*. This clenching increases the resistance to blood flow and sends the blood pressure up, just as screwing down the nozzle on a hose builds up pressure in the line. The heart must now work harder to force blood through. Over a period of time, the stepped-up pumping effort may cause the heart muscle to thicken and enlarge, much as the arm muscles do on a weight lifter. Eventually, the overworked circulatory system may break down, with resultant failure of the heart or kidneys, or the onset of stroke. The constant hammering of blood under high pressure on the walls of the arteries also accelerates the development of atherosclerosis and heart attacks.

How Blood Pressure Is Measured

Blood pressure is measured in millimeters of mercury with an instrument called a *sphygmomanometer*. The device consists of an inflatable cuff attached to a mercury meter. The physician wraps the cuff around the arm and inflates it with air from a squeeze-bulb. This drives the mercury column up towards the top of the gauge while shutting off blood flow through the brachial artery in the arm. With a stethoscope placed just below the cuff, the physician releases the air and listens for the first thudding sounds that signal the return of blood flow as the blood pressure on the wall of the artery equals the air pressure in the cuff. He records this mercury meter reading. This number represents the *systolic* pressure, the force developed by the heart when it contracts.

By continuing to let air out, the physician reaches a point where he can no longer hear the pulsing sounds of flowing blood. He marks the gauge reading as the *diastolic* pressure, the pressure on the artery when the heart is relaxing between beats. Thus, two numbers are used to record blood pressure, the systolic followed by the diastolic.

Recorded when the patient is relaxed, normal systolic pressure for most adults is between 100 and 140, and diastolic between 60 and 90. Many factors, such as age and sex, account for the wide variations in normal readings from individual to individual. Systolic blood pressure, for example, tends to increase with age.

Normally, blood pressure goes up during periods of excitement and physical labor. Hypertension is the diagnosis when repeated measurements show a persistent elevated pressure—160 or higher for systolic and 95 or more for diastolic.

In addition to the sphygmomanometer reading in the examination for high blood pressure, the physician shines a bright light in the patient's eyes so that he can look at the blood vessels in the retina, the only blood vessels that are readily observable. Any damage there resulting from hypertension is usually a good index of the severity of the disease and its effects elsewhere in the body.

An electrocardiogram and X ray may be in order to determine if and how much the heart has been damaged. The physician may also perform some tests of kidney function to ascertain whether hypertension, if detected, is of the essential or secondary kind, and if there has been damage to the kidneys as well.

Causes

About 85 percent of all hypertension cases are classified as *essential*. This simply means that no single cause can be defined. Rather, pressure is up because a number of factors—none of which has yet been firmly implicated—are operating in some complex interplay.

One theory holds that hypertension arises from excessive activity of the sympathetic nervous system, which helps regulate blood vessel response. This notion could help explain why tense individuals are susceptible to hypertension. Emotional reactions to unpleasant events or other mental stresses prompt the cardiovascular system to react as it might to exercise, including widespread constric-

tion of small blood vessels and increased heart rate.

The theory suggests that repeated episodes of stress may ultimately affect pressure-sensitive cells called *baroreceptors*. Situated in strategic places in the arterial system, these sensing centers are thought to be preset to help maintain normal blood pressure, just as a thermostat works to keep a house at a preset temperature. Exposure to regularly recurrent elevated blood pressure episodes may bring about a resetting of the baroreceptors—or *barostats*—to a new, higher normal. Once reset, the barostats operate to sustain hypertension.

Symptoms

Essential hypertension usually first occurs when a person is in his thirties. In the early stages, one may pass through a transitional or prehypertensive phase lasting a few years in which blood pressure rises above normal only occasionally, and then more and more often until finally it remains at these elevated levels.

Symptoms, if they exist at all, are likely to be something as nonspecific as headaches, dizziness, or nausea. As a result, without a physical examination to reveal its presence, a person may have the disease for years without being aware of it. That can be dangerous, because the longer hypertension is left untreated, the greater the likelihood that the heart will be affected.

About 15 percent of cases fall under the *secondary hypertension* classification, because they arise as a consequence of another known disorder. Curing the underlying disorder also cures the hypertension. Usually it is brought on by an obstruction of normal blood flow to the kidney because of atherosclerotic deposits in one or both of its major supply lines, the

renal arteries. Many patients can be cured or substantially improved through surgery.

Treatment

The outlook is good for almost all patients with essential hypertension, whether mild or severe, because of the large arsenal of antihypertensive drugs now at the physician's disposal. Not all drugs will benefit all patients, but where one fails another or several in combination will almost invariably succeed. Even the usually lethal and hard-to-treat form of essential hypertension described as *malignant* is beginning to respond to new medications. *Malignant hypertension,* which may strike as many as five percent of hypertensive victims, does not refer to cancer, but rather describes the rapid, galloping way blood pressure rises.

Mild hypertension often may be readily treated with tranquilizers and mild sedatives, particularly if the patient is tense, or with one of a broad family of agents known as *diuretics*. These drugs flush the body of excess salt, which appears to have some direct though poorly-understood role in hypertension.

Against more severe forms, there are a large number of drugs which work in a variety of ways to offset or curb the activity of the sympathetic nervous system so that it relaxes its hold on the constricted arterioles.

Rheumatic Fever and Rheumatic Heart Disease

Rheumatic heart disease is the possible sequel of rheumatic fever. Triggered by streptococcal attacks in childhood and adolescence, rheumatic fever may leave permanent heart scars. The heart structures most often affected are the valves.

Causes

The cause of rheumatic fever is still not entirely understood. It is known that rheumatic fever is always preceded by an invasion of bacteria belonging to the group A beta hemolytic streptococcus family. Sooner or later, everybody has a strep infection, such as a strep throat or scarlet fever. Most of us get over it without any complications. But in 1 out of every 100 children the strep infection produces rheumatic fever a few weeks later, even after the strep attack has long since subsided. The figure may rise to 3 per 100 during epidemics in closed communities, such as a children's camp.

The invasion of strep sparks the production of protective agents called antibodies. For some reason, in a kind of biological double cross, the antibodies attack not only the strep but also make war on the body's own tissues—the very tissues they are called upon to protect.

Researchers are now suggesting the possible reason, although all the evidence is not yet in. According to a widely-held theory, the strep germ possesses constituents (*antigens*) that are similar in structure to components of normal, healthy cartilage and connective tissues—found abundantly in joints, tendons, and heart valves—in susceptible individuals. Failing to distinguish between them, the antibodies attack both. The result: rheumatic fever, involving joint and valve inflammation and, perhaps, permanent scarring.

Prevention

The development of antibiotics has made rheumatic fever preventable. These drugs can knock out the strep before the germs get a chance to set off the inflammatory defense network sequences, but early detection is necessary. Among the symptoms of strep are a sore throat that comes on suddenly, with redness and swelling; rapidly acquired high fever; nausea and headaches. The only sure way to tell, however, is to have a throat swab taken by passing a sterile piece of cotton over the inflamed area. This culture is then exposed for 24 hours to a laboratory dish containing a substance that enhances strep growth. A positive identification calls for prompt treatment to kill the germs before the complications of rheumatic fever have a chance to set in.

Unfortunately, many strep infections may be mild enough to escape detection. The child may recover so quickly that the parents neglect to take the necessary precautions, but the insidious processes may still be going on in the apparently healthy child. This is a major reason why rheumatic fever is still with us, though in severe decline.

Symptoms

Rheumatic fever itself is not always easy to diagnose. The physician must detect at least one of five symptoms, derived by the American Heart Association from the work of the late Dr. T. Duckett Jones. The so-called Jones criteria include:

- Swelling or tenderness in one or more joints; usually, several joints are involved, not simultaneously but one after the other in migratory fashion

- Carditis or heart inflammation

- Heart murmur

- An unusual skin rash, which often disappears in 24 to 48 hours

- Chorea, or St. Vitus's dance, so-called because of the uncoordinated, jerky and involuntary motions of the arms, legs, or face, which result from rheumatic inflammation of brain tissue; (it may last six to eight weeks and even longer, but when symptoms disappear there is never any permanent damage and the brain and nervous system return to normal)

- Hard lumps, under the skin and over the inflamed joints, usually indicating severe heart inflammation

Confirmation of rheumatic fever also requires other clinical and laboratory tests, to determine, for example, the presence of strep antibodies in the patient's blood. Rheumatic fever does not always involve the heart; even when it does, permanent damage is not inevitable. Nor does the severity of the attack have any relationship to the development of rheumatic heart disease.

The real danger arises when heart valve tissue becomes inflamed. When the acute attack has passed and the inflammation finally subsides, the valves begin to heal, with scar tissue forming.

Scar tissue may cause portions of the affected valve leaflets to fuse together. (*Leaflets* are the flaps of the heart valves.) This restricts leaflet motion, impeding the full swing action and thereby blood flow through the valve. This condition is called valvular *stenosis*. The leaflets may become shrunken or deformed by healing tissue, causing *regurgitation* or backspill because the valve fails to close completely.

Both stenosis and regurgitation are often present. Most susceptible are the *mitral valve*, which regulates flow from the upper to the lower left chambers of the heart, and the *aortic valve*, the gateway between the left ventricle and the general circulation. Rarely attacked are the two valves in the right chambers.

Treatment

During the acute stages of rheumatic

fever, the patient is given heavy doses of antibiotics to rid the body of all strep traces, aspirin to control swelling and fever, and sometimes such hormones as ACTH and cortisone to reduce inflammation.

In the past, rheumatic fever spelled mandatory bed rest for months. Now the routine is to get the patient up and about as soon as the acute episode is over to avert the problem of psychological invalidism. The biggest restriction, especially for young people, is that no participation in competitive sports or other severely taxing exercises is allowed for two to three months while a close watch is kept on cardiac status.

The patient with valve damage can in many cases be treated medically, without the need for surgical intervention. He may, of course, have to desist from certain strenuous activities, but in all other ways he can lead a relatively normal life. Surgical relief or cure is available, however, for patients with severe damage or those who may, with age, develop progressive narrowing or leakage of the valves.

Surgery

Stenotic valves can be scraped clear of excess scar tissues, thereby returning the leaflets to more normal operation. In some cases individually scarred leaflets are replaced with synthetic substitutes. The correction of severe valvular regurgitation requires replacement of the entire valve with an artificial substitute, or, as some surgeons prefer, with a healthy valve taken from a human donor dying of other causes.

Heart Murmurs and Recurrences of Rheumatic Fever

The prime sign that rheumatic heart disease has developed is a heart mur-

mur—although a heart murmur does not always mean heart disease. The murmur may be only temporary, ceasing once the rheumatic fever attack subsides and the stretched and swollen valves return to normal. To complicate matters more, many heart murmurs are harmless. Such functional murmurs may appear in 30 to 50 percent of normal children at one time or another.

As many as three in five patients with rheumatic fever may develop murmurs characteristic of scarred valves—sounds of blood flowing through ailing valves that fail to open and close normally.

Anyone who has had an attack of rheumatic fever has about a 50–50 chance of having one again unless safeguards are taken. As a result, all patients are placed on a daily or monthly regimen of antibiotics. The preventive dose, although smaller

than that given to quell an in-progress infection, is enough to sabotage any attempts on the part of the strep germs to mount an attack.

There is some encouraging evidence that rheumatic fever patients who escape heart damage the first time around will do so again should a repeat attack occur. On the other hand, those with damaged valves will probably sustain more damage with subsequent strep-initiated attacks.

Endocarditis

One of the additional bonuses of antibiotic therapy is that it has all but eliminated an invariably fatal complication to which rheumatic patients were especially vulnerable—an infection of the heart's inner lining, or *endocardium,* called *subacute bacterial endocarditis.* The scar tissue provides an excellent nesting site for bacteria to grow.

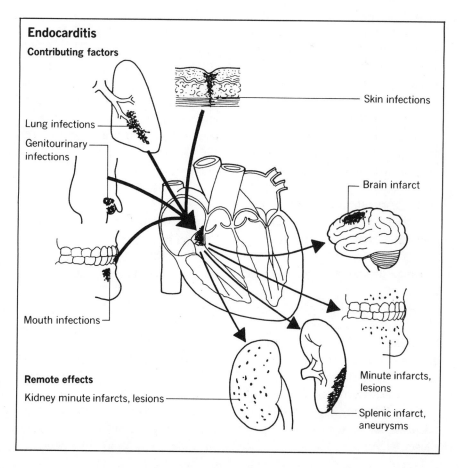

The responsible germs are found in almost everyone's mouth and usually invade the bloodstream after dental surgery. Fortunately, it is easy to prevent or cure because the germs offer little resistance to antibiotics. As a precaution, dentists are usually advised to give rheumatic fever patients larger doses of penicillin (or other antibiotics to those allergic to penicillin) before, during, and after dental work.

Congenital Heart Disease

There are some 35 recognized types of congenital heart malformations. Most—including all of the 15 most common types—can be either corrected or alleviated by surgery. The defects result from a failure of the infant's heart to mature normally during development in the womb.

The term *blue baby* refers to the infant born with a heart impairment that prevents blood from getting enough oxygen. Because blood low in oxygen is dark bluish red, it imparts a blue tinge to the skin and lips.

The cause of inborn heart abnormalities is not known in most cases. Some defects can be traced to maternal virus infection, such as German measles (rubella), during the first three months of pregnancy when the fetus' heart is growing rapidly. Certain drugs, vitamin deficiencies, or excessive exposure to radiation are among other environmental factors known to be associated with such defects.

Heart abnormalities may come singly or in combination. There may be, for example, a hole in the walls separating the right and left heart chambers or a narrowing of a valve or blood vessel which obstructs blood flow, or a mixup in major blood vessel connections—or a combination of all of these.

Diagnosis

A skilled cardiologist often can make a reasonably complete diagnosis on the basis of a conventional physical examination, including visual inspection of the infant's general condition, blood pressure reading, X ray, blood tests, and electrocardiogram. For more complex diagnosis, the physician may call for either *angiography* or *cardiac catheterization.* The former, a variation of coronary arteriography, allows direct X-ray visualization of the heart chambers and major blood vessels. In cardiac catheterization, a thin plastic tube or catheter is inserted into an arm or leg vein. While the physician watches with special X-ray equipment, the tube is advanced carefully through the vein until it reaches the heart chambers, there to provide information about the nature of the defect.

Advanced techniques known as computed tomography (CT), positron emission tomography (PET), and nuclear magnetic resonance (NMR) may also be used. Both the CT and PET scanners require injection of a contrast fluid so that a "picture" can be taken. The CT scanner takes X-ray images of "slices" of the patient's body with the aid of a computer. The PET scanner works on an electronic principle, with detectors located in a circle around the subject. Also computerized, NMR diagnoses by employing magnetic forces to "see" through bones and revealing such details as the differences between healthy and diseased tissues.

Treatment

From these tests, the cardiologist together with a surgeon can decide for or against surgery. Depending on the severity of the disease, some conditions may require an immediate operation, even on days-old infants. In other conditions, the specialists

may instead recommend waiting until the infant is older and stronger before surgery is undertaken. In a number of instances, the defect may not require surgery at all.

Open-heart surgery in infants with inborn heart defects carries a higher risk than does the same surgery in older children. Risks must be taken often, however, because about one-third will die in the first month if untreated, and more than half within the first year.

Refinements in surgical techniques and postoperative care have given surgeons the confidence to operate on infants who are merely hours old with remarkable success. Specially adapted miniature heart-lung machines may also chill the blood to produce *hypothermia,* or body cooling. This slows metabolism and reduces tissue oxygen needs so that the heart and brain can withstand short periods of interrupted blood flow.

A good deal has been learned, too, about the delicate medical management required by infants during the surgical recovery period. All of this accounts for the admirable record of salvage among infants who would have been given up for lost only a few years ago.

Congestive Heart Failure

Heart failure may be found in conjunction with any disease of the heart—coronary artery disease, hypertension, rheumatic heart disease, or congenital defects. It occurs when the heart's ability to pump blood has been weakened by disease. To say the heart has failed, however, does not mean it has stopped beating. The heart muscle continues to contract, but it lacks the strength to keep blood circulating normally throughout the body. Physicians sometimes refer to the condition as cardiac insufficiency or *dropsy,* although the latter term is seldom heard anymore.

When the heart fails to pump efficiently, the flow slows down, causing blood returning to the heart through the veins to back up. Some of the fluid in the blood is forced out through the thin walls of smaller blood vessels into surrounding tissues. Here the fluid piles up, or congests.

The result may be swelling, or *edema,* which can occur in many parts of the body but is most commonly seen in the legs and ankles. Fluids sometimes collect in the lungs, interfering with breathing and making the person short of breath. Heart failure also affects the ability of the kidneys to rid the body of sodium and water. Fluid retained in this way adds to the edema.

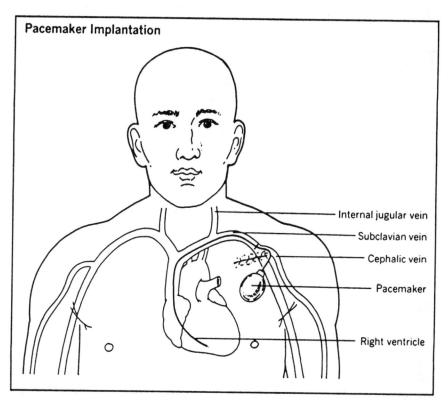

Pacemaker Implantation

Internal jugular vein
Subclavian vein
Cephalic vein
Pacemaker
Right ventricle

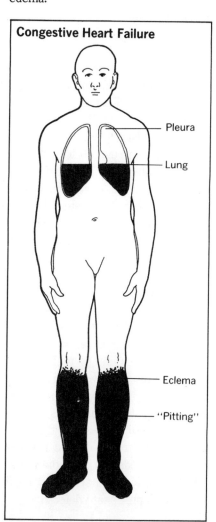

Congestive Heart Failure

Pleura
Lung
Eclema
"Pitting"

Treatment

Treatment usually includes a combination of rest, drugs, diet, and restricted daily activity. *Digitalis,* in one of its many forms, is usually given to strengthen the action of the heart muscle. It also slows a rapid heartbeat, helps decrease heart enlargement, and promotes secretion of excess fluids. Care must be taken to find the right dose, because this will vary from person to person. When edema is present, diuretics are prescribed to speed up the elimination of excess salt and water. Many improved diuretics are available today. A sodium-restricted diet is generally necessary to reduce or prevent edema. Patients will also probably need bed rest for a while, with a gradual return to slower-paced activity.

Most important, however, is the adequate treatment of the underlying disease that led to heart failure in the first place.

Heart Block

Sometimes the scars resulting from

rheumatic fever, heart attack, or surgical repair of the heart may damage the electrical network in a way that blocks normal transmission of the signal between the upper and lower chambers. The disruption, called *atrioventricular block,* may so severely slow down the rate at which the ventricles beat that blood flow is seriously affected, especially to the brain. Blackouts and convulsions may ensue.

For less serious slowdown, there are nervous system stimulants to keep the heart from lagging. In the case of *Stokes-Adams syndrome*—where the ventricles may not beat from four to ten seconds—drugs are not enough. An artificial electronic pacemaker, implanted in the body and connected to the heart by wires, has been successfully applied to many thousands of people throughout the world. This pacemaker fires electrical shocks into the ventricle wall to make it beat at the proper rate. Most devices are powered by tiny batteries which must be replaced on the average every three to five years.

11

Diseases of the Digestive System

Digestive Functions and Organs

The function of the digestive system is to accept food and water through the mouth, to break down the food's chemical structure so that its nutrients can be absorbed into the body, a process called *digestion,* and to expel undigested particles. This process takes place as the food passes through the entire *alimentary tract.* This tract, also called the *gastrointestinal tract,* is a long, hollow passageway that begins at the mouth and continues on through the esophagus, the stomach, the small intestine, the large intestine, the rectum, and the anus. The salivary glands, the stomach glands, the liver, the gallbladder, and the pancreas release substances into the gastrointestinal tract that help the digestion of various food substances.

Digestion

Digestion begins in the mouth where food is shredded by chewing and mixed with saliva, which helps break down starch into sugars and lubricates the food so that it can be swallowed easily. The food then enters the *esophagus,* a muscular tube that for-cibly squeezes the food down toward the stomach, past the *cardiac sphincter,* a ring of muscle at the entrance of the stomach that opens to allow food into the stomach.

The stomach acts as a reservoir for food, churns the food, mixes it with gastric juices, and gradually releases the food into the small intestine. Some water, alcohol, and glucose are absorbed directly through the stomach into the bloodstream. Enzymes secreted by the stomach help break down proteins and fats into simpler substances. Hydrochloric acid secreted by the stomach kills bacteria and prepares some minerals for absorption in the small intestine. Some food may leave the stomach one minute after it enters, while other parts of a meal may remain in the stomach for as long as five hours.

The food passes from the stomach to the first section of the small intestine, the *duodenum,* where it is acted on by pancreatic enzymes that help break down fats, starches, proteins, and other substances. While the food is in the duodenum it is also digested by *bile,* which is produced by the liver and stored in the gallbladder. During a meal, the gallbladder discharges its bile into the duodenum. The bile promotes the absorption of fats and vitamins.

The semidigested food is squeezed down the entire length of the intestines by a wavelike motion of the intestinal muscles called *peristalsis.* Digestion is largely completed as the food passes through 20 feet of small intestine, which absorbs the digested food substances and water and passes them into the bloodstream. The food nutrients are distributed by the bloodstream throughout the body and used by the body cells.

Those parts of the food that are indigestible, such as the skins of fruits, pass into the large intestine, or *colon,* along with bacteria, bile, some minerals, various cells, and mucus. This combination of substances makes up the *feces,* which are stored in the colon until *defecation.* Some water and salts in the feces are absorbed through the walls of the colon into the bloodstream. This conserves the body's fluids and dries the feces. The formation of a semisolid fecal mass helps precipitate defecation.

The Oral Cavity

The Salivary Glands

The smell of food triggers the salivary glands to pour saliva into the mouth; that is what is meant by "mouth-watering" odors. During a meal, saliva is released into the mouth to soften the food as it is chewed.

Stones

Stones will sometimes form in the salivary glands or ducts, blocking the ducts and preventing the free flow of saliva into the mouth. After a meal, the swollen saliva-filled glands and ducts slowly empty. The swelling may sometimes be complicated by infection. Surgical removal of the stones is the usual treatment; sometimes the entire gland is removed.

Tumors

Tumors sometimes invade the salivary gland. An enlarged gland may press on the auditory canal and cause deafness, or it may result in stiffness of the jaw and mild facial palsy. The tumors can grow large enough to be felt by the fingers, and surgery is required to remove them.

Inflammation of the Parotid Glands

Inflammation of the upper (*parotid*) salivary glands may be caused by an infection in the oral cavity, by liver disease, or by malnutrition.

Mumps

One of the commonest inflammations of the salivary glands, called *mumps,* occurs especially in children. It is a highly contagious virus disease characterized by inflammation and swelling of one or both parotid salivary

glands, and can have serious complications in adults. See "Alphabetic Guide to Child Care" in Ch. 2, *The First Dozen Years,* for a fuller discussion of mumps.

Bad Breath (Halitosis)

Poor oral hygiene is the principal cause of offensive mouth odor, or *halitosis*. It can result from oral tumors, abscesses from decaying teeth, and gum disease or infection. The foul smell is primarily a result of cell decay, and the odors are characteristic of the growth of some microorganisms.

When halitosis results from poor

oral sanitation, the treatment is obvious—regular daily tooth brushing and the use of an antiseptic mouthwash. If the halitosis is because of disease of the oral cavity, alimentary tract, or respiratory system, the cure will depend on eradicating the primary cause.

Nonmalignant Lesions

The oral cavity is prone to invasion by several types of microorganisms that cause nonmalignant lesions. The most prominent follow.

Canker Sores

These are of unknown origin and

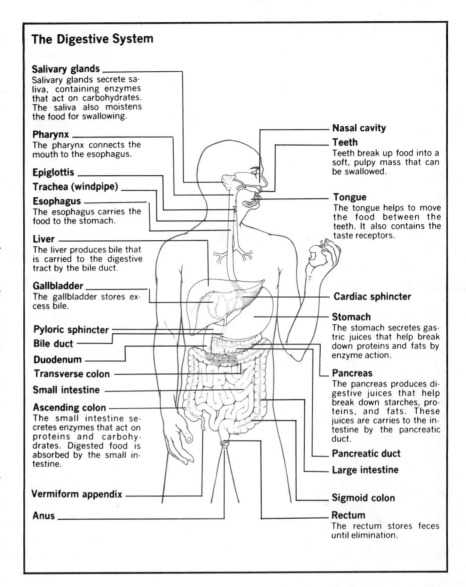

The Digestive System

Salivary glands
Salivary glands secrete saliva, containing enzymes that act on carbohydrates. The saliva also moistens the food for swallowing.

Pharynx
The pharynx connects the mouth to the esophagus.

Epiglottis

Trachea (windpipe)

Esophagus
The esophagus carries the food to the stomach.

Liver
The liver produces bile that is carried to the digestive tract by the bile duct.

Gallbladder
The gallbladder stores excess bile.

Pyloric sphincter

Bile duct

Duodenum

Transverse colon

Small intestine

Ascending colon
The small intestine secretes enzymes that act on proteins and carbohydrates. Digested food is absorbed by the small intestine.

Vermiform appendix

Anus

Nasal cavity

Teeth
Teeth break up food into a soft, pulpy mass that can be swallowed.

Tongue
The tongue helps to move the food between the teeth. It also contains the taste receptors.

Cardiac sphincter

Stomach
The stomach secretes gastric juices that help break down proteins and fats by enzyme action.

Pancreas
The pancreas produces digestive juices that help break down starches, proteins, and fats. These juices are carries to the intestine by the pancreatic duct.

Pancreatic duct

Large intestine

Sigmoid colon

Rectum
The rectum stores feces until elimination.

show up as single or multiple small sores near the molar teeth, inside the lips, or in the lining of the mouth. They can be painful but usually heal in a few days.

Fungus Infections

Thrush is the most common oral fungus infection and appears as white round patches inside the cheeks of infants, small children, and sometimes adults. The lesions may involve the entire mouth, tongue, and pharynx. In advanced stages the lesions turn yellow. Malnutrition, especially lack of adequate vitamin B, is the principal cause. Thrush is also one of the opportunistic infections commonly found in persons with AIDS. See also "AIDS" in Ch. 19, *Other Diseases of Major Importance*. Fungus growth may be aided by the use of antibiotic lozenges, which kill normal oral bacteria and permit fungi to flourish.

Tooth Decay and Vitamin Deficiencies

Lack of adequate vitamins in the daily diet is responsible for some types of lesions in the oral cavity. Insufficient vitamin A in children under five may be the cause of malformation in the crown, dentin, and enamel of the teeth. Lack of adequate vitamin C results in bleeding gums. Vitamin D insufficiency may lead to slow tooth development.

An inadequate and improper diet supports tooth decay, which in turn may be complicated by ulcers in the gums and abscesses in the roots of the decaying teeth. A diet with an adequate supply of the deficient vitamins will cause the symptoms to disappear. Infections, abscesses, cysts, or tumors in the mouth require the attention of a physician, dentist, or dental surgeon. See Ch. 22, *The Teeth and Gums*.

Chancres

These are primary syphilis lesions, which commonly develop at the lips and tongue. They appear as small, eroding red ulcers that exude yellow matter. They can invade the mouth, tonsils, and pharynx. Penicillin therapy is usually required.

The Esophagus

Varices

Varices (singular: *varix*) are enlarged and congested veins that appear in the esophagus because of increased blood pressure to the liver in patients with liver cirrhosis. This disease is most common in chronic alcoholics. Esophageal varices can be complicated by erosion of the mucous lining of the esophagus as a result of inflammation or vomiting. This causes hemorrhaging of the thin-walled veins, which can be fatal.

Bleeding esophageal varices may require hospitalization, immediate blood transfusions, and surgery.

Hiatus Hernia

The lower end of the esophagus or part of the stomach can sometimes protrude through the diaphragm. This *hiatus hernia*, sometimes referred to as a *diaphragmatic hernia*, can be a result of congenital malformation; in adults, the principal cause is weakness of the muscles around the opening of the esophagus leading into the stomach.

In individuals who are obese and who have large stomachs, the stomach contents may be forced back into the lower esophagus, causing this area to herniate. Other causes include stooping, bending, or kneeling, which increases pressure in the stomach. Pregnancy may increase abdominal pressure in the same manner as obesity.

Typical symptoms are vomiting when the stomach is full, heartburn with pain spreading to the ears, neck, and arms, swallowing difficulty with the food sometimes sticking in the esophagus, and a swollen abdomen. The vomiting may occur at night, with relief obtained by getting up and walking about for a few minutes. Belching will relieve the distension, and *antacids* (acid neutralizers) may be prescribed to counter gastric hyperacidity.

Conservative treatment involves

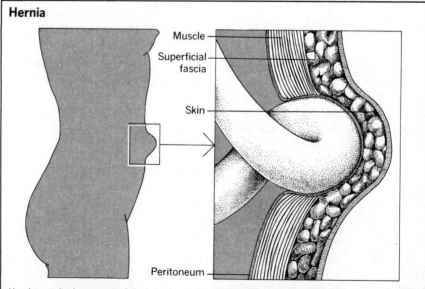

Hernia

Muscle

Superficial fascia

Skin

Peritoneum

Hernias result when a part of the intestine pushes through layers of muscle against the body's layers of skin.

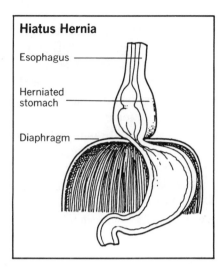

Hiatus Hernia

Esophagus

Herniated
stomach

Diaphragm

eating small portions at frequent intervals. Dieting and a reduction in weight cause the symptoms to disappear. When the symptoms are due to pregnancy, they disappear after delivery. When medical management is not successful, surgical repair of the hernia is necessary. See also "Hernias" later in this chapter.

Achalasia

Achalasia is abnormal dilation of the lower esophagus caused by failure of the cardiac sphincter to relax and allow food to enter the stomach. Food collects in the esophagus and does not flow into the stomach. The patient feels as though the food is sticking in the middle of his chest wall. Small amounts of food may eventually pass into the stomach, and the mild pain or discomfort disappears.

If the condition persists, the pain may increase to become a continuous burning sensation at each meal, due to inflammation of the esophagus by accumulated food. If the patient lies down, some of this esophageal content will regurgitate and enter the pharynx. If the vomitus gets into the lungs, the end result may be *aspiration pneumonia,* a form of pneumonia caused by inhaling particles of foreign matter.

The disease is difficult to control,

and the condition tends to return, so that surgery is often used to create a permanent opening between the esophagus and stomach.

Swallowing Difficulty

Difficulty in swallowing is called *dysphagia,* which should not be confused with *dysphasia,* a speech impairment. Dysphagia may be caused by lesions in the mouth and tongue, acute inflammatory conditions in the oral cavity and pharynx (mumps, tonsillitis, laryngitis, pharyngitis), lesions, cancers, or foreign bodies in the esophagus. Strictures in the esophagus— from esophageal ulcers or from swallowing corrosive liquids—will also impair swallowing.

Stomach and Intestines

Indigestion (Dyspepsia)

There are times when the gastrointestinal tract fails to carry out its normal digestive function. The resulting indigestion, or *dyspepsia,* generates a variety of symptoms, such as heartburn, nausea, pain in the upper abdomen, gases in the stomach (*flatulence*), belching, and a feeling of fullness after eating.

Indigestion can be caused by ulcers of the stomach or duodenum and by excessive or too rapid eating or drinking. It may also be caused by emotional disturbance.

Constipation

Constipation is the difficult or infrequent evacuation of feces. The urge to defecate is normally triggered by the pressure of feces on the rectum and by the intake of food into the stomach. On the toilet, the anal sphincter is relaxed voluntarily, and the fecal material is expelled. The

need to defecate should be attended to as soon as possible. Habitual disregard of the desire to empty the bowels reduces intestinal motion and leads to constipation.

Daily or regular bowel movements are not necessary for good health. Normal bowel movements may occur at irregular intervals due to variations in diet, mental stress, and physical activity. For some individuals, normal defecation may take place as infrequently as once every four days.

Simple Constipation

In simple constipation, the patient may have to practice good bowel movement habits, which include a trip to the toilet once daily, preferably after breakfast. Adequate fluid intake and proper diet, including fresh fruits and green vegetables, can help restore regular bowel movement. Laxatives can provide temporary relief, but they inhibit normal bowel function and lead to dependence. When toilet-training young children, parents should encourage but never force them to have regular bowel movements, preferably after breakfast.

Chronic Constipation

Chronic constipation can cause feces to accumulate in the rectum and *sigmoid,* the terminal section of the colon. The colonic fluid is absorbed and a mass of hard fecal material remains. Such impacted feces often prevent further passage of bowel contents. The individual suffers from abdominal pain with distension and sometimes vomiting. A cleansing enema will relieve the fecal impaction and related symptoms.

In the overall treatment of constipation, the principal cause must be identified and corrected so that normal evacuation can return.

Intestinal Obstructions

Obstruction to the free flow of digestive products may exist either in the stomach or in the small and large intestines. The typical symptoms of intestinal obstruction are constipation, painful abdominal distension, and vomiting. Intestinal obstruction can be caused by the bowel's looping or twisting around itself, forming what is known as a *volvulus*. Malignant tumors can either block the intestine or press it closed.

In infants, especially boys, a common form of intestinal obstruction occurs when a segment of the intestine folds into the section below it. This condition is known as *intussusception,* and can significantly reduce the blood supply to the lower bowel segment. The cause may be traced to viral infection, injury to the abdomen, hard food, or a foreign body in the gastrointestinal tract.

The presence of intestinal obstructions is generally determined by consideration of the clinical symptoms, as well as X-ray examinations of the abdomen. Hospitalization is required, since intestinal obstruction has a high fatality rate if proper medical care is not administered. Surgery may be needed to remove the obstruction.

Diarrhea

Diarrhea is the frequent and repeated passage of liquid stools. It is usually accompanied by intestinal inflammation, and sometimes by the passing of mucus or blood.

The principal cause of diarrhea is infection in the intestinal tract by microorganisms. Chemical and food poisoning also brings on spasms of diarrhea. Long-standing episodes of diarrhea have been traced to inflammation of the intestinal mucosa, tumors, ulcers, allergies, vitamin deficiency, and in some cases emotional stress. Diarrhea, in conjunction with

other symptoms, can also indicate infection with human immunodeficiency virus (HIV), the suspected cause of AIDS. See "AIDS" in Ch. 19, *Other Diseases of Major Importance.*

Patients with diarrhea commonly suffer abdominal cramps, lose weight from chronic attacks, or have vomiting spells. A physician must always be consulted for proper diagnosis and treatment; this is especially important if the attacks continue for more than two or three days. Untreated diarrhea can lead to dehydration and malnutrition; it may be fatal, especially in infants.

Dysentery

Dysentery is caused by microorganisms that thrive in the intestines of infected individuals. Most common are *amoebic dysentery,* caused by amoebae, and *bacillary dysentery,* caused by bacteria. The symptoms are diarrhea with blood and pus in the stools, cramps, and fever. The infection is spread from person to person through infected excrement that contaminates food or water. The bacteria and amoebae responsible can also be spread by houseflies which feed on feces as well as on human foods. It is

a common tropical disease and can occur wherever human excrement is not disposed of in a sanitary manner.

Dysentery must be treated early to avoid erosion of the intestinal wall. In bacillary dysentery, bed rest and hospitalization are recommended, especially for infants and the aged. Antibiotic drugs may be administered.

In most cases the disease can be spread by healthy human carriers who must be treated to check further spread.

Typhoid

Enteric fever or *typhoid* is an acute, highly communicable disease caused by the organism *Salmonella typhosa.* It is sometimes regarded as a tropical disease because epidemic outbreaks are common in tropical areas where careless disposal of feces and urine contaminates food, milk, and water supplies. In any location, tropical or temperate, where unsanitary living predominates, there is always the possibility that the disease can occur. Flies can transmit the disease, as can shellfish that live in typhoid-infested waters.

The typhoid bacilli do their damage to the mucosa of the small intestines.

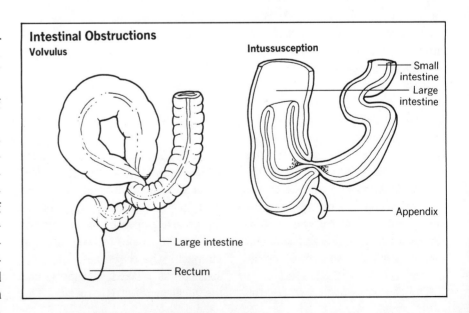

Intestinal Obstructions
Volvulus

Intussusception

Small intestine
Large intestine

Appendix

Large intestine

Rectum

They enter via the oral cavity and stomach and finally reach the lymph nodes and blood vessels in the small bowel.

Symptoms

Following an incubation period of about ten days, general bodily discomfort, fever, headache, nausea, and vomiting are experienced. Other clinical manifestations include abdominal pain with tenderness, greenish diarrhea (or constipation), bloody stools, and mental confusion. It is not unusual for red spots to appear on the body.

If untreated, typhoid victims die within 21 days of the onset of the disease. The cause of death may be perforation of the small bowel, abdominal hemorrhage, toxemia, or other complications such as intestinal inflammation and pneumonia.

Treatment and Prevention

A person can best recover from typhoid if he receives diligent medical and nursing care. He should be isolated in a hospital on complete bed rest. Diet should be restricted to highly nutritious liquids or preferably intravenous feeding. Destruction of the bacilli is achieved by antibiotic therapy, usually with Chloromycetin.

The best way to prevent the spread of typhoid is to disinfect all body refuse, clothing, and utensils of the person infected. Isolation techniques practiced in hospitals prevent local spread. Milk and milk products should always be pasteurized; drinking water should be chlorinated.

Human beings can carry the disease and infect others without themselves becoming ill; they are usually not aware that they are carriers. Within recent years, a vaccination effective for a year has been developed.

People traveling to areas where sanitation practices may be conducive to typhoid should receive this vaccination. In such areas, it is usually a good practice to boil drinking water as well.

Foreign Bodies in the Alimentary Tract

Anyone who accidentally swallows a foreign body should seek immediate medical aid, preferably in a hospital. Foreign bodies that enter the gastrointestinal tract may cause obstruction anywhere along the tract, including the esophagus. For emergency procedures, see "Obstruction of the Windpipe" in Ch. 31. *Medical Emergencies.*

Dental plates and large chunks of meat have been known to cause fatal choking. A foreign body in the esophagus may set off a reflex mechanism that causes the trachea to close. The windpipe may have to be opened by means of a *tracheostomy* (incision in the windpipe) to restore breathing. If the object swallowed is long and sharp-pointed, it may perforate the tract.

Foreign bodies in the esophagus are usually the most troublesome. Small fish bones may stick to the walls of the esophagus; large pieces of meat may block the tract. X-ray studies aid the physician in locating the swallowed object and in determining how best to deal with it.

Small objects like coins and paper clips may pass through the digestive tract without causing serious problems. Their progress may be checked by X rays of the abdomen. Examination of stools will indicate whether or not the entire object has been expelled. With larger objects, the problem of blockage must be considered. It is sometimes necessary for a surgeon to open the stomach in a hospital operating room and remove the foreign object.

Ulcers

A *peptic ulcer* is an eroded area of the mucous membrane of the digestive tract. The most common gastrointestinal ulcers are found in the lower end of the esophagus, stomach, or duodenum and are caused by the excessive secretion of gastric acid which erodes the lining membrane in these areas.

The cause of ulcers is obscure, but any factor that increases the gastric acidity may contribute to the condition. Mental stress or conflict, excessive food intake, alcohol, and caffeine all cause the stomach to increase its output of hydrochloric acid.

The disease is sometimes considered to be hereditary, especially among persons with type O blood. Symptoms usually appear in individuals of the 20-to-40 age group, with the highest incidence in persons over age 45. Peptic ulcers of the stomach (*gastric ulcers*) and duodenal ulcers occur more frequently in men than in women. Ulcers are common in patients with arthritis and chronic lung disease.

Symptoms

Early ulcer symptoms are gastric hyperacidity and burning abdominal pain that is relieved by eating, vomiting, or the use of antacids. The pain may occur as a dull ache, especially when one's stomach is empty, or it may be sharp and knifelike.

Other manifestations of a peptic ulcer are the following: nausea, associated with heartburn and regurgitation of gastric juice into the esophagus and mouth; excessive gas; poor appetite with undernourishment and weakness in older victims; and black stools resulting from a bleeding ulcer.

The immediate goal of ulcer therapy is to heal the ulcer; the long-term goal is to prevent its recurrence. An ulcer normally heals through the formation of scar tissue in the ulcer crater. The healing process, under proper medical care, may take several weeks. The disappearance of pain does not necessarily indicate that the ulcer has healed completely, or even partially. The pain and the ulcerative process may recur at regular intervals over periods of weeks or months.

Although treatment can result in complete healing and recovery, some victims of chronic peptic ulcers have a 20-to-30-year history of periodic recurrences. For such patients, ulcer therapy may have to be extended indefinitely to avoid serious complications. If a recurrent ulcer perforates the stomach or intestine, or if it bleeds excessively, it can be quickly fatal. Emergency surgery is always required when perforation and persistent bleeding occur.

Treatment

The basic principles of ulcer therapy are diet, rest, and the suppression of stomach acidity. A patient with an active gastric ulcer is generally hospitalized for three weeks to make certain that he receives the proper diet and to remove him from sources of emotional stress, such as business or family problems. During hospitalization the healing process is monitored by X-ray examination. If there is no evidence of healing within three to four weeks, surgery may be advisable. For patients with duodenal ulcers, a week or two of rest at home with proper diet may be sufficient.

Ulcer diets consist of low-residue bland foods taken in small amounts at frequent intervals, as often as once an hour when pain is severe. The preferred foods are milk, soft eggs, jellies, custards, creams, and cooked cereals. See "Minimal Residue Diet" in Ch. 27, *Nutrition and Weight Control*. Because ulcer diets often lack some essential nutrients, prolonged

dietary treatment may have to be augmented with daily vitamin capsules. Antispasmodic medication may be prescribed to reduce contractions of the stomach, decrease the stomach's production of acid, and slow down digestion. Antacids, such as the combination of aluminum hydroxide and magnesium trisilicate, may be required after meals and between feedings. Spicy foods, alcohol, coffee, cola and other caffeine-containing drinks, large meals, and smoking should be strictly avoided.

In addition to common antacids, some new drugs have been introduced to help treat ulcers and other digestive disorders. Tagamet in particular, a brand name for the drug cimetidine, has been found to be effective in treating duodenal ulcers. It has also been used to prevent ulcer-related stomach, esophagus, and duodenal problems. The drug acts primarily to reduce secretions of gastric acid. But side effects have been reported, some of them serious. These include mental confusion, fever, slowed pulse, and others. Metiamide, another drug used to control the production of gastric acids in the digestive system, has been found to attack the leukocytes or white cells of the blood. Other problems have been reported with metiamide.

If the ulcer does not respond to medical therapy, or if pain persists, surgery may be the preferred treatment. Such surgery is elective surgery, a matter of choice, as opposed to the emergency surgery required by large, bleeding, or perforated ulcers. After the removal of the acid-producing section of the stomach, some patients may develop weakness and nausea as their digestive system adjusts to the reduced size of their stomach. A proper diet of special foods and fluids, plus sedatives, can alleviate the condition. The chances for complete recovery are good. For

a full description of surgical treatment of peptic ulcers, see "Peptic Ulcers" in Ch. 20, *Surgery*.

Diverticula

A *diverticulum* is an abnormal pouch caused by herniation of the mucous membrane of the digestive tract. The pouch has a narrow neck and a bulging round end. Diverticula are found in the esophagus, stomach, duodenum, colon, and other parts of the digestive tract.

The presence of diverticula in any segment of the digestive tract is referred to as *diverticulosis*. When diverticula become inflamed the condition is known as *diverticulitis*. The latter is a common form of disease of the sigmoid colon and is found in persons past the age of 45.

In mild cases, there may be no symptoms. On the other hand, a diverticulum may sometimes rupture and produce the same symptoms as an acute attack of appendicitis—vomiting and pain with tenderness in the right lower portion of the abdomen. Other symptoms are intermittent constipation and diarrhea, and abdominal pain.

Diverticulosis is treated by bed rest, restriction of solid food and increase of fluid intake, and administration of antibiotics. Surgery is recommended when diverticulosis causes obstruction of the colon or creates an

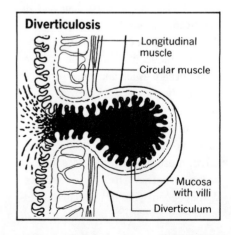

Diverticulosis

Longitudinal muscle
Circular muscle
Mucosa with villi
Diverticulum

opening between the colon and the bladder, or when one or more diverticula rupture and perforate the colon. The outlook for recovery following surgery is good.

Hemorrhoids (Piles)

Hemorrhoids, or *piles,* are round, purplish protuberances at the anus. They are the results of rectal veins that become dilated and rupture. Hemorrhoids are very common and are often caused by straining because of constipation, pregnancy, or diarrhea.

Hemorrhoids may appear on the external side of the anus or on the internal side; they may or may not be painful. Rectal bleeding and tenderness are common. It is important to emphasize, however, that not all rectal bleeding results from hemorrhoids. Small hemorrhoids are best left untreated; large painful ones may be surgically reduced or removed. *Prolapsed* piles—those that have slipped forward—are treated by gentle pressure to return the hemorrhoidal mass into the rectum. The rectal and anal opening must be lubricated to keep the area soft. Other conditions in the large bowel can simulate hemorrhoids and need to be adequately investigated.

Hernias

Hernias in the digestive tract occur

Hemorrhoids

Internal
External

when there is muscular weakness in surrounding body structures. Pressure from the gastrointestinal tract may cause a protrusion or *herniation* of the gut through the weakened wall. Such hernias exist in the diaphragmatic area (*hiatus hernias,* discussed above), in the anterior abdomen (*ventral hernias*), or in the region of the groin (*inguinal hernias*). Apart from hiatus hernias, inguinal hernias are by far the most common.

One of the causes of intestinal obstruction is a *strangulated hernia.* A loop of herniated bowel becomes

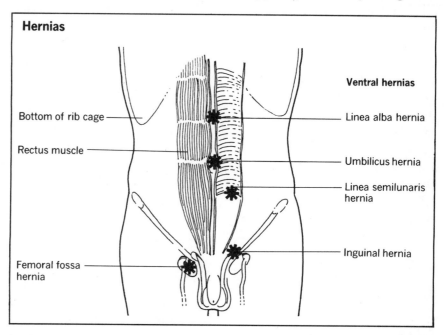

Hernias

Bottom of rib cage
Rectus muscle
Femoral fossa hernia

Ventral hernias
Linea alba hernia
Umbilicus hernia
Linea semilunaris hernia
Inguinal hernia

tightly constricted, blood supply is cut off, and the loop becomes gangrenous. Immediate surgery is required since life is threatened from further complications.

Except for hiatus hernias, diagnosis is usually made simple by the plainly visible herniated part. In men, an enlarged scrotum may be present in untreated inguinal hernias. The herniating bowel can be reduced, that is, manipulated back into position, and a truss worn to support the reduced hernia and provide temporary relief. In all hernias, however, surgical repair is the usual treatment.

Gastritis

Gastritis is inflammation of the mucosa of the stomach. The patient complains of *epigastric* pain—in the middle of the upper abdomen—with distension of the stomach, loss of appetite, nausea, and vomiting.

Attacks of acute gastritis can be traced to bacterial action, food poisoning, peptic ulcer, the presence of alcohol in the stomach, the ingestion of highly spiced foods, or overeating and drinking. Occasional gastritis, though painful, is not serious and may disappear spontaneously. The general treatment for gastritis is similar to the treatment of a gastric ulcer.

Enteritis

Enteritis, sometimes referred to as *regional enteritis,* is a chronic inflammatory condition of unknown origin that affects the small intestine. It is called regional because the disease most often involves the terminal ileum, even though any segment of the digestive tract can be involved. The diseased bowel becomes involved with multiple ulcer craters and ultimately stiffens because of fibrous healing of the ulcers.

Regional enteritis occurs most often in males from adolescence to middle age. The symptoms may exist for a long period before the disease is recognized. Intermittent bloody diarrhea, general weakness, and lassitude are the early manifestations. Later stages of the disease are marked by fever, increased bouts of diarrhea with resultant weight loss, and sharp lower abdominal pain on the right side. This last symptom sometimes causes the disease to be confused with appendicitis, because in both conditions there is nausea and vomiting. Occasionally in women there may be episodes of painful menstruation.

Treatment involves either surgical removal of the diseased bowel or conservative medical management and drug therapy. In acute attacks of enteritis, bed rest and intravenous fluids are two important aspects of treatment. Medical management in less severe occurrences includes a daily diet rich in proteins and vitamins, excluding harder foods such as fresh fruits and vegetables. Antibiotics are prescribed to combat bacterial invasion.

Colitis

Colitis is an inflammatory condition of the colon, of uncertain origin, and often chronic. It may result from a nervous predisposition which leads to bacterial or viral infection. The inflammation can cause spasms that damage the colon, or can lead to bleeding ulcers that may be fatal.

In milder forms, colitis first appears with diarrhea in which red bloody streaks can be observed. The symptoms may come and go for weeks before the effects become very significant. As the disease process advances, the diarrhea episodes become more frequent; more blood

and mucus are present in the feces. These are combined with abdominal pain, nausea, and vomiting. Because of the loss of blood, the patient often becomes anemic and thin. If there are ulcer craters in the mucosa, the disease is called *ulcerative colitis.*

Hospitalization is necessary in order to provide proper treatment that will have a long-term effect. Surgery is sometimes necessary if an acute attack has been complicated by perforation of the intestines or if chronic colitis fails to respond to medical management.

Nonoperative treatment includes control of diarrhea and vomiting by drug therapy. Antibiotics are given to control infection and reduce fever, which always accompanies infection. A high protein and vitamin diet is necessary. But if the diarrhea and vomiting persist, intravenous feeding becomes a must. Blood transfusions may be required for individuals who have had severe rectal bleeding. Because there is no absolute cure, the disease may recur.

Appendicitis

The *vermiform appendix* is a narrow tubular attachment to the colon. It can become obstructed by the presence of undigested food such as small seeds from fruits or by hard bits of feces. This irritates the appendix and causes inflammation to set in. If it is obstructed, pressure builds within the appendix because of increasing secretions, a situation that can result in rupture of the appendix. A ruptured appendix can be rapidly fatal if *peritonitis,* inflammation of the peritoneal cavity, sets in.

In most cases the onset of appendicitis is heralded by an acute attack of pain in the center of the abdomen. The pain intensity increases, shifts to the right lower abdomen with nausea, vomiting, and fever as added symp-

toms. Some individuals, however, suffer from recurrent attacks of dull pain without other signs of gastrointestinal disease, and these may not be significant enough to warrant immediate hospitalization.

Diagnosis of appendicitis is usually dependent on the above symptoms, along with tenderness in the appendix area, increased pulse rate, and decreasing blood pressure. The last two are very significant if the appendix ruptures and peritonitis sets in. Whenever these symptoms are observed, the patient should be rushed to the nearest hospital.

Immediate surgical removal of the diseased appendix by means of a small incision is necessary in all nonperforated acute cases. This type of operation (*appendectomy*) is no longer considered major surgery. If the appendix ruptures and peritonitis is evident, emergency major surgery is necessary to drain the infection and remove the appendix. In the absence of postoperative complications, the patient recovers completely. One of the major problems of appendicitis is early diagnosis to prevent dangerous complications.

Intestinal Parasites

Not all the diseases of man are caused by microscopic organisms. Some are caused by parasitic worms, *helminths,* which invade the digestive tract, most often via food and water. In recent years government health agencies have largely eliminated the prime sources of worm infection: unwholesome meat or untreated sewage that finds its way into drinking water. Nevertheless, helminths still exist. Drugs used to expel worms are called *vermifuges* or *anthelmintics.*

The following are among the major intestinal parasites.

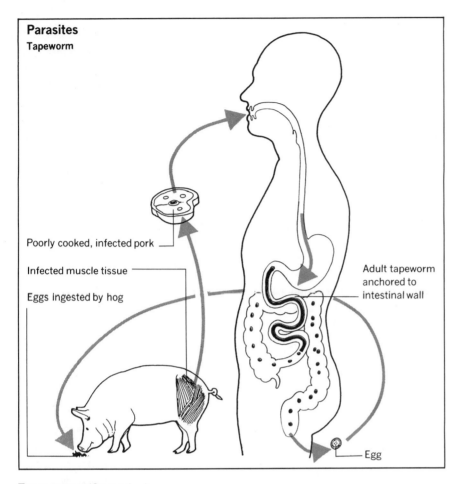

Parasites
Tapeworm

Poorly cooked, infected pork

Infected muscle tissue

Eggs ingested by hog

Adult tapeworm anchored to intestinal wall

Egg

Tapeworms (Cestodes)

These ribbon-shaped flatworms are found primarily in beef, fish, and pork that have not been thoroughly cooked. There are several species ranging from inch-long worms to tapeworms that grow to about 30 feet and live for as long as 16 years.

Tapeworms attach themselves to intestinal mucosa and periodically expel their eggs in excreta. If such feces are carelessly disposed of, the eggs can reach drinking water and be taken in by fish or ingested by grazing cattle. The eggs hatch in the animal's large bowel and find their way into the bloodstream by boring through the intestinal wall. Once in the blood they eventually adhere to muscles and live a dormant life in a capsule.

People who eat raw or partially cooked meat and fish that are infested with tapeworms become infected. The worms enter the bowel, where they feed, grow, and produce eggs. When the egg-filled segments are excreted, the cycle begins anew. Tapeworm infection is usually asymptomatic. It is discovered when egg-laden segments in feces are recognized as such.

Medication must be given on an empty stomach, followed later by a laxative. This will dislodge the worms and enable the body to purge itself of them. A weekly check of stools for segments of the worms may be necessary to confirm that the host is free of the parasites.

Hookworms

There are many species of these tiny, threadlike worms which are usually less than one centimeter long. They are found principally in tropical and subtropical areas of China, North Africa, Europe, Central America, and the West Indies, but they are by no means extinct in the United States.

The eggs are excreted in the feces of infected individuals, and if fecal materials are not well disposed of, the eggs may be found on the ground of unsanitary areas. In warm, moist conditions they hatch into larvae that penetrate the skin, especially the feet of people who walk around barefooted. The larvae can also be swallowed in impure water.

Hookworm-infected individuals, most often children, may experience an inflammatory itch in the area where the larvae entered. The host becomes anemic from blood loss, due to parasitic feeding of the worms, develops a cough, and experiences abdominal pain with diarrhea. Sometimes there is nausea or a distended abdomen. Diagnosis is confirmed by laboratory analysis of feces for the presence of eggs.

Successful treatment requires administration of anthelmintic drugs, preferably before breakfast, to destroy the worms. Weekly laboratory examination of the feces for evidence of hookworm eggs is a necessary precaution in ascertaining that the disease has been eradicated. Untreated hookworm infestation often leads to small bowel obstruction.

Trichinosis

This sometimes fatal disease is caused by a tiny worm, *Trichinella spiralis*, which is spread to man by eating improperly cooked pork containing the tiny worms in a capsulated form. After they are ingested the worms are set free to attach themselves to the mucosa of the small intestines. Here they mature in a few days and mate; the male dies and the female lays eggs that reach the muscles via the vascular system.

Trichinella organisms cause irritation of the intestinal mucosa. The infected individual suffers from abdominal pains with diarrhea, nausea, and vomiting. Later stages of the disease are marked by stiffness, pain, and swelling in the muscles, fever with sweating, respiratory distress, insomnia, and swelling of the face and eyelids. Death may result from complications such as pneumonia, heart damage, or respiratory failure. Despite government inspection of meats, all pork should be well-cooked before eating.

Threadworms (Nematodes)

These worms, also called pinworms, infect children more often than adults. Infection occurs by way of the mouth. The worms live in the bowel and sometimes journey through the anus, where they cause intense itching. The eggs are laid at the anal opening, and can be blown about in the air and spread in that manner. The entire family must be medically treated to kill the egg-laying females, and soothing ointment should be applied at the rectal area to relieve the itching. Good personal hygiene, especially hand washing after toilet use, is an essential part of the treatment.

Roundworms (Ascaris)

These intestinal parasites closely resemble earthworms. The eggs enter the digestive tract and hatch in the small bowel. The young parasites then penetrate the walls of the bowel, enter the bloodstream, and find their way to the liver, heart, and lungs.

Untreated roundworm infestation leads to intestinal obstruction or blockage of pancreatic and bile ducts caused by the masses of roundworms, which usually exist in the hundreds. Ingestion of vermifuge drugs is the required treatment.

Food Poisoning

Acute gastrointestinal illnesses may result from eating food that is itself poisonous, from ingesting chemical poisons, or from bacterial sources. The bacteria can either manufacture *toxins* (poisonous substances) or cause infection. Improperly canned fish, meats, and vegetables may encourage the growth of certain toxin-manufacturing organisms that resist the action of gastric juice when ingested. A person who eats such foods may contract a type of food poisoning known as *botulism*. The symptoms include indigestion and abdominal pain, nausea and vomiting, blurred vision, dryness in the mouth and throat, and poor muscular coordination.

If the toxins become fixed in the central nervous system, they may cause death. Emergency hospitalization is required, where antitoxins are administered intravenously and other measures are taken to combat the effects of botulism.

Salmonella food poisoning is caused by a species of bacteria of that name and is spread by eating contaminated meat, or by eating fish, egg, and milk products that have not been properly cooked or stored or have been inadequately refrigerated. The organisms are also transmitted by individuals who handle well-prepared food with dirty hands. Victims suffer from vomiting, diarrhea, abdominal pain, and fever. This type of food poisoning can be fatal in children and the aged, especially if the latter are ailing. Medical treatment with hospitalization, administration of broad-spectrum antibiotics, and intravenous fluids (to replace water loss due to vomiting) is required.

Some people develop allergic reactions to certain foods and break out in severe rashes after a meal containing any of these foods. Among such foods are fruits, eggs, and milk or milk products. Vomiting or diarrhea may also occur. The best treatment is to avoid eating such foods and, when necessary, supplement the diet with manufactured protein and vitamins.

Liver Disease

Cirrhosis

Chronic disease of the liver with the destruction of liver cells is known as *cirrhosis*. A common cause is excessive intake of alcoholic beverages along with malnutrition. However, there are other predisposing factors, such as inflammation of the liver (*hepatitis*), syphilis, intestinal worms, jaundice or biliary tract inflammation, and disorders in blood circulation to the liver.

Victims of cirrhosis are usually anemic and have an elevated temperature, around 100° F. Alcoholics very often lose weight, suffer from indigestion, and have distended abdomens.

Accurate diagnosis of cirrhosis depends on complex laboratory tests of liver function, urine, and blood. If liver damage is not too far advanced, treatment of the complications and underlying causes can aid the liver cells in the process of regeneration. In long-standing chronic disease, liver damage may be irreversible. Alcoholics who forgo alcohol may be restored to health, depending on the extent of liver damage, with a proper diet rich in proteins and vitamins.

Successful treatment of liver cirrhosis may require long hospitalization with drug therapy and blood transfusions. During alcoholic withdrawal, the patient may require close medical observation and psychiatric help. If the patient's jaundice improves and his appetite returns, recovery in milder cirrhosis cases is possible.

Jaundice

In diseases of the liver and biliary tract, excessive bile pigment (*bilirubin*) is recirculated into the bloodstream. It enters the mucous membranes and skin, giving them the characteristic yellow pigmentation of the disease.

Gallstones or tumors that obstruct the free flow of bile are one cause of jaundice. Other causes include hepatitis, overproduction of bile pigments with resultant accumulation of bile within the liver, cirrhosis, and congenital closure of the bile ducts, the last a common cause of jaundice in infancy.

Apart from the typical yellow appearance of the skin, jaundice generates such symptoms as body itching, vomiting with bile (indicated by the green appearance and bitter taste), diarrhea with undigested fats present in the stools, and enlargement of the liver with pain and tenderness in the right upper abdomen.

Treatment of jaundice requires continued medical care with hospitalization. Surgery may be necessary to remove stones in the biliary tract or other obstructions. If there is bacterial infection, antibiotic therapy is necessary.

Hepatitis

Inflammation of the liver results in the disease known as *hepatitis*. The most common cause is an infectious process brought on by viruses, jaundice, or high fevers. Other causes of hepatitis include intestinal parasites, circulatory disturbances (such as congestive heart failure), hypersensitivity to drugs, damage to the liver or kidneys, or bacterial infection elsewhere in the body.

One common form of this disease is *infectious hepatitis*, a highly contagious viral infection that often attacks children and young adults, especially those who congregate in large groups. Infectious hepatitis has been known to break out as an epidemic in schools, summer camps, music festivals, and military installations.

The virus is spread by food and water contaminated by feces from infected individuals; good sanitation thus becomes a vital preventive factor. Whole blood used in transfusions can transmit the organisms if the donor is infected. This form of the disease is known as *serum hepatitis* or *hepatitis B*. With the great increase in the use of blood transfusions in recent years in complex surgery, the danger of transmitting hepatitis B by infected blood or infected syringes has become correspondingly greater. Drug addicts are particularly vulnerable to hepatitis B from the use of shared, infected needles.

Symptoms

The incubation period of infectious hepatitis lasts from one to six weeks—that of hepatitis B is longer—followed by fever with headache, loss of appetite (especially for fatty foods), and gastrointestinal distress (nausea, vomiting, diarrhea, or constipation). As the disease progresses, the liver becomes enlarged and the patient jaundiced. There may be some pain in the right upper abdomen.

Treatment

Bed rest, preferably hospital isolation, is a necessary step in the initial treatment stages. Drug therapy with steroids may hasten the recovery process, which may take three to four weeks. When discharged from the hospital, the patient is usually very weak.

Untreated hepatitis causes severe liver damage and may result in coma resulting from liver failure. Sometimes death occurs. Several assaults on the liver reduce the regeneration process and promote cirrhosis. Persons who may have been exposed to the causative virus can receive temporary immunity if they are given an injection of gamma globulin, especially if there is an epidemic. Recent research directed toward the development of a vaccine against serum hepatitis has been very encouraging, and gives rise to the hope that some day wide-scale outbreaks of this disease may become a thing of the past.

Research directed toward the development of a vaccine against hepatitis B, one of three forms of the disease, resulted in the first genetically engineered vaccine. Called Recombivax HB, the vaccine opened a new era in disease prevention. Scientists genetically altered a special type of brewers' yeast to produce a part of the hepatitis B virus. Injected into humans, the vaccine carrying the virus touches off a protective immune system response. Researchers believed similar methods could lead to the development of other vaccines.

An older vaccine for hepatitis B was made from the blood plasma of people infected with the hepatitis B virus. Because the vaccine derived from human blood, there was a small possibility that the vaccine could transmit acquired immune deficiency syndrome (AIDS). The new vaccine eliminates that danger.

Gallbladder Disease

The biliary tract is very often plagued by the presence of stones, either in the gallbladder or in one of the bile ducts. Gallstones are mostly a mixture of calcium carbonate, cholesterol, and bile salts, and can occur either as one large stone, a few smaller ones, or several very small stones.

When fats from the daily diet enter

the small intestines, the concentrated bile from the gallbladder is poured into the duodenum via the bile ducts. Bile is necessary if fats are to be digested and absorbed. If stones are present in the biliary tract, the gallbladder will contract, but little or no bile will reach the fats in the small bowel.

A sharp pain to the right of the stomach is usually the first warning sign of gallstones, especially if the pain is felt soon after a meal of fatty foods—eggs, pork, mayonnaise, or fried foods. The presence of stones very often causes inflammation of the gallbladder and such symptoms as occasional diarrhea and nausea with vomiting and belching. The abdominal area near the gallbladder is usually very tender.

Untreated gallbladder disease leads to several possible complications. The obstructed bile pigments may be recirculated in the bloodstream, causing jaundice. Obstruction of the ducts causes increased pressure and may also result in perforation of the gallbladder or ducts. Acute inflammation of the biliary tract is always a possibility due to the irritation caused by the concentrated bile.

A gallbladder that is full of stones or badly diseased must be surgically removed for the patient's health to improve. In milder cases, other treatment and special diet can prevent attacks.

Treatment and Diagnosis of Gastrointestinal Disorders

Some medications used in treating gastrointestinal disorders, such as antacids and laxatives, can be purchased without prescription. Such medications should be taken only upon a physician's advice.

Treatment of gastrointestinal diseases may require low-residue diets—that is, a diet of foods that pass through the digestive tract very readily without a large amount of solid fecal residue. Included are low-fat meals, liquids, and finely crushed foods. Diagnostic tests may require overnight fasting, fat-free meals, or eating specific foods. Bland meals are vital in the treatment of peptic ulcers and should consist of unspiced soft foods and milk. Raw fruits and vegetables, salads, alcohol, and coffee do not belong in a bland diet. See under Ch. 27, *Nutrition and Weight Control,* for further information on special diets.

X-ray examinations play an important role in diagnosis of gastrointes-tinal disorders, such as ulcers, diverticula, foreign bodies, malignant lesions, obstruction, achalasia of the esophagus, and varices.

Plain film radiographs are used in initial studies in cases where intestinal obstruction or perforation is suspected. Metallic foreign bodies are easily demonstrated on plain X rays of the digestive tract.

GI Series

By filling the digestive tract with *barium sulfate,* a substance opaque to X rays, a radiologist can locate areas of abnormality. Barium sulfate can be mixed as a thin liquid or paste and be swallowed by the patient during studies of the esophagus, stomach, and small intestines. The type of radiological examination that utilizes such a barium meal is known as a *GI* (gastrointestinal) *series*. The large bowel is examined with the barium mixture administered through the rectum like a standard enema, known as a *barium enema*. This procedure makes it possible to visualize the inner walls of the colon. For further information on diagnostic procedures, see Ch. 26, *Physicians and Diagnostic Procedures*.

12

Diseases of the Respiratory System

The human body cannot survive for more than a very few minutes in an environment that lacks oxygen. Oxygen is required for the normal functioning of all living body cells. This vital gas reaches the body cells via the bloodstream; each red blood cell transports oxygen molecules to the body tissues. The oxygen comes from the atmosphere one breathes, and it enters the bloodstream through the very thin membrane walls of the lung tissue, a fresh supply of oxygen entering the bloodstream each time a person inhales. As the red blood cells circulating through the walls of the lung tissue pick up their fresh supply of oxygen, they release molecules of carbon dioxide given off by the body cells as a waste product of metabolism. When a person exhales, the lungs are squeezed somewhat like a bellows, and the carbon dioxide is expelled from the lungs.

The automatic action of breathing in and out is caused by the alternate contraction and relaxation of several muscle groups. The main muscle of breathing is the *diaphragm,* a layer of muscle fibers that separates the organs of the chest from the organs of the abdomen. Other muscles of respiration are located between the ribs, in the neck, and in the abdomen. As the diaphragm contracts to let the lungs expand, the other muscles increase the capacity of the *thorax,* or chest cavity, when one inhales. The muscles literally squeeze the lungs and chest when an individual exhales.

Any disease of the muscles and bones of the chest wall or of the passages leading from the nose to the lung tissue—containing the small air sacs where the gases are actually exchanged—will interfere to some extent with normal function. As with any organ of the body, there is a great reserve built into the lungs that assures that small to even moderate amounts of diseased tissue can exist without compromising their ability to sustain life. However, when disease of the lungs, air passages, thoracic (rib) cage, or any combination of these parts decreases the capacity of the reserve areas, then the oxygen supply to all the organs and tissues of the body becomes deficient, and they become incapable of performing their vital functions.

Diseases of the thoracic cage are relatively uncommon. Certain forms of arthritis cause fixation of the bony cage and limit expansion when breathing. Various muscle and nervous system diseases weaken the muscles used to expand the chest for breathing.

Diseases of the *bronchi* or air passages tend to narrow those tubes and thereby limit the amount of air that can pass through to the tiny *alveoli,* or air sacs. Other conditions affect the alveoli themselves, and, if widespread enough, allow no place for the oxygen and carbon dioxide to be exchanged.

The most common forms of lung disease are infections caused by vi-

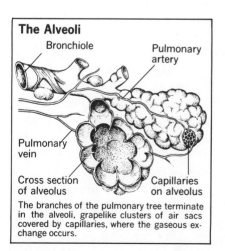

The Alveoli

Bronchiole

Pulmonary artery

Pulmonary vein

Cross section of alveolus

Capillaries on alveolus

The branches of the pulmonary tree terminate in the alveoli, grapelike clusters of air sacs covered by capillaries, where the gaseous exchange occurs.

Interaction between Heart and Lungs

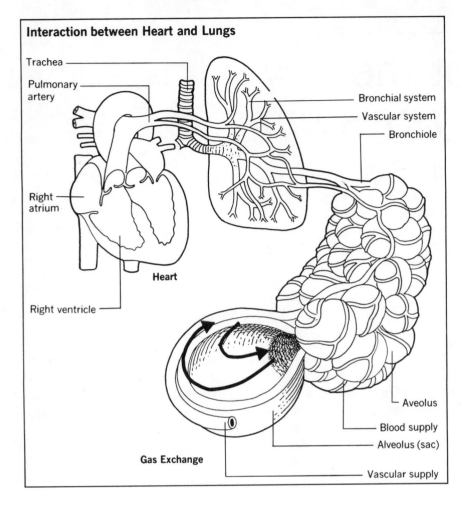

Trachea

Pulmonary artery

Right atrium

Right ventricle

Heart

Bronchial system

Vascular system

Bronchiole

Aveolus

Blood supply

Alveolus (sac)

Vascular supply

Gas Exchange

weather, fatigue, and other factors.

For years it has been felt that chilling plays a role in causing the common cold, and, although difficult to prove, there is almost certainly some truth to the idea. By some as yet unclear process, chilling probably causes certain changes in our respiratory passages that make them susceptible to viruses that otherwise would be harmless.

The common cold affects only the upper respiratory passages: the nose, sinuses, and throat. It sometimes is associated with fever. Several viruses have been implicated as the cause for the common cold. But in the study centers that investigate this illness, isolation of a cold virus is only achieved in about one half of the cases. These viruses are not known to produce any other significant illnesses. Most likely they inhabit the nose and throat, often without producing any illness at all.

Symptoms

The major part of the illness consists of about three days of nasal congestion, possibly a mild sore throat, some sneezing and irritation of the eyes (though not as severe as in hay fever), and a general feeling of ill health often associated with some muscle fatigue and aching. After three days the symptoms abate, but there is usually some degree of nasal congestion for another ten days.

Prevention is difficult, and there is no specific treatment. The natural defenses of the body usually are capable of resolving the infection. Attention should be paid to avoiding further chilling of the body, exhausting activity, and late hours that can further lower the defenses and lead to complications.

Complications

Ear infection may develop because of

ruses, bacteria, or fungi. Infection is always a potential threat to the lung because this organ is in constant contact with the outside air and therefore constantly exposed to infectious agents. It is only through elaborate defenses that the body is able to maintain normal functions without interference by these agents.

The major defenses are simply mechanical and consist mainly of the hairs in the nose and a mucous blanket coating the inside of the bronchi. The very small hairs (called *cilia*) in the breathing passage act as a filtering system; mucous membranes of the bronchi help to intercept small particles as they are swept along by the action of the cilia. Whenever these structures are diseased, as in chronic bronchitis, there is a much greater likelihood of acquiring infection.

The Common Cold, Influenza, and Other Viral Infections

The Common Cold

The common cold is the most prevalent illness known to mankind. It accounts for more time lost from work than any other single condition. The infection rate varies from one individual to another.

Surveys indicate that about 25 percent of the population experience four or more infections a year, 50 percent experience two or three a year, and the remaining 25 percent have one or no infections in a year. There is also some variation from year to year for each person, explained often by the amount of exposure to young children, frequent extreme changes in blockage of the *Eustachian tube,* which leads from the back of the throat to the inner part of the ear. That complication is heralded by pain in the ear. Bronchitis and pneumonia may be recognized early by the development of cough and production of *sputum* (phlegm). *Sinusitis* develops when the sinus passages are obstructed so that the infected mucus cannot drain into the pharynx (as in postnasal drip). The pain develops near the sinus cavity involved. These complications can and should be treated with specific drugs, and, if they develop, a physician should be consulted.

Influenza

A number of other viruses cause respiratory illness similar to the common cold, but are much more severe in intensity and with frequently serious, and even fatal, complications. The best known member of the group is the *influenza* (flu) virus. It can cause mild symptoms that are indistinguishable from those of the common cold, but in the more easily recognizable form it is ushered in by fever, cough, and what physicians refer to as *malaise*—chills, muscle ache, and fatigue.

The symptoms of influenza appear quickly; they develop within hours and generally last in severe form from four to seven days. The disease gradually recedes over the following week. The severity of the local respiratory and generalized symptoms usually forces the influenza patient to stay in bed.

Not only is the individual case often severe, but an outbreak of influenza can easily spread to epidemic proportions in whole population groups, closing factories, schools, and hospitals in its wake. There have been 31 very severe *pandemics* (epidemics that sweep many countries) that have occurred since 1510. The most devastating of these pandemics occurred in 1918; it led to the death of 20 million people around the world. Rarely is death directly attributable to the influenza virus itself, but rather to complicating bacterial pneumonia or to the failure of vital organs previously weakened by chronic disease.

Flu Shots

Inoculation is fairly effective in preventing influenza, but is not long-lasting and has to be renewed each year. Unfortunately, there are several different types of influenza virus, and a slightly different vaccine is needed to provide immunity to each type of infection. Each recent epidemic in the United States has been the result of a different strain, and although there have been several months' warning before the epidemics started, it has been difficult to mass-produce a vaccine in time to use it before the epidemic developed.

Treatment

Once acquired, there is no cure for influenza, but the body defenses are usually capable of destroying the virus if given the necessary time and if the defenses are not depressed by other illness. Fluids, aspirin, and bed rest help relieve the symptoms. Special attention should be paid to sudden worsening of fever after seeming recovery, or the onset of sputum production. In elderly people more intensive medical care is often necessary, including hospitalization for some.

Pneumonia

Pneumonia might be defined as any inflammation of the lung tissue itself, but the term is generally applied only to infections of an acute or rapidly developing nature caused by certain bacteria or viruses. The term is generally not used for tuberculous or fungal infections. The most common severe pneumonia is that caused by the *pneumococcus bacterium.*

Pneumonia develops from inhaling infected mucus into the lower respiratory passages. The pneumococcus is often present in the nasal or throat secretions of healthy people, and it tends to be present even more often in the same secretions of an individual with a cold. Under certain conditions these secretions may be *aspirated,* or inhaled, into the lung. There the bacteria rapidly multiply and spread within hours to infect a sizable area. As with the common cold, chilling and fatigue often play a role in making this sequence possible. Any chronic debilitating illness also makes one very susceptible to pneumonia.

Symptoms

Pneumonia develops very suddenly with the onset of high fever, shaking chills, chest pain, and a very definite feeling of total sickness or malaise. Within hours enough pus is produced within the lung for the patient to start coughing up thick yellow or greenish sputum that often may be tinged or streaked with blood. The patient has no problem in recognizing that he has suddenly become extremely ill.

Prior to penicillin the illness tended to last about seven days, at which time it would often suddenly resolve almost as quickly as it started, leaving a healthy but exhausted patient. But it also could frequently lead to death or to serious complications, such as abscess formation within the chest wall, meningitis, or abscess of the brain. Because penicillin is so very effective in curing this illness today, physicians rarely see those complications.

Treatment

The response of pneumococcal pneumonia to penicillin is at times one of the most dramatic therapeutic events in medicine. After only several hours of illness the patient presents himself to the hospital with a fever of 104° F, feeling so miserable that he does not want to eat, talk, or do anything but lie still in bed. Within four to six hours after being given penicillin he may have lost his fever and be sitting up in bed eating a meal. Not everyone responds this dramatically, but when someone does, it is striking.

Prevention

There is no guaranteed way to prevent pneumonia. The advice to avoid chilling temperatures, overexertion, and fatigue when one has a cold is directed principally toward avoiding pneumonia. Anybody exposed to the elements, especially when fatigued and wearing damp clothing, is particularly susceptible to pneumonia; this explains its frequent occurrence among army recruits and combat troops. The elderly and debilitated become more susceptible when exposed to extremes of temperature and dampness.

Pneumonia is not really a contagious illness except in very special circumstances, so that isolation of patients is not necessary. In fact, all of us carry the pneumococcus in our noses and throats, but we rarely have the constellation of circumstances that lead to infection. It is the added physical insults that allow pneumonia to take hold.

Other Kinds of Pneumonia

All bacteria are capable of causing pneumonia and they do so in the same manner, via the inhalation of infected upper airway secretions. Some diseases, such as alcoholism, tend to predispose to certain bacterial pneumonias. Usually these are not as dramatic as those caused by the pneumococcus, but they may be much more difficult to treat and thereby can often be more serious.

Far less severe are the pneumonias caused by certain viruses or a recently discovered organism that seems to be intermediate between a virus and a bacterium. The term *walking pneumonia* is often applied to this type, because the patient is often so little incapacitated that he is walking about and not in bed. These pneumonias apparently occur in the same way as the bacterial pneumonias, but the difference is that the infecting agent is not capable of producing such severe destruction. These pneumonias are usually associated with only mild temperature elevation, scant amount of sputum production, and fewer general body symptoms. They should be suspected when coughing dominates the symptoms of a cold, especially if it turns from a dry or nonproductive cough to one that produces sputum. Antibiotic therapy tends to hasten recovery and prevent the complication of bacterial pneumonia.

Pleurisy

No discussion of pneumonia is complete without mention of *pleurisy*. This term refers to any inflammation of the lining between the chest wall and the lung. Infection is only one of the causes, but probably the most common, of inflammation of the *pleura*. Pleurisy is almost always painful, the pain being felt on inhaling and exhaling but not when the breath is quietly held for a brief period. It is a symptom that always deserves the attention of a physician and investigation of its cause. The same type of pain on breathing can often be mimicked by a strain of the chest wall muscles, but the difference can usually be determined by a physician's examination. If not, a chest X ray will help to reveal the cause of the pain.

Tuberculosis

At the turn of the century *tuberculosis* was the leading cause of death in the world; now it is eighteenth. The change in status is due both to the discovery of antibiotics and to modern preventive measures. In this century most other infectious diseases have likewise decreased in incidence and severity for similar reasons. The general decline leaves tuberculosis still at the top of the list as the leading cause of death among infectious diseases. And tuberculosis remains a very serious health problem, accounting for 40,000 new illnesses every year in the United States. In contrast to a disease like influenza, physicians already have the tools with which to eliminate tuberculosis. But many factors, primarily social, make that a very distant possibility.

Tuberculosis is caused by one specific type of bacterium. Certain ethnic groups seem particularly susceptible to the disease, but the reasons are unclear. The American Indian and the Eskimo are two susceptible groups. However, there is no recognized hereditary factor. The disease is different from many commonly known infections in several ways. Unlike pneumonia, tuberculosis is a chronic and painless infection, measured more in months than in days. Because of this pattern, it not only takes a long time to develop serious disease, but it also takes a long time to effect a cure.

Another very important difference between tuberculosis and many other infections is its ability to infect individuals without causing symptoms of illness, but then to lie dormant as a potential threat to that person for the rest of his life. The early stages of the disease do not produce any symptoms. Consequently a patient develops large areas of diseased tissue before he begins to feel sick. Screening procedures, therefore, are very important in detecting early disease in patients who feel perfectly healthy. Another is the skin testing of schoolchildren, which is carried out routinely in many communities today.

How Tuberculosis Spreads

Tuberculosis is contracted by inhaling into the lungs bacteria that have been coughed into the air by a person with advanced disease. It is, therefore, contagious, but not as contagious as measles, mumps, or chicken pox. Unlike those illnesses, it usually requires fairly close and prolonged contact with a tuberculous patient before the infection is passed on. Once the bacteria are inhaled, the body defenses are usually capable of isolating them into small areas within the tissues, thereby preventing any significant destruction or disease. However, though defenses are able to isolate the bacteria, they are not able to destroy all of them. Some bacteria persist in a state in which they are unable to break out and destroy tissue, but they always maintain the potential to do so at a time when the body defenses are impaired.

In about 20 percent of individuals the body defenses are not initially capable of isolating the tubercle bacilli. These individuals, mostly children, develop progressive tuberculosis directly following their initial contact. Others are successful in preventing actual disease at the time of initial contact, but they join a large group with the potential for active disease at some time in the future. Most of the new cases of active tuberculosis come

from this second group; their defenses break down years after the initial contact and resultant infection.

Weight loss, malnutrition, alcoholism, diabetes, and certain other chronic illnesses are particularly likely to lead to deterioration of the defense mechanisms holding the tuberculosis organisms in check. Still other individuals develop active disease with no recognizable condition to account for the loss of defenses. In fact, the most likely age group to develop active disease as a result of breakdown of past infection is the 20- to 30-year-old group.

Once active disease has appeared it usually involves the chest, although it can develop anywhere in the body. There is gradual spread of inflammation within lung tissue until large areas are involved. Holes, or cavities, are formed as a result of tissue destruction. These contain large numbers of tuberculosis organisms and continue to enlarge as new tissue is destroyed at the edges. At any stage of this development organisms may find their way into the bloodstream and new foci of disease can spring up throughout the body. The sputum becomes loaded with organisms that are coughed into the air and go on to infect other individuals. The infected sputum from one area of the lung may gain access to other areas and cause development of diseased tissue there as well.

Treatment

Before the modern era of drug treatment all these events followed an inexorable course to death in 85 percent of people with active tuberculosis. Only a lucky few were able to survive as cured, usually because their disease was found at an early stage. That survival was often at the expense of years confined to a sanatorium. Because of its almost uniform

outcome and the required separation from family and home, tuberculosis was formerly looked upon with quite as much dread as cancer is today.

The sanatorium rest cure of tuberculosis was first developed in the mid-nineteenth century at a time when the cause of the disease was unknown. In 1882, Robert Koch first demonstrated the tuberculosis organism, thereby proving the disease was an infection. As the twentieth century progressed, general public health measures helped limit the number of new cases, and new surgical procedures were developed to treat the disease. These measures were effective enough to arrest tuberculosis in another 25 percent of cases, brightening somewhat the dismal outlook of the past century.

But the discovery of specific antibiotics in the 1940s made the real difference in tuberculosis. Because of drug treatment, surgery is rarely resorted to today, although it still may be helpful in certain patients. Now patients with tuberculosis can face a relatively bright future without having to be hospitalized for prolonged periods or enduring periods of endless disability.

Tuberculosis Control

People still contract tuberculosis, and people still die from it. Two of the principal causes of death are delayed therapy and interruptions in therapy, the latter leading to the development of tuberculosis organisms that are unaffected by drugs. Both of these causes are often under the control of the patient. The first can be avoided by seeing a physician whenever one develops a cough that lasts more than two weeks, especially when it is not associated with the typical symptoms of a cold at the outset. The other symptoms of developing tuberculosis are also seen in other illnesses, and should always lead one to recognize that he is sick and needs to consult his physician. These symptoms are weight loss, loss of appetite, fever, and night sweats. When tuberculosis is diagnosed, the patient must follow carefully the directions regarding medication, which is always continued for a long time after the patient has regained his feeling of well-being.

There are other ways, however, to attack tuberculosis, even before one becomes sick. Once a person has had contact with tuberculosis, even though he usually does not develop active disease, he produces antibodies against the bacteria. A person with such antibodies can be recognized by injecting under the skin specially prepared material from dead tuberculosis bacteria, which gives rise to a reaction within the skin after two days. This material is called *tuberculin* and the test is known as the *tuberculin test.*

There are now many mass screening programs of tuberculin testing for schoolchildren, hospital personnel, and industrial groups. Those with positive skin test reactions are screened further for the presence of active disease. If they are found to be active cases, they are treated during what is usually an early and not very severe stage of the disease. The other people with positive tuberculin tests, without any evidence of active disease, are candidates for *prophylactic* (preventive) *therapy.* This therapy employs *isoniazid (INH)*, the most effective of many drugs for the treatment of tuberculosis and one that has virtually no side effects. Treatment for one year has been shown to reduce greatly the chance of future progress from the merely infected state to the state of active disease.

The goal of prophylactic therapy is chiefly to prevent the far more serious development of active disease. But in addition, by preventing disease

before it develops, physicians can prevent the infection of others, since the typical patient with tuberculosis has already infected some of those living with him before he becomes ill and seeks medical attention. The surface has just been scratched in this regard, however, as there are estimated to be 25 million people in the United States who would demonstrate reactions to tuberculin tests. Many of these people have never been tested and are not aware of the potential threat within them.

In most foreign countries the tuberculosis problem is much more serious. An estimated 80 percent of the populations of the countries of Asia, Africa, and South America would show positive tuberculin skin tests, with the number of active cases and deaths being proportionately high.

Sarcoidosis

Sarcoidosis (or *Boeck's sarcoid*), a disease that affects black people more often than whites, has symptoms closely resembling those of tuberculosis and other diseases. The most obvious symptom is the formation of skin nodules, often of the face, but the nodules, called *granulomas* (small tumors composed chiefly of granulation tissue), commonly occur in many other places as well, especially in the lungs and lymph nodes. They can occur also in the liver, bones, eyes, and other tissues.

Although sarcoidosis occurs all over the world, it is more common in temperate regions, and in the United States occurs more frequently in the southeastern states than elsewhere. Men and women are about equally affected. The onset of the disease occurs usually in the third or fourth decade of life.

Diagnosis and Treatment

The disease is diagnosed by an ex-

amination of chest X rays, which will show the proliferation of nodules in the lungs. Surgical biopsy and microscopic examination of skin tissue or tissue from a lymph node is usually necessary to confirm the presence of the disease.

There is no specific treatment for sarcoidosis, and in spite of its similarities in some respects to tuberculosis, no connection between the two disorders has been established. Steroids are sometimes used to treat the skin lesions, but in many cases the skin nodules clear up eventually without any treatment. About half of the patients, however, do not recover completely, and the disease becomes chronic—though of varying severity. Ultimately the granulomas can change into fibrous scars that may pose serious threats to the patient, depending upon where the scarring occurs. Respiratory distress, heart failure, and glaucoma, for example, can result from tissue changes in the lungs, heart, and eyes, respectively.

Respiratory Diseases Caused by Fungi

Two fungal diseases affecting respiration are of great importance in particular regions of the United States. They are both caused by types of fungi capable of growing within mammalian tissue, thereby infecting and destroying it. Both cause chronic diseases very similar to tuberculosis and may lead to death, though that is a far less common outcome—even when untreated—than in tuberculosis.

The spores of the fungi are inhaled from the air, and the response of the body is similar to that in tuberculosis in that most people become merely infected (the spores being contained by body defenses) while a few develop progressive disease. The body also produces anitbodies, and consequently skin tests similar to the tuberculin test can identify infected individuals.

Histoplasmosis (named for a fungus called *histoplasma*) organisms are prevalent in the Midwest, generally in the areas of the Ohio, Mississippi, and Missouri rivers. Largely unknown prior to World War II, histoplasmosis has been studied extensively since. Local epidemics have brought it to public attention on several occasions. The fungus grows readily in soil containing large amounts of bird (chickens, pigeons, starlings) or bat excrement. One of the better ways to assure exposure is to clean out an old chicken coop. The concentration of organisms may reach such high levels in bat caves that entry by spelunkers may prove fatal. In contrast to tuberculosis, the amount of exposure seems to play a very important role in determining the extent of the disease. There also seem to be few cases of late breakdown (the rule in tuberculosis). Most people develop the active disease, if at all, at the time of their initial exposure.

Coccidioidomycosis (for *Coccidioides* fungus) also generates in the soil, in this case in California, the southwest United States, and Mexico. It grows best in hot, dry soil. The common names for this disease are *desert rheumatism* or *valley fever*. Infection and disease occur in a similar pattern to that of histoplasmosis. Skin testing of large population groups for both these fungi in the appropriate geographical areas indicates that the majority of exposed individuals quite adequately contain the initial infection and never develop any illness or active disease.

Because Americans travel into infected regions, these diseases are being seen more frequently in people who do not live where the fungi are found. Both conditions, fortunately, are often self-limited, even when active disease develops. For more se-

vere cases there is a drug, *amphotericin-B,* which is quite effective; however, because it is also quite toxic to the patient, it must be given in progressive doses starting with a small initial dose, to permit the body's tolerance to build up. It is hoped that less toxic agents will be found in the future that will be just as effective against the fungus.

Allergic Respiratory Diseases

Hay fever (*allergic rhinitis*) and *asthma* are two very common allergic diseases of the respiratory tract. The two have much in common as to age at onset, seasonal manifestations, and causation. Hay fever involves the *mucosa,* or lining, of the upper respiratory tract only, whereas asthma is confined to the bronchial tubes of the lower respiratory tract. Physicians usually distinguish two main types of asthma, allergic and infectious. The infectious type of asthma resembles bronchitis, with cough and much wheezing as well. The discussion here will be confined to the allergic form of asthma.

In hay fever and asthma the allergenic substance causing the reaction is usually airborne, though it can be a food. In most cases the offender is pollen from a plant. The pollen is inhaled into the nostrils and alights upon the lining of the respiratory passages. In the allergic individual, antibodies react with the proteins in the pollen and cause various substances to be released from the tissue and blood cells in the immediate area. These substances, in turn, produce vessel enlargement in the area and an outpouring of mucus, plus certain irritating symptoms that result in a stuffy or runny nose and itchy eyes. The same reactions occur in the bronchial lining in asthma, but the substances released there also cause constriction of the bronchial muscle and conse-

quent narrowing of the passages. This muscular effect and the narrowing caused by greatly increased amounts of mucus in the passages are both responsible for the wheezing in asthma.

Hay Fever

Hay fever is never a threat to life, but in severe cases it can upset one's life patterns immensely. For unknown reasons it is more common in childhood, where it is often seen in conjunction with eczema or asthma. The tendency to develop hay fever, eczema, and asthma is hereditary. The transmission of the hereditary factors is complex, so that within a family group any number of individuals or none at all may exhibit the trait.

Most people with hay fever have their only or greatest difficulty in the summer months because of the airborne pollens from trees, grasses, flowers, and molds that are prevalent then. The most notorious of all pollens is the ragweed pollen. This weed pollinates around August 15 and continues to fill the air until late September. In many cities an official pollen count is issued every day, and those with severe difficulty can avoid some trouble by staying outside as little as possible on high-count days. *Antihistamine* drugs are used to counteract the nasal engorgement in hay fever. These drugs counteract the effect of *histamine,* which is one of the major substances released by the allergic reaction.

Allergic Asthma

Allergic asthma is the result of the allergic reaction taking place in the bronchial mucosal lining rather than in the nasal lining. A person may suffer from both asthma and hay fever. The common inciting factors are pollens, hair from pets (especially cats), house dust, molds, and certain foods (especially shellfish). When foods are responsible, the reaction initially occurs within the bloodstream, but the major effect is felt within the lung, which is spoken of as the target organ.

Most allergic asthma is seen in children. For unclear reasons it usually disappears spontaneously at puberty. In those who continue to have difficulty after puberty, the role of infection as a cause for the asthma usually becomes more prominent. Allergic asthma attacks start abruptly and can usually be aborted rather easily with medication.

People with asthma are symptom-free much of the time. When exposed to high concentrations of pollen they begin wheezing and producing sputum. Wheezing refers to the high-pitched squeaking sound that is made by people exhaling through narrowed bronchi. Associated with the wheezing and sputum is a distinct sensation of shortness of breath that varies in severity according to the nature of the attack. Milder attacks of asthma often subside spontaneously, merely with relaxation. This is especially true when the wheezing is induced by non-specific factors, such as a cloud of dust, cold air, or exercise. Asthmatic individuals have more sensitive air passages and they are more easily bothered by these nonspecific irritants.

Treatment

For more severe attacks of asthma there are several types of treatment.

There are oral medications that dilate the bronchi and offset the effects of the allergic reaction. (Antihistamines, however, exert no effect on asthma and may even worsen the condition.) Also available are injectable medications, such as adrenaline, and sprays that contain substances similar to adrenaline and that can be inhaled. Any or all of these methods may be employed by the physician. During times of high exposure it is often helpful to take one of the oral medications on a regular basis, thereby avoiding minor episodes of wheezing.

A recently discovered remedy for asthma is particularly useful to persons—primarily infants and small children, who cannot swallow tablets. The remedy comes in capsules containing tiny pellets of the drug theophylline. Once the capsule is twisted open, the pellets can be sprinkled on soft foods, including strained baby food, applesauce, pudding, or hot or cold cereal. The pellets give relief for about 12 hours, long enough to protect children during sleep.

The best therapy for asthma and hay fever is avoidance of the allergen responsible for attacks. Obviously, cats and certain foods can be avoided more readily than pollens and other airborne substances. The first requisite, however, is to identify the offender. The most important method of identification is the patient's medical history. Sometimes the problem is easy, as when the patient states that he only has trouble during the ragweed season. At other times a great amount of detective work may be required. Skin testing is used to complement the history. The skin test merely involves the introduction under the skin (usually within a tiny scratch) of various materials suspected of being allergens. If the individual has antibodies to these substances he will form a hive at the site of introduction. That he reacts does not necessarily mean that his asthma is due to that test substance, because many people have reactions but no hay fever or asthma. The skin test results need to be interpreted in the light of the history of exposure.

If the substance so identified cannot be avoided, then hyposensitization may prove useful. This form of treatment is based on the useful fact that the human body varies its ability to react depending upon the degree and the frequency of exposure. In a hyposensitizing program small amounts of pollen or other extract are injected frequently. Gradually the dose of extract is increased. By this technique many allergic individuals become able to tolerate moderate exposure to their offending material with few or no symptoms. Hyposensitization does not succeed in everyone, but it is usually worth attempting if other approaches are unsuccessful. For more information see Ch. 21, *Allergies and Hypersensitivities.*

13

Lung Disease

Two present-day problems of major proportions are not diseases in themselves, but both are detrimental to health. These are smoking and air pollution. The former is a habit that, in some users, can produce as serious results as narcotics or alcohol addiction. Knowledge of air pollution has grown with the increased public awareness of our environment. It is quite clear that there are many serious consequences produced by the products with which we foul our air. Both tobacco and air pollution are controllable: one by individual will, the other by public effort.

Smoking

Eighty-five million Americans smoke, and the vast majority of these people smoke cigarettes. This discussion will therefore center on cigarettes. The number of new smokers is increasing, which offsets the number of quitters, thereby producing a new gain in smokers each year. There was a temporary absolute decline in 1964 when the first U.S. Surgeon General's report on smoking outlined the many hazards, but that trend quickly reversed itself. The tobacco industry

spends $280 million per year to promote smoking. The U.S. Public Health Service and several volunteer agencies spend $8 million in a contrary campaign to discourage smoking.

Dangers of Smoking

Scientists know much about the ways in which smoking produces health dangers. As they burn, cigarettes release more than 4,000 different substances into the atmosphere. Carried in the cigarette smoke, these substances enter the smoker's lungs or simply dissipate in the air. Three of the substances, carbon monoxide, "tar," and nicotine, are the primary threats to health.

Smoking has "mainstream" effects on the smoker who inhales. But there are "sidestream" effects as well. For example, persons who habitually breathe the smoke from others' cigarettes may be inhaling higher concentrations of possibly harmful chemicals than the smokers themselves. These nonsmokers may experience such unpleasant symptoms as watery eyes and headaches. If they have lung or heart diseases, suffer from asthma or some allergies, or wear contact

lenses, the nonsmokers may find that their symptoms are worsening.

Some of the direct effects of breathing tobacco smoke suggest its capacity for producing disease in the smoker. Smoking lowers skin temperature, often by several degrees, principally through the constricting effect of nicotine on blood vessels. Carbon monoxide levels rise in the blood when a person is smoking. Even a single cigarette may impair somewhat the smoker's ability to expel air from the lungs. Adverse changes in the activity of several important chemicals in the body can be demonstrated after smoking.

Smoking has been strongly implicated in bronchitis and emphysema, lung and other cancers, heart disease, and peripheral vascular disease. Cigarette smoking causes more "preventable" deaths in the United States than any other single factor. Of the five leading causes of American deaths, smoking is related to four. According to verified statistics, a smoker faces a 70 percent greater risk of dying prematurely than a nonsmoker of comparable age. Smoking-related diseases take six times as many American lives annually as automobile accidents.

Lungs

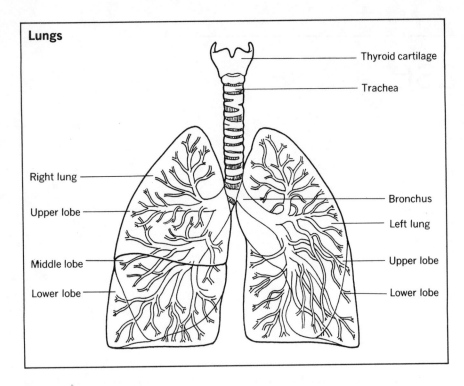

Thyroid cartilage

Trachea

Right lung

Upper lobe

Middle lobe

Lower lobe

Bronchus

Left lung

Upper lobe

Lower lobe

A Cause of Cancer

Lung cancer takes more American lives annually than any other type of cancer. Some 80 percent of all lung cancer deaths, over 90,000 in a typical year, may be attributed to cigarette smoking. On average, 7 in 10 lung cancer patients die within a year of diagnosis.

The cigarette smoker's risks are not confined to lung cancer. Such serious and sometimes fatal diseases as cancers of the mouth, pharynx, larynx, and esophagus may also be smoking-related. Of all cancer deaths, 30 percent are related to smoking. Smoking leads to 10 times as many cancer deaths as all other reliably identified cancer causes combined.

Heart Disease

Heart disease caused by smoking cigarettes takes more American lives than does cancer. But smoking is implicated in about 30 percent of all deaths resulting from coronary heart disease, the most common cause of American deaths. In 1982, about

170,000 U.S. citizens died of heart disease resulting from smoking.

In the mid-1980s, statistics showed that one living American in every 10 would die prematurely as a result of smoking-related heart disease. The smoker who refused to give up smoking after a heart attack was inviting a second attack to a significant degree. But the person who quit smoking would after some 10 years face a heart-disease risk about equal to that of a nonsmoker.

Women and Smoking

Where women accounted for one lung cancer death in six in 1968, one-fourth of all such deaths occurred among women in 1979. Those figures suggest what later statistics have borne out: that lung cancer would soon replace breast cancer as the leading cause of cancer death among women.

Women were once thought to be less susceptible to smoking-related diseases than men. But later epide-

miological studies have proved the opposite. When the earlier studies were conducted, women had simply not been smoking as long as men, or in such numbers. As the picture has changed, the statistics have changed. Like men, women smokers who experience other heart disease risk factors, including hypertension and high serum cholesterol levels, face a greatly increased risk of coronary heart disease.

The Dose-Response Relationship

The number of cigarettes an individual smokes is one of the determinants of eventual damage even though individual susceptibility is also important. Thus a definite dose-response relationship exists between smoking and disease. If a person smokes one pack a day for one year he has smoked one pack-year; if he smokes one pack a day for two years or two packs a day for one year, he has smoked two pack-years, and so on. Calculating by pack-years, it appears that 40 pack-years is a crucial time period above which the incidence of cancer of the lung, emphysema, and other serious consequences rises rapidly. Smoking three packs a day, it takes only about 13 years to reach this critical level.

Breaking the Smoking Habit

Obviously, the best way not to smoke is never to start. Unfortunately, young people are continuing to join the smoking ranks at a rapid rate. The teenager often is one of the hardest persons to convince of the hazards of smoking. He is healthy, suffers less from fatigue, headaches, breathlessness, and other immediate effects of smoking, and he often feels the need to smoke to keep up with his peers. Once he starts, it is not long before he becomes addicted. The addiction to cigarettes is very real. It is more psychological dependency than the physical addiction associated with narcotics, but there are definite physical addiction aspects to smoking that are mostly noted when one stops.

For most people it is quite a challenge to stop smoking. There are many avenues to travel and many sources now available to aid one on the way. They include smoking clinics that offer group support and medical guidance to those anxious to quit. The clinics vary in their format but basically depend on the support given the smoker by finding other individuals with the same problems and overcoming the problems as a group. The medical guidance helps people recognize and deal with withdrawal symptoms as well as helping them with weight control.

Withdrawal Symptoms

Withdrawal symptoms vary from person to person and include many symptoms other than just a craving for a cigarette. Many people who stop smoking become jittery and sleepless, start coughing more than usual, and often develop an increased appetite. This last withdrawal effect is especially disturbing to women, and the need to prevent weight gain is all too often used as a simple excuse to avoid stopping the cigarette habit or to start smoking again. The weight gained is usually not too great, and one generally stops gaining after a few weeks. Once the cigarette smoking problem is controlled, then efforts can be turned to weight reduction. Being overweight is also a threat to health, but ten extra pounds, even if maintained, do not represent nearly the threat that confirmed smoking does.

Despite all efforts, many individuals who would like to stop smoking fail in their attempts. The best advice

for them is to keep trying. Continued effort will at least tend to decrease the amount of smoking and often leads to eventual abstinence, even after years of trying. If a three-pack-per-day smoker can decrease to one pack a day or less, he has helped himself even though he is still doing some damage. For prospective quitters it is important to remember that cigarette smoking is an acquired habit, and that the learning process can be reversed. The problem most people have is too little knowledge of the dangers and too much willingness to believe that disease and disability cannot strike them, just the other fellow.

Air Pollution

While 85 million Americans pollute the air they breathe individually with cigarettes, all 210 million of us collectively pollute the atmosphere we all breathe. Some people are obviously more responsible than others, but air, water, and land pollution is a disease of society and can only be solved through a concerted effort by the whole society. Pollution has always been a problem to man. As we have become more urbanized the problem has grown. It has now reached what many consider to be crisis proportions in our large cities and even in some of our smaller ones.

We have had ample warning. In 1948 a killer smog engulfed Donora, Pennsylvania, killing 20 persons and producing serious illness in 6,000 more. In 1952 a lingering smog over London was blamed for 4,000 deaths in a few weeks. New York City has had several serious encounters with critical smog conditions that have accounted for many illnesses and deaths. The exteriors of many buildings in our cities are showing signs of vastly increased rates of decay due to the noxious substances in the air. It

is estimated that air pollution costs the United States $11 billion a year in damage, illness, and in other ways. Even if all this loss of life and property were not a result it would clearly be more pleasant to live in a clean atmosphere than in a foul one.

Emphysema and Bronchitis

Emphysema and chronic bronchitis are diseases that involve the whole lung. They can be of varying severity, and both are characterized by the gradual progression of breathlessness.

Because chronic bronchitis is almost invariably associated with pulmonary emphysema, the combined disorder frequently is called *obstructive-airway disease*. The disease involves damage to the lung tissue, with a loss of normal elasticity of the air sacs (*emphysema*), as well as damage to the *bronchi*, the main air passages to the lungs. In addition, chronic bronchitis is marked by a thickening of the walls of the bronchi with increased mucus production and difficulty in expelling these secretions. This results in coughing and sputum production.

The condition known as *acute bronchitis* is an acute process generally caused by a sudden infection, such as a cold, with an exaggeration of bronchitis symptoms. If a spasm of the bronchi occurs, accompanied by wheezing, the ailment is called infectious or nonallergic asthma.

Obstructive-airway disease is very insidious, and characteristically people do not, or will not, notice that they are sick until they suddenly are very sick. This is partly because of chronic denial of the morning cough and breathlessness, but also because we are fashioned in such a way as to have great reserve strength in our organs. As the disease progresses one starts using up his reserve for exertion. Be-

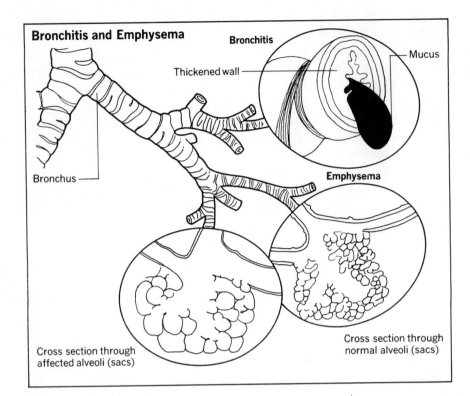

Bronchitis and Emphysema

Bronchitis

Thickened wall

Mucus

Bronchus

Emphysema

Cross section through affected alveoli (sacs)

Cross section through normal alveoli (sacs)

cause most people's life styles allow them to avoid exertion easily, the victim of this disease may have only rare chances to notice his breathlessness. Then, suddenly, within a period of a few months he becomes breathless with ordinary activity because he has used up and surpassed all his reserve. He goes to a physician thinking he has just become sick. Usually this event occurs when the patient is in his fifties or sixties and little can be done to correct the damage. The time for prevention was in the previous 30 years when elimination of smoking could have prevented much or all of the illness.

Chronic cough and breathlessness are the two earliest signs of chronic bronchitis and emphysema. A smoker's cough is not an insignificant symptom. It indicates that very definite irritation of the bronchi has developed and it should be respected early. Along with the cough there is often production of phlegm or sputum, especially in the morning, because of less effective emptying of the bronchial tree during the relatively

motionless period of sleep. Another early manifestation of disease is the tendency to develop chest infections along with what would otherwise be simple head colds. With these chest infections there is often a tightness or dull pain in the middle chest region, production of sputum and sometimes wheezing.

Treatment

Once emphysema or bronchitis are diagnosed there are many forms of therapy that can help. Stopping smoking is the most important measure, and will in itself often produce dramatic effects. The more bronchitis the patient has, the more noticeable the effect, as the bronchial irritation and mucous production decrease, cough lessens, and a greater sense of well-being ensues. The emphysema component does not change, as the damage to the air sacs is irreversible, but the progression may be greatly slowed. When chest infections develop they can be treated with antibiotics.

For more severe disease a program of breathing exercises and graded exertion may be beneficial. When these people develop heart trouble as a result of the strain on the heart, a treatment to strengthen the heart is rewarding. For those with the most advanced stage of the disease new methods of treatment have been devised in recent years. One of the most encouraging is the use of controlled oxygen administration, treatment that can sometimes allow a patient to return to an active working life from an otherwise helpless bed-and-chair existence. But it must be remembered that all these measures produce little effect if the patient continues to smoke.

Vaporizers, Nebulizers, IPPB

Mechanical methods have been developed to help control emphysema, bronchitis, acute and chronic asthma, and other respiratory disorders. These methods include the use of vaporizers, nebulizers, and intermittent positive pressure breathing (IPPB).

The vaporizer is a device that increases the moisture content of a home or room. In doing so, the vaporizer relieves the chronic condition that makes breathing difficult: the increased humidity loosens mucus and reduces nasal or bronchial congestion. One simple type of vaporizer or humidifier is the "croup kettle" or hot-steam type that releases steam into the air when heated on the stove or electrical unit. A more formal type of vaporizer is the electric humidifier that converts water into a spray. In dispersing the spray into the atmosphere, the vaporizer raises the humidity level without increasing the temperature.

The nebulizer also converts liquid into fine spray. But the nebulizer dispenses medications, such as isoproterenol hydrochloride, directly into the throat through a mouthpiece and pressure-injector apparatus like an atomizer. Used in limited doses according to a physician's instructions, nebulization can relieve the labored or difficult breathing symptoms common to various respiratory diseases, among them asthma and bronchitis. The patient controls the dosage while using the nebulizer simply by employing finger pressure and obeying instructions.

In IPPB, a mask and ventilator are used to force air into the lungs and enable the patient to breathe more deeply. The ventilator supplies intermittent positive air pressure. The IPPB method of treatment has been used to help persons suffering from chronic pulmonary disease that makes breathing difficult. But IPPB may also be used with patients who cannot cough effectively; these patients include those who have recently undergone surgery. Newer IPPB units are highly portable; but they must be cleaned carefully with an antibacterial solution before use, and should always be used carefully to avoid producing breathing difficulties or aggravating heart problems.

Smoking and Obstructive Diseases

The problems encountered by patients with obstructive disease do not encompass merely that disease alone. Because of their smoking history these patients are also prone to develop lung cancer. All too often a person with a potentially curable form of lung cancer is unable to undergo surgery because his lungs will not tolerate the added strain of surgery. Patients with obstructive disease are also more prone to pneumonia and other infectious pulmonary conditions. When these develop in the already compromised lung, it may be impossible for the patient to maintain adequate oxygen supply to his vital

tissues. If oxygen insufficiency is severe and prolonged enough, the patient dies from pulmonary failure.

Despite the emphasis placed on smoking as the predominant factor for the development of obstructive disease, there are people with the disease who have never smoked. For many of these individuals there is no known cause for their disease. However, a group of younger people with obstructive disease has been found to be deficient in a particular enzyme. (Enzymes are agents that are necessary for certain chemical reactions.) Individuals with this deficiency develop a particularly severe form of emphysema, become symptomatic in their third or fourth decade, and die at a young age. They may not smoke, but if they do, the disease is much more severe. Just how the enzyme deficiency leads to emphysema is not clear, but a great amount of research is being conducted on this new link to try to learn more about the causes of emphysema.

The Pneumoconioses

Pneumoconiosis is a chronic reaction of the lung to any of several types of inhaled dust particles. The reaction varies somewhat but generally consists of initial inflammation about the inhaled particle followed by the development of scar tissue. The pneumoconioses develop predominantly from various occupational exposures to high concentrations of certain inorganic compounds that cannot be broken down by the cells of the body. The severity of the disease is proportional to the amount of dust retained in the lung.

Silica is the most notorious of these substances. People who work in mining, steel production, and any occupation involved with chipping stone, such as manufacturing monuments, are exposed to silica dust. Many of the practices associated with these occupations have been altered over the years because of the recognition of the hazard to workers. Other important pneumoconioses involve talc and asbestos particles, cotton fibers, and coal dust. Coal dust has gained wide attention in recent years with the heightened awareness of *black lung,* a condition seen in varying degrees in coal miners. The attention has resulted in a federal black lung disease law under which more than 135,000 miners have filed for compensation.

Although there are individual dif-

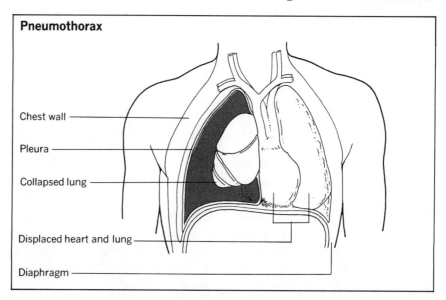

Pneumothorax

Chest wall

Pleura

Collapsed lung

Displaced heart and lung

Diaphragm

ferences in reaction to the varied forms of pneumoconiosis, the ultimate hazard is the loss of functioning lung tissue. When enough tissue becomes scarred, there is interference with oxygenation. Those people with pneumoconiosis who smoke are in great danger of compounding their problem by adding obstructive disease as well.

Prevention

Once the scarring has taken place there is no way to reverse the process. Therefore, the answer to the pneumoconioses is to prevent the exposure. Attention to occupational diseases in the United States has lagged about 30 years behind Europe, so that we are just now beginning to show concern about certain industrial practices condemned as hazardous in many European countries in the 1940s. New lung diseases caused by inhaled substances are discovered every year, and more will undoubtedly be found in the future. People in industries in which there is exposure to industrial dust should be aware of the potential danger and should be prepared to promote the maintenance of protective practices and the investigation of new ideas and devices. Where masks have been supplied, the workers should wear them, a practice too often neglected.

Pulmonary Embolism

Pulmonary embolism is a condition in which a part of a blood clot in a vein breaks away and travels through the heart and into the pulmonary circulatory system. Here the vessels leading from the heart branch like a tree, gradually becoming smaller until finally they form *capillaries,* the smallest blood vessels. Depending on its size, the clot will at some point reach a vessel through which it cannot pass, and there will lodge itself. The clot disrupts the blood supply to the area supplied by that vessel. The larger the clot, the greater is the area of lung that loses its blood supply, and the more drastic the results to the patient.

This condition develops most commonly in association with inflammation of the veins of the legs (*thrombophlebitis*). People with varicose veins are particularly susceptible to thrombophlebitis. Because of constrictions produced by garters or rolled stockings, or just sitting with crossed legs for a long time, the sluggish blood flow already present is aggravated, and a clot may form in a vessel. Some people without varicose veins can also develop clots under the same conditions. The body often responds to the clot with the reaction of inflammation, which is painful. However, when there is no inflammatory response, there is no warning to tell that a clot has formed. In either situation there is always a chance that a piece may break off the main clot and travel to the lung. Of recent concern in this regard are studies that appear to link oral contraceptives with the incidence of clotting, thereby leading to pulmonary embolism. The number of women affected in this way by the use of oral contraceptives is small, but enough to be of concern.

The symptoms of pulmonary embolism are varied and may be minor or major. Most common are pleurisy—marked by chest pain during breathing—shortness of breath, and cough with the production of blood. Once the pulmonary embolism is diagnosed the treatment is simple in the less severe cases, which are the majority. But in cases of large clots and great areas of lung deprived of blood supply there may be catastrophic effects on the heart and general circulation.

Prevention

Certain preventive measures are worthwhile for all people. Stockings should not be rolled, because that produces a constricting band about the leg that impairs blood flow and predisposes to clot formation. Especially when taking long automobile or airplane rides one should be sure to stretch the legs periodically. Individuals with varicose veins or a history of thrombophlebitis should take these precautions more seriously. People who stand still for long periods during the day should wear elastic support stockings regularly and elevate their feet part of the day and at night.

When considering the use of oral contraceptives the physician must weigh the risks of developing clots from the drug against the psychological, social, and physical risks of pregnancy. The risk from oral contraceptives is lessened if the woman does not have high blood pressure. Any persistent pain in the leg, especially in the calf or behind the knee, deserves the attention of a physician. Anyone with varicose veins or anyone taking oral contraceptives should be especially attentive to these symptoms.

Pneumothorax

Another less common lung condition is spontaneous *pneumothorax* or collapse of a lung. This most commonly occurs in the second and third decade of life and presents itself with the sudden development of pain in the chest and breathlessness. The collapse occurs because of a sudden leak of air from the lung into the chest cavity.

The lung is ordinarily maintained in an expanded state by the rigid bony thorax, but if air leaks out into the space between the thorax and the lung, the lung collapses. This condition is rarely very serious but the patient needs to be observed to be sure that the air leak does not become greater with further lung collapse.

Treatment

Often a tube has to be placed in the chest, attached to a suction pump, and the air pumped out from the space where it has collected. When the air is removed the lung expands to fill the thoracic cage again. Some individuals tend to have several recurrences. Because the reason for the collapse is poorly understood, there is no satisfactory method of preventing these recurrences except by surgery. This is rarely required. In a person with a proven propensity for recurrence it is usually advisable to open the chest and produce scarring of the lung surface so that it becomes fixed to the thoracic cage. Although it is usually successful, even this procedure does not always solve this bothersome problem.

14

Diseases of the Endocrine Glands

Glands are organs that produce and secrete substances essential for normal body functioning. There are two main types of glands: the *endocrine* and the *exocrine*. The endocrines, or *ductless,* glands send their secretions directly into the bloodstream. These secretions, which are biochemically related to each other, are called *hormones*. The exocrines, such as the sebaceous or sweat glands, the mammary (or milk) glands, and the lachrymal (or tear) glands, have ducts that carry their secretions to specific locations for specific purposes.

The exocrine glands are individually discussed elsewhere in connection with the various parts of the body where they are found. This section is devoted to diseases of the ductless glands, which include:

- The *pituitary,* which controls growth and the activity of the adrenal, thyroid, and sex glands

- The *thyroid,* which controls the rate of the body's chemical activity or metabolism

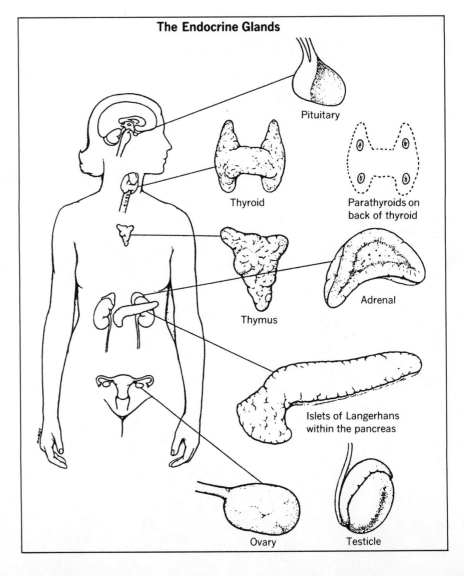

The Endocrine Glands

Pituitary

Thyroid

Parathyroids on back of thyroid

Thymus

Adrenal

Islets of Langerhans within the pancreas

Ovary

Testicle

- The *adrenals,* which affect metabolism and sex characteristics

- The *male gonads* or testicles and the *female gonads* or ovaries

- The *parathyroids,* which regulate bone metabolism

Unlike the exocrine glands, which can function independently of one another, the endocrines form an interrelated system. Thus a disorder in one of them is likely to affect the way the others behave. Glandular disorder can sometimes be anatomical, but it is usually functional. Functional disease can result in the production and release of too little or too much of a particular secretion.

When too much of a hormone is being secreted, the prefix *hyper-* is used for the condition, as in *hyperthyroidism.* When too little is being secreted, the prefix *hypo-* is used, as in the word *hypofunction,* to indicate that a gland operates below normal.

Abnormalities of the endocrine glands that cause changes in their functioning are responsible for a wide variety of illnesses. These illnesses are almost always accompanied by symptoms that can be recognized as distinctly abnormal. Prompt and accurate diagnosis can usually prevent the occurrence of irreversible damage. For many people with glandular disorders, treatment may have to be lifelong. They can feel well and function almost normally, but they must follow a program of regulated medication taken under a physician's supervision.

Anterior Pituitary Gland

The anterior pituitary gland, also called the *hypophysis,* is located in the center of the brain. It produces two types of secretions: a growth hor-

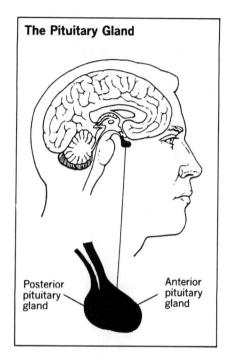

The Pituitary Gland

Posterior pituitary gland

Anterior pituitary gland

mone and hormones that stimulate certain other glands.

The anterior pituitary gland is subject to neurochemical stimulation by

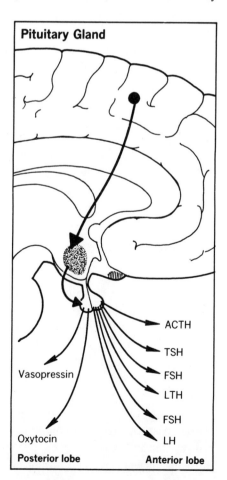

Pituitary Gland

Vasopressin

Oxytocin

Posterior lobe

ACTH

TSH

FSH

LTH

FSH

LH

Anterior lobe

the *hypothalamus,* a nearby part of the brain. This stimulation results in the production of the hormones that promote testicular and ovarian functioning, and does not occur normally until around 12 years of age in girls and 14 in boys. The beginning of this glandular activity is known as the onset of *puberty.*

Puberty is sometimes delayed for no apparent reason until age 16 or 17. Because the hypothalamus is affected by emotional factors, all of the endocrine glands governed by the anterior pituitary can also be affected by feelings. Psychological factors can therefore upset the relationships in the glandular system and produce the physical symptoms of endocrine disorders.

It is extremely rare for the anterior pituitary to produce too much or too little of its hormones, but sometimes hypofunction may follow pregnancy because of thrombosis or changes in the blood vessels.

A truly hypofunctioning anterior pituitary gland can cause many serious disturbances: extreme thinness, growth failure, sexual aberration, and intolerance for normal variations in temperature. When appropriate diagnostic tests determine the deficiency, the patient is given the missing hormones in pill form.

Absence of the growth hormone alone is unknown. Most cases of *dwarfism* result from other causes. However, excess production of the growth hormone alone does occur, but only rarely. If it begins before puberty when the long bones are still growing, the child with the disorder will grow into a well-proportioned giant. When it begins after puberty, the head, hands, feet, and most body organs except the brain slowly enlarge. This condition is called *acromegaly.* The cause of both disorders is usually a tumor, and radiation is the usual treatment.

The thyroid, adrenal cortex, testicles, ovaries, and pancreatic glands are target glands for the anterior pituitary's stimulating hormones, which are specific for the functioning of each of these glands. Therefore, a disorder of any of the target organs could be caused either by an excess or a deficiency of a stimulating hormone, creating a so-called *secondary disease.* There are various tests that can be given to differentiate primary from secondary disorders.

The Thyroid Gland

The thyroid gland is located in the front of the neck just above its base. Normal amounts of *thyroxin,* the hormone secreted by the thyroid, are necessary for the proper functioning of almost all bodily activities. When this hormone is deficient in infancy, growth and mental development are impaired and *cretinism* results.

Hypothyroidism

In adulthood, a deficiency of thyroxin hormone is caused primarily by a lack of sufficient iodine in the diet. In *hypothyroidism,* the disorder resulting from such a deficiency, the metabolic rate is slower than normal, the patient has no energy, his expression is dull, his skin is thick, and he has an intolerance to cold weather.

Treatment consists of increasing the amount of iodine in the diet if it is deficient or giving thyroid hormone medication. Normal metabolic functioning usually follows, especially if treatment is begun soon after the symptoms appear.

Hyperthyroidism

An excess amount of thyroid hormone secretion is called *hyperthyroidism* and may relate to emotional stress. It causes physical fatigue but mental alertness, a staring quality in the eyes, tremor of the hands, weight loss with increased appetite, rapid pulse, sweating, and intolerance to hot weather.

Long-term treatment is aimed at decreasing hormone production with the use of a special medicine that inhibits it. In some cases, part of the gland may be removed by surgery; in others, radiation treatment with radioactive iodine is effective.

Hyperthyroidism may recur long after successful treatment. Both hypothyroidism and hyperthyroidism are common disorders, especially in women.

Other Thyroid Disorders

Enlargement of part or all of the thyroid gland occurs fairly often. It may be a simple enlargement of the gland itself caused by the lack of iodine, as in *goiter,* or it may be caused by a tumor or a nonspecific inflammation. Goiter is often treated with thyroxin, but it is easily prevented altogether by the regular use of iodized table and cooking salt. Treatment of other problems varies, but surgery is usually recommended for a tumor, especially if the surrounding organs are being obstructed.

The Adrenal Glands

The adrenals are paired glands located just above each kidney. Their outer part is called the *cortex.* The inner part is called the *medulla* and is not governed by the anterior pituitary. The cortex produces several hormones that affect the metabolism of salt, water, carbohydrate, fat, and protein, as well as secondary sex characteristics, skin pigmentation, and resistance to infection.

An insufficiency of these hormones

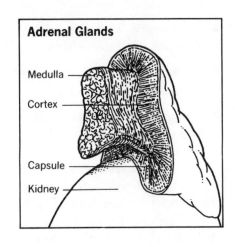

Adrenal Glands

Medulla

Cortex

Capsule

Kidney

can be caused by bacterial infection of the cortex, especially by *meningococcus;* by a hemorrhage into it; by an obstruction of blood flow into it; by its destruction because of tuberculosis; or by one of several unusual diseases.

In one type of sudden or acute underfunctioning of the cortex, the patient has a high fever, mental confusion, and circulatory collapse. Unless treated promptly, the disorder is likely to be fatal. When it persists after treatment, or when it develops gradually, it is called *Addison's disease* and is usually chronic. The patient suffers from weakness, loss of body hair, and increased skin pigmentation. Hormone-replacement treatment is essential, along with added salt for as long as hypofunction persists.

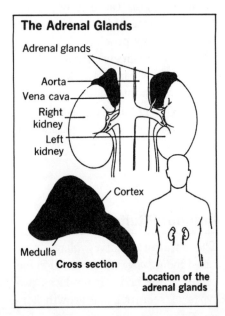

The Adrenal Glands

Adrenal glands

Aorta

Vena cava

Right kidney

Left kidney

Cortex

Medulla

Cross section

Location of the adrenal glands

The formation of an excess of certain cortical hormones (i.e., hormones produced in the adrenal cortex)—a disorder known as *Cushing's syndrome*—may be caused by a tumor of the anterior pituitary gland, which produces too much specific stimulating hormone, or by a tumor of one or both of the adrenal glands. It is a rare disease, more common in women, especially following pregnancy. Symptoms include weakness, loss of muscle tissue, the appearance of purple streaks in the skin, and an oval or "moon" face.

Treatment involves eliminating the overproducing tissue either by surgery or irradiation and then replacing any hormonal deficiencies with proper medication.

An excess of certain other cortical hormones because of an increase in cortical tissue or a tumor can result in the early onset of puberty in boys, or in an increase in the sexuality of females of any age. Surgical removal of the overproducing tissue is the only treatment.

The Adrenal Medulla

The medulla of the adrenal glands secretes two hormones: *epinephrine* (or *adrenaline*) and *norepinephrine*. Although they contribute to the proper functioning of the heart and blood vessels, neither one is absolutely indispensable. Disease caused by hypofunction of the medulla is unknown. Hyperfunction is a rare cause of sustained high blood pressure. Even more rarely, it causes episodic or paroxysmal high blood pressure accompanied by such symptoms as throbbing headache, profuse perspiration, and severe anxiety. The disorder is caused by a tumor effectively treated by surgical removal. Cancer of the adrenal medulla is extremely rare and virtually incurable.

Changes in hormone production

can be caused by many intangible factors and are often temporary disorders. However, persistent or recurrent symptoms should be brought to a physician's attention. The accurate diagnosis of an endocrine disease depends on careful professional evaluation of specific laboratory tests, individual medical history, and thorough examination. No one should take hormones or medicines that affect hormone production without this type of evaluation, since their misuse can cause major problems.

Male Sex Glands

The male sex glands, or *gonads,* are the two testicles normally located in the *scrotum.* In addition to producing sperm, the testicles also manufacture the male hormone called *testosterone.* This hormone is responsible for the development and maintenance of secondary sex characteristics as well as for the male *libido,* or sexual impulse. Only one normal testicle is needed for full function.

Testicular Hypofunction

Hypofunction of one or both of the testicles can result from an abnor-

mality in prenatal development, from infections such as mumps or tuberculosis, from injury, or from the increased temperature to which undescended testicles are exposed.

When hypofunction occurs before puberty, there is failure in the development of secondary sex characteristics. The sex organs do not enlarge; facial, pubic, and armpit hair fails to appear; and the normal voice change does not occur. Fertility and libido also fail to develop. A person with this combination of abnormalities is called a *eunuch.*

If the disorder is secondary to anterior pituitary disease, it is called *Froehlich's syndrome.* When it occurs after puberty, the body changes are less striking, but there may be a loss of fertility and libido. The primary disease is usually treated by surgery, and testosterone may be given. If the disorder is secondary to anterior pituitary disease, the gonad-stimulating hormone should be administered.

Testicular hypofunction is rare because it results only when both testicles are damaged in some way. Although mumps may involve the testicles, it is rarely the cause of sterility, even though this is greatly

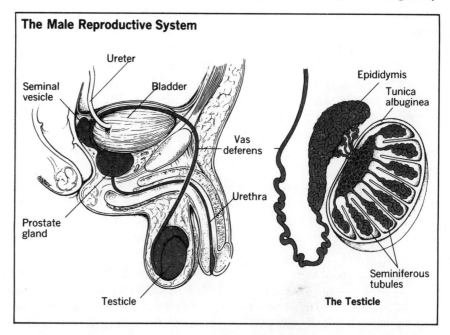

The Male Reproductive System

Ureter

Seminal vesicle

Bladder

Vas deferens

Urethra

Prostate gland

Testicle

Epididymis

Tunica albuginea

Seminiferous tubules

The Testicle

feared. Even so, everyone should be immunized against mumps in infancy.

It is advisable to wear an appropriate athletic supporter to protect the testicles when engaged in strenuous athletics or when there is a possibility that they might be injured. However, nothing that restricts scrotal movement should be worn regularly, since movement is essential for the maintenance of constant testicular temperature.

A sudden decrease in sexual drive or performance may be caused by disease, trauma, or emotional factors. In certain cases administering male hormones may relieve the condition. However, a decrease in sexual drive is one of the natural consequences of aging. It is not a disease and should not be treated with testosterone.

Testicular Hyperfunction

Testicular hyperfunction is extremely rare and is usually caused by a tumor. Before puberty, the condition results in the precocious development of secondary sex characteristics; after puberty, in the accentuation of these characteristics. Such a tumor must be removed surgically or destroyed by irradiation.

Cancer can develop in a testicle without causing any functional change. It is relatively uncommon. When it appears, it shows up first as a painless enlargement. The cancer cells then usually spread quickly to other organs and have a fatal result. Prompt treatment by surgery and irradiation can sometimes arrest the condition.

Because an undescended testicle may become cancerous, it should be repositioned into the scrotum by surgery or removed.

Female Sex Glands

The female gonads are the *ovaries,* situated on each side of and close to

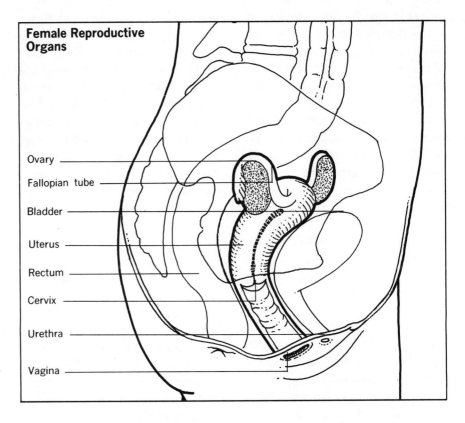

Female Reproductive Organs

Ovary

Fallopian tube

Bladder

Uterus

Rectum

Cervix

Urethra

Vagina

the uterus or womb. In addition to producing an *ovum* or egg each month, they manufacture the female hormones *estrogen* and *progesterone,* each making its special contribution to the menstrual cycle and to the many changes that go on during pregnancy. Estrogen regulates the secondary sex characteristics such as breast development and the appearance of pubic and axillary hair.

The periodicity of the menstrual cycle depends on a very complicated relationship between the ovaries and the anterior pituitary. Birth control pills, most of which contain estrogen and progesterone, interrupt this relationship in such a way that no ovum is produced and pregnancy therefore should not occur.

Changes in normal ovarian hormone function create problems similar to changes in normal testicular hormone function, except of course

for the female–male differences. In general, the diseases responsible for these changes are the same in males and females. However, changes in female hormone function are very often caused by emotional stress or by other unspecific circumstances.

Ovarian Hypofunction

Hypofunction of the ovaries may cause failure to menstruate at all or with reasonable regularity. A disruption of the menstrual cycle is an obvious indication to the woman past puberty that something is wrong. Less obvious is the reduction or complete loss of fertility that may accompany the disorder.

Both menstrual and infertility problems should be evaluated by a trained specialist, preferably a gynecologist, to find out their cause. If it should be hormonal deficiency, treatment may consist of replacement hormone therapy. In many cases, however, effective treatment consists of eliminating the emotional stress that has affected the stimulation relationship between the anterior pituitary and the ovaries, thereby inhibiting hormone production. Occasionally, hormone treatment for infertility causes several ova to be produced in the same month, increasing the possibility of a multiple pregnancy.

Menopause

All women eventually develop spontaneous ovarian hypofunction. This usually happens between the ages of 45 and 50 and is called the *climacteric* or *menopause*. When it happens before the age of 35, it is called premature menopause.

Normal menopause results from the gradual burning out of the ovaries so that estrogen is deficient or absent altogether. Most women experience very few changes or symptoms at this time other than the cessation of menstruation, usually preceded by progressive irregularity and reduction of flow.

A few women become excessively irritable, have hot flashes, perspire a great deal, gain weight, and develop facial hair. Such women, as well as those who have premature menopause, are likely to benefit greatly from estrogen replacement therapy for a few years. However, because recent statistical studies have implicated sustained use of estrogen therapy as increasing the risk of uterine cancer in postmenopausal women, the American Cancer Society has cautioned physicians to supervise such women closely. At the present time, most physicians feel that the treatment should be given temporarily and only when menopause symptoms are causing special discomfort.

Ovarian Hyperfunction

Hyperfunction of the ovaries after puberty is one cause of increased menstrual flow during or at the end of each cycle. This is called functional bleeding and is caused by excess estrogen. The disorder is treated with progesterone, which slows down estrogen production. In cases where this treatment fails, it is sometimes necessary to remove the uterus by an operation called a *hysterectomy*.

Some diseases of the ovaries, such as infections, cysts, and tumors, do not necessarily cause functional changes, but they may call attention to themselves by being painful, or a physician may discover them during a pelvic examination. Treatment may be medical, surgical, or by irradiation, depending on the nature of the disorder. See Ch. 25, *Women's Health,* for fuller treatment of ovarian and other disorders affecting women.

A rather common cause of short-lived ovarian pain is connected with *ovulation,* which occurs about 14 days before the next expected menstrual period. This discomfort is called *mittelschmerz,* which is German for "middle pain," and can be treated with aspirin or any other simple analgesic.

The Pancreas

The pancreas, a combined duct and endocrine gland, is to some extent regulated by the anterior pituitary. See Ch. 15, *Diabetes Mellitus,* for a discussion of the pancreas and diabetes.

Posterior Pituitary Gland

The posterior lobe of the pituitary gland, the parathyroid glands, and the adrenal medulla are not governed by the anterior pituitary gland. The posterior pituitary produces a secretion called *antidiuretic hormone* which acts on the kidneys to control the amount

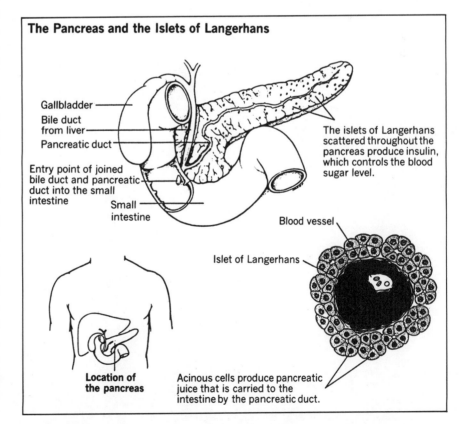

The Pancreas and the Islets of Langerhans

Gallbladder

Bile duct from liver

Pancreatic duct

Entry point of joined bile duct and pancreatic duct into the small intestine

Small intestine

The islets of Langerhans scattered throughout the pancreas produce insulin, which controls the blood sugar level.

Blood vessel

Islet of Langerhans

Location of the pancreas

Acinous cells produce pancreatic juice that is carried to the intestine by the pancreatic duct.

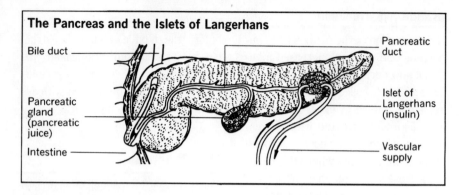

The Pancreas and the Islets of Langerhans

Bile duct

Pancreatic
gland
(pancreatic
juice)

Intestine

Pancreatic
duct

Islet of
Langerhans
(insulin)

Vascular
supply

of urine produced. A deficiency of this hormone causes *diabetes insipidus,* which results in the production of an excessive amount of urine, sometimes as much as 25 quarts a day. (A normal amount is about one quart.) The natural consequence of this disorder is an unquenchable thirst. It is an extremely rare disease, the cause of which is often unknown, although it may result from a brain injury or tumor. Treatment involves curing the cause if it is known. If not, the patient is given an antidiuretic hormone.

The Parathyroid Glands

The parathyroid glands are located in or near the thyroid, usually two on each side. They are important in the regulation of blood calcium and phosphorus levels and therefore of bone metabolism. Hypofunction of these glands almost never occurs except when they have been removed surgically, usually inadvertently during a thyroid operation. In underfunctioning of the parathyroids, blood calcium levels fall and muscle spasm results. The patient is usually given calcium and replacement therapy with parathyroid hormone to correct the disorder.

Hyperfunction is rare and is slightly more common in women. A benign tumor, or *adenoma,* is the usual cause. The amount of calcium in the blood rises as calcium is removed from the bones, which then weaken and may break easily. The excess calcium is excreted in the urine and may coalesce into kidney stones, causing severe pain. Treatment for hyperfunction of the parathyroids consists of surgical removal of the affected glands.

15

Diabetes Mellitus

A lot of people have diabetes and they live a long time with it. In the United States there are around four million diabetics, or people who have diabetes. About a third of them at any one time are undiagnosed. This figure constitutes about two percent of the population, and ranges from one one-hundredth percent of people under 24 years of age to seven percent of those over 64.

Diabetes can develop at any age. Susceptibility gradually increases up to age 40, and then rapidly increases. After age 30 it more commonly affects women than men.

History of Diabetes

Diabetes has been known for several thousand years. Because people with this disease, when untreated, may urinate frequently and copiously, the Greeks named it diabetes, meaning "siphon." In the late seventeenth century the name *mellitus*, meaning "sweet", was added. In early days, diagnosis was made by tasting the urine. The sweetness is caused by the presence of sugar (*glucose*) in the urine; its presence distinguishes diabetes mellitus from the much rarer

diabetes insipidus, an entirely different problem. See under Ch. 14, *Diseases of the Endocrine Glands,* for a discussion of diabetes insipidus.

Discovery of Insulin

Late in the nineteenth century, when diabetes was well recognized as an abnormality in carbohydrate metabolism, several scientists discovered that the experimental removal of certain cells, the *islets of Langerhans,* from the pancreas, produced diabetes in dogs. This observation led to the 1921 discovery and isolation of insulin by two Canadian doctors, Frederick Banting and Charles Best. Insulin is a hormone produced by these islets. Injection of insulin proved to be the first and remains the most effective means of treating diabetes. And so began a real revolution in improving the outcome of this disease. Previously death occurred in a few years for almost every diabetic. Often death was much quicker, especially for people who were under 30 years of age when they developed diabetes—because this age group tends to have a more severe form of the disease. Since 1921 new knowledge and techniques have made it possible to do more and

more for diabetics.

An early pioneer in the treatment of diabetes with insulin was Dr. Elliott Joslin of Boston. Dr. Joslin realized that the diabetic patient needed to have a full understanding of his disease so that he could take care of himself. He knew that the diabetic, with the chronic abnormality of a delicate and dynamic metabolic process, could not be cared for successfully solely by knowledgeable physicians. The patient and his family had to be informed about the disease and had to make day-to-day decisions about managing it.

In many ways this marked the beginning of what have become ever-increasing efforts to educate patients about all their diseases, especially chronic ones. The results have been rather remarkable.

Characteristics of Diabetes

The fundamental problem in diabetes is the body's inability to metabolize glucose, a common form of sugar, fully and continually. This is a vital process in creating body cell energy. Glucose is a chemical derivative of the carbohydrate in foods after they have been ingested. Carbohydrates are mostly of plant origin and may be called starch, saccharide, sucrose, or simply sugar. Glucose is stored under normal conditions in the form of *glycogen,* or animal starch, in the liver and muscles for later use, at which time it is reconverted to glucose.

Need for Insulin

Insulin is necessary for both the storage and reconversion of glucose. The metabolic failure may come about because of an insufficiency of insulin, an inability of the body to respond normally to it for a number of complex chemical reasons, or a combination of both factors. In any event, the failure to metabolize glucose results in an abnormal accumulation of sugar in the bloodstream.

This failure is somewhat similar to starvation. A starved person eats no food, whereas the diabetic eats food but cannot use the carbohydrate in it and cannot get sufficient energy from the protein and fat content of food. After the starving person has used his previously stored glycogen, which the diabetic without insulin cannot do, the body has to metabolize its stored fat for energy. This results in a loss of weight and is often an early indication of diabetes.

A by-product of fat metabolism is the formation of *ketone bodies* (chemical compounds) which, when excessive, cause a condition known as diabetic *acidosis.* This can cause coma and death if not treated with insulin and the right kind of intravenous fluids. Before insulin was discovered, this was the way most diabetics died.

Excess Urine Production

As glucose accumulates above normal levels in the diabetic's bloodstream it is filtered by his kidneys and remains in the urine. Additional amounts of u-rine are produced to contain the excess glucose. This situation results in copious and frequent urination that in turn causes dehydration and an often insatiable thirst. These are classically the first signs of the presence of diabetes.

This is diabetes described largely in terms of changes in carbohydrate metabolism. But protein and fat metabolism are also involved, as are almost invariably some changes in the nerves, muscles, eyes, kidneys, and blood vessels.

No one knows why diabetes develops. In some ways diabetes resembles premature aging, and the causes of diabetes, if known, might shed some light on the causes of aging.

The body's need to obtain energy from glucose and to convert glucose to glycogen and vice versa is continuous but always changing quantitatively. Meeting these needs requires constantly fluctuating amounts of effective insulin. Nondiabetics produce these amounts no matter what they eat or do, thus maintaining a steady state of metabolism. Diabetics, however, cannot achieve this steady state simply by taking insulin; they must also control their diets and their activities. They may have to change the amounts of their medications from time to time.

Diabetes is not an all-or-nothing phenomenon. It can be mild, moderate, or severe, and can fluctuate in degree in any one individual over a long period of time, or even from day to day. Very little is known about the reasons for these differences and changes. It is known, however, that diabetes generally gets worse in the presence of illness, particularly infections (even colds). It is also affected adversely by hyperfunctioning diseases of the anterior pituitary, thyroid, and adrenal glands, by emotional and physical stress, and during pregnancy.

Diabetes Diagnosis

The diagnosis of diabetes is not ordinarily a difficult one. Especially in children, the symptoms of rapid weight loss, extreme hunger, generalized weakness, frequent and copious urination, and insatiable thirst make it easy to recognize. Finding glucose in the urine along with increased levels of glucose in the blood generally confirms the diagnosis. However, glucose in the urine does not always indicate the presence of diabetes. A few people with unusual kidney function have glucose in their urine with normal blood levels, a condition known as *renal glycosuria.*

Moreover, an adult with diabetes may not have such a definite set of symptoms for months or years after he has actually developed the disease. Instead he may have vague fatigue or persistent skin infections. A woman may have a persistent genital itch that a physician might suspect is due to diabetes. Proof is provided by urine and blood tests. Glucose in the urine at the time of a routine physical examination might provide the first clue. Once diagnosed, treatment should be begun.

Treatment of Diabetes

Diet

The diet of a diabetic, although a major part of his treatment, is similar to what a normal person of the same age should eat. However, some radical dietary changes may be ordered if the previous diet has not been a proper one. This is particularly true in regard to reducing the calories in food eaten by overweight diabetics.

Diet is the only treatment needed by many adult diabetics, particularly those who are obese when they develop the disease, provided they can lose and not regain their excess weight. Because obese people are more likely to develop diabetes, they should have urine or blood sugar tests yearly after the age of 40. But it is more important for them to make every effort to lose weight before they become diabetics.

Individualized Diets

Each diabetic's diet has to be individualized to a certain extent. This is done originally by the physician when the diagnosis is made and periodically thereafter. The physician must learn the eating habits, customs, and preferences of his diabetic patient. Because eating is so much a part of the patient's personality and has such great psychological importance, its pattern should be changed radically only when necessary.

Certain principles that may not involve major changes should be kept in mind. For example, the diet should conform to the patient's customary cultural and ethnic pattern. It should not make him feel weak and without energy. If it does, he needs more food and more insulin.

Some nonobese diabetics, especially elderly ones, need only to eliminate sugar, soft drinks, and pastry from their diets. A mild diabetic often needs only to reduce the amount of carbohydrate in his diet and replace it with fats and proteins. Alcohol can be a part of a diabetic's diet under certain circumstances, which he should discuss with his physician. Sugar-free foods and beverages enable a diabetic to enjoy some of life's minor luxuries.

Children should, if possible, have diets that are similar to those of their friends, although they must be helped to understand that they should avoid eating foods containing concentrated sugars, like soda pop, candy, jams, and jellies.

Diet Guides

Most physicians have available printed diet guides to help their patients adjust their diets as needed. These indicate the number of calories and amount of protein, carbohydrate, and fat per household measure in all foods. See also Ch. 27, *Nutrition and Weight Control,* for additional reading on this subject.

When to eat is another matter, and this often necessitates some changes in eating habit patterns, especially for people taking insulin. Most important is regularity in relation to the patient's rest-activity time patterns. In general, almost half of the day's carbohydrates should be eaten at lunch because this is usually when activity and energy expenditure are greatest. The remainder should be divided between breakfast and dinner.

Insulin

Until recent years, insulin was prepared commercially in the United States from beef or pork pancreas. More recently, researchers have developed an insulin drug that is manufactured with a synthetic duplicate of human genes. Until this drug, called Humulin, appeared diabetics who were allergic to insulin products made from animal cells had to resort to more complex drugs such as steroids. Unlike animal insulins, Humulin, the first consumer health product made with DNA (*deoxyribonucleic acid*), can be produced in unlimited quantities.

Insulin has to be given by injection, usually *subcutaneous injection,* just beneath the skin, because it is destroyed by gastric secretions when taken orally.

The method of preparation also determines the timing of its action, and it is classified into three basic types:

TYPE OF INSULIN	TIME (HOURS) OF ACTION AFTER INJECTION		
	Onset	Peak	Duration
Rapid	½–1	2–8	4–14
Intermediate	2–4	6–12	10–26
Prolonged	4–8	12–24	24–36

There are two or three different insulin preparations for each type—rapid, intermediate, and prolonged.

Ideally, insulin injected once a day should more or less mimic the normal insulin action of a nondiabetic. That is the purpose of the intermediate and long-acting insulins, with which a rapid insulin is sometimes combined. Many diabetics are able to take insulin only once a day, particularly when their diet and activity pattern is sufficiently constant. Others, however, require two or more injections. The usual time to take insulin is before breakfast. This should be the same time every day. Second injections are often taken at suppertime.

A diabetic's basic insulin dose has to be established initially according to the severity of his disease. The dose is determined largely by his blood and urine glucose levels, the physician's judgment, and trial and error. Once established, the dosage has to be assessed daily and adjusted as necessary on the basis of the amount of sugar in the urine, diet, activity, and other factors.

Many diabetics take the same dose daily for years; others need to readjust theirs constantly. The number of units taken per day varies greatly from person to person, but probably most diabetics take between 10 and 40 units a day. The cost generally is less than one cent a unit. Insulin comes in 10-cc vials that must be refrigerated until first used. Thereafter they can be kept at room temperature.

Self-medication

Most diabetics self-inject their insulin. One can learn the technique of self-injection by practicing injecting an orange before trying it on oneself. The needle should always be sharp. It is important to change the exact site of the injection from day to day. Too frequent use of the same site may impair insulin absorption. The specially calibrated syringe and the needle can be either presterilized and discarded after one use, or they can be reused after resterilization by boiling for five minutes.

Insulin Shock

When injected insulin is active in the body system it must be matched by a sufficient amount of blood sugar. If not matched because of too much insulin, too much exercise, or too little ingested carbohydrate, the blood sugar level falls, a condition known as *hypoglycemia,* and the brain is deprived of an essential source of energy. This is most apt to occur at the time of the insulin's peak activity.

The first sign of an insulin reaction or *insulin shock* is usually mild hunger. Then come, and rather quickly, sweating, dizziness, palpitation, shallow breathing, trembling, mental confusion, strange behavior, and finally loss of consciousness. Prompt treatment is important. A lump of sugar or a piece of candy taken when symptoms first begin to appear will usually provide enough glucose to abort the reaction.

It is sometimes necessary to give intravenous glucose to counter insulin shock. This terminates the reaction almost immediately. Diabetics who use insulin should always have a lump or two of sugar or some candy with them and learn to recognize an oncoming insulin reaction. In general they should eat a small snack of glu-

Injection of Insulin Dose

1. Wipe site of injection with cotton swab dipped in alcohol.
2. With one hand, pinch up skin at injection site. Place syringe perpendicularly to the skin and quickly insert needle for its entire length in order to insure injection of sufficient depth *(see illustration).* The more rapidly the needle is inserted, the less the pain will be. Stainless steel needles are preferred.
3. Inject insulin dose.

Sites of Insulin Injections

It is important to change the site of injection daily for best absorption of insulin.

cose of some sort about the time their insulin activity reaches its peak.

Insulin reaction or shock can happen to any diabetic taking insulin. It is one of the liabilities of insulin therapy. Repeated and prolonged episodes of insulin reaction can be damaging to the brain. All diabetics, and especially those taking insulin, should have an identification bracelet or necklace indicating they have diabetes so that anyone examining them in an unconscious state can quickly realize the probable cause of their uncon-

sciousness. This can be supplemented by a card in the wallet or purse with additional details. These are available from the Medic Alert Foundation, Turlock, CA 95380, at a very modest cost. It is also vital that at least a few persons with whom the diabetic regularly associates know about his disease so that they can take prompt action if they see problems developing.

The Insulin Pump

Development of a pump for infusion of insulin into the body may offer a better method of treating diabetics with keto-acidosis, or ketosis. The pump method of continuous intravenous (IV) infusion has been used with moderate success in such cases.

Some advantages have been noted. A reduced amount of hypoglycemia has been reported, for example. Because the insulin is injected directly into the bloodstream, a smaller amount is required for control. Shots, or injections, under the skin have not been necessary while the patient has been receiving infusion treatment. Some physicians believe, however, that the older method of administering insulin by injection will remain useful. These physicians point out that better control of the treatment results when shots are given and the amount of urine glucose is monitored closely. Also, patients can observe how the insulin is given when the needle is used.

The insulin pump system generally includes a reservoir for the insulin; a peristaltic pump, one that impels the fluid by contracting and expanding; and a "power pack" containing batteries that activate the pump. The entire assembly, with associated tubings, typically weighs about 1.5 pounds (525 grams). The system is rugged enough to withstand rough treatment under difficult weather and environmental conditions.

If widely accepted and used, the insulin pump system may answer a basic need for improved ways to introduce drugs into the body. Earlier methods, including the subcutaneous, or needle, technique, have been described as faulty because they are "nonphysiologic"—they do not deliver the drugs where they can be used immediately by the body.

Oral Drugs

Oral *hypoglycemic drugs* have been available since the late 1950s. They are mainly helpful in controlling mild diabetes that develops in people 45 and over. However, younger people can occasionally be maintained on these drugs rather than on insulin. They stimulate the release of *endogenous* (self-produced) *insulin* from the pancreas or foster insulin activity in other ways. Chemically composed of *sulfonylurea,* they are remotely related to sulfa drugs but are not true sulfas. An entirely different oral hypoglycemic agent is *DBI* (*phenformin*). Some physicians urge that such drugs be prescribed only in cases that cannot be controlled effectively by other techniques.

For these drugs to work, some of the islet cells must be producing insulin or be capable of producing it. They either work well or not at all. The dose varies from one to eight tablets taken before meals and throughout the day. They cost a few cents a tablet. Insulin reactions do not occur although some diabetics take insulin also and are thereby vulnerable to insulin reactions. The decision about treating a given diabetic with these pills, insulin, or both has to be left to the patient's physician.

Diabetic Coma

Prolonged *hyperglycemia,* or excess sugar in the blood, from insufficient insulin activity can cause *diabetic coma.* This condition involves the increasing buildup of ketone bodies, the by-product of fat metabolism, which creates an *acidotic* condition (chemical imbalance in the blood, marked by an excess of acid). When this has been present for several days, perhaps a week or longer, symptoms begin to develop that are similar to those associated with the onset of diabetes. They include excessive urination and thirst, dry and hot skin, drowsiness, and finally, coma. The earliest stage of the problem is called *diabetic ketosis;* a slightly later stage is known as *diabetic acidosis.* From the beginning there are increasing amounts of glucose as well as ketone bodies in the urine. The unconscious patient will have deep, labored breathing, and a fruity odor to his breath.

Diabetic acidosis resembles an insulin reaction, although they can be distinguished from each other. If you find a diabetic in coma and you do not know the cause, assume the cause is an insulin reaction and treat him initially with sugar. This will give immediate relief to an insulin reaction but will not affect diabetic acidosis.

Diabetic acidosis occurs for many reasons. The patient does not take his insulin or oral hypoglycemic drugs for several days. He may take too little insulin because he is confused about the dosage. He may overeat or underexercise for a number of days, perhaps because he feels ill or has a cold.

Treatment

In its early stages ketosis generally can be treated by the patient himself with directions from his physician, usually by telephone. The fundamentals of this treatment involve taking rapid-acting insulin—every diabetic should keep a bottle of this on hand—every three or four hours until the urine has less glucose and no longer contains ketone bodies. Ketone bodies can be tested in the urine along with glucose. If there is a treatable underlying cause for the acidosis, such as an infection, it should be treated as well. In the later stages, hospital treatment with larger amounts of insulin, often given intravenously, and specific intravenous fluid therapy is essential.

Diabetes Control

An occasional insulin reaction is almost unavoidable, but diabetic acidosis occurs mainly because the diabetes was not well controlled. Good control means feeling well with only small amounts of sugar, or none, in the urine. This is possible for most but not all diabetics. A few diabetics can never achieve good control for a variety of reasons relating largely to the vagaries of this disease.

Personal Glucose Tests

The amount of glucose in the urine provides a kind of barometer of diabetic control. The amount in the blood at a given point in time provides a better barometer but is more difficult to check for obvious reasons. Therefore all diabetics should test their urine daily and sometimes more often, particularly in the beginning or when they are having control problems.

The ordinary urine specimen contains urine collected in the bladder over a period of several hours or overnight. The glucose in it is an average indication of what the blood sugar has been during a previous period. To get an idea of the blood sugar level at the time of the urine test, the urine that has accumulated in the bladder must first be discarded. Then a second specimen of urine should be passed about a half hour later and that specimen tested for glucose.

Several types of tests are available for this purpose. Some utilize chemically treated paper which, when dipped in urine, turns different colors to indicate varying amounts of glucose in the urine. Others use tablets that change to different colors when dropped into small amounts of urine. Adjustments in diet, activity, and insulin or oral hypoglycemic agents can be made on the basis of these test results. It costs a few cents to do each test.

Making Lifelong Adjustments

Once a diabetic has learned the fundamentals of his diet, his insulin or oral hypoglycemic agent medication, and has stabilized sufficiently his daily physical activities, he is well on his way to leading a normal life. There are, however, still a few psychological roadblocks.

First is the hard business of adjusting to the disease and coming to accept the fact that it can be lived with even though there is no cure. Initial depression is understandable and common. It does not persist. Then comes the often difficult task of regularizing one's life in terms of eating schedules, taking insulin, testing the urine, and exercising regularly.

Not many diabetics can maintain good control if they go to a Saturday night party, postpone their dinner time by four or five hours, and sleep until noon on Sunday. Maintaining one's usual schedule while traveling is another obstacle. The diabetic may feel that people treat him differently from the way they used to treat him or from the way they treat others. He will have to get used to seeing his physician frequently and regularly and having blood drawn to determine his blood sugar. He will have to spend a certain amount of money for insulin or oral hypoglycemic drugs, syringes and needles, urine-testing materials,

special sugar-free foods, and medical care.

Self-pity and then rebellion against these factors are not unusual, especially in children. And with rebellion comes an increased likelihood of insulin reactions or diabetic ketosis. Some diabetics use their disease as a way to manipulate others and thus create trying interpersonal relationships. The sensitive physician is aware of all of this and will give his patient the opportunity to verbalize his feelings.

Those with whom the diabetic lives—parents, siblings, spouse, and children—are also affected in various ways. The family's food style may be changed to some extent. Parents may have a sense of guilt about what they erroneously presume to be their part in the child's development of diabetes. They may have difficulty differentiating normal adolescent moods from those associated with the diabetic's fluctuating carbohydrate metabolism. They may become controlling and coddling or rejecting and resentful. Either reaction pattern will affect the child adversely. Parents should be helped to understand the disease as well as its effect on their child.

Juvenile Insulin Dependent Diabetes (JIDD)

Boys and girls develop diabetes in approximately equal numbers. For both sexes, the average age of onset is about eight years. For both sexes, too, diabetes may be discovered in the first hours or days of life. More frequently, diabetes appears at the age of puberty.

In severe cases, the youthful victim of diabetes suffers from a critical shortage of insulin. Acidosis may occur. The child in this situation usually has what is known as juvenile insulin dependent diabetes (JIDD). Insulin therapy may be required throughout the young person's life.

Therapy need not adversely affect the child's activities, growth rate, or psychological or intellectual development. The young person on continuous insulin therapy can usually be allowed to eat as much as he or she wants; but if abnormally large quantities of food are consumed, or if hunger continues even after meals, a physician should be consulted.

What kind of diet is best for the child with juvenile insulin dependent diabetes? High-carbohydrate diets appear to meet this child's need best. But animal fats should be restricted; ice cream in particular should be avoided. Ice milk may serve as a substitute. The rule restricting the intake of animal fats also means that commercially baked cookies, candy containing fat, including chocolate mixtures, and similar foods are unsuitable.

Some kinds of candy, fruit juices, meat, and eggs may be included in the young JIDD child's diet. "Permissible" candy may contain honey, or it may be made from sorbitol. Some health-food shops stock sesame crunch that the diabetic child can enjoy. Because they contain protein and vegetable oil, nuts make good snack foods.

Fruit juices, meat, and eggs supply a number of nutrients that the diabetic child needs. Orange and grapefruit juices, for example, contain potassium, fructose, and vitamins C and A. Meat provides protein, and should be included in the diet. Eggs supply lecithin, which keeps cholesterol from building up in blood vessels, and amino acids, essential to body-building. Eggs should be soft- or hard-boiled or poached, not fried in butter or other kinds of fat.

Fresh fish, chicken, and turkey belong properly in the diabetic child's diet, as do peanut butter and jelly sandwiches. Peanut butter made from fresh-ground nuts is preferred, but cannot be obtained in all stores. For essential whole grains, the child should eat whole wheat bread, millet, oatmeal, and other cereals—but dried cereals should be ruled out. Fresh vegetables may be served if the child does not like cooked vegetables.

Adequate amounts of sugar and starches will usually prevent hypoglycemic reactions in the JIDD child. But where such a reaction does set in, the child should drink fruit juice or some kind of rapidly digestible carbohydrate. The prepared child always carries hard candy or a box of raisins. Both help terminate hypoglycemic attacks.

Pregnancy and Diabetes

Pregnancy is a very special time in any woman's life, but it is particularly special for a diabetic and her unborn child. Diabetes is not a factor of any magnitude as far as conception is concerned, but pregnancy affects the diabetic's carbohydrate metabolism dramatically. In general there is an increase in blood glucose levels and an ever-increasing need for insulin. However, there can be periodic and unpredictable reductions in insulin need. Therefore, urine glucose and blood glucose need to be tested more frequently than under ordinary circumstances.

The urine should be tested three or four times a day and the blood glucose at every visit to the obstetrician. With good management during a diabetic's pregnancy, her baby has an excellent chance of being as normal and healthy as that of the nondiabetic mother.

Diabetes in Later Life

The association between aging and diabetes relates largely to a gradual loss of elasticity in the cells of the blood vessels, kidneys, eyegrounds (the inner sides of the backs of the eyeballs), and nerve tissues. These cellular changes may not become apparent for many years after the development of diabetes. However, occasionally they are present before or appear several years after the diabetes is recognized. This is particularly apt to be true in older people who develop diabetes.

The nerve-tissue changes can cause a diminished sensation to touch and pain and sometimes a loss of motor function of the extremities as well as sexual impotence. The eyeground changes damage the retina in various ways and can cause varying degrees of loss of vision. In about eight percent of cases this progresses to blindness.

The changes in the kidneys affect their filtration functions, causing *albuminuria,* a loss of protein from the blood serum into the urine and the development of high blood pressure in roughly 23 percent of diabetics. The vascular changes, which are rather diffuse, contribute to the specific organ changes noted above, and frequently cause a reduction in blood supply to the legs and heart muscle. This ultimately causes heart damage in perhaps 20 percent of diabetics. Medicine can do much to reduce the effects of these many changes but cannot cure them.

Some degree of prevention is possible, and good diabetic control generally is thought to contribute to a reduction and delay in the development of these complications. Because the nerve and vascular changes make the feet particularly vulnerable to infections that can be serious and even lead to amputation—gangrene occurs in about three percent of diabetics— proper and daily care of the feet is essential to prevent the development of infections. The older diabetic should be careful to keep his feet clean and dry and cut his toenails frequently and evenly. Some physicians recommend that diabetics have their toenails cut only by a podiatrist.

Early Detection

Anyone who does not have diabetes might very well wonder whether he or she is at all likely to get it, and, if so, what can be done to prevent it. One answer is clear. If you are obese, whatever your age, try to lose weight. This is especially important if you have grandparents, parents, brothers, sisters, or children who developed diabetes in middle age or earlier. It is important also if you are a mother who has had babies weighing nine or more pounds at birth.

A fairly simple laboratory test, called a *glucose tolerance test* (GTT), has been developed to identify a person who is prediabetic. The subject either swallows a drink containing 100 grams of glucose or is given the same amount intravenously. Thereafter his blood sugar is determined at set intervals over a three-to-six-hour period. If his blood sugar level remains abnormally high for too long, he is said to be a prediabetic or to have *chemical diabetes.*

All adults should have their urine tested at least once a year for the presence of sugar. Some adults and younger persons should have more frequent urine tests and perhaps periodic glucose tolerance tests.

Genetically, diabetes has many characteristics of a Mendelian recessive inherited disease. Theoretically the chances are one in four of a child developing diabetes if one parent has the disease; it is almost inevitable if both have it. These are obviously important factors for diabetics to consider before they have children, particularly when both prospective parents have diabetes.

16

Diseases of the Eye and Ear

Most people never experience any impairment of the senses of smell, taste, and touch. But it is indeed lucky and unusual to reach old age without having some problems connected with sight or with hearing or both.

The Eyes

All sensations must be processed in the brain by a normally functioning central nervous system for their proper perception. In addition, each sensation is perceived through a specific sense organ. Thus, sight is dependent on at least one functioning eye.

The eye is an optical system that can be compared to a camera, because the human lens perceives and the retina receives an image in the same way that a camera and its film does. Defects in this optical system are called errors in refraction and are the most common type of sight problem.

Myopia

Nearsightedness or *myopia* is a refractive error that causes faraway objects to be seen as blurred and indistinct. The degree of nearsightedness can be measured by testing each eye with a Snellen Test Chart. Normal vision is called 20/20. This means that at 20 feet the eye sees an image clearly and accurately.

Eyesight of less-than-normal acuity is designated as 20/50 or 20/100 and so on. This means that what the deficient eye can see accurately at a distance of 20 feet or less, the normal eye can see accurately at 50 or 100 feet.

Myopia is the most common of all the refractive errors and usually results from an elongation of the eyeball. The cause of this abnormality is unknown, but it prevents the image from being focused on the retina. Those who are affected by myopia usually develop it between the ages of 6 and 15. They are likely to become aware of the condition when they can no longer see as well as they used to in school or at the movies or as well as their friends can. Individually prescribed eyeglasses or contact lenses can correct the refractive error and produce normal vision.

Farsightedness and Astigmatism

The opposite of myopia is *hyperopia,* or farsightedness, which results from a shortening of the eyeball. The two conditions may be combined with *astigmatism,* in which vertical and horizontal images do not focus on the same point, mainly because of some abnormality of the front surface of the cornea. Properly fitted glasses can correct all of these deficiencies.

Presbyopia

A fourth refractive error combines with the other three to make up about 80 percent of all visual defects. It is known as *presbyopia,* or old-sight, and results from an inability of the lens to focus on near objects. Almost everyone is affected by presbyopia some time after the age of 40, because of the aging of the lens itself or the muscles which expand and contract it. The condition is usually noticed when it becomes necessary to hold a book or newspaper farther and farther away from the eyes in order to be able to read it. Although presbyopia is a nuisance, it can be easily corrected with glasses.

All these conditions represent variations in the sight of one or both eyes from what is considered the norm.

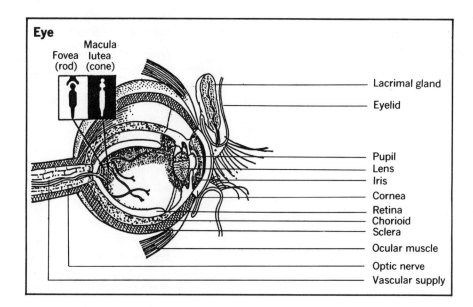

Eye

Fovea (rod)
Macula lutea (cone)

Lacrimal gland
Eyelid

Pupil
Lens
Iris
Cornea
Retina
Chorioid
Sclera
Ocular muscle
Optic nerve
Vascular supply

Because seating distance from a school blackboard, the size of print, and the distance at which signs must be read are all based on what is considered to be normal vision, eye defects are handicaps, some mild and some severe.

Many people can function normally without glasses if the defects are minor. But because uncorrected refractive errors can cause headaches and general fatigue as well as eye aches and eye fatigue, they should receive prompt medical attention.

Color Blindness

Color blindness is a visual defect that occurs in about eight percent of men but is extremely rare in women. It is hereditary, and usually involves an inability to differentiate clearly between red, green, and blue. It is a handicap for which there is no known cure at the present time.

Glaucoma

Glaucoma is a serious problem that affects about two percent of those people who are over 40. It is caused not only by the aging process, but also and more importantly by anatomical changes inside the eye that pre-

vent the normal drainage of fluid. The pressure inside the eye is therefore increased, and this pressure causes further anatomical change that can lead to blindness.

Glaucoma may begin with occasional eye pain or blurred vision, or it may be very insidious, cause no symptoms for years, and be discov-

ered only at an eye examination. Glaucoma is the number one cause of blindness, and an annual check for its onset by a specialist is particularly recommended for everyone over 40. The test is quick, easy, and painless, and should symptoms appear, early treatment, either medical or surgical or both, can reduce the likelihood of partial or complete loss of sight.

Cataracts

Another serious eye problem is the development of *cataracts*. These are areas in the lens that are no longer transparent. The so-called *senile cataract* is common among elderly people because of degenerative changes in the lens. The condition causes varying degrees of loss of vision which are readily noticed by the patient. If the vision is reduced a great deal, the entire lens can be removed surgically and appropriate glasses or contact lenses can be provided.

Focusing

Distant vision
Object
Pupil
Iris
Lens

Radial muscle
Pupil
Circular muscle

Near vision
Object
Pupil
Iris
Lens

Radial muscle
Pupil
Circular muscle

When viewing a distant object (more than 20 feet away), the lens flattens and the pupil dilates, allowing more light to enter the eye. The pupil is dilated by the action of the outer radial muscles of the iris, which contract and thus stretch the previously contracted circular muscles. When viewing a near object, the lens becomes more oval and the pupil contracts as more light enters the eye. This prevents overstimulation of the retina. The pupil is reduced in size by the contraction of the inner circular muscles, which serve to stretch the previously contracted radial muscles.

Eye Surgery

Eye muscle
Catarct
Cornea transplant

Lens

Cornea
Iris

Corneal transplant

Cornea

Cataract

Vitreous humor

Retinal vessels

Canal

Laser

Retina

Aqueous humor

Retinal detachment

Glaucoma

Detached Retina

Among the most serious eye disorders is the condition known as *separated* or *detached retina*. It occurs when fluid from inside the eye gets under the retina (the inner membrane at the back of the eye, on which the image is focused) and separates it from its bed, thus breaking the connections that are essential for normal vision. The most common cause of the detachment is the formation of a hole or tear in the retina. However, the condition may also develop following a blow to the head or to the eye, or because of a tumor, nephritis, or high blood pressure.

The symptoms of the onset of retinal separation are showers of drifting black spots and frequent flashes of light shaped like pinwheels that interfere with vision. These disturbances are usually followed by a dark shadow in the area of sight closest to the nose.

A retinal detachment is treated by surgical techniques in which the accumulated fluid is drained off and the hole in the tissue is sealed. About 60 percent of all cases are cured or considerably improved after surgery. The earlier the diagnosis, the more favorable is the outcome. Proper postoperative care usually involves several weeks of immobilization of the head so that the retinal tissue can heal without disturbance.

Trauma

Like any other part of the body, the eye can be injured by a major accident or *trauma*, although it is somewhat protected by the bones surrounding it. Trauma can cause most of the problems previously described. In addition, small objects can get into the eye easily, and particles of soot and other wind-borne dirt can cause great discomfort. The tearing that results

from the irritation usually floats foreign substances away, but occasionally they have to be removed by an instrument.

When a particle in the eye or under the eyelid is not easily dislodged and begins to cause redness, it should be removed by someone qualified to do so. The eye should never be poked at or into by untrained hands.

Leaving contact lenses in the eye for too long can cause discomfort that lasts for quite a while even after they have been taken out. Bacterial or viral infections of the outer surface of the eye such as *conjunctivitis* or *pinkeye,* or of the eyelids, are quite common and should be treated by a physician if they are extensive or chronic.

Contact Lenses

Contact lenses, which are fitted directly over the iris and pupil of the eye in contact with the cornea (the tissue covering the outer, visible surface of the eye), are preferred by some people for the correction of vision defects. In some cases of severe astigmatism or nearsightedness, or following cataract surgery, contact lenses can be more effective and comfortable than eyeglasses. But the chief reason for their popularity has been cosmetic. They are practically invisible.

Hard contact lenses adhere to the eye by suction; a partial vacuum is created between the inner surface of the lens and the outer surface of the eyeball.

Soft plastic contact lenses are *hydrophilic* (literally, water-loving) and adapt their shape to the shape of the moist cornea, to which they adhere. Thus they are relatively easily fitted, and patients seldom experience discomfort in adjusting to them. It is virtually impossible for dust particles to get under them. Many ophthalmologists, however, advise that the soft lens be sterilized daily.

The soft lens has proved valuable in the treatment of some eye disorders. But it often leads to problems among wearers. It may scratch or tear, for example, and generally it has

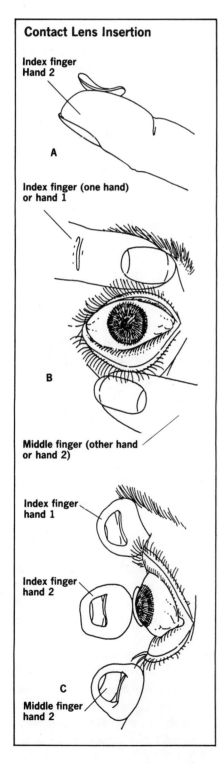

Contact Lens Insertion

Index finger
Hand 2

A

Index finger (one hand)
or hand 1

B

Middle finger (other hand
or hand 2)

Index finger
hand 1

Index finger
hand 2

C

Middle finger
hand 2

been limited to the correction of certain kinds of nearsightedness and farsightedness.

Extended wear lenses (EWLs) were introduced in the 1970s. Made of soft plastic like the older lenses, but thinner and more porous, they could be worn as long as 30 days. But wearing EWLs too long was found to cause such problems as scarring of the cornea; neurovascularization, the growth of tiny blood vessels that can cloud the vision and in extreme cases threaten the wearer's sight; the development of microcysts during sleep; and bacterial infections of the eye or eyelid, such as *Acanthamoeba keratitis.*

Disposable lenses and cosmetic contacts appeared in the late 1980s. Worn for a week and then discarded, disposable lenses reduce the danger of keratitis and other infections. But they cost about 50 percent more than the regular EWLs. Cosmetic contacts simply change the color of the eyes. Disposables should not be worn longer than prescribed, and cosmetic lenses should not be shared to prevent the spread of eye diseases and other infections. Clean the lenses according to instructions and seek medical help quickly if problems arise.

Diseases That Affect Vision

In addition to the various disorders involving only the eye, there are a number of generalized diseases that affect vision. Among these are arteriosclerosis, diabetes mellitus, and hypertension or high blood pressure, which often cause abnormalities in the blood vessels of various parts of the eye. These abnormalities can lead to tissue changes that cause the patient to see spots or to notice that his vision is defective.

Diseases of the brain, such as mul-

tiple sclerosis, tumors, and abscesses, although rare, can result in double vision or loss of lateral or central vision. Any sudden or gradual changes in vision should be brought to a physician's attention promptly, since early diagnosis and treatment is usually effective and can prevent serious deterioration.

The Ears

The ear, like the eye, is a complicated structure. Its major parts consist of the auditory canal, middle ear, and inner ear. Hearing results from the perception of sound waves whose loudness can be measured in decibels and whose highness or lowness of pitch can be measured by their frequency in cycles per second.

Sound waves usually travel through the auditory canal to the eardrum or *tympanic membrane,* vibrating it in such a way as to carry the vibrations to and along the three interlocking small bones in the middle ear to the inner ear. Here the vibrations are carried to the auditory nerve through a fluid-filled labyrinth called the communicating channel.

An abnormality at any of these points can produce a hearing deficiency. Normal hearing means the ability to hear the spoken voice in a relatively quiet room at a distance of about 18 feet. How well a person hears can be tested by an audiometer, which measures decibels and frequency of sound.

Wax Accumulation

A very common cause of hearing deficiency is the excessive accumulation of wax in the auditory canal, where it is continually being secreted. When the excess that blocks the passage of sound waves is removed—sometimes by professional instrumenta-

Ear

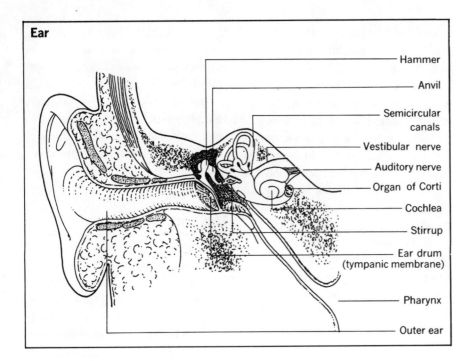

Hammer

Anvil

Semicircular canals

Vestibular nerve

Auditory nerve

Organ of Corti

Cochlea

Stirrup

Ear drum (tympanic membrane)

Pharynx

Outer ear

tion—hearing returns to normal. Anyone whose hearing is temporarily impaired in this way should avoid the use of rigid or pointed objects for cleaning out the accumulated wax.

Infection

Infections or other diseases of the skin that lines the auditory canal can sometimes cause a kind of local swelling that blocks the canal and interferes with hearing. Although such a condition can be painful, proper treatment, usually with antibiotics, generally results in a complete cure.

A major cause of hearing deficiency acquired after birth is recurrent bacterial infection of the middle ear. The infecting organisms commonly get to the middle ear through the *Eustachian tube,* which connects the middle ear to the upper throat, or through the eardrum if it has been perforated by injury or by previous infection.

The infection can cause hearing loss, either because it becomes chronic or because the tissues become scarred. Such infections are usually painful, but ever since treatment with antibiotics has become pos-

sible, they rarely spread to the mastoid bone as they used to in the past.

Disorders Caused by Pressure

The Eustachian tube usually permits the air pressure on either side of the eardrum to equalize. When the pressure inside the drum is less than that outside—as occurs during descent in an airplane or elevator, or when riding through an underwater tunnel, or during skin diving—the eardrum is pushed inward. This causes a noticeable hearing loss or a stuffy feeling in the ear that subsides as soon as the pressure equalizes again. Yawning or swallowing usually speeds up the return to normal.

When the unequal pressure continues for several days because the Eustachian tube is blocked, fluid begins to collect in the middle ear. This is called *serous* (or *nonsuppurative*) *otitis media* and can cause permanent hearing damage.

Eustachian tube blockage is more commonly the result of swelling around its *nasopharyngeal* end because of a throat infection, a cold, or an allergy. Nose drops help to open

up the tube, but sometimes it may be necessary to drain the ear through the eardrum or treat the disorder with other surgical procedures.

Otosclerosis

A very common cause of hearing loss that affects about 1 in 200 adults—usually women—is *otosclerosis.* This disorder is the result of a sort of freezing of the bones in the middle ear caused by an overgrowth of tissue. The onset of the disorder usually occurs before age 30 among about 70 percent of the people who will be affected. Only one ear may be involved, but the condition does get progressively worse. Although heredity is an important factor, the specific cause of otosclerosis is unknown. In some cases, surgery can be helpful.

Injury

A blow to the head, or a loud noise close to the ear such as the sound of a gunshot or a jet engine, especially when repeated often, can cause temporary and sometimes permanent hearing defects. Anyone who expects to be exposed to damaging noise should wear protective earmuffs. Injury to the auditory nerve by chemicals or by medicines such as streptomycin can also cause loss of hearing.

Ringing in the Ears

Sometimes people complain of hearing noises unrelated to the reception of sound waves from an outside source. This phenomenon is called *tinnitus* and occurs in the form of a buzzing, ringing, or hissing sound.

It may be caused by some of the conditions described above and may be relieved by proper treatment. In many cases, however, the cause is unknown and the patient simply has to learn to live with the sounds and ignore them.

Impairment of Balance

The *labyrinths* of the inner ear are involved not only in hearing but also in controlling postural balance. When the labyrinths are diseased, the result can be a feeling of *vertigo* or true dizziness. This sensation of being unable to maintain balance is quite different from feeling lightheaded or giddy.

Vertigo can be an incapacitating disorder. Sometimes it is caused by diseases of the central nervous system such as epilepsy or brain hemorrhage, but more often by inflammation sometimes caused by infection of the labyrinth. It can be sudden and recurrent as in *Ménière's disease,* or somewhat gradual and nonrecurrent. It may or may not be accompanied by vomiting or hearing loss. Treatment for the condition varies depending on the cause.

Deafness

Deafness at birth or in a very young baby is an especially difficult problem because hearing is necessary for the development of speech. Although the deafness itself may be impossible to correct, its early recognition and management can usually prevent muteness from developing.

Many communities now have special schools for deaf children, and new techniques and machines are constantly being devised for helping them to learn how to speak, even if imperfectly. Any doubt about an infant's ability to hear should therefore be brought to a physician's attention immediately.

Deafness at birth can be caused by a maternal infection such as rubella (German measles) during pregnancy. Because children are often the ones who spread this disease, youngsters should be immunized against it.

Hearing Aids

Hearing loss that cannot be treated medically or surgically can often be compensated for by an accurately fitted hearing aid. This device, which now comes in many sizes, shapes, and types, converts sound waves into electrical impulses, amplifies them, and reconverts them into sound waves. A hearing aid can be placed in the auditory canal for air conduction of sound waves, or it can be worn behind the ear for bone conduction. See under "Hearing Loss" in Ch. 6, *The Later Years,* for further information about hearing aids.

17

Diseases of the Urinogenital System

The parts of the urinogenital tract that produce and get rid of urine are the same for men and women: the kidneys, ureters, bladder, and urethra. To understand some of the problems that can arise from diseases of the urinary tract, it is necessary to know a few facts about the anatomy and function of these parts.

The two kidneys are located on either side of the spinal column in the back portion of the abdomen between the last rib and the third lumbar vertebra of the spine. They are shaped like the beans named after them but are considerably larger.

Their function is to filter and cleanse the blood of waste substances produced in the course of normal living and, together with some other organs, to maintain a proper balance of body fluids. The kidneys do this job by filtering the fluid portion of the blood as it passes through them, returning the necessary solids and water to the bloodstream, and removing waste products and excess water, called *urine*. These products then flow into the *ureters,* the ducts that connect the kidneys and bladder.

The *bladder* holds the urine until voiding occurs. The duct from the bladder to the urinary opening is called the *urethra*. In the male, it passes through the penis; in the female, in front of the anterior wall of the vagina.

Symptoms of Kidney Disorders

Normal kidney function can be disrupted by bacterial or viral infection, by tumors, by external injury, or by congenital defects. Some of the common symptoms that may result under these circumstances are:

- *Anuria:* inability to produce or void urine

- *Dysuria:* pain, often of a burning quality, during urination

- Frequency: abnormally frequent urination, often of unusually small amounts

- Hesitancy: difficulty in starting urination

- Urgency: a very strong urge to urinate, often strong enough to cause loss of urine

- *Oliguria:* reduced production of urine

- *Polyuria:* voiding larger than normal amounts of urine

- *Nocturia:* frequent voiding at night

- *Hematuria:* voiding blood in the urine

Because any of these symptoms may indicate a disease of the urinary tract, their appearance should be brought to the attention of a physician without delay.

Kidney Failure

Kidney failure can occur gradually—either from kidney disease or as a secondary condition resulting from another disease—or suddenly, as from an infection.

Acute Kidney Failure

The sudden loss of kidney function over a period of minutes to several days is known as acute kidney failure. It may be caused by impairment of blood supply to the kidneys, by severe infection, by nephritis (discussed below), by poisons, and by various other conditions that injure both kidneys.

Urogenital Systems

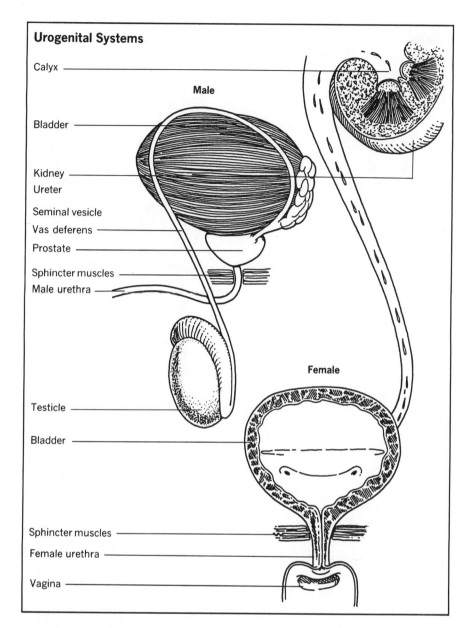

Calyx

Male

Bladder

Kidney

Ureter

Seminal vesicle

Vas deferens

Prostate

Sphincter muscles

Male urethra

Testicle

Bladder

Female

Sphincter muscles

Female urethra

Vagina

The body can function adequately throughout a normal lifespan with only one healthy kidney, but if both are impaired sufficiently over a short period of time, there will be symptoms of acute kidney failure: production of a decreased amount of urine (*oliguria*) sometimes with blood in it; fluid retention in body tissues, a condition known as *edema;* increasing fatigue and weakness; nausea and loss of appetite.

If damage to the kidneys has not been too severe, the patient begins to have a *diuresis,* or greater than normal urine output. When this hap-

pens—usually after one or two weeks of reduced urine output—he is kept on a restricted diet and reduced fluid intake after recovery until normal kidney function returns.

Causes

Heredity is rarely a factor in acute kidney failure, although people born with one kidney or with congenital defects of the urinary tract may lack the normal reserve capacity to prevent it. It is also unusual for external injury to result in a loss of function in both kidneys. However, severe internal

shock accompanied by a reduction of blood flow to the kidneys can cause acute kidney failure.

Prevention and Treatment

Acute kidney failure can occur at any age. Prevention hinges on the proper control of its many causes. About 50 percent of patients with this disease may succumb to it; in cases of severe kidney failure involving widespread destruction of tissue, mortality may be almost 100 percent.

When acute kidney failure occurs as a complication of another serious illness, its prevention and treatment are usually managed by physicians in a hospital. If the patient is not already under a physician's supervision when he has the characteristic symptoms, he should immediately be brought to a medical facility for diagnosis and treatment.

Chronic Kidney Failure and Uremia

Many progressive kidney diseases can eventually lead to a group of symptoms called *uremia.* Other diseases, such as severe high blood pressure, diabetes, and those leading to widespread damage of kidney tissue, can also cause uremia.

In this condition, as in acute kidney failure, waste products and excess fluid accumulate in the body and cause the symptoms of chronic kidney failure. Certain congenital defects in the urinogenital system such as *polycystic kidney disease,* in which cysts in the kidneys enlarge slowly and destroy normal kidney tissue, may lead to uremia. Hereditary diseases such as hereditary nephritis may cause chronic kidney failure, but this is uncommon. Injury is also rarely the cause of uremia.

Although kidney failure is more likely to occur in older people because of the decreased capacity of the body to respond to stress, uremia can occur in any age group if kidney damage is severe enough. The onset of uremia may be so gradual that it goes unnoticed until the patient is weak and seems chronically ill. Voiding unusually large amounts of urine and voiding during the night are early symptoms.

Sleepiness and increasing fatigue set in as the kidney failure progresses, and there is a loss of appetite accompanied sometimes by nausea and hiccups. As the disease gets more serious, increasing weakness, anemia, muscle twitching, and sometimes internal bleeding may occur. High blood pressure is another characteristic symptom. Because of fluid retention, there will often be marked signs of facial puffiness and swelling of the legs.

Kidney damage that leads to chronic kidney failure is irreversible and the outlook for the victim of uremia is poor. The technique of dialysis (discussed below) has, however, prolonged many lives and continues to be a life-saving procedure for many.

Dialysis

An effective method of treatment of kidney failure developed in the 1960s is based on an artificial kidney that cleanses the patient's blood if his own kidneys are not functioning properly. The procedure, known as *dialysis* (or *hemodialysis*), removes dangerous waste products and excess fluids from the patient's bloodstream. It is the accumulation of waste products and fluids that probably causes the symptoms of acute kidney failure and that can be fatal if not reversed in one way or another.

Dialysis for Chronic Kidney Failure

For patients suffering chronic kidney failure or uremia, dialysis is a life-preserving but unfortunately expensive

Dialysis

Intermediate mechanical support system

Circulating blood

Inflow

Outflow

Vein

Artery

Supporting mesh

Flat tubing

Washing solution

To drain pump

procedure. The patient must be dialyzed with the artificial kidney unit two or three times a week, usually for six to eight hours at a time. Although the technique does not cure uremia, it can keep the patient comfortable provided that his diet is carefully restricted and supervised.

Dialysis in the Home

One approach that promises to be helpful in reducing the excessive cost is the development of home dialysis programs prepared with the cooperation of hospitals having departments specializing in kidney disease. Home dialysis is not suitable for everyone; the patient must be mature and stable enough to be relied on to undertake the procedure on schedule and in the prescribed manner. The overall costs of home dialysis, however, are about one-third those of in-hospital dialysis.

Medicare Coverage

Medicare coverage is now available for a part of the costs for dialysis maintenance for those suffering from permanent kidney failure, even if they are under 65 years of age. Coverage includes training in self-dialysis and the cost of dialysis equipment and applies to dialysis done in the home as well as in hospitals or other approved facilities. For details of this coverage, see your local social security office or write for the free booklet, *Medicare Coverage for Kidney Dialysis and Kidney Transplant Services,* published by the Social Security Administration.

Kidney Transplant Surgery

Some people suffering from kidney disease may benefit greatly from the surgical transplant of a donor's kidney. The donor kidney may be taken from a live relative or from someone recently deceased. The organ is removed from the donor's abdomen, usually flushed with a salt solution, and then reattached to a large artery and vein in the recipient's abdomen and to his ureter.

The successfully transplanted kidney functions just as the patient's own did when he was healthy, removing wastes and excess fluids from his bloodstream and excreting the resulting urine through the bladder. The recipient of a kidney transplant must take special medication to prevent the rejection of the newly installed organ by his own body tissues. With proper medical care, recipients have lived for many years with their transplanted organs.

Medicare Coverage

Medicare coverage is now available for a part of the costs of kidney transplant surgery for those under 65 as well as those over 65. This coverage includes hospital charges for costs incurred by the donor. For details of this coverage, see your local social security office or write for the free booklet, *Medicare Coverage of Kidney Dialysis and Kidney Transplant Services,* published by the Social Security Administration.

Nephritis

Nephritis is a disorder characterized by inflammation of the *glomeruli* of the kidneys. The glomeruli are tiny coiled blood vessels through which the liquid portion of the blood is filtered as it enters the outer structure of the kidneys. There are about one million of these tiny blood vessels in each kidney. The fluid from the blood passes from them into many little ducts called *tubules.* Water and various substances are secreted into and absorbed from the liquid in the tubules. The final product of this passage of filtered fluid from the glomeruli through the tubules to the ureters and then to the bladder is urine. It contains the excess fluid and waste products produced by the body during normal functioning.

When the glomeruli become inflamed, the resulting disease is called *glomerulonephritis.* There are several forms of this disease. One type is thought to be caused by the body's allergic reaction to infection by certain streptococcal bacteria. Another type sometimes accompanies infection of the valves of the heart. The relationship between glomerulonephritis and strep infections is not fully understood at present, and the same may be said for nephritis, which is associated with allergic reaction to certain drugs and to heart valve infections.

Glomerulonephritis may occur ten days to two weeks after a severe strep throat infection. For this reason, any severe sore throat accompanied by a high fever should be seen and diagnosed by a physician. Prompt treatment with antibiotics may decrease the possibility of kidney involvement.

Nephritis Symptoms

The inflammation and swelling of the glomeruli cause a decrease in the amount of blood that the kidney is able to filter. As a result of the slowing down of this kidney function, the waste products of metabolism as well as excess fluid accumulate in the body instead of being eliminated at the normal rate.

In a typical case, a person will develop a severe sore throat with fever and a general feeling of sickness. These symptoms will disappear, but after one or two weeks, there will be a return of weakness and loss of appetite. The eyes and the face may become puffy, the legs may swell, and there may be shortness of breath—all because of the retention of excess fluid in the body. The amount of urine is small and the color is dark brown, somewhat like coffee. Abdominal pain, nausea, and vomiting may occur, always accompanied by fatigue. In most cases, the blood pressure increases, leading to headaches.

Although there is a hereditary type of nephritis, the more common types of the disease have other causes. When the disease is suspected, the physician examines a specimen of urine under a microscope and looks for red blood cells. These cells, which usually do not pass through the walls of the normal glomerulus in large numbers, do pass through the damaged walls of the inflamed blood vessels characteristic of nephritis. Evidence of decreased kidney function is also found by special blood tests.

Nephritis occurs in all age groups. Children under ten have an excellent chance of recovery, about 98 percent. In adults, from 20 to 50 percent of the cases may be fatal or may progress to chronic nephritis, which often leads to uremia and death.

Treatment

It is absolutely essential for anyone with a streptococcal infection, which may lead to acute glomerulonephritis, to receive prompt and proper treatment. Penicillin is considered the most effective antibiotic at present.

Once acute nephritis is present, the treatment consists of bed rest, some fluid restriction, and protein restriction if kidney failure occurs. If there is a total loss of kidney function, a specially restricted diet is prescribed. Complete lack of urine output—*anuria*— may last as long as ten days, but the patient can still make a full recovery if the treatment is right. Usually a gradual return of kidney function occurs over a period of several months.

Nephrosis

The *nephrotic syndrome,* commonly referred to as *nephrosis,* is a disease in which abnormal amounts of protein in the form of *albumin* are lost in the urine. Albumin consists of microscopic particles of protein present in the blood. These particles are important in maintaining the proper volume of fluids in the body, and they have other complicated functions as well. The loss of albumin in the urine affects the amount that remains in the blood, and it is this imbalance, together with other body changes, that results in the retention of excess fluid in the tissues, thus causing facial puffiness and swelling of the legs.

The disease is caused by damage to the glomeruli, but at the present time the exact nature of the damage is uncertain. It may be caused by an allergic reaction, by inflammation, or it may be a complication of diabetes. The nephrotic syndrome may also appear because of blood clots in the veins that drain the kidneys.

Although the disease is more common among children than among adults, it may affect a person of any age. The main symptom is painless swelling of the face, legs, and sometimes of the entire body. There is also loss of appetite, a tired, rundown feeling, and sometimes abdominal pain, vomiting, and diarrhea.

Recovery from nephrosis varies with age. More than 50 percent of child patients are completely free of kidney ailments after the first attack. Adults are more likely to develop some impairment of kidney function, or the disease may become chronic, with accompanying high blood pressure. In some people, protein loss may continue over the years, although the kidneys function in an apparently normal manner without any visible symptoms.

Treatment

Treatment of the nephrotic syndrome has been greatly helped by the use of the adrenal hormones known as *steroids*. The treatment is effective for about two-thirds of child patients and for about one-fourth to one-third of adults. Some patients may relapse after therapy is completed, sometimes years after such therapy has been discontinued. For this reason, steroids are sometimes continued after initial treatment but in reduced dosage, to avoid some of the unpleasant side effects such as acne and facial swelling.

Unlike the dietary treatment for uremia, a high protein diet is used with nephrotic patients so that the protein loss can be replaced. Salt intake is usually restricted because salt contributes to fluid retention and may cause high blood pressure or heart failure. If fluid retention doesn't respond to steroid treatment, other medicines called *diuretics,* which increase urinary output, are used.

Anyone with unusual swelling of the face, limbs, or abdomen should see a physician promptly. Even though the swelling is painless, it may be the first sign of the onset of a serious kidney problem.

Infection in the Urinary Tract

Infection in the urinary tract is a common disorder that can be serious if the kidneys themselves are involved.

Cystitis

Infection of the bladder is called *cystitis*. The symptoms include a burning sensation when urine is passed, the frequent need to urinate, occasionally blood in the urine, and sometimes difficulty in starting to urinate. Cystitis is rarely accompanied by high fever.

The problem may be recurrent and is more usual with women than men, probably because the female urethra is shorter and closer to the rectum, permitting bacteria to enter the bladder more easily. These bacteria multiply in the urine contained in the bladder, causing irritation to the bladder walls and producing the symptoms described above.

Cystitis should be treated promptly because the infection in the bladder can easily spread to the kidneys, with serious consequences. Treatment usually consists of antibiotics after urine analysis and culture have determined the type of bacteria causing the infection. Cystitis and other kidney infections are especially common during pregnancy because of the body changes that occur at this time. At no time is cystitis itself a serious disease, but it must be diagnosed and treated promptly to avoid complications.

Other Causes of Infection

Infection of the bladder and kidneys may occur because of poor hygiene in the area of the urethra, especially in women. It is also caused by some congenital defects in the urinary tract or by the insertion of instruments used to diagnose a urinary problem.

Sometimes bacteria in the bloodstream can settle in and infect the kidneys. Patients with diabetes seem to be more prone to urinary infections—indeed to infections generally—than other people. Any obstruction to the flow of urine in the urinary tract, such as a kidney stone, increases the possibility of infection in the area behind the obstruction. Damage to the nerves controlling the bladder is another condition that increases the chances of infection in that area.

Pyelonephritis

Infection in the kidneys is called *pyelonephritis*. Although it sometimes occurs without any symptoms, a first attack usually causes an aching pain in the lower back, probably due to the swelling of the kidneys, as well as nausea, vomiting, diarrhea, and sometimes severe pain in the front of the abdomen on one or both sides, depending on whether one or both kidneys are involved. Fever may be quite high, ranging from 103° F to 105° F, often accompanied by chills.

Although the symptoms of pyelonephritis may disappear in a few days without treatment, bacterial destruction of the kidney tissue may be going on. This silent type of infection may eventually disrupt normal kidney function and result in a chronic form of the disease, which in turn can lead to uremia. If the disease is not halted before this, it can be fatal.

Anyone with symptoms of acute pyelonephritis must have prompt medical attention. To diagnose the disease properly, the urine is analyzed and the number and type of bacteria in the urine are determined. The disease is brought under control by the right antibiotics and by administering large amounts of fluids to flush out the kidneys and urinary tract, thus decreasing the number of bacteria in the urine. In its chronic form the disease is much more difficult to cure because bacteria that are lodged deep in the kidney tissue do not seem to be susceptible to antibiotics and are therefore almost impossible to get rid of.

Kidney Stones

Another cause of infection in the bladder and kidneys is obstruction in the urinary tract by *kidney stones*. These stones, crystallizations of salts that form in the kidney tissue, may be quite small, but they can grow large enough to occupy a considerable part of one or both of the kidneys. The smaller ones often pass from the kidney through the ureters to the bladder, from which they are voided through the urethra. However, obstruction of the flow of urine behind a kidney stone anywhere in the urinary tract usually leads to infection in the urine. This type of infection may lead to attacks of acute pyelonephritis.

Removal of Stones

Kidney stones must be removed unless they cause no symptoms of infection. Removal may be accomplished by flushing out the urinary tract with large fluid intake, by surgical methods, or by lithotripsy, a method of dissolving the stones with electrical shock waves so that the fragments can be flushed out of the body. Any accompanying infection may be treated with antibiotics. A drug, *potassium citrate*, may also be used to keep kidney stones from forming. See "Urinary Stones" in Ch. 20, *Surgery*.

Why kidney stones form in some people and not in others is not clearly understood. Because of metabolic disorders, certain substances may build up in the body. The increased excretion of these substances in the urine as well as excessive amounts of calcium in the blood may encourage kidney stone formation. People who have gout are also likely to develop them.

Renal Colic

Sometimes the formation and passage of stones cause no symptoms. However, when symptoms do occur with the passage of a kidney stone, they can be uncomfortably severe. The pain that results from the passage of a stone through the ureter, referred

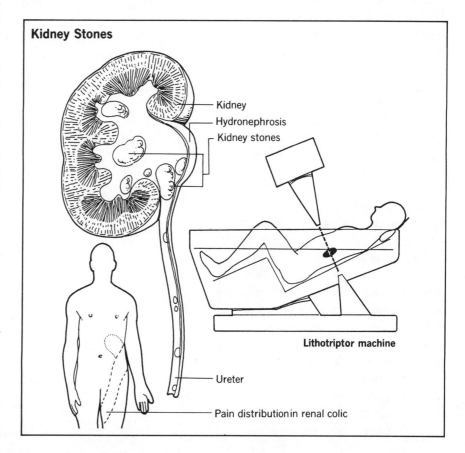

Kidney Stones

Kidney
Hydronephrosis
Kidney stones

Lithotriptor machine

Ureter

Pain distribution in renal colic

to as *renal colic,* is usually like an intense cramp. It begins in the side or back and moves toward the lower abdomen, the genital region, and the inner thigh on the affected side. The attack may last for a few minutes or for several hours. Sometimes bloody urine may be passed accompanied by a burning sensation.

Kidney stones are more likely to form in middle-aged and older people than in young ones. A history of stones is sometimes found in several generations of a family, since the metabolic disorders encouraging their formation have a hereditary basis.

Treatment for an acute attack of renal colic usually relieves the pain several hours after the patient has taken medication and fluids. If they are not promptly treated, kidney stones may lead to serious infection and eventual impairment of function.

Tumors of the Urinary Tract

Benign and malignant tumors of the kidney are not common problems. However, anyone with pain in the midback, blood in the urine, or a mass in the abdomen should have the symptoms diagnosed. If a malignant tumor is discovered early enough, it can be removed with the affected kidney, and normal function can be maintained by the healthy kidney that remains.

Malignant kidney tumors are most often found in children or adults over 40, and more often in men than in women. A tumor of any type can usually be diagnosed by X-ray studies. Where this technique is inadequate, an operation is necessary to search for the suspected growth. About one-fourth of all patients with a malignant kidney tumor live for more than ten years after surgery.

A malignant tumor of the bladder is a serious problem because it obstructs kidney drainage and may cause death from uremia. The main symptom is the painless appearance of blood in the urine, although sometimes a burning sensation and a frequent need to urinate are also present. Treatment usually includes surgical removal of the bladder followed by radiation treatment of the affected area to destroy any malignant cells that remain after the operation.

Some malignant bladder tumors grow very slowly and do not invade the bladder wall extensively. Surgical treatment for this type, called *papillary tumors,* is likely to be more successful than for tumors of the more invasive kind.

The Prostate Gland

The *prostate gland,* which contributes to the production of semen, encircles the base of the male urethra where it joins the bladder. When it begins to enlarge, it compresses the urethra and causes difficulty in voiding. Urination may be difficult to start, and when the urine stream appears it may be thinner than normal.

Because urine may remain in the bladder, there is the possibility of local infection that may spread to the kidneys. If the kidneys become enlarged because of this type of obstruction, a condition of *hydronephrosis* is said to exist. This disease can cause impaired kidney function and lead to uremia.

Benign Prostatic Enlargement

Enlargement of the prostate gland occurs in about half the male population over 50, and the incidence increases with increasing age. The condition is called *benign prostatic enlargement* and must be treated surgically if sufficient obstruction is present. For temporary relief, a catheter can be inserted into the bladder through the urethra, allowing the urine to drain through the catheter and out of the body. If surgery is necessary, the entire prostate may be removed or only that part of it that surrounds the urethra.

Symptoms of benign prostatic enlargement are quite distinctive: increased difficulty in voiding; an urge to continue to urinate after voiding has been completed; burning and frequent urination, caused in part by infection from urine retained in the bladder.

The cause of benign prostatic en-

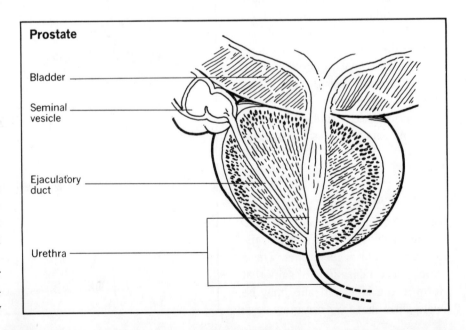

Prostate

Bladder

Seminal vesicle

Ejaculatory duct

Urethra

largement is thought to be a change during the aging process in the hormones that affect prostate tissue, but the exact nature of the change and its effect is not clear. It is likely that hormone-containing medicines will eventually be developed that will prevent or reverse prostate tissue growth.

Acute Prostatitis

Acute prostatitis occurs typically in young men. Symptoms include pain on urinating, sometimes a discharge of pus from the penis, pain in the lower back or abdomen indicating a tender and enlarged prostate, and fever. It is caused by a bacterial infection and usually responds promptly to antibiotics.

Cancer of the Prostate

Cancer of the prostate is a common type of malignancy in older men. It accounts for about 10 percent of male deaths from cancer in the United States. The disease may be present without any symptoms or interference with normal function and is therefore difficult to diagnose. A very high proportion of men over 80—probably more than 50 percent—has been found to have had cancer of the prostate at autopsy.

When symptoms are present, they are likely to be the same as those of benign prostatic enlargement. The disease can be diagnosed only by a biopsy examination of a tissue sample taken from the prostate during surgery. If malignancy is found, the gland is surgically removed when feasible to do so; the testes are removed too so that the level of male hormones in the body is lowered.

Male hormones increase the growth of malignant prostate tissue, but because female hormones slow it down, they may be administered after a diagnosis of prostate malignancy. If the tumor has spread to bone tissue,

radiation treatment of the affected areas may slow down cancerous growth and relieve pain.

Men over 40 should have a rectal examination once a year, since tumors of the prostate and benign prostatic enlargement can often be diagnosed early in this way.

Bedwetting

Enuresis, the medical term for bedwetting, is the unintentional loss of urine, usually during sleep at night. Infants do not have sufficiently developed nervous systems to control urination voluntarily until they are about two-and-a-half or three years old. Controlling urination through the night may not occur until after the age of three. A child who wets his bed recurrently after he has learned to control urination has the problem of enuresis.

There are many causes of enuresis. It may occur because of a delay in normal development or as a result of emotional stress. About 15 percent of boys and 10 percent of girls are bedwetters at the age of 5. By 9, about 5 percent of all children still have the problem, but most children outgrow it by the time they reach puberty.

Children who are bedwetters should be examined to rule out any physical abnormality in the urinary tract. Obstruction at the neck of the bladder where it joins the urethra or obstruction at the end of the urethra may cause uncontrollable dribbling of urine, but this usually occurs during the day as well as at night.

Disease of the nerves controlling the bladder, sometimes hereditary, can cause loss of urine. It can also occur in children who are mentally retarded or mentally ill, or because of an acute or chronic illness. In the latter cases, the problem disappears when the child regains his health.

Emotional Problems

If all physical abnormalities for bedwetting have been explored and eliminated as possible causes, the emotional problems of the child and his family should be examined. An understanding attitude rather than a hostile or punitive one on the part of the parents is extremely important in helping a child who is a bedwetter. He may be anxious about school or angry at a favored younger child, or he may feel insecure about parental acceptance. In such cases, an effort to bring the child's hidden feelings into the open and to deal with them sympathetically usually causes the problem to disappear.

Sexually Transmitted Diseases

The name of Venus, the Roman goddess of love, is preserved in the term *venereal disease* because they are transmitted by sexual contact. But today the broader phrase *sexually transmitted disease* (STD) is more commonly used to refer to both venereal and other diseases that may be passed from one person to another during sexual activity. STDs include some diseases, among them *acquired immunodeficiency syndrome,* or AIDS (see "AIDS" in Ch. 19, *Other Diseases of Major Importance*), that had not been identified as separate disorders until the 1970s or 1980s.

Sexually transmitted diseases were spreading at epidemic rates by the middle 1980s. Because all are contagious by definition, and can often cause serious complications, the symptoms should be treated without delay. At least two of the STDs, AIDS and genital herpes, or herpes simplex type II, are incurable. Some drugs and medications can, however, ameliorate specific symptoms of both diseases.

Except for pelvic inflammatory disease (PID), a serious complication among women, STDs afflict both men and women. Of the 11 most common STDs, chlamydia is the most prevalent. Public health officials believe the disease has spread because it has no obvious symptoms and victims can live for years without realizing they have it.

AIDS

While neither a disease of the urinogenital system nor an STD, strictly speaking, acquired immunodeficiency syndrome (AIDS) ranks as one of the most feared diseases today. Because the disease may be transmitted by intravenous needles that are shared by drug abusers as well as through sexual contact and contaminated blood it cannot strictly be called an STD. The disease strips the body of its acquired immunity against infection and leaves its victims susceptible to a variety of opportunistic infections. These include a rare form of pneumonia and Karposi's sarcoma, a rare type of cancer. AIDS is uniformly fatal.

A virus called the *human immunodeficiency virus* (HIV) is thought to be the cause of AIDS. Researchers speculate, however, that more than one virus may be the causative agent in AIDS. Exposure to the disease does not mean inevitably that a person will contract AIDS. Perhaps no more than 10 to 20 percent of the individuals who have been exposed to HIV will develop full-blown cases of AIDS. Many will develop what has been termed ARC, AIDS-related complex, which is less often fatal and not considered by authorities to be AIDS per se.

Diagnosis

No simple means of diagnosing AIDS exists. Physicians can test for certain opportunistic infections. They also study symptoms as reported by individuals. Damage to white blood cells (specifically the T-cells), revealed by tests, may indicate the presence of the disease. The only test available now, commonly called the "AIDS test," can only test for the presence of antibodies. These antibodies are indicative of exposure to HIV and do not indicate the presence of the virus itself. Because the test was developed for blood donor screening its use by individuals concerned about possible exposure to HIV is not advocated by most health professionals. A positive test showing AIDS antibodies does not necessarily mean that the person will contract the disease, nor does a negative test mean the person has not become infected. The present blood screening test has a relatively high degree of unreliability and so should therefore not be relied upon as the sole indicator of exposure to AIDS.

The symptoms of AIDS range across a broad grouping of complaints that are common to various illnesses. Because these complaints are so common, diagnosis becomes even more difficult. The symptoms include night sweats, diarrhea, fatigue, weight loss of 10 or more pounds over a short period, swollen lymph nodes, fever, and loss of appetite. The symptoms may appear from six months to five years or more after infection.

Treatment

There is no treatment for AIDS as yet; therefore, physicians can only treat the specific symptoms that occur from the various opportunistic diseases that attack AIDS patients. Also, an antiserum has been found to keep the AIDS virus from invading human cells in laboratory tests. The antiserum, a blood substance, reacts with a thymus gland hormone called thymosin alpha 1. Researchers hope the antiserum will eventually lead to development of an AIDS vaccine. The development of such a vaccine, however, is thought to be some years away.

Chlamydia

Chlamydia is a bacterial infection that can cause sterility in men and women and has been called "the disease of the '80s." Most women with the disease have no obvious symptoms. For that reason, physicians suggest that sexually active women undergo tests for chlamydia at least once a year. The disease is spreading more rapidly than any other STD.

Persons at highest risk of contracting chlamydia are under 35 years of age. A bacterium, *Chlamydia trachomatis,* causes the disease, which is spread to adults during sexual contact and to babies of infected mothers during birth. Complications affect both sexes: both men and women may become infertile, and women may have pregnancy problems that could kill a fetus. In some cases the disease may be fatal for the mother. Babies infected during birth may develop infections of the eyes, ears, or lungs.

Diagnosis

A new diagnostic technique has led to hope that chlamydia can be brought under control. The technique, *antigen detection testing,* is a relatively simple and painless laboratory procedure.

Symptoms that indicate the possibility of chlamydia may or may not appear. Men may experience a discharge from the penis or a burning sensation while urinating. Women may have vaginal itching, bleeding between menstrual periods, and chronic abdominal pain. The symptoms may appear two to four weeks after infection.

Treatment

Even though chlamydia is spreading more rapidly than other STDs, it ranks among the lesser STD threats. Treatments involve drug therapies with tetracycline or doxycycline. Erythromycin has also been used successfully. The drugs usually take effect in about seven days. The partner of a person who is undergoing treatment for chlamydia should also be treated.

Gonorrhea

The second most common STD, *gonorrhea,* has afflicted mankind for centuries. Gonorrhea, caused by the bacteria gonococcus, lives in the mucous membranes of the body, including the vagina, rectum, throat, or hollow of the cheek. Cervical, penile, or rectal gonorrhea are contracted through intercourse; oral sex may lead to throat gonorrhea. Women may acquire gonorrhea in a single contact with an infected male; but men face only about a 20 to 40 percent risk of contracting the disease from a female.

Untreated, gonorrhea can lead to various complications. Women can suffer from pelvic inflammatory disease. In relatively unusual cases gonococci can enter the bloodstream and cause blood poisoning. The babies of infected mothers may be born blind. Gonococci settling in joints may cause arthritis. Very rarely the disease leads to *endocarditis,* an inflammation of the lining of the heart, or to *meningitis,* an inflammation that destroys the membrane surrounding the brain and spinal cord.

Except for PID, men experience most of the basic symptoms of untreated gonorrhea. Thus male problems can range from back pains to sterility.

Diagnosis

Anyone suspecting the presence of gonorrhea should arrange for a medical examination as quickly as possible. A test "just in case" may be advisable if, for example, a sex partner indicates that he or she has contracted the disease. Women are cautioned against douching before a visit to a physician or public health clinic; nor should self-treatment with antibiotics be attempted. In either case diagnosis may become more difficult.

Gonorrhea is more difficult to detect in women than in men. As many as four out of five women infected with cervical gonorrhea may not realize for days or weeks that they have the disease. When symptoms do appear, they include vaginal discharges and discomfort when urinating. These symptoms, appearing three to eleven days after exposure, may become steadily worse. Urinating may become extremely painful. With rectal gonorrhea, burning sensations, bleeding or mucous discharges may accompany defecation. Approximately nine of ten males know within a week to ten days that they have been infected. Male symptoms are, commonly, a puslike discharge from the penis and a burning sensation while urinating.

Treatment

Penicillin is the most effective treatment for gonorrhea. For persons allergic to penicillin, physicians usually prescribe tetracycline or erythromycin in oral doses. All three drugs are effective in most cases.

Researchers believe the possibility that they will find a vaccine for gonorrhea is strong. Experimental vaccines have been successfully tested on laboratory animals.

Genital Herpes

Genital herpes, or herpes simplex type II, is transmitted by physical—usually sexual—contact. The virus is one of the herpesviruses that also cause shingles, mononucleosis, or chicken pox. The disease is transmitted through skin-to-skin contact with herpes sores or the secretions of an infected person. The virus enters the body through the mucous membranes of the genitals, mouth, or anus.

The first attack of genital herpes usually occurs one to two weeks after exposure. Sores may appear; the afflicted person may have difficulty urinating or defecating. The symptoms usually disappear in ten days to three weeks, but for most herpes victims a recurrence can be expected within six months. Later attacks may be milder, but the disease is incurable and can be transmitted even when no symptoms are visible.

Stress and depression, authorities say, can trigger herpes attacks. Women suffering from the disease face increased risks of cervical cancer. They may also pass the virus to babies during delivery. So exposed, the babies may die within a few weeks; some newborns are deformed, blind, or mentally handicapped. Because of the danger that the herpesvirus poses to newborns, women with genital herpes should alert their obstetricians so that delivery can be by cesarian section. By avoiding vaginal mucous membranes, the infant will not be exposed to the virus.

Diagnosis

Physicians can usually diagnose herpes by visual examination while the characteristic sores are evident. A physician may also take a herpes culture from the base of the lesion.

Treatment

While no cure for genital herpes exists, the drug acyclovir has been found to reduce the severity of the flareups. Acyclovir is applied as a topical ointment, usually for initial outbreaks. In an oral form the drug alleviates subsequent attacks. The oral preparation has been reported to be effective in about seven cases out of ten.

Whether treated or not, later outbreaks of herpes are generally shorter and less severe than the first. Physicians agree that acyclovir effects improvement in the majority of cases, but some reserve judgment concerning the drug's long-term effects.

Trichomoniasis

A type of leukorrhea, *trichomoniasis* is caused by the *Trichomonas vaginalis,* an organism that causes an irritating itching condition in women. Men usually have no symptoms. The organism, a parasite, favors warm, moist areas, such as genital tissues; but some experts believe it can sometimes survive in damp cloths, douching syringes, towels, around toilet seats, on beaches, and around swimming pools. Thus the disease can, it is believed, be spread without sexual contact.

Complications can follow trichomoniasis. Women victims experience discomfort and pain. Chronic infection, according to some researchers, may make a woman more susceptible to cervical cancer. Constant irritation of the cervix is said to produce such susceptibility.

Diagnosis

The trichomoniasis leukorrhea consists of a yellow to green frothy discharge. The itching that accompanies the infection tends to begin or worsen immediately after a menstrual period. Some women report a burning sensation when they urinate. In diagnosis the physician uses a test similar to a Pap smear (see "Pap Smear" in Ch.

25, *Women's Health*), made with a specimen taken from the vagina. Under a microscope the trichomonas organisms are easy to identify because they are pear-shaped and have three to five whiplike tails.

Treatment

Several drugs are available for treating trichomoniasis. They include tablets taken orally and suppositories inserted in the vagina. Most commonly prescribed is metronidazole. Cures may be effected quickly. One dose of two grams (eight 250 mg tablets) may be adequate for both the victim and his or her partner. The oral medication may, however, be continued for weeks or months if the infection resists the drug.

Trichomoniasis victims have reported such side effects as nausea, depression, and hives. Because many persons are allergic to metronidazole, physicians may suggest the use of vaginal douches made up of vinegar and water, or of vaginal suppositories. The latter relieve trichomoniasis symptoms, but do not cure the disease.

Venereal Warts

Venereal warts, also called *genital warts,* may be painless but they can be serious and thus require medical attention. If left untreated, researchers say, venereal warts can increase the risk of penile cancer in men and cervical cancer in women. A pregnant woman with these growths may transmit the virus to her infant during delivery. Warts may then develop in the newborn's windpipe, causing later breathing problems.

The *human papilloma viruses* cause venereal warts, which may appear in a variety of places in the pubic area. The growths are usually small pink bumps, but they can grow to-

gether to resemble tiny cauliflowers. In most cases, the growths itch and produce a foul-smelling discharge.

Diagnosis

A physician can usually diagnose venereal warts from their external appearance. To make certain that the warts are not syphilis growths, however, the physician may take a biopsy. A tiny part of the wart is removed for study under a microscope. The papilloma virus can then be identified.

Women with external venereal warts may also have the growths on the cervix. A Pap test is required for detection of these internal warts.

Treatment

The drug podophyllin can be used in solution to remove venereal warts. The solution is painted on the growths, left for six hours, then washed off. The warts usually disappear within a few days. The treatment may have to be repeated several times. If any wart cells remain, the problem will most likely recur.

Podophyllin is not effective in all cases. Where it cannot achieve a cure, other methods, including surgery, may have to be attempted. Among these other methods, which are not always successful, are freezing and burning of the growths. Some studies have indicated that the hormone interferon can prevent recurrences of the disease. Interferon therapy may, however, produce such flulike side effects as fatigue and fever.

Syphilis

Historically, syphilis has ranked among mankind's chief health scourges. Modern medicine has brought it largely under control, but it can still be life-threatening.

Syphilis strikes men about three times as often as women. Approximately half of the male victims are homosexuals. A spiral-shaped bacterium called *Treponema pallidum* causes the disease. Transmittal takes place during sex with a person in the infectious stage in which open sores or rashes are typical symptoms. The *Treponema* bacteria fill the sores and in infecting another person invade the mucous membranes of the genitals, mouth, or rectum. The *spirochete,* or spiral bacterium, succumbs to heat, dryness, ordinary antiseptics, or even soap and water. But it can tolerate cold and survive freezing.

Stages

Unless it is treated early, syphilis progresses from a primary to secondary and sometimes tertiary stages. In the primary stage, the victim may have a painless chancre, or ulcer, that may be small, single, or multiple and that may look like any common skin ulcer. The reddish-brown ulcers generally appear between ten days and three months after exposure to the disease, with a typical incubation time of three weeks.

The secondary and latent stages of syphilis can lead to serious complications unless treatment is undertaken. A month to six weeks after the first ulcers appear, secondary lesions may develop, taking the form of a rash or almost any other kind of skin eruption. The lesions may appear on the trunk of the body, on the face, the arms and legs, or the palms of the hands and soles of the feet. The lesions may or may not itch, and they may not appear at all. The victim may, however, experience fevers and flu symptoms as well as hair loss. A latent stage of many years' duration follows untreated secondary syphilis. In this stage only a blood test can reveal

the presence of the bacteria in the body.

If still untreated, late or tertiary-stage syphilis follows the secondary and latent stages in about one case in four. Tertiary syphilis involves the gradual destruction of the central nervous system, the heart, the bones, the liver, the stomach, or other organs. The bacteria can cause paralysis, convulsions, heart failure, insanity, and even death. Attacking the circulatory system, syphilis can cause an *aneurysm,* dilated section, of the aorta just above the heart. The blood flow to the heart is reduced; a ruptured aneurysm can produce a fatal hemorrhage. While gummas, rubbery syphilitic tumors inside organs, may respond to antibiotics in the late stage of syphilis, damage to the heart valves and arteries may be irreversible.

General Paresis

Permanent tissue damage to the brain and nerves can result from syphilitic invasion of the central nervous system; this the chronic, progressive form of syphilis known as *general paresis.* The damage occurs gradually, and early symptoms may include headaches, a tendency to forget things, or difficulty in concentrating. Mental effects may progress from memory loss to psychotic symptoms of delusions of grandeur.

Tabes Dorsalis

Late syphilis involving deterioration of the sheaths of spinal nerves (demyelination) and other destructive changes in the spinal cord is known as *tabes dorsalis.* The patient may become uncoordinated in movement. Tremors of the hands and fingers may be noticed, as well as tremors of the lips and tongue. Vision may be affected, and sensory effects can range

from sharp sudden pains to a loss of feeling. The patient may lose control of bladder function or the ability to walk.

Congenital Syphilis

The latent syphilitic condition is not uncommon, and it is a period of great danger to the fetus if an infected woman, especially a recently infected woman, becomes pregnant at this time. The fetus can acquire syphilis through the placenta and be born with congenital syphilis. Or it can be still-born or die shortly after birth. Some of the signs of syphilis in an infant born with the congenital form of the disease are similar to those of secondary syphilis. Others are very different, more closely resembling tertiary syphilis. Because of the hazards to the child, most physicians test the mother's blood for the presence of the spirochete during the first three months of pregnancy and during the last three months; syphilis acquired during pregnancy is especially likely to affect the fetus. Treatment of the mother has the added benefit of treating the fetus. Treatment begun before the eighteenth week of pregnancy will prevent syphilis from developing; treatment begun after the eighteenth week will cure the fetus of syphilis.

Diagnosis

Because the symptoms of syphilis may appear sporadically or not at all, and because they so closely resemble the symptoms of other diseases, diagnosis usually calls for a blood test. If a chancre has developed, the physician may take a scraping from the lesion and order a special microscopic examination.

Treatment

Long-lasting penicillin, given by intravenous injection, usually cures syphilis. But the disease can, as noted, cause irreversible damage if allowed to spread unchecked. For persons who are allergic to penicillin, physicians may prescribe tetracycline or erythromycin. Both are effective as treatments.

Pelvic Inflammatory Disease

Pelvic inflammatory disease (PID) is a serious complication of STDs. It affects women as a result of infection from a number of diseases including chlamydia and gonorrhea. To produce PID, a disease has to progress to the point where it leads to inflammation and abscesses of a victim's Fallopian tubes, ovaries, and pelvis.

One woman in about seven who contract PID becomes infertile. On the average, three of four women experiencing attacks of the disease will be unable to conceive.

Diagnosis and Treatment

Physicians can diagnose PID by conducting abdominal and pelvic examinations as well as various laboratory tests.

Antibiotics are prescribed in some cases. In more severe cases, surgery may be necessary. The surgery usually results in infertility.

Lymphogranuloma Venereum

This disease, also known as LGV and *lymphogranuloma inguinale*, is a venereal disease that produces a primary lesion like a small blister, which ruptures to form a small ulcer. It is caused by a virus that is spread by sexual intercourse, although sexual contact is not necessary for transmission of the disease. It can be acquired by contact with the fluid excreted by a lesion.

The primary lesion usually appears in the genital area within one to three weeks after contact with an infected person. It may appear only briefly or be so small as to go unnoticed. But the disease spreads to neighboring lymph nodes, where the next sign of the disorder appears 10 days to a month later. The swelling of the lymph nodes (forming *buboes*) is often the first symptom to be noted by the patient; the lymph nodes become matted together and hard, forming channels (or *fistulas*) through which pus drains to the surface of the skin. Enlargement of the lymph nodes may produce painful swelling of the external genitalia. The lymph-node involvement may spread to the anal region, leading to rectal constriction and painful bowel movements.

Diagnosis and Treatment

Because the lesions of lymphogranuloma venereum may resemble those of syphilis, chancroid, or certain nonvenereal diseases, physicians usually make a number of tests to determine whether or not the condition is, in fact, LGV. Therapy includes administration of antibiotics and sulfa drugs for a period of about a week to a month, depending on the severity of the infection.

Chancroid

Chancroid, or *soft chancre,* is a venereal disease transmitted by a bacterium that causes a tender, painful ulcer. The ulcer, which may erode deeply into the tissues, follows the formation of a primary pustule at the site of infection. The pustule appears within five days after contact with an infected person. While essentially a venereal disease, like other venereal diseases it is transmissible without sexual intercourse. Physicians, for

example, have been known to develop a soft chancre on a finger after examining an infected patient.

Diagnosis and Treatment

Physicians usually do tests to make sure that the lesion is not a syphilitic chancre. Although the disease can spread from the genital region to other parts of the body, the soft chancre generally is self-limiting. Therapy consists of administration of sulfa drugs or tetracycline.

Granuloma Inguinale

Granuloma inguinale, also called *granuloma venereum,* is not the same, in spite of the similarity in name, as lymphogranuloma venereum. The former is an insidious, chronic venereal disease that produces lesions on the skin or mucous membrane of the genital or anal regions. The first sign of the infection may be a painless papule or nodule that leaves an ulcer with a reddish granular base. If untreated, the lesions tend to spread to the lower abdomen and thighs. In time, the sores produce a sour, pungent odor.

Treatment

Antibiotics such as streptomycin and tetracycline are prescribed. Relapses may occur and cure may be slow, especially in cases of long standing.

External Venereal Maladies

The two conditions described below, one related to viruses and one a parasitic infestation, may generally be considered sources of discomfort and disfigurement rather than threats to general health. Both of these STDs are transmissible by other means besides sexual contact.

Molluscum Contagiosum

A viral disease transmitted during sexual intercourse is known by the medical term *molluscum contagiosum*. The disease can also be transmitted by ordinary person-to-person contact, as between members of a family or children in a classroom. The virus causes raised lesions containing a waxy white material. The lesions, which may be very small or as large as an inch in diameter, occur on the skin or mucous membranes, commonly in the anal or genital area but sometimes on the face or torso. The lesions may last for several months or several years, then disappear spontaneously, or they may be removed by medications or surgery.

Pubic Lice

Infestations of pubic lice constitute a unique kind of venereal disease. Pubic lice, known popularly as crabs, are a species somewhat larger than body and head lice but still almost invisible to the naked eye. These whitish, oval parasites usually remain in the hair of the anal and genital regions, but they may sometimes be found attached to the skin at the base of any body hair, including eyelashes and scalp. A very few pubic lice in the anal and genital areas can cause intense irritation and itching. The itching results in scratching which, in turn, produces abrasions of the skin. The lice may also produce patches of bluish spots on the skin of the inner thighs and lower abdomen. Another sign of their presence is the appearance of tiny brown specks deposited by the lice on the inside of undergarments.

Pubic lice are commonly spread by sexual contact, but they can be acquired from toilet seats, clothing, towels, bedclothes, combs, or any article of intimate use. Creams or ointments containing various parasiticides are available for disinfestation. They are applied every night for several nights, but overuse should be avoided because of the danger of injury to the tender tissues of the genital and anal region. Some physicians recommend soaking the infested part of the body several times daily in a mild solution of potassium permanganate. Lice on the eyebrows and eyelashes may have to be removed individually with a pair of tweezers. Treatment must be repeated after one week to kill the nits (eggs) that have hatched since the first treatment. Clothing and other contaminated materials must be cleaned to prevent reinfestation.

Complications of an infestation of pubic lice include intense itching (known medically as *pruritus*) and secondary infections from scratching. These may require special medical care and administration of antibiotics, corticosteroid creams, or other appropriate remedies.

18

Cancer

Cancer has always figured uniquely in the diseases of mankind. For centuries people spoke of it only in whispers, or not at all, as if the disease were not only dreadful but somehow shameful as well. Today, the picture is changing and rapidly. This decade may see the time—undreamt of only scant years ago—when half of those stricken by cancer will survive its ravages. And much of the mystery that cloaked the disease in an awful shroud has been dissipated, although the last veils remain to be stripped away.

Of course, cancer remains a formidable enemy. More than a million Americans are under medical care for cancer; an estimated 385,000 will die of it each year. Of all Americans now alive, some 55 million—one in four—will be stricken; and some 36 million will die of the disease. Cancer is the greatest cause of lost working years among women and ranks third after heart disease and accidents in denying men working years.

But in context, the picture is not as bleak as it might seem. At the beginning of the twentieth century, survival from cancer was relatively rare. At the end of the 1930s, the five-year

survival rate (alive after five years) was one in five or fewer. Ten years later it had shot up to one in four, and in the mid-fifties to one in three. This figure has remained relatively stable because the survival rate for some of the more widespread cancers has leveled off despite the best efforts of physicians to devise better forms of treatment. For such cancers, which include those of the breast, colon, and rectum, improvements will come through earlier detection and even prevention. Dr. Richard S. Doll, Professor of Medicine at Oxford University, has said that we could prevent 40 percent of men's cancer deaths and 10 percent of women's simply by applying what we already know. For example, according to the American Cancer Society, the risk of death from lung cancer is 15 to 20 times greater among men who smoke cigarettes than among men who have never smoked. The relative risk of lung cancer among women smokers is five times that of women who have never smoked.

Considerable progress is being made on many fronts in the war against cancer. It ranges from advances in early detection to breakthroughs in treatment. The past 25 years have seen a 50 percent dip in the death rate from cervical cancer, mostly because of increasing acceptance of the Pap test, which can detect the disease at a very early stage. At the same time, children with acute lymphocytic leukemia, which used to be invariably fatal in weeks or months, have benefited from new therapies, with at least half now surviving three years, some more than five years, and a few on the verge of being pronounced cured. Similar advances in the treatment of a cancer of the lymph system called *Hodgkin's disease* have improved the five-year survival rate from 25 percent at the end of World War II to about 55 percent today.

What Is Cancer?

Cancer would surely be easier to detect and treat if it were a single entity with a single simple cause. But it is not. Experts agree that there are actually some 200 different diseases that can be called cancers. They have different causes, originate in different tissues, develop for different reasons

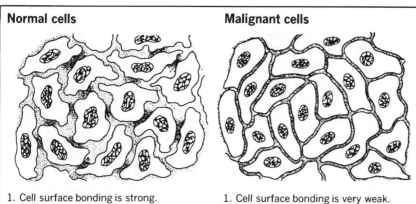

Normal cells	Malignant cells
1. Cell surface bonding is strong.	1. Cell surface bonding is very weak.
2. Cells remain in place.	2. Cells spread and invade normal tissue.
3. Electrical voltage level is high.	3. Electrical voltage level is low.
4. Cells divide at a low rate.	4. Cells divide at a rapid pace.

and in different ways, and demand vastly different kinds of treatment. All have one fatal element in common, however; in every case, normal cells have gone wild and lost their growth and development controls.

Initial Stages

The cancer may start with just one or a few cells somewhere in the body that undergo a change and become malignant, or cancerous. The cells divide and reproduce themselves, and the cancer grows.

Most cancers arise on the surface of a tissue, such as the skin, the lining of the uterus, mouth, stomach, bowel, bladder, or bronchial tube in the lung, or inside a duct in the breast, prostate gland, or other site. Eventually, they grow from a microscopic clump to a visible mass, then begin to invade underlying tissues. As long as the cells remain in one mass, however, the cancer is localized.

Later Stages

At some later phase, in a process called *metastasis,* some of the cancer cells split off and are swept into the lymph channels or bloodstream to other parts of the body. They may be captured for a while in a nearby lymph node (a stage called *regional involve-*

ment), but unless the disease is arrested, it will rapidly invade the rest of the body, with death the almost certain result. Some cancers grow with a malevolent rapidity; some are dormant by comparison. Some respond to various therapies, such as radiation therapy; others do not. About half of the known types of cancer are incurable at any stage. Of the remaining half, it is obviously imperative to diagnose and treat them as early as possible.

How Cancers Are Classified

The cancers described above, arising in *epithelial* (covering or lining) tissue, are called *carcinomas* as a group. Another class of malignant tumors, similar in most basic respects, is the *sarcomas,* which originate in connective tissue, such as bones and muscles. A third group of cancers—*leukemia* and the *lymphomas*—includes diseases of the blood-forming organs and the lymphatic system, respectively, and does not produce tumors. They arise and spread in a basically different way.

What Causes Cancer?

In its battle with cancer, medical science devotes constant attention to a search for those factors in our environment that can produce cancer in human beings. They include a large

number of chemical agents such as those in tobacco smoke, and including asbestos fibers and other occupational chemical hazards; ionizing radiation such as that from X rays, nuclear bombs, and sunlight; injury or repeated irritation; metal or plastic implants; flaws in the body's immune reaction; genetic mistakes; parasites; and—many scientists believe—viruses.

It is this last factor that is generating perhaps the most interest among medical scientists today. It has been shown that viruses cause a variety of cancers in animals; yet they have never been proved responsible in human cancer, although they have been linked to at least six different ones. Recently, researchers discovered an enzyme in a virus believed to cause cancer and also in the tissues of leukemia patients. This enzyme may be the key to the mechanism by which a virus induces a malignant change in normal cells.

Scientists have also discovered that certain substances in the environment which by themselves may not stimulate the growth of a cancer can be dangerously activated to become carcinogenic by the presence of one or more other substances. Each of these potential cancer-causing agents is called a *cocarcinogen.* It is possible that some cocarcinogens are present in ordinary fruits and vegetables, in certain food additives, and in such other substances as the synthetic estrogen diethylstilbestrol (DES). For more information on DES, see Ch. 25, *Women's Health.*

Major Forms of Cancer

The following material includes

discussions of the major forms of cancer with the exception of those cancers that affect women only. Cancers affecting women are discussed under *Women's Health,* Ch. 25. See especially "Cancers of the Reproductive System" and "Cancer of the Breast."

For additional information on many kinds of tumors for which surgery may be indicated, see also Ch. 20, *Surgery.*

Lung Cancer

Lung cancer kills more Americans than any other cancer. The average annual death toll for recent years is almost 70,000 men and over 20,000 women. It represents 22 percent of all cancers in men, 6 percent of all cancers in women. And there has been a steady increase in the incidence of lung cancer in both men and women over the past 35 years—especially so in men, among whom the mortality rate has gone up 15 times. In 1965, women accounted for one in eight lung cancer mortalities; the figure now is almost one in four. The current chance of being cured of this disease where there is regional involvement is no greater than 10 percent.

Symptoms

Although some early lung cancers do not show up on an X-ray film, they are the ones that usually produce cough as an early symptom. For this reason, any cough that lasts more than two or three weeks—even if it seems to accompany a cold or bronchitis—should be regarded as suspicious and investigated in that light. Blood in the sputum is another early warning sign that must be investigated immediately; so should wheezing when breathing. Later symptoms include shortness of breath, pain in the chest, fever, and night sweats.

Detection

If many lives could be saved by preventing lung cancer in the first place, others could be saved by early detection. By the time most lung cancers are diagnosed, it is too late even for the most radical approach to cure—removal of the afflicted lung. Experts estimate that up to five times the present cure rate of 10 percent could be achieved if very early lung cancers could be spotted. They therefore recommend a routine chest X ray every six months for everyone over 45.

Causes

Lung cancer is one of the most preventable of all malignancies. Most cases, the majority of medical experts agree, are caused by smoking cigarettes. The U.S. Public Health Service has indicted smoking as "the main cause of lung cancer in men." Even when other agents are known to produce lung cancers—uranium ore dust or asbestos fibers, for example—cigarette smoking enormously boosts the risk among uranium miners and asbestos workers.

Various theories have been proposed to explain the mechanism by which smoking causes cancer in human beings; none has been proved. But it is known that the lungs of some cigarette smokers show tissue changes before cancer appears, changes apparently caused by irritation of the lining of the *bronchi*—the large air tubes in the lung. Physicians believe these changes can be reversed before the onset of cancer if the source of irritation—smoking—is removed. This is why a heavy smoker who has been puffing away for many years but then stops smoking has a better chance of avoiding lung cancer than one who continues smoking.

Until recently, the evidence linking cigarette smoking and lung cancer was purely statistical, although overwhelming. No one had succeeded in producing lung cancer in laboratory animals by having them ingest smoke. However, lung cancer has been induced in dogs specially trained to inhale cigarette smoke, as reported by the American Cancer Society.

Cigarette smoking has also been implicated in other kinds of lung disease, including the often-fatal emphysema, and in cardiovascular diseases. To any sensible person, then, the options would seem clear: If you don't smoke, don't start. If you do smoke, stop. If you can't stop, cut down, and switch to a brand low in tars and nicotine—suspected but not proved to be the principal harmful agents in cigarette smoke.

Colon-Rectum Cancer

Cancer of the colon (large intestine) and rectum is the second leading cause of cancer death in the United States. Each year it claims an estimated 50,000 lives, and produces about 100,000 new cases—more than any other kind of cancer except skin cancer. It afflicts men and women about equally. The five-year survival rate from this form of cancer, usually after surgery, is 71 percent where the cancer was localized and 43 percent where there was regional involvement. However, authorities now believe that this rate could be upped substantially through early diagnosis and prompt treatment.

Symptoms

It is important, then, to be alert to the early symptoms of these cancers. Cancers of the colon often produce changes in bowel habits that persist longer than normal. The change may be constipation or diarrhea, or even both alternating. Cancers of the colon also often produce large quantities of gas, which cause abdominal discomfort ranging from a feeling of overfullness to pain, intermittent at first and then coming as regular cramps.

Both colon cancer and rectal cancer may also cause bleeding. Sometimes such bleeding is evidenced in the stool or on the tissue (the most frequent first sign of rectal cancer); but if the bleeding is slight and occurs high enough up the colon, it may not be visible at all. After a period of weeks, however, the persistent bleeding causes anemia in the patient.

All such symptoms should be investigated promptly. Unfortunately, many persons tend to ignore them. Chronic constipation, for example, or gas, is easy to dismiss for the nuisance that it usually is. Even rectal bleeding, which demands immediate medical consultation, is often ignored by hemorrhoid sufferers, who fail to realize that hemorrhoids and cancer, though unrelated, can and sometimes do exist in the same persons at the same time.

Detection

For these reasons, the key to successful and early diagnosis of colon and rectum cancer lies in making a *proctoscopy* part of the regular annual health checkup. In this procedure, performed in a physician's office, a lighted tube called a *proctoscope* is passed into the rectum. Through it, the physician can examine the walls visually for signs of tumor. If the physician thinks it advisable to check the sigmoid colon also, the procedure is called a *proctosigmoidoscopy*, and a similar instrument called a *sigmoidoscope* is used. The American Cancer Society now recommends that everyone over age 40 have a proctoscopy or proctosigmoidoscopy in routine annual checkups.

Therapy

The indicated treatment for colon-rectum cancer is surgical removal of the affected part of the bowel. Adjacent portions and related lymph nodes may also be removed, and if the surgeon sees that the cancer is widespread, he may have to perform extensive surgery. This may require that he create a *colostomy*—a temporary or permanent opening in the abdominal wall through which solid wastes may pass. Although this method of voiding the bowels is somewhat inconvenient at first, most colostomy patients adjust to it very easily and lead perfectly normal, active, and healthy lives. The wall of prudish silence that used to surround the disease and the colostomy is fortunately crumbling. An organization for colostomy patients called the United Ostomy Association keeps up with current information on diet, colostomy equipment, and other problems the members have in common.

Radiotherapy is sometimes used before the operation (occasionally to make surgery possible) and sometimes afterward to treat recurrence of the cancer. Various chemical agents have been found useful in treating colon-rectum cancer that has spread to the lymph nodes or more widely.

Skin Cancer

With as many as 500,000 new cases occurring annually, skin cancer is the largest single source of malignancy in the United States. An estimated 6,000 persons die of this disease each year. Since 1980, the number of cases of malignant melanoma, the most deadly form of skin cancer, has risen by more than 90 percent.

Experts believe that many cases of skin cancer could be prevented if more people avoided exposure to the sun. Radiation in sunlight not only burns and dries the skin; it also is thought to suppress the human immune system and thus contribute indirectly to skin problems. Long and continued exposure to the sun has been associated with cataracts as well as with skin aging and wrinkling.

Symptoms

Persons with skin problems should report promptly to their physicians any sores that refuse to heal, or changes in warts or moles. Pimples that itch and recur may also be symptoms of skin cancer.

Therapy

Most skin cancers remain localized. They can usually be removed by excisional surgery, with an electric needle, or by cryosurgery (freezing). X-ray irradiation and chemotherapy may also be used.

Causes

Most skin cancers appear after the age of 40. Scientists point to the ultraviolet radiation in sunlight as the primary cause, with ultraviolet-B (UV-B), the shorter wavelength band, as the more dangerous. But dermatologists recommend that ultraviolet-A (UV-A), used often in high-intensity sunlamps, be avoided as well. While UV-A is spread more evenly throughout the day, UV-B is largely concentrated around midday.

Fair-skinned individuals who burn readily, rather than tanning, are more vulnerable to radiation-caused cancer than darker-skinned persons. Geographic location is also important. Skin cancer occurs more frequently in the southern belt of states, particularly in the sunny Southwest.

Chemicals, too, can cause skin cancer. Before the relationship was discovered, skin cancer was an occupational hazard for many thousands of unprotected workers who dealt with arsenic and various derivatives of coal and petroleum.

Kinds

Of the three primary kinds of skin cancer, two are both common and relatively curable. These are basal-cell and squamous-cell *carcinoma*. Early detection almost ensures that a cure can be effected.

A *melanoma,* or so-called *black cancer,* is a malignant tumor that arises from a mole. The moles may begin as flat, soft, brown, and hairless protrusions, but they can change suddenly into darker, larger growths that itch and bleed. They can also metastasize, spreading cancer cells to other parts of the body through the bloodstream and the lymphatic system.

Unlike other types of skin cancer, melanomas may grow in skin areas not usually exposed to the sun, such as the feet, in the genital area, or under the belt or collar. Chronic irritation from tight clothing is one suspected cause. Melanomas rarely occur before middle age; nearly three-fourths of the victims are women.

Oral Cancer

Cancers of the mouth and lips strike an estimated 24,000 persons in the United States each year and kill a shocking 8,500. Shocking because anyone with the aid of a mirror and a good light can see into his mouth and therefore spot even very small cancers early in their development.

Symptoms

Any sore, lump, or lesion of the mouth or lips should be regarded as suspicious if it persists more than two weeks without healing, and a physi-

cian or dentist should then be consulted without delay. The five-year survival rate for localized mouth cancers—when they are usually no larger than the little fingernail—is 67 percent—about two out of three. But if regional involvement occurs, the rate falls to 30 percent—fewer than one out of three.

Detection

Just as the Pap test screens for cervical cancer by scraping up sloughed-off cells that are then examined under a microscope, so one day your dentist may routinely scrape mouth cells to detect oral cancer. When more than 40,000 patients were screened over a five-and-one-half-year period at the Western Tennessee Cancer Clinic, about 230 cases of oral cancer were diagnosed, of which 35 percent would have been missed otherwise.

Right now, a weekly or monthly personal inspection of your mouth is the best detective method available. The American Cancer Society has materials explaining the best way to conduct such an examination.

Therapy

Oral cancers are treated by surgical removal or by irradiation.

Causes

No one can pinpoint the causes of oral cancer definitely, but there are a number of leading suspects. They are smoking, in all its forms; exposure to wind and sun (for lip cancer); poor mouth hygiene; sharp or rough-edged teeth or improperly fitted, irritating dentures; dietary inadequacies, and constant consumption of very hot foods and liquids.

Stomach Cancer

Before World War II, cancer of the stomach was the most common type

of cancer among men and women in the United States. The death rate from stomach cancer in the 1930s was about 30 per 100,000 population. In recent years, stomach cancer has declined in proportion to other forms of the disease, such as lung, breast, and uterine cancer. However, stomach cancer is still one of the more frequently diagnosed types of cancer and the death rate is relatively high, at nearly 10 per 100,000 population.

Today, men are twice as likely to be victims of stomach cancer as women. The disease is seldom found in persons under 30 years of age, but after that age the incidence increases steadily, reaching a peak before the age of 60. One of the disease's mysterious incidental factors is its peculiar geographical distribution, the highest rates of occurrence being in Japan, Chile, Iceland, northern Russia, and the Scandinavian countries.

Symptoms

Stomach cancer seems to develop slowly and insidiously, with initial symptoms that may be disregarded by the patient because they mimic ordinary gastric distress. The victim may experience a distaste for foods, particularly meats, and display a slow but progressive loss of weight. There may be sensations of fullness, bloating, or pain after meals. The same

---

**Cancer's Seven
Warning Signals***

1. Change in bowel or bladder habits
2. A sore that does not heal
3. Unusual bleeding or discharge
4. Thickening or lump in breast or elsewhere
5. Indigestion or difficulty in swallowing
6. Obvious change in wart or mole
7. Nagging cough or hoarseness

**If you have a warning signal,
see your doctor without delay.**

*from the American Cancer Society

symptoms may be noted between meals and be aggravated by eating. The pain may vary from intermittent stomachaches to intense pain that seems to extend into the patient's back. The patient also experiences fatigue or weakness and anemia, and, as the cancerous condition progresses, may have periods of vomiting. The vomitus is dark, much like the color of coffee grounds, and there may be other signs of bleeding in the patient's stools.

Detection

X rays of the stomach and examination of the stomach interior by gastroscopy usually locate and define the cancerous area; they may also reveal another cause of the symptoms, such as a peptic ulcer. During the physical examination, the physician may find a tissue mass and tenderness in the stomach area. The laboratory report usually will show signs of anemia from blood loss, the presence of blood in a stool sample, and the level of hydrochloric acid in the stomach; a lack of hydrochloric acid is found in more than half the stomach cancer patients. A biopsy study of the suspected tissue usually completes the diagnosis.

Therapy

Unfortunately, because of the insidious nature of stomach cancer, the disease becomes easier to diagnose as it progresses. By the time cancer has been confirmed, the most expedient form of treatment is surgery to remove the affected area of the stomach. If the cancer is small and has not spread by metastasis to lymph nodes in the region, the chances are relatively good that the patient will survive five years or more; the odds against surviving five years without surgery are, by comparison, about 50 to 1 at best. Chemotherapy treat-

ments may be used in cases where surgery is not feasible, but the use of medicines instead of surgery for stomach cancer is not a routine procedure and generally is not recommended.

Occasionally, a stomach tumor is found to be noncancerous. The tumor may be a polyp, a *leiomyoma* (a growth consisting of smooth muscle tissue), or a *pseudotumor* (false tumor), such as an inflammatory fibroid growth. Such benign tumors produce symptoms ranging from gastric upset to internal bleeding and should be removed by surgery.

Causes

Many possible factors have been suggested as causes of stomach cancer. Dietary factors include hot food and beverages, as well as fish and smoked foods. Food additives have been implicated despite the fact that the incidence of stomach cancer has been declining during the period in which the use of additives has been increasing. Cured meats and cheeses, preserved with nitrites to retard spoilage, reportedly foster the development of carcinogenic chemical compounds in the digestive tract.

On the other hand, the widespread use of refrigeration has been offered as an explanation for the declining incidence of stomach cancer, since refrigeration reduces the need for chemical food preservatives.

Beyond the influence of diet, medical epidemiologists have found that genetic factors may play a role in the development of stomach cancer. Statistical analysis of large population studies of stomach cancer shows a tendency for the disease to occur in persons with blood type A, or with below-normal levels of hydrochloric acid in the stomach, or with inherited variations in the stomach lining. There also seems to be a good pos-

sibility that stomach cancers evolve from noncancerous changes in the stomach lining, as from polyps or peptic ulcers.

Bladder Cancer

As with stomach cancer, the incidence of cancer of the bladder rises progressively with age and occurs much more frequently in men than in women. Extensive occurrence of bladder cancer is commonly associated with industrial growth, but internationally its incidence ranges from a high rate in England to a low one in Japan; in the United States, the highest incidence of bladder cancer is in southern New Jersey. A study by the Roswell Park Memorial Institute, a cancer research center in Buffalo, New York, found that persons of Italian-American parentage were more likely to have bladder cancer than those of different parentage, and that women living in urban areas were more likely to develop the disease than their country cousins. American blacks have less bladder cancer than American whites.

Bladder cancer appears at an annual rate of about 30,000 new cases each year in the United States. Worldwide, it causes more than 7,000 deaths annually.

Symptoms

A change in bladder habits is among the first signs of bladder cancer. The change might be the presence of pain while urinating, a noticeable difficulty in urinating, or a difference in the frequency of urination.

Another symptom of the disease is the appearance of blood in the urine. The degree of blood coloration is not necessarily related to the severity of the cancer; any sign of blood in the urine should be investigated. Nor should the absence of pain be allowed to minimize the seriousness of urinary bleeding as a symptom of a diseased bladder. Even without pain, the presence of blood can indicate a problem such as an obstruction to the urinary flow that can lead to uremia, a toxic condition caused by retention of urinary waste products in the system.

Detection

Cancer of the bladder is frequently diagnosed from common signs and symptoms, particularly the appearance of blood in the urine. A laboratory examination of the patient's urine may also reveal the presence of cancer cells that have been washed out of the bladder. The disease can be detected by a *pyelogram*—a kind of X-ray picture made by filling the urinary system with a fluid that makes tissue details appear in sharp contrast—and by examination of the membrane lining the bladder. The bladder lining may be examined by surgical biopsy or by *cystoscopy,* the viewing of the interior of the bladder by means of a device inserted in the urethra—or both.

Examination of the bladder lining is needed to determine the type of tumor that may be the cause of the symptoms. One type, called a *papillary tumor,* or *papilloma,* is relatively harmless and usually does not invade the wall of the bladder as does the more dangerous type, sometimes described as a solid lesion. The degree of invasion of the bladder tissues by the infiltrating mass determines the type of treatment recommended. However, any tumor found in the lining of the bladder must be removed, because the papillary type can progress into a solid lesion if not treated.

Therapy

The cure of a bladder tumor can be approached in several ways, the choice of treatments depending upon the size and type of growth, the location of the tumor, and so on. Chemotherapy, using drugs such as thiotepa, has been successful in treating papillary bladder tumors; the chemical is applied directly to the bladder lining. A kind of electric cautery known as *fulguration* also may be used to destroy the tissue growth; it may be employed by cystoscopy or as part of a surgical approach. Radiation therapy also may be used by implanting radium needles in the affected bladder tissue. Surgical excision of the cancerous area, with or without radiation, chemotherapy, or cautery, may be the procedure chosen. In advanced cases of bladder cancer, the bladder may be removed and its function performed by the construction of a substitute organ from other tissues or by the relocation of the upper ends of the ureters at other urine-collecting points.

Causes

Cancer of the bladder may be caused by irritation from bladder stones or by toxic chemicals excreted from the kidneys. A high incidence of bladder cancer has been found among persons who are heavy cigarette smokers; a possible explanation is that certain carcinogenic tobacco-burning by-products are absorbed into the blood and excreted through the kidneys. The evidence includes studies showing that when such patients quit smoking, the carcinogens no longer appear in their urine.

Occupational factors have been associated with cancer of the bladder since 1895, when it was discovered that persons who worked with aniline chemical dyes were among those most likely to develop the disease. The incidence of the disease among chemical workers was found to be 30 times greater than that of the general population. The aniline dye workers developed bladder cancer at an average age 15 years younger than among the general population. The effect of the chemical dyes was verified by the development of cancer in the bladders of laboratory animals exposed to the dyes. In recent years, it has been found that many other chemicals can cause bladder cancer.

Besides the influence of industrial environmental factors, bladder cancer is associated with *schistosomiasis,* a disease occurring in Africa, Asia, South America, and other regions. Schistosomiasis develops after bathing or wading in water infested by a blood fluke. The organisms penetrate the skin and migrate to the intestines or urinary bladder, producing an inflammation that eventually leads to cancer. See Ch. 19, *Other Diseases of Major Importance,* for a fuller description of the disease.

Cancer of the Prostate

Cancer of the prostate is one of the most common cancers among men and is second only to lung cancer as a lethal type of tumor for men. The death rate has been around 14 per 100,000. The incidence increases with advancing age from the fifth decade of life, when prostatic cancer cells are found in nearly 20 percent of all men examined, to those in their 70s, an age when 60 percent of the men have been found to have cancer cells in their prostate glands. Fortunately, only 15 percent of the men with evidence of latent carcinoma of the prostate ever develop clinical symptoms of cancer before death. But after the age of 75, there are almost as many deaths, due to prostatic cancer as to lung cancer.

Symptoms

Cancer of the prostate is a disease noted for its secondary symptoms. It usually is detected because a physician begins analyzing symptoms that could suggest other disorders. There may, for example, be blood in the urine, indicating a serious problem that could be located anywhere along the urinary tract. Because the prostate encircles the urethra, which is the outlet from the bladder, any prostatic problem can cause disturbances in the normal passage of urine, including increased frequency of urination or discomfort in urinating. However, these also could be the symptoms of ailments other than cancer of the prostate.

Detection

Diagnosis of prostatic cancer usually begins with an examination of the prostate through the wall of the rectum. This technique is a regular part of a physical examination for men over the age of 40. If during the examination of the prostate the physician feels a lump or hardened area, further tests are ordered. The presence of a lump in the prostate need not be evidence of cancer; about half of the lumps and nodules are caused by fibrosis, calcium deposits, or other noncancerous bodies.

Additional tests may include examination by a cystoscope, which is inserted through the urethra to provide a view of the tissues of the area, plus a laboratory examination of tissue samples and prostatic fluid samples. A microscopic study of the samples may reveal the presence of cancer cells. The examination of prostatic cells for signs of cancer is similar to the technique used in the Pap test for cancer of the cervix in women.

In the search for evidence of cancer of the prostate, diagnostic clues may be found in blood chemistry tests and by the examination of a urinary pyelogram that could indicate obstructions from the prostate walls. Additional information may be forthcoming from an evaluation of the patient's medical history; low back pain complaints, for example, may result from prostate disorders.

Therapy

Surgery is the usual treatment for cancer of the prostate when the tumor is confined to the prostate gland. The surgical removal of the prostate may be supplemented by the administration of estrogens, or hormone therapy. If the cancer has spread to other areas, a frequent complication of prostatic cancer, an additional form of therapy could be the administration of radioactive drugs or some other form of radiation. An additional measure may be *orchiectomy,* the surgical removal of the testicles, performed because of the close physiological relationship between the testicles and the prostate.

Causes

Cancer of the prostate seems to be associated with activity of the sex hormones in men. It has been reported that all patients with prostatic cancer previously had a normal history of sex-hormone activity. The cancer symptoms begin to appear at a period of life when male sex-hormone activity is waning. Laboratory studies of the urine of patients show a decrease in levels of male sex hormones after the age of 40. As in female breast cancer, which also is related to sex-hormone activity, there are certain tissues of the body that appear to be more sensitive to influences of hormones. Changes in hormonal activity lead to increasing numbers of cells in those tissues and abnormal tissue growth.

Cancer of the Kidney

Cancer of the kidneys is most likely to occur in young children or in adults over the age of 40. The most common form of kidney cancer in children is known as *Wilms' tumor.* In adults, kidney cancer is usually in the form of a growth called *Grawitz's tumor,* or *hypernephroma,* a malignant growth that occurs chiefly among men.

Wilms' Tumor

Wilms' tumor, also called *nephroblastoma,* accounts for perhaps 25 percent of all cancers in children. About 90 percent of the cases develop before the age of seven; it has been diagnosed in infants less than five months old.

Symptoms

The symptoms can include fever, abdominal pain, weight loss, lack of appetite, blood in the urine, and an abdominal mass that may grow quickly to enormous size. The growth may be accompanied by symptoms of hypertension.

Detection

Examination of the patient may show the tumor to be on either the left or the right kidney. In a small percentage of the cases both kidneys are affected. A biopsy usually is performed in order to verify the presence of cancer cells in the growth.

Therapy

Treatment is most effective when the disease is diagnosed before the age of two. Surgery, radiation, and chemotherapy may be employed. The choice of chemotherapeutic agents may be varied as follow-up examinations reveal side effects or tumor resistance to one of the previously administered medications.

The five-year survival rate for victims of Wilms' tumor is about 65 percent when surgery and other measures are employed at an early stage. If not controlled, the cancer cells from Wilms' tumor tend to spread by metastasis to the lungs, liver, and other organs.

Causes

Wilms' tumor is believed to be congenital in nature. Studies of the tumor cells indicate that it may develop from embryonic kidney tissue that fails to evolve as a normal part of that organ.

Grawitz's Tumor

In about half of the cases of Grawitz's tumor, the common adult kidney cancer, the disease manifests itself through a combination of three symptoms: abdominal mass, pain in the area of the kidneys, and blood in the urine. In the other half of the cases, the cancer has metastasized and is found in the brain, lung, liver, or bone.

Detection

The physician may get important information about the seriousness of the tumor through laboratory studies of blood and urine samples; these can indicate the presence of substances that appear in body fluids when cancer cells are active.

Information can also be obtained by angiogram studies. An angiogram is an X-ray picture of an organ that has been injected with a dye to make the blood vessels, which carry the dye, markedly visible. A kidney angiogram shows different dye patterns for a normal organ, a kidney with a cyst, or a kidney with a tumor. The diagnosis usually is confirmed by biopsy or surgical exploration.

Therapy

Surgery and radiation treatment are the usual forms of therapy for adult kidney tumors, and the chances of ten-year survival, even after removal of a cancerous kidney, are fairly good.

Causes

Causes of adult kidney tumors remain largely unknown, but they have been thought to be associated with other disorders, such as infections or the presence of kidney stones.

Cancer of the Pancreas

Pancreatic cancer affects men about twice as frequently as women and accounts for about five percent of the cancer deaths. It is most likely to develop after the age of 40, and persons who are diabetic seem to be particularly susceptible to the disease.

Symptoms

The pancreatic cancer patient complains of apparent digestive disorders, such as abdominal pain, nausea, loss of appetite, and perhaps constipation. The abdominal distress may improve or worsen after eating and the pain may increase when the patient lies on his back. He will suffer weight loss and there will be jaundice. Many victims of pancreatic cancer also complain of itching sensations. Abdominal pain is usually persistent.

Detection

Along with signs of jaundice and scratching, the examining physician will evaluate laboratory reports of urine, blood, and stool analyses. Glucose tolerance tests and bilirubin levels are helpful in defining the source of the disorder. Negative findings of X-ray studies of the gastrointestinal tract, kidney-bladder area, and gallbladder can suggest a pancreatic disorder; by their normal condition, the physician can conclude that the disease is elsewhere in the abdominal region.

Therapy

Surgery is the usual treatment recommended for cancer of the pancreas; the precise location of the tumor within the pancreas may determine the exact surgical procedure to be undertaken. Removal of the tumor surgically has a more hopeful outcome if it is located at the head of the pancreas; cancers in the body or tail of the pancreas usually are not detected until the disease has spread to other parts of the body. Radiation and chemotherapy are not as effective in the treatment of pancreatic cancer as in controlling cancer in other organs.

Cancer of the Liver

Cancer of the liver is commonly found to be the result of metastasis from other parts of the body. Cancers that originate in the liver (primary cancers) account for less than 2 percent of the cancers reported in the United States. Primary cancers of the liver occur more frequently in men than in women and appear most frequently after the age of 40.

Symptoms

Weakness, weight loss, and pain in the upper abdomen or right side of the chest are among the symptoms of liver cancer. A fever apparently unrelated to any infection also may mark the onset of liver cancer.

Detection

An enlarged liver with masses of abnormal tissue may be detected by an examining physician. Laboratory tests usually reveal alterations in metabolism that are associated with changes in the liver cells caused by the cancer growth. A biopsy test of the abnormal liver tissue may confirm the presence of cancer. A more direct approach is to perform exploratory surgery for examination of the liver.

Therapy

If the tumor is located during exploratory surgery and the area can be excised, part of the liver is removed. Chemotherapy may also be used. The age of the patient and his general good health are important in making a successful recovery.

Researchers in 1985 announced a nonsurgical therapy for liver cancer involving the use of so-called "radiolabeled antibodies." To these molecules of antibodies, the defensive compounds of the body, radioactive substances are attached. The antibodies then seek out the cancer cells, and the radioactivity helps them destroy the cancer. The procedure has been used experimentally on patients whose tumors were too large for surgical instruments.

Causes

While the exact cause of primary liver cancer is unknown, a large proportion of cases is associated with cirrhosis of the liver. In recent years, some types of liver cancer have been traced to exposure of industrial workers to chemicals known to be carcinogenic. The high incidence of primary liver cancer in Asia and Africa is related to *aflatoxins* in grains and legumes, such as peanuts; the aflatoxin molds grow rapidly in warm, moist climates where the foods are not protected against natural hazards of the environment.

Secondary cancers of the liver are the result of primary cancers in other body areas; the liver is vulnerable to metastasis from cancers in every organ except the brain because of the pattern of blood circulation that carries cancer cells through the body.

Cancer of the Brain

Cancers in the brain tissue frequently are the result of metastasis from other body organs. They travel through the bloodstream, primarily from cancers of the lung, kidney, gastrointestinal tract, and breast. They become implanted in both the cerebrum and cerebellum, and, although there is wide distribution of the cancer cells, they are clustered mainly near the surfaces of the brain tissues. Primary brain tumors are more common among children than among adults; in children, other cancer sites are not likely to have had time to develop to the stage of metastasis required for the transmission of malignant cells to the brain.

A cancer that seems to originate in the brain tissues is known as *glioblastoma multiforme,* a malignant growth that may strike at any age but is more likely to occur during middle age. The glioblastoma may develop in nearly any part of the brain structure, including the brain stem, and spread extensively into a large tumorous mass.

Symptoms

Symptoms of brain cancer may be varied and misleading. They include headache, dizziness, nervousness, depression, mental confusion, vomiting, and paralysis. The symptoms sometimes are interpreted as those of a psychiatric disorder, and treatment of the organic disease may be postponed until too late.

Detection

Diagnosis may be difficult and the physician must evaluate the symptoms in terms of other findings from laboratory tests, X rays, and other techniques. In some cases, cancer cells may be detected in samples of spinal fluid.

Therapy

Treatment of brain cancers usually requires surgery or radiation or both, depending upon the type of tumor, its location, and other factors. Whether or not the brain tumor is a true cancer is not as important as early treatment, because any kind of abnormal tissue growth in the brain causes destructive pressure against vital tissues.

Cancer of the Larynx

Cancer of the larynx is chiefly a disease of men; about eight times as many men as women are stricken with this form of cancer, which usually makes its appearance around the age of 60. It is not one of the major types of cancer, with about 9,000 new cases appearing each year in the United States; but more than 35 percent of these cases are fatal. About 70 percent involve tumors on the vocal cords and are classed as *intrinsic* cancers of the larynx—that is, cancers originating with the larynx. The remainder of the cases involve tissues originating outside the vocal cords and are designated as *extrinsic.*

Symptoms

One of the first symptoms of intrinsic cancer of the larynx is hoarseness. Later the patient loses his ability to speak and experiences difficulty in breathing. The same series of symptoms occurs in cases of extrinsic cancer except that in extrinsic cancer there is an initial period of pain or discomfort in the throat before hoarseness begins. *Adenopathy,* or swelling of the lymph nodes in the area, also may be an early symptom of extrinsic cancer of the larynx.

Detection

Diagnosis of cancer of the larynx is relatively simple because the throat's interior can be examined by a physician and tissue samples can be removed for biopsy study. Detection of extrinsic cancer may be complicated by the fact that it is more likely to metastasize than intrinsic forms.

Therapy

In early cases of intrinsic cancer, treatment may require only radiation. Radiation also may be the therapy of choice for small lesions that appear in the middle of the vocal cords.

Surgery may be required for more serious cases, with radiation treatments before or after surgery, or both. The surgery, called a *laryngectomy,* may involve partial or total removal of the larynx. If a partial laryngectomy is performed, an effort is made to save as much of the vocal cords as possible. The voice will be changed after surgery, but it will be functional. The respiratory tract will be preserved. When total laryngectomy is required, the entire larynx is removed and the neck is dissected to determine if cancer cells have migrated to the lymph nodes in the neck. A new trachea is constructed by plastic surgery to permit normal or nearly normal respiration.

Thyroid Cancer

Cancer of the thyroid gland is relatively uncommon, with fewer than three new cases per 100,000 population per year. The death rate is even less, about one thyroid-cancer death per year per 200,000 persons. One reason for the low death rate is that many of the cancers are detected during examination or surgery for goiter or other throat symptoms.

Symptoms

These include rapid growth of the thyroid gland, hoarseness, paralysis of nerves in the larynx, and enlarged lymph nodes in the neck and surrounding area. Diagnosis is aided by the rate at which suspected areas of cancer in the thyroid gland absorb radioactive iodine; the pattern of radioactive uptake helps pinpoint tissue abnormalities, including cysts and noncancerous tumors as well as cancerous growths.

Therapy

Treatment may include surgery to remove the cancer and part of the surrounding tissue, plus removal of lymph nodes that may contain cancer cells that have metastasized from the thyroid tumor. In addition, surgeons may recommend removal of other lymph nodes that are in the path of drainage from the thyroid gland. Surgery usually is more successful in the treatment of young patients than in older persons. Radiation sometimes is used, either from an external source or by injection of large doses of radioactive chemicals.

Causes

Among causes of cancer of the thyroid gland is exposure of children and young adults to radiation therapy of the head and neck region; many such patients later develop thyroid cancer.

Hodgkin's Disease

Hodgkin's disease is one of the *lymphomas*—cancers of the lymphatic system. It occurs most commonly among young adults, although it can appear at any age. Men are more likely to be victims than are women.

Symptoms

One of the first symptoms of Hodgkin's disease is a painless enlargement of a lymph node, usually in the area of the neck. The enlarged lymph nodes usually are firm and rubbery at first. The patient may experience a severe and persistent itching for several weeks or months before the first enlarged lymph node appears.

Other symptoms may include shortness of breath, fever, weight loss, anemia, and some pressure or pain as the disease progresses and nerve tissue becomes involved. As the disease progresses, the lymph nodes that originally were separate and movable become matted and fixed, and sometimes become inflamed. Over a period of months to years, the disease spreads through other parts of the body.

Therapy

The presence of Hodgkin's disease is ordinarily confirmed by removal of an affected lymph node for biopsy study. If the disease is limited to one or two localized areas the usual therapy is radiation treatments. Surgical excision of the nodes may be employed in special cases, as when a mass of nodes threatens a vital organ. But intense radiation exposure is generally more effective than surgery in controlling the disease. Radiation treatments when properly applied may have a cure rate of as high as 95 percent at the site treated. In cases where the disease has spread over a large area of the body, the treatment of choice may be chemotherapy utilizing nitrogen mustard, steroid drugs, and other substances.

Causes

The cause of Hodgkin's disease is unknown. Experiments involving efforts to transmit the disease by injecting ground bits of excised nodes into animals have not been successful. The nodes also have failed to yield any bacteria that can be identified with the disease. However, because of the fever and other symptoms associated with the disorder, and because it appears to occur more frequently among members of the same family or community than in the population as a whole, it has been suggested that Hodgkin's disease is a viral disease that has a malignant effect on the human lymphatic system.

Leukemia

Because leukemia involves blood cells circulating through the body rather than a fixed mass of tissue, as in skin or stomach cancer, the classification of leukemia as a true cancer is occasionally challenged. However, leukemia cells, when studied under the microscope and in cell cultures, behave like cancer cells found in tumors. They have a nucleus and cytoplasm that are abnormal and tend to multiply in a prolific and erratic manner.

Medical scientists frequently refer to the disease in the plural, as leukemias, because there are at least ten different kinds of blood cells that have been identified with various forms of the disease. In addition, there are both acute and chronic forms of leukemia, such as *acute granulocytic leukemia* and *chronic lymphocytic leukemia,* named after the particular kind of white blood cells that are most affected.

Leukemia affects the blood-forming tissues, such as the bone marrow, resulting in an overproduction of white blood cells. The disease is particularly lethal to children under the age of 15; more than ten percent of the leukemia deaths each year are among children. The incidence by age group varies according to the specific type of leukemia, however; one variety of acute granulocytic leukemia can occur at any age, but chronic lymphocytic leukemia usually does not appear before the age of 40. Men are more likely than women to be the victims of one of the various forms of leukemia.

Symptoms

There are several symptoms that the different leukemias have in common. These include fever, weight loss, fatigue, bone pain, anemia as expressed in paleness, and an enlarged spleen or masses under the skin caused by an accumulation of leukemic cells. There may be skin lesions and, as the disease advances, a tendency to bleed. Infections may become more common and less responsive to treatment because of a loss of the normal blood cells needed to resist disease.

Detection

Diagnosis of leukemia from early symptoms may be difficult because they resemble those of mononucleosis and other infections. Biopsies of bone marrow and careful blood studies usually identify the disease.

Therapy

Treatment usually is directed toward reducing the size of the spleen and the number of white cells in the blood, and increasing the level of blood hemoglobin to counteract the effects of anemia. Antibiotics may be included

to help control infections when natural resistance to disease has been lowered. X-ray treatments, radioactive phosphorus, anticancer drugs, and steroid hormone medications are administered according to the needs of the individual patient and the type of leukemia being treated.

Acute leukemia may be fatal within a few weeks of the onset of symptoms. But chronic cases receiving proper treatment have been known to survive more than a quarter of a century with the disease. In recent years remission rates have improved, partly because of new drugs and methods of treatment. The new chemotherapeutic approaches include the following:

- For acute leukemia in children, *methotrexate* has been used with increasing success. One of the antimetabolites, the family of drugs that interfere with development of essential cell components, methotrexate reduces the production in the blood of folic acid. In that way the drug competes with the cancer cells for the vital enzyme folic reductase—and inhibits the cancer's growth.

- In adults, chronic and acute forms of leukemia may be treated with *chlorambucil* or *cyclophosphamide.* Both drugs are types of nitrogen mustard. Both may produce such side effects as suppression of bone marrow, loss of hair, nausea, dizziness, and vomiting.

- In cases of acute leukemia in childhood, the vinca alkaloid drugs have proved valuable. These drugs, such as *vincristine sulfate,* are extremely powerful. They attack active cancer cells more directly than they attack normal cells. They may lead to such side effects as headaches, convulsions, and loss of some muscular control.

Other drugs in the alkaloid and other drug families have been used to treat leukemia. The others include *cytosine arabinoside,* which works to prevent cell synthesis—including cancer-cell synthesis; 6-Mercotopurine, which inhibits some metabolic processes; and *busulfan* and similar drugs, which work against multiplication of the cancer cells. Antitumor antibiotics that prevent growth of cancer cells include daunoribicin, doxorubicin, and bleomycin.

Causes

There is no general theory about the cause of leukemia. Animals, including mice and poultry, are known to be susceptible to a form of leukemia transmitted by virus, but there is no solid evidence that human leukemias are caused by viral infections. Survivors of nuclear explosions in Hiroshima and Nagasaki, as well as persons exposed to large doses of X rays, have developed leukemia at a higher-than-normal rate than other people. There is evidence that at least one type of acute leukemia may be a result of an inherited genetic defect.

Other Cancers

Lymphosarcoma

Another of the cancers that involve the lymphatic system is called *lymphosarcoma*—a malignant lymphoma that tends to metastasize in lymphatic tissue. The most common first symptom is a swelling of the lymph nodes, and the diagnosis and treatment are similar to those of Hodgkin's disease. Lymphosarcoma can occur at any stage of life and make its appearance in any part of the body where there is lymphatic tissue, including the gastrointestinal tract, the tonsils, the tongue, or the nasopharynx area.

Reticulum-Cell Sarcoma

The lymphomas also include *reticulum-cell sarcoma.* (A sarcoma is a malignant tumor in the connective tissue. Reticulum cells are a particular kind of connective tissue.) The disease is marked by the invasion of normal tissue by increased numbers of reticulum cells or fibers. As in the treatment of leukemia, it is important to know which of the various types of cancer has affected the lymphatic system, because each of the lymphomas responds to a different therapeutic routine.

Myeloma and Multiple Myeloma

Myelomas, once considered rare but now reported in increasing numbers, are cancerous growths that seem to originate in the bone marrow. (*Myelos* is the Greek word for "marrow.") The disease is seldom found in persons younger than 40; the average age at onset is about 65. Men are twice as likely as women to be victims of myelomas.

The disease is marked by bone destruction, mainly in the pelvis, ribs, and spine. The bones break easily, sometimes causing collapse of the spinal column and pressure on the spinal cord. There also may be anemia, kidney damage, and changes in the blood chemistry. When the myelomas occur at numerous sites in the bone marrow throughout the body, the disease is known as *multiple myeloma.*

Treatment

Various methods of treating lymphomas have evolved despite serious difficulties. Lymphomas appear in many different forms, and can change form in the process of spreading to another part of the body. Different types may be found in a single lymph gland.

Despite these difficulties, many chemotherapeutic agents have been found useful in treatment of lymphomas. To an extent, the preferred drugs fall in the same categories as those used in treating leukemia. The principal drugs, thus, include:

- alkalyting agents, such as nitrogen mustard, cyclophosphamide, and chlorambucil;

- vinca alkaloids, among them vincristine and vinblastine;

- procarbazine, which works like the alkalyting agents;

- antibiotics, which work to reduce or eliminate tumors, including Adriamycin and actinomycin D; and

- the corticosteroids, combinations of agents including hormones, acids, and other body elements.

These and other drugs have been used in various combinations in the treatment of lymphomas. One of the more successful has been named for the four drugs that are included in the protocol, or treatment series. The four are nitrogen mustard, vincristine (Oncovin), Procarbazine, and Prednisone; the combination treatment is known as MOPP. The treatment is used at certain stages of lymphoma, and has encouraged medical specialists to consider lymphoma as potentially curable.

In addition to drug therapy, methods of treating lymphomas include irradiation therapy, or radiotherapy, and a combination of drugs and radiotherapy.

19

Other Diseases of Major Importance

This chapter discusses a number of diseases of major importance that are not dealt with elsewhere: acquired immune deficiency syndrome (AIDS), a disease characterized by a defect in the body's natural immune system; plague, of great historical importance but fortunately now uncommon in the United States; two infectious diseases—tularemia and Rocky Mountain Spotted Fever; and seven tropical diseases that afflict millions of people in the warmer regions of the world and that occasionally occur elsewhere—malaria and yellow fever, leishmaniasis, trypanosomiasis, filariasis, schistosomiasis, and leprosy.

AIDS

First reported widely in 1981, AIDS has become a priority of the U.S. Public Health Service. Researchers have isolated a virus, the *human immunodeficiency virus* (*HIV*), that they believe causes AIDS. This virus was initially called the *human T-cell leukemia virus III* (*HTLV-III*). Persons with AIDS (PWAs) are susceptible to a variety of unusual or rare illnesses called *opportunistic diseases*. These include *Pneumocystis carinii* pneu-

monia (PCP); Kaposi's sarcoma; thrush, or *Candida albicans*; dementia (AIDS dementia complex or ADC); herpes simplex; and meningitis.

Groups at highest risk of contracting AIDS include homo- and bisexual men and intravenous drug users in large cities; hemophiliacs; female prostitutes; heterosexuals with multiple partners in areas where AIDS is common; and recipients of multiple blood transfusions from areas where the disease was common between 1983 and 1985. Evidence suggests that the HIV virus may also be affecting more and more young people, particularly runaways. In "passive transmission," a mother can pass AIDS to her child before or during birth.

Increasingly, medical authorities view AIDS as a disease with which victims may live for years. But AIDS is incurable. No treatment has successfully restored the immune system of an AIDS patient to normal functioning. Making the task of researching AIDS more difficult, the virus can lie inactive in the human body for as long as 10 years without causing any symptoms. Where this occurs, a "carrier" of AIDS can infect others with the disease.

Symptoms

Once infection with AIDS occurs, the human body may take from six weeks to a year or more to produce antibodies. These appear in response to the virus's invasion of the blood stream. The symptoms that can follow may resemble those of flu or even the common cold. Symptoms may include swollen glands, or enlarged lymph nodes, in the neck, armpits, or groin; night sweats; fever; unexplained rapid weight loss; chronic, unexplained diarrhea; fatigue; loss of appetite, and bruising and bleeding that do not heal.

Prevention

To prevent the spread of AIDS, the U.S. Public Health Service has recommended that persons at risk of contracting the disease should:

- Not donate blood or plasma, sperm, body organs, or other tissues

- Limit sexual contacts and be assertive with sexual partners about engaging only in safe sexual practices

- Not engage in sexual acts in which

exchange of body fluids, including semen, takes place

- Refrain from sharing toothbrushes, razors, or other implements that could be contaminated with blood

- If a drug user, limit drug use, do not let others use needles you have used, and do not leave needles or other drug paraphernalia where others might find and use them

- If a woman who has had a positive antibody test (see below), or who is the sexual partner of a man with a positive antibody test, avoid or postpone pregnancy

The Public Health Service has reported that no evidence indicates that the AIDS virus can be transmitted through casual kissing or other casual social contacts. But persons who have had positive antibody tests should let their physicians and dentists know about the test results. The physician and dentist can then cooperate in preventing the spread of the virus if the patient has become infected. There has been no risk of contracting AIDS through blood donations or transfusions since the introduction of blood-screening procedures in 1985.

Treatment

Although there is no known cure, a blood test called the *ELISA* (enzyme-linked immunosorbent assay) test has been developed to detect the presence of antibodies to the AIDS virus in human blood. The test has helped to eliminate nearly all questionable blood and plasma from the nation's blood supply—not to diagnose individuals. Laboratories have also used the Western Blot test to verify positive results from ELISA. In 1989, the FDA approved marketing of the HIVAG-1 test, the first designed to help physicians detect the AIDS virus

and to monitor its development in the human body. Already in use, a rapid screening test, the Recombigen HIV-1 Latex Agglutination test, can detect AIDS virus antibodies in five minutes.

More than 50 pharmaceutical companies have begun to develop vaccines, antiviral drugs, and other diagnostic tests for AIDS patients. The drugs in use include zidovudine, or AZT, the only compound proven effective against AIDS; alpha interferon, used to treat AIDS-generated cancer; and aerosolized pentamidine, approved in 1989 for broadened use with patients afflicted at least once with Pneumocystis pneumonia. AZT offered hope to some 600,000 Americans infected with AIDS after it was discovered that the drug can delay the onset of active symptoms.

At least 25 potential anti-HIV compounds were in various stages of testing in the late 1980s. The drugs worked in different ways. Researchers believed some of the agents might be most effective when used in combination. For example, alpha interferon has been combined in tests with AZT to reduce AZT's toxic effects, including anemia and liver problems. Various experimental drugs are designed to prevent the AIDS virus from binding to body cells, from entering into cells, or from developing into "virus factories" once inside human cells. Still others are designed to combat groups of AIDS symptoms, known as AIDS-Related Complex (ARC). Among the test drugs were several natural human products that bolster the immune system or antiviral defenses, including Imreg-2, interleukin-2, and virus-fighting interferons.

The FDA has taken steps to reduce the time elapsing between testing of drugs for treating life-threatening diseases and introduction of those compounds into the marketplace. The goal is to make possible

decisions on the approvability of various drugs much sooner than would once have been possible. In line with this program, the FDA approved expanded studies of the drugs foscarnet and ganciclovir, both of them potential compounds for the prevention of AIDS-related blindness.

Plague

Bubonic plague, one of the many diseases transmitted to humans through direct or indirect contact with animals, usually is listed among the scourges of past centuries. At least three great epidemics of bubonic plague have been recorded, including the Black Death of the 14th century, when the disease claimed at least 50 million lives. The most recent worldwide epidemic of the plague occurred in the 1800s. While recent cases of the plague in North America have been relatively rare, the disease organism is still carried by rodents, including squirrels, rats, and rabbits; and cases of the plague still occur in the western United States. Increased activity in western areas by hunters, campers, and other outdoor enthusiasts has resulted in a higher incidence of the disease among humans in recent years. The disease also is fairly common in Asia, Africa, and South America.

Symptoms

The infection is transmitted from animals to man through the bite of a flea carrying the disease organism. Symptoms usually develop in several days but may take as long as two weeks after the flea bite. The victim experiences chills and fever, with the temperature rising above 102° F. He may experience headaches, a rapid heart beat, and difficulty walking. Vomiting and delirium also are among the symptoms of plague. There may be pain and tenderness of the lymph nodes, which become inflamed and swollen; the enlarged lymph nodes are known as *buboes,* a term that gives its name to the type of plague involved. The buboes occur most frequently in the legs and groin because these are the most frequent sites for flea bites.

The site of the flea bite may or may not be found after the symptoms develop. If present, it may be marked by a swollen, pus-filled area of the skin.

Diagnosis of plague can be confirmed by laboratory tests that might include examination of the bacteria taken in samples from buboes or other diseased areas of the body, inoculation of laboratory animals with suspected disease organisms, and studies of the white blood cells of the patient.

Complications can include pneumonia and hemorrhages, with bleeding from the nose or mouth or through the gastrointestinal or urinary tracts, and abscesses and ulcerations. The pneumonic form of plague can be transmitted from one person to another like colds or other infectious diseases; in other words, plague organisms are spread by being exhaled by one person and inhaled by another.

Treatment and Prevention

As in other infectious diseases, early treatment is most effective. Antibiotics are administered every day for a period of one to two weeks, and buboes are treated with hot, moist applications. The buboes may be drained if necessary after the patient has responded to antibiotic medications. Antibiotics have reduced the fatality rate from plague infections from a high of 90 percent to a maximum of about 10 percent. Vaccines are available but are of limited and temporary

value. Prevention requires eradication of rats and other possibly infected rodents (some 200 species are known to carry the disease), use of insecticides to control fleas, and avoidance of contact with wild animals in areas where plague is known to exist. Domestic animals also should be protected from contact with possibly infected wild animals.

Tularemia

An infectious disease known as *tularemia,* sometimes called *rabbit fever,* is transmitted from animals to humans who come in contact with the animal tissues. It also can be transmitted through the bites of ticks or flies or by drinking contaminated water. Like the plague-disease organism, tularemia can be transmitted by inhalation of infected particles from the lungs of a diseased person, although such occurrences are rare.

Symptoms

Within a couple of days to perhaps two weeks after exposure to the tularemia germ, the patient develops chills and a fever with temperatures rising to 103° F. or higher. Other symptoms include headache, nausea and vomiting, extreme weakness, and drenching sweats. Lymph nodes become enlarged and a pus-filled lesion develops at the site of the infection. Usually only one pustular papule develops on a finger or other skin area, marking the point of the insect bite or contact with infected animal tissues; but there may be several such sores in the membranes of the mouth if that is the point of infection. It is not uncommon for the eyes or lungs to become involved.

Laboratory tests, along with a record of contact with wild animals or game birds, eating improperly cooked

meats, being bitten by deer flies or ticks, or drinking water from ponds or streams, usually helps verify the cause of the symptoms as tularemia. In some cases the contact with the disease organism can be made through bites or scratches of infected dogs or cats, but most frequently the disease of humans originates through handling of the meat or fur of wild animals or by camping or hiking in areas where the disease is endemic.

Treatment

Treatment includes bed rest and administration of antibiotics. Adequate fluid intake is important and oxygen may be required. Aspirin usually is given also, to relieve headache and muscle aches. Hot compresses are applied to the enlarged lymph node areas; it may be necessary to drain the swollen, infected nodes. If the disease is complicated by pneumonic tularemia or infection of the eye, the patient usually is hospitalized. Success of the therapy depends upon early and adequate treatment. The disease is rarely fatal when properly treated with antibiotics, but it can be lethal if the symptoms are ignored. Anyone who develops the symptoms of tularemia after handling wild animals or being exposed to biting insects or contaminated water in rural or rugged country should seek immediate medical help.

Hunters, campers, hikers, and others venturing into the great outdoors should protect their bodies against invasion by ticks by wearing long-sleeved shirts and long trousers with cuffs securely fastened. Regular checks should be made of the scalp, groin, and armpits for ticks. Any ticks found should be detached quickly and the bite area cleansed with soap and water, followed by an alcohol cleansing. If the head of the tick breaks off, it can be removed by the same techniques used to remove a splinter from the skin. Raw water from ponds and streams should be boiled or disinfected with chemicals before using. Rubber gloves should be worn while dressing the meat of wild game or birds, and the meat should be thoroughly cooked. On the positive side, once the disease occurs, the recovered patient develops immunity to tularemia.

Rocky Mountain Spotted Fever

The name of an increasingly common tick-borne disease, *Rocky Mountain spotted fever,* is misleading, because humans are most likely to become infected in regions far from the Rocky Mountains. The disease, also known as *tick fever,* has become most prevalent in rural and suburban areas of the southern and eastern United States. It is caused by a rickettsial organism transmitted by a tick bite. Wild rodents are a reservoir of the infected ticks that carry the disease.

Symptoms

Rocky Mountain spotted fever may be relatively mild or dangerously severe. The symptoms of headache, chills, and fever may begin suddenly and persist for a period of two or three weeks. Fever temperatures may reach 104° F and may be accompanied by nausea and occasional vomiting. Headaches have been described in some cases as excruciating, with the pain most intense along the forehead. Muscles of the legs, back, and abdomen may ache and feel tender. The most serious cases seem to develop within a few days after a tick bite; milder cases usually are slower to develop. A rash usually develops a few days after the onset of other symptoms and is most likely to be concentrated on the forearm, ankles, feet,

wrists, and hands. If untreated, Rocky Mountain spotted fever symptoms may abate in two weeks, but the infection can be fatal, particularly in persons over the age of 40.

Treatment

Treatment includes administration of antibiotics and, in some cases, steroid hormones. Careful nursing care and adequate intake of protein foods and liquids also are needed.

Preventive measures are similar to those recommended to guard against tularemia. Wear adequate protective clothing that forms a barrier against tick invasion of the skin surfaces, check the scalp and other hairy body areas regularly for ticks, and remove and destroy any ticks found. In addition, ground areas known to be inhabited by wood ticks should be sprayed with an effective insecticide safe for humans; insect repellents also should be applied to clothing and exposed skin surfaces when venturing into wooded or brushy areas. Ticks may become attached to dogs and other animals and care should be used in removing them from the pets, because the disease organism can enter the body through minor cuts and scratches on the skin. A vaccine is available for protection of persons who are likely to use possibly infested tick areas for work or recreation. Immunity usually is established by two inoculations, about a month apart, and booster shots as needed.

Tropical Diseases

Most people living in the temperate climates of North America and Europe are spared the ravages of

some of the most lethal and debilitating diseases known to mankind. They include malaria, which probably has killed more people than any other disease in history, yellow fever, leishmaniasis, trypanosomiasis, filariasis, schistosomiasis, and leprosy.

While many persons probably have never heard of some of these diseases and at least a few doctors might have trouble in diagnosing the symptoms, they affect hundreds of millions of people each year and could pose a threat to persons living in any part of the world. They are generally classed as tropical diseases, but so-called tropical or exotic diseases have been prevented from spreading into temperate regions partly because of alert medical care and preventive measures by public health experts. Malaria, for example, has been found as far north as the Arctic Circle, as far south as the tip of South America, and at one time was a disease of epidemic proportions in such northern cities as Philadelphia and London. These diseases have altered the course of history, ending the life of Alexander the Great as he tried to conquer the world, nipping in the bud Napoleon's plans to retake Canada from the English, defeating French efforts to build the Panama Canal, and contributing to the black-slave trade between Africa and the Americas.

The major tropical diseases are caused by a variety of organisms, including viruses, protozoa, and worms. Some are transmitted by insect bites, some by contact with contaminated water, and others, like leprosy, are spread by means that remain a mystery despite centuries of medical experience with millions of cases of the disease. Space does not permit detailed discussion of all tropical diseases; only those regarded by medical authorities as among the most significant to world health are described in this chapter.

Malaria

Malaria, one of the most common diseases in the world, gets its name from an Italian word for "bad air" because of an ancient belief that a mysterious substance in the air was the cause of the ailment. It is now known that the disease is caused by any of at least four parasites carried by Anopheles mosquitoes. According to the World Health Organization (WHO), some 200 million persons are affected by the disease, including one-fourth of the adult population on the continent of Africa. WHO estimates that at least one million children die each year of malaria. The disease was relatively rare in the United States until the 1960s, when hundreds of cases began to appear among military personnel who apparently contracted the disease in southeast Asia but did not develop symptoms until they returned to the United States; the disease later occurred in soldiers who had never left the United States, apparently transmitted by domestic Anopheles mosquitoes that had become infested with the malaria parasites.

Symptoms

The symptoms of malaria differ somewhat among various patients because the four known kinds of plasmodia, or protozoa, that cause the infection do not produce the same specific effects. However, the general symptoms common to all forms of malaria are fever, chills, headache, muscle pains, and, in some cases, skin disorders such as cold sores, hives, or a rash. A malaria attack may begin with a severe chill that lasts from twenty minutes to an hour, followed by a fever lasting from three to eight hours with temperature rising to more than 104° F. The fever usually is accompanied by profuse sweating, and the afflicted person is left exhausted by the cycle of chills and fever. The attacks become more or less successively milder, less frequent, and more irregular, and finally cease, although there may be relapses.

One kind of malarial organism seems to cause attacks that occur every other day, while another type produces attacks that appear quite regularly on every third day; still another type of malaria plasmodium seems to cause a fever that is continuous. While the liver seems to be a favored target organ, other body systems can be involved, with related complications. If the organism reaches the brain, the patient may suffer convulsions, delirium, partial paralysis, or coma. If the organism invades the lungs, there may be coughing symptoms and blood-stained sputum. In some cases, there may be gastrointestinal symptoms with abdominal pain, vomiting, or diarrhea.

Medical examination of malaria patients frequently reveals signs of anemia, an enlarged spleen, liver abnormalities, and edema, or swelling because of fluid accumulation. Blood studies may show the malaria parasites in the blood, damaged red blood cells, and an abnormal white blood cell count. The four species of malaria organism are distinctive enough to be identified in laboratory tests.

Treatment

Treatment includes administration of antimalarial drugs such as quinine, chloroquine, or primaquine. Newer antimalarial drugs are sometimes used in combinations because of the development of drug-resistant strains of the organism in South America and Asia. There is no vaccine that protects against malaria.

Causes

The protozoa that cause malaria are carried by the Anopheles mosquito,

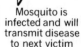

How Malaria Is Transmitted

Infected mosquito

Protozoa multiply in human bloodstream

Mosquito is infected and will transmit disease to next victim

A mosquito infected with malaria protozoa bites a human. The protozoa produce daughter cells within the human bloodstream. These cells are transmitted to another mosquito that bites the infected human. This mosquito will infect the next human it bites, thus perpetuating the malaria cycle.

but humans are the intermediate host. This means that both infected humans and infected mosquitoes are needed to continue the life cycle of the organism. The disease therefore can be controlled if Anopheles mosquito populations are eradicated and humans are not carrying the protozoa in their blood. When these organisms get into human blood, they invade the red blood cells and multiply until the blood cells rupture to release offspring called *daughter cells*. When the mosquito bites a human for a blood meal, the daughter cells enter the mosquito stomach, where they complete their life cycle and migrate to the mosquito's salivary gland to be injected into the next human, and so on. It takes from ten days to six weeks following a mosquito bite for the first malaria symptoms to develop, the time differences varying with the species of protozoa involved. The malaria mosquito in recent years has developed resistance to insecticides, and areas of infestation have spread in some countries where irrigation for farming has been expanded.

Yellow Fever

Yellow fever, which sometimes produces symptoms similar to those of malaria, also is transmitted by a mosquito. But yellow fever is a virus disease carried by the Aedes mosquito.

Yellow fever also can be harbored by other animals, while the malaria organism that affects humans is not transmitted between humans and lower animals. Like malaria, yellow fever has in past years spread deeply into North America with cases reported along the Gulf Coast, the Mississippi River Valley, and as far north as Boston. A vaccine is available for protection against yellow fever.

Leishmaniasis

Leishmaniasis is similar to malaria in that the disease organisms are protozoa transmitted to humans by an insect bite, but the insect in this case is the sandfly. There are several forms that leishmaniasis can take. The kind considered most lethal, with a mortality rate of up to 95 percent of untreated adults, is known as *kala-azar*, a term derived from the Hindi language meaning "black disease". Kala-azar also is known as *black fever, dumdum fever,* and *visceral leishmaniasis*. It occurs from China through Russia and India to North Africa, the Mediterranean countries of Europe, and in parts of Central and South America. Kala-azar has appeared in the United States in cases contracted overseas.

Symptoms

The symptoms may not appear for a period of from ten days to more than three months after the bite of a sandfly, although the disease organism may be found in blood tests before the first symptoms occur. Symptoms include a fever that reaches a peak twice a day for a period of perhaps several weeks, then recurs at irregular intervals while the patient experiences progressive weakness, loss of weight, loss of skin color, and a rapid heartbeat. In some cases, de-

pending upon the type of infection, there may be gastrointestinal complaints and bleeding of the mucous membranes, particularly around the teeth. There also can be edema, an accumulation of fluid in the tissues that conceals the actual loss of body tissue. Physical examination shows an enlarged spleen and liver plus abnormal findings in blood and urine tests.

American Cutaneous Leishmaniasis

The American cutaneous form of leishmaniasis usually begins with one or more skin ulcers resulting from sandfly bites, with the skin of the ear the target site of the insect in many cases. The skin lesion may enlarge, with or without secondary infection by other disease organisms, and spread into the lymphatic system of the body. From the lymph system, the infecting protozoa may invade the mouth and nose, producing painful and mutilating skin ulcers and other destructive changes in the tissues. Bacterial infections and respiratory problems can lead to the death of the patient. In some areas of Central and South America, more than 10 percent of the population suffer from the disfiguring effects of leishmaniasis. Diagnosis usually is confirmed by medical tests that identify the leishmaniasis organism in the patient's tissues.

Old World Cutaneous Leishmaniasis

A milder form, sometimes known as Old World cutaneous leishmaniasis, occurs from India westward to the Mediterranean countries and North Africa. An ulcer appears at the site of a sandfly bite, usually several weeks after the bite, but it heals during a period of from three months to a year. A large pitted scar frequently remains to mark the site of the ulceration, but the invading organism does not

spread deeply into the body tissues as in the severe types of leishmaniasis.

Treatment

Therapy for leishmaniasis cases includes administration of various medications containing antimony, along with antibiotics for the control of secondary infections. Bed rest, proper diet, and, in severe cases, blood transfusions also are advised.

Causes

The leishmaniasis organisms injected into the human body by the sandfly bite multiply through parasitic invasion of the tissue cells, particularly blood cells that usually resist infection. They may invade the lymph nodes, spleen, liver, and bone marrow, causing anemia and other symptoms. In populated areas, sandflies can be eradicated by insecticides. Unfortunately, rodents and other wild and domestic animals serve as a reservoir for the leishmaniasis protozoa and tend to perpetuate the disease in rural and jungle areas of warm climates.

Trypanosomiasis

Trypanosomiasis is a group of diseases caused by similar kinds of parasitic protozoa. The diseases, which include two kinds of African *sleeping sickness* and *Chagas' disease* of Central and South America, affect about 10 million people. The sleeping-sickness forms of trypanosomiasis are transmitted by species of the tsetse fly, while Chagas' disease is carried by insects known as *assassin bugs* or *kissing bugs*. Besides affecting humans, the trypanosomiasis organisms infect other animals, including cattle, horses, dogs, and donkeys, and have made an area of nearly four million square miles of Africa uninhabitable. According to the World Health Organization, the African land devastated by trypanosomiasis contains large fertile areas capable of supporting 125 million cattle, but domestic animals cannot survive the infestation of tsetse flies.

Sleeping Sickness

The two kinds of African sleeping sickness, Gambian and Rhodesian, are similar. Gambian, or mid-African, sleeping sickness is transmitted by a tsetse fly that lives near water; Rhodesian, or East African, sleeping sickness is carried by a woodland species of tsetse fly that uses antelopes as a reservoir of the infectious organism. The most likely victims of tsetse fly bites are young men, probably because they are more likely to be exposed to the insects.

Symptoms

The symptoms of trypanosomiasis infections from tsetse fly bites can vary considerably according to various factors, such as the general health of the victim. A small area of inflammation, called a *chancre,* appears at the site of the tsetse fly bite about two days after the incident; some patients complain of pain and irritation in the area around the bite for several weeks, but others have no symptoms. Then, for a period of perhaps several months, episodes of fever occur, with temperatures rising to 106° F. The bouts of fever may be accompanied by skin rashes, severe headaches, and heart palpitations. Loss of appetite and weight follow, with insomnia, an inability to concentrate, tremors, and difficulty in speaking and walking. There also may be signs of anemia and delayed reaction to a painful stim-

ulus. Eventually, the protozoa can invade the central nervous system, producing convulsions, coma, and death.

Sleeping sickness, which may progress gradually, gets its name from the appearance of the patient, who develops a vacant expression and drooping eyelids, along with blurred speech, general lethargy, and occasional periods of paralysis.

Gambian and Rhodesian Varieties

A major difference between the Gambian and Rhodesian forms of African sleeping sickness is that the Rhodesian variety, which has similar symptoms, is more acute and progresses more rapidly than the Gambian. The fevers are higher, weight losses greater, the disease more resistant to treatment, and the span of time from first symptoms to death much shorter. Even with intensive treatment, Rhodesian sleeping sickness patients have only a 50–50 chance of survival, while 90 to 95 percent of the Gambian sleeping sickness patients recover when properly treated for the disease.

Treatment

Several chemotherapeutic agents are available for treatment of Gambian and Rhodesian sleeping sickness; they include suramin, pentamidine, and tryparsamide given by injection. Good nutrition, good nursing care, and treatment of secondary infections are additional therapeutic measures.

Chagas' Disease

Chagas' disease, or American trypanosomiasis, is a primary cause of heart disease from Mexico through much of South America. The protozoan infection is rare in the United

States, but cases have been reported. The first symptoms may be edema of the face. The accumulation of fluid occuring in the area of the eyelids, conjunctivitis, hard reddish nodules on the skin, along with the fever and involvement of the heart, brain, and liver tissues. The assassin or kissing bugs by which the disease is spread tend to bite the face, especially around the lips or eyelids, accounting for the swelling of those facial areas. The bite may be painful, or if the victim is sleeping at the time, it may not be noticed at all.

Symptoms

The protozoa multiply rapidly at the site of the bug bite, frequently producing symptoms resembling those of leishmaniasis—intermittent fever, swollen spleen, and enlarged liver, after signs of an insect bite. After several days, the trypanosomiasis organisms spread from the site of infection into other tissues, especially the heart and brain, where they cause tissue destruction, inflammation, and often death.

Treatment

There is no specific treatment for Chagas' disease, and, except for experimental drugs, most therapeutic measures are intended to treat the symptoms.

Like the African sleeping sickness forms of trypanosomiasis, the American type can involve reservoirs of wild and domestic animals; the disease has been found in cats and dogs as well as in opossums and armadillos. Persons traveling in endemic areas should use preventive measures that are appropriate, such as insect sprays and repellents. Efforts to eradicate large areas of insects carrying the trypanosomiasis organisms have been futile; in some instances it has been found to be more effective to move villages away from the insects than to try to remove the insects from the villages.

Filariasis

The species of mosquitoes that transmit malaria and yellow fever, diseases caused by protozoa and viruses, also transmit *filariasis,* caused by a parasitic worm—a nematode or roundworm. Filariasis affects 300 million people living in tropical and subtropical areas of the world. The worm invades the subcutaneous tissues and lymph system of the human body, blocking the flow of lymph and producing symptoms of inflammation, edema, abscesses, and, in one form of the disease, blindness. Filariasis is not unknown to Americans; some 15,000 soldiers contracted the disease during World War II fighting in the Pacific Theater, and cases have been reported along the Carolina coast area. But most of the victims of filariasis live in a region extending from Africa through Asia to the islands of New Guinea and Borneo.

Symptoms

Symptoms of filariasis can develop insidiously during an incubation period that may last from three months to a year after infection. There can be brief attacks of a low-grade fever, with chills and sweating, headache, nausea, and muscle pain. The patient also may feel sensitive to bright lights. Signs and symptoms more specifically related to filariasis are the appearance of red, swollen skin areas with tender spots that indicate the spread of the threadlike worms through the lymphatic system. Most likely sites for the first signs of filariasis are the lymph vessels of the legs, with later involvement of the

groin and abdomen, producing the swollen lower frontal effect known as *elephantiasis.* Diagnosis of the disease is confirmed by finding the tiny worms in the lymph; the infecting organism also may be found in blood tests, but only at certain times. The worms of one form of the disease are only 35 to 90 millimeters long in the adult stage, and those of a second type of the disease are only half that size. Larvae, or embryos, of the worms may be only 200 microns (one-fifth of a millimeter) in size.

Treatment

An oral medication, diethylcarbamazine, is available to kill the larvae in the system; the drug has only limited value in destroying the adult worms. The drug is taken orally for three weeks, but courses may have to be repeated over a period of two years because relapses can occur. Other therapeutic measures include bed rest during periods of fever and inflammation, antibiotics to control secondary infections, and, occasionally, surgery to remove damaged tissues that may interfere with normal working activities following recovery.

Onchocerciasis

The type of filariasis that causes blindness is transmitted by a species of blackfly that introduces or picks up the worm larvae while biting. As in mosquito-transmitted filariasis, the worms work their way through the skin to the lymphatic system but tend to migrate to eye structures. Blackfly filariasis, also called *onchocerciasis,* occurs most frequently in Africa and from southern Mexico to northern South America. More than one million cases of onchocerciasis have been found in the upper basin of the Volta River of Africa, with thousands of patients already blinded by the infection.

Loiasis

A third variation of filariasis is called *loiasis.* It is carried from man to monkey or from monkey to man by a biting fly. The larvae develop into adult worms that migrate under the skin and sometimes through the eye. Migration of a worm through the skin causes swelling, irritation, and redness. The disease is treated with drugs to kill the larvae, as well as by antihistamines and, occasionally, surgery to remove the adult worms.

Control of filariasis requires eradication of the flies and mosquitoes that transmit the parasitic worms and perhaps the wild animals that can serve as reservoirs. As in the examples of other tropical diseases, it frequently is easier to separate the humans from the areas infested by the insects than to eradicate the insects.

Schistosomiasis

A worm of a different sort—the trematode, a flatworm of the class *Trematoda,* which includes the flukes—is responsible for *schistosomiasis.* This disease occurs in various forms in Africa, Asia, South America, and the Caribbean, including Puerto Rico. About 200 million people are infected with schistosomiasis, also called *bilharziasis.*

Life Cycle of the Fluke Parasite

The process of infection by one kind of fluke involves free-swimming larvae that penetrate the skin of a human who has entered waters containing the organism. The larvae follow the human bloodstream to the liver, where they develop into adult worms. The adult worms then move into the blood vessels of the host and lay eggs. Some of the eggs find their way into the intestine or urinary bladder and are excreted with the urine or feces of the host. If they find their way to fresh water, the eggs hatch and the released organisms find their way to the body of a snail. Inside the snail they multiply into thousands of new larvae over a period of one or two months, after which they return to the water and invade the skin of another human. In this manner the fluke worm continues its life cycle, infecting more humans who venture into the contaminated waters.

Symptoms

Skin rashes and itching, loss of appetite, abdominal discomfort, and diarrhea are among early symptoms of schistosomiasis infections. There also may be fever and generalized aches and pains. During a period of from one to two or more months after the initial infection, more severe symptoms may occur as a result of a growing number of adult worms and eggs in the body, which produce allergic reactions. Those symptoms may include diarrhea, abdominal pain, coughing spells, and high fever and chills. Medical examination may reveal a tender and enlarged liver plus signs of bleeding in the intestinal tract. Complications may result from obstruction by masses of worms and eggs or by rupturing of the walls of body organs during migration of the organisms. Diagnosis usually can be confirmed by examination of the victim's stools or of the lining of the rectum for the presence of eggs of the fluke worms.

Treatment

Therapy may consist of administration of antimony-based drugs, tartar emetic, measures to relieve the symptoms, and, when deemed necessary, surgery. In some cases, a medication may be administered to flush the eggs of the fluke worm through a specific part of the circulatory system during a surgical procedure in which a filter is inserted in a vein to trap the eggs; thousands of fluke worms can be removed by this technique. Some of the medications used in treating schistosomiasis can have serious side effects and are used cautiously. However, the alternative may be prolonged emaciation of the victim, with a bloated abdomen and early death by cancer or other causes related to the infection. The female fluke worm has been known to continue depositing eggs during a life span of 30 years, causing frequent recurrence of acute symptoms.

Other Forms of Schistosomiasis

There are several other forms of schistosomiasis that cause variations in symptoms. One kind involves the liver and central nervous system, resulting in death of the victims within as little as two years after infection. Another form seems to involve the urinary bladder, causing frequent, painful, and blood-tinged urination with bacterial infection as a complication.

Swimmer's Itch

A mild form of schistosomiasis is known by the popular name *swimmer's itch*. It can occur anywhere from Asia to South America and as far north as Canada and western Europe, affecting bathers in both fresh water and sea water. As in the severe forms of schistosomiasis, snails are the intermediate hosts, and wild animals and birds provide a reservoir of the organism. The effects are treated as a skin allergy, and shallow local waters used for swimming are treated with chemicals to eradicate the snails. Careful drying and examination of the skin after swimming in possibly infected waters can control to some degree the invasion of the skin by fluke larvae. A chemical skin cream that tends to repel fluke larvae also is available as a protective measure.

Leprosy

More than 10 million people are victims of *leprosy,* an infectious disorder also known as *Hansen's disease.* Although leprosy is more common in tropical regions, where up to 10 percent of some population groups may be affected, the disease also occurs in several northern countries, including the United States, where the disease is found in coastal states from California through Texas and Louisiana, and from Florida to New York. Ancient medical writings indicate that leprosy was known in China and India about 3,000 years ago but did not spread to the eastern Mediterranean until A.D. 500 or 600. Thus, the disease described in the Bible as leprosy probably was not the same disease known today by that name.

Symptoms

The manifestations of leprosy resemble those of several other diseases, including syphilis, sarcoidosis, and vitiligo, a skin disease marked by patches where pigmentation has been lost. The lesions of leprosy, which may begin as pale or reddish areas of from one-half inch to three or four inches in diameter, appear on body surfaces where the temperature is cooler than other body areas. These cooler surfaces include the skin, nose and throat, eyes, and testicles. The early cosmetic symptoms are followed gradually by a loss of feeling in the affected areas because of involvement of the nerve endings in those tissues. At first the patient may notice a loss of ability to distinguish hot and cold sensations in the diseased area.

Then there may be a loss of tactile sensation. Finally, there is a loss of pain sensation in the affected tissues.

A case of leprosy may progress into one of two major forms, *tuberculoid leprosy* or *lepromatous leprosy,* or a combination of the two forms. The advanced symptoms can include more severe nerve damage and muscular atrophy with foot drop and contracted hands, plus damage to body areas from burns and injuries that are not felt but that can become infected. Damage to nose tissues can lead to breathing difficulties and speech problems. Crippling and blinding are not uncommon in untreated causes of leprosy, and death may occur as a result of secondary infections.

Treatment

A number of different sulfone drugs have been found effective against the mycobacterium that apparently causes leprosy, but the drugs also produce such side effects as fever and anemia. When intolerance to sulfones occurs, other medications are offered, including thiourea, mercaptan, and streptomycin. Steroid hormones are used to help control adverse reactions.

Causes

The disease organism, *Mycobacterium leprae,* or *Hansen's bacillus,* is believed to enter the skin or the respiratory system of the victim, probably during childhood. It rarely infects adults except under unusual circumstances, as through skin tattooing. Some medical scientists believe the infection may be transmitted through an insect bite, since the disease organism has been found in insects. However, the true process of leprosy infection remains unknown, and efforts to cultivate the mycobacterium in laboratory tissue cultures have been futile, although the disease can be induced in the footpads of experimental animals. Doctors have not found it necessary to isolate patients with the disease except during the period when treatments begin. Regular and thorough skin examinations of persons who have been in contact with leprosy patients and early detection and treatment of the disease by specialists are the recommended means of control.

20
Surgery

What You Should Know Before Undergoing Surgery

Almost everyone can expect to be wheeled into an operating room at some point in his lifetime. The range of surgical procedures performed every year is vast—correction of broken bones, organ transplants, facial uplifts, hernia repairs, hysterectomies, caesarian sections, vasectomies, appendectomies, and so on. It is obviously impossible for a work of this sort to describe more than a fraction of the thousands of surgical procedures and their variations that are widely performed. For a representative sampling of some specific surgical procedures, see "Common Surgical Procedures" later in this chapter.

The seriousness of surgical procedures within the same category can vary widely. For example, one case of inguinal hernia may be repaired quickly and simply in a young man physically able to leave the hospital on the same day he arrived. Another inguinal hernia case could be a real emergency if a portion of the small intestine were to become trapped in the hernia sac protruding into the abdominal wall, resulting in the death of

the bowel-tissue cells. Easy generalizations about the seriousness of a given procedure are simply not warranted.

Types of Surgery

Surgery is sometimes categorized according to whether it is vital to life, necessary for continued health, or desirable for medical or personal reasons. Although there are many ways in which surgical procedures are classified, the following breakdown is one that is widely accepted among surgeons.

Emergency Surgery

Most disorders requiring surgery do not improve by delaying the trip to the hospital. Some can be planned and scheduled so as to coincide with periods in which a few days in the hospital will be unlikely to interfere with job or family responsibilities. But, unfortunately, there are also unpredictable events that precipitate an immediate need for surgery. An

automobile accident, a fire, a violent crime, or even a sudden change in a chronic medical problem, like a perforated ulcer or a strangulated hernia, can create situations in which the life of the patient depends upon the time it takes to get the victim into the hands of a trained surgeon. Emergency surgery cases typically involve the treatment of gunshot and stab wounds, fractures of the skull and other major bones, severe eye injuries, or life-threatening situations, such as obstruction of the windpipe caused by choking on a piece of food.

Emergency surgery may be one of the most common routes for patients entering the operating room. Accident patients, according to one estimate, require four times as many hospital beds as cancer patients and more hospital beds than all heart patients. They account for more than a half-million deaths and disabilities in America each year. They present tremendous challenges to surgeons, because emergency room patients frequently have multiple injuries involving several organ systems.

Such victims are often unconscious or otherwise unable to communicate coherently about their injuries, and there may be little or no time to obtain medical histories or information about their blood types, allergies to medicines, etc.

When possible, vital information about the patient and the circumstances surrounding the injury or sudden need for surgery is obtained by medical personnel who question anybody who might provide one or more clues. Efforts to maintain life are begun even while blood samples are taken for laboratory analysis and X-ray photographs made of the chest, abdomen, and other body areas that may be involved. Many *heroic* measures—extreme measures taken when life is in immediate peril—may be used in critical cases; for example, resuscitation, induction of anesthesia, and surgery might proceed simultaneously as soon as a diagnosis is made. When several teams are working on the patient at the same time, a general surgeon may be called upon to coordinate the multiple operating room procedures.

Urgent Surgery

Next in priority for the surgeon are cases in which an operation is vital but can be postponed for a few days. A person injured in an automobile accident but conscious and suffering a minor bone fracture may be classed as an urgent rather than emergency surgery case, and the delay would give surgeons and other medical personnel time to study X rays carefully, evaluate blood tests and other diagnostic data, and otherwise plan corrective therapy while under less pressure. A penetrating ulcer of the stomach likely would be classed as urgent surgery, but the ulcer case would become emergency surgery if it were to rupture through the stomach wall. An

acute, inflamed gall bladder, kidney stones, or cancer of a vital organ would be examples of urgent surgery cases.

Elective Surgery

Elective surgery is usually subdivided into three categories: required, selective, and optional.

Required Surgery

Physical ailments that are serious enough to need corrective surgery but that can be scheduled a matter of weeks or months in advance generally are designated as required surgery cases. Conditions such as a chronically inflamed gall bladder, cataracts, bone deformities, or diseased tonsils and adenoids would be examples of conditions that require surgery. Also in this classification might be cases of uncomplicated inguinal hernia, hiatal hernia, and surgery of the reproductive organs which do not need immediate attention.

Selective Surgery

Selective surgery covers a broad range of conditions that are of no real threat to the health of the patient but nevertheless should be corrected by surgery in order to improve his comfort and well-being. Certain congenital defects such as cleft lip (harelip) and cleft palate would be included in this classification, as well as removal of certain cysts and nonmalignant fatty or fibrous tumors. Selective surgery also might include operations to correct crossed eyes in children so that normal binocular vision can develop properly.

Optional Surgery

Of the lowest priority are operations

that are primarily of cosmetic benefit, such as removal of warts and other nonmalignant growths on the skin, blemishes of the skin, and certain cases of varicose veins. Optional surgery also includes various kinds of plastic surgery undertaken for cosmetic effect. Among popular types of plastic surgery are operations to change the shape of female breasts; this would include the correction of unusually large or pendulous breasts as well as the enlargement of unusually small breasts. Other common plastic surgery procedures are *rhinoplasty*, or nose shaping; *otoplasty*, the correction of protruding ears; *blepharoplasty*, the removal of bags under the eyes; and *rhytidoplasty*, known popularly as a facelift. Rhytidoplasty is relatively simple, virtually painless, and effective; because the benefits usually are temporary, it is an operation that many patients volunteer to undergo more than once. For fuller information on these procedures, see "Plastic and Cosmetic Surgery" later in this chapter.

Since the end of World War II, there has been a proliferation of surgical specialties. The general surgeon of past eras who handled all kinds of operations is gradually being replaced by a battery of highly specialized experts who may work only on the nervous system, the eye, the ear, the bones and muscles, and so on. When warranted, a patient's case may be handled by several different surgical specialists. The result has been safer, more effective surgical treatment for the average patient.

Laser Surgery

Advancing technology has made laser surgery an accepted method of treating a growing number of physical disorders (see sections in this chapter titled "Cataract"; "Glaucoma"; "Retinal Detachment or Disease"; and

"Brain Tumor"). Surgeons have found that laser beams provide a noninvasive operating technique, or a less invasive one than the traditional method. The laser promotes coagulation of vessels, including blood vessels, while also keeping the operating area sterile. The laser can reach otherwise inaccessible body parts. Because of this flexibility, repair of many organs is possible without removing them.

An acronym for **L**ight **A**mplification by **S**timulated **E**mission of **R**adiation, the laser is a precisely controlled light beam that is narrowly focused and that can be aimed at a minute target. In each laser, the light is all one frequency, or wavelength, and contains only one color. The color determines how the beam will interact with particular kinds of tissue, and may be different for different kinds of surgery. Lasers may function continuously or in pulsed bursts. The type of laser determines the number of pulses per second and the duration of the pulses.

Three kinds of lasers have been found to be of special value as surgical tools:

The *argon laser,* functioning in the blue-green frequencies, utilizes a very high electric current passed through argon gas. Because it readily coagulates the blood in the operating area, the argon laser has been especially useful in the fields of ophthalmology, plastic surgery, and dermatology.

The *carbon dioxide laser,* with a wavelength in the far infrared spectrum, penetrates tissue to a depth of only one millimeter. Utilizing a gas mixture of CO_2, nitrogen, and helium, the carbon dioxide laser can cut tissue to a precisely controlled depth. It has thus been used widely as a surgical scalpel to treat some types of cancer, gynecological disorders, and brain tumors.

The *neodymium YAG laser* (YAG representing "yttrium-aluminum garnet") has a wavelength in the near infrared spectrum. Applications of the YAG laser include the treatment of bleeding in the esophagus and digestive tract, treatment of some cancers and glaucoma, burn therapy, and some types of neurosurgery.

Preoperative Procedures

Preparation of a patient for surgery involves a variety of procedures determined by the urgency of the operation, the anatomical area involved, the nature of the disease or injury requiring surgery, the general condition of the patient, and other factors. Emergency surgery of an accident victim in critical condition obviously requires a greatly accelerated pace of preparing the patient for the operating room; medical personnel may cut away the clothing of the victim in order to save precious minutes. An operation on the intestine, on the other hand, may require a full week of preparation, including the five or so days needed to sterilize the bowel with drugs and evaluate laboratory tests. However, most *preop* procedures, as they are commonly called, generally follow a similar pattern designed to insure a safe and sound operation. Even in a case of emergency surgery, certain information must be compiled to help guide the surgeon and other hospital staff personnel in making the right decisions affecting proper care of the patient during and after the operation.

Medical History

This pattern begins with a medical history of the patient. The medical history should reveal the general health of the patient and any factors that might increase the risk of surgery. Perhaps one of his parents or another close relative suffered from heart disease or diabetes; such facts might suggest a predisposition of the patient to problems associated with those disorders. The data should also show whether the patient has a tendency to bleed easily and whether he has been following a special diet, such as a sodium-restricted diet.

It is important that the patient reveal quite frankly to his own physician, the surgeon, and the anesthetist the names of any drugs or other medications used. It also is vital that the medical personnel have a complete record of any patient experiences, including allergic reactions to certain drugs, that might help predict drug sensitivities that could complicate the surgery. The simple fact that a patient suffers from asthma or hay fever might indicate that he may be more sensitive than other individuals to drugs that might be administered.

Allergic Reactions

Some patients are allergic to penicillin or other antibiotics. Others may be sensitive to aspirin or serums. Still others could be allergic to iodine, Merthiolate, or even adhesive tape. All of these factors if they are known and if they apply to the patient about to undergo surgery, should be brought to the attention of the medical staff.

Medications Currently Being Used

Among medications routinely used by the patient that should be brought to the attention of the surgeon and anesthetist are insulin for diabetes, digitalis drugs for heart diseases, and cortisone for arthritis. Depending upon various factors relating to the individual case, the patient may be directed to continue using the medication as usual, change the size of the dose before or after surgery, or discontinue the drug entirely for a while.

A patient who has been taking certain sedatives or drinking alcoholic beverages regularly for a prolonged period before surgery may have developed a tolerance for the anesthetic used, which means that he would require a larger than usual dose to get the desired effect. A patient who has been using epinephrine-type eye drops for glaucoma may be asked to increase the dosage before surgery as an adjustment to one of the drugs used in conjunction with a general anesthetic.

Diuretics, tranquilizers, and anticoagulant drugs are among other medications commonly used by patients that could affect the manner in which a surgical procedure is carried out. When possible, the patient should take a sample of the medication, a copy of the prescription, or the pharmacist's label from a container of the medication to the hospital so the medical staff can verify the type of drug used.

Psychological Evaluation

Of increasing importance in recent years has been a psychological evaluation of the patient. Individuals with a past history of mental disease or patients whose complaints may be based on psychoneurotic factors may react differently to surgery than persons who could be described as psychologically well balanced. The preoperative interviews also may seek to obtain information about the patient's use of drugs of abuse or alcohol; a patient who has developed a physical dependence upon alcohol could develop withdrawal symptoms after suddenly being separated from alcoholic beverages during his hospital stay.

Physical Examination

In addition to the medical history evaluation, the surgeon will need vital information about the physical condition of the patient. This requires a complete physical examination, including a chest X ray, an electrocardiogram of the heart activity, a neurological examination, and a check of the condition of the blood vessels in various areas of the body. Other body areas may be checked as warranted by complaints of the patient or by the type of surgery to be performed. An examination of the rectum and colon may be suggested, for example, if the medical history includes problems related to the digestive tract. Adult women patients usually receive a Pap test and possibly a pelvic examination. Samples of blood and urine are taken for laboratory analysis, including blood typing in the event a transfusion is needed. The laboratory tests for older patients frequently are more detailed and may include an examination of a stool sample.

Many hospitals and surgeons will accept information obtained from a preop examination conducted several days or more before admission to the hospital for surgery, especially for elective surgery. By completing the blood and urine tests, physical examination, X rays, electrocardiograms, and medical history interview in advance of the trip to the hospital, the patient can reduce the length of the hospital stay. In some instances, the patient may be able to report to the hospital the night before the surgery is scheduled or even a few hours ahead of actual surgery. However, additional blood and urine samples may be taken immediately after admission to recheck the body chemistry, and a brief physical examination may be made to make sure the patient does not have any open wounds or infections that might complicate the chances of recovery or introduce a dangerous strain of bacteria into the sterile environment of the operating room.

Preparation for Anesthesia

After the patient is settled in his assigned bed, he is visited by the anesthetist who will be working with the surgeon. The anesthetist usually has an advance copy of all the information obtained by the surgeon and other physicians who have examined the patient, along with laboratory reports of blood chemistry, etc. He may want to review the information with the patient and examine him briefly to learn more about his particular problem. If the patient uses a medication that might interfere with the intended effects of the anesthetic to be used, the anesthetist will make a decision regarding the best way to avoid a possible chemical conflict during surgery.

Other Preparations

In a typical case of elective surgery, the patient can expect to experience the actual preoperative preparations on the afternoon or evening before surgery is scheduled. If blood transfusions may be required, there will be a final check by the hospital staff to make sure enough units of the correct cross-matched type are available.

If the surgery involves the lower digestive tract, or is an abdominal operation that may result in a disturbance of normal bowel function, the patient can expect to be given an enema. However, enemas are not administered routinely to surgery patients who are being prepared for other kinds of operations. An exception to the rule would be patients who complain of constipation.

Legal Authorization

Before the preoperative preparations are completed, chances are good that a member of the hospital staff will make sure that the patient has signed a permit authorizing the operation. The permit is a legal form describing the operation to be performed, or a special diagnostic or therapeutic procedure other than surgery if that is the purpose of the hospitalization. The statement may be signed by a close relative or legal guardian if for some reason the patient is unable to take responsibility for this action. For example, a parent will be asked to sign a permit authorizing an operation on his or her child.

Exceptions may be made in cases of emergency surgery where the patient is unable to sign a permit and a relative or guardian cannot be located in time. But there are in-house procedures of consultation among staff members who accept the responsibility. Laws regarding permission to perform surgery may vary locally; and in some communities, for example, a married patient cannot authorize surgery that may affect his or her reproductive organs without consent of the spouse. Abortion, likewise, may be illegal in some areas without the husband's consent.

Preop Meals

A light but adequate evening meal is served if the surgery is scheduled for the following morning, but no solid food is permitted for 12 hours before surgery. No fluids are allowed during the eight hours before surgery. Children and patients with certain diseases, such as diabetes, may be given special orders regarding nutrients. An infant, for example, may be allowed sweetened orange juice up to four hours before surgery in order to prevent the child from developing restless anxiety because of hunger.

Preparation of the Skin Area

The area of the skin around the surgery site is carefully prepared beginning the evening before the operation. A member of the hospital staff may assist or direct the cleaning of the area with soap and warm water. The cleansing may be done in a shower or tub, or simply with a pan of water and soap brought to the patient's bedside. The cleaned skin area is usually scrubbed again in the operating room as further protection against possible infection.

Shaving

Whether or not the skin area is to be shaved depends upon the amount of hair present. If there is no hair, the tiny nicks or cuts made by a razor would constitute an unnecessary hazard of infection. Where hair is present, however, shaving is essential in order to make available a very clean skin surface. Also, it is important that no hair or hair fragments be close enough to the surgical incision to fall beneath the skin; the bit of hair beneath the skin could cause a serious infection after surgery. Thus, to clean an area for an inguinal hernia, the patient's abdomen may be shaved and scrubbed from a point above the navel down to the mid-thigh level.

Sedation

After all these preop steps have been completed, the patient usually is given a bedtime sedative or other medication and additional sedatives plus special medications in the morning, about 30 minutes to an hour before surgery is scheduled to begin.

The Surgical Team

Most surgical operations are performed not by the surgeon alone but by a surgical team. Depending upon the complexity of the surgical procedure involved, the surgeon may have one or more assistants working with him. The assistants may be interns or hospital residents who participate in the operation as a part of their advanced training in surgical techniques, or they may be other surgeons who are specialists in a particular field. An abdominal surgeon or orthopedic surgeon, for example, may be assisted by a neurosurgeon if the operation is likely to require a special knowledge of the nervous system as it affects another organ system.

The Anesthetist

The anesthetist, who is also likely to be a physician, specializes in maintaining the proper degree of anesthesia in the patient, while also helping to maintain the body's life systems. The job of the anesthetist is more complicated than one might suppose, because in addition to making the patient unaware of pain during the operation—sometimes by making him unconscious, sometimes without affecting consciousness—the muscles and nervous reflexes must be kept in proper state for the type of surgery to be performed. Each of the various functions—muscle relaxation, reflex paralysis, etc.—requires a different anesthetic drug. Their performance must be perfectly coordinated to prevent complications during the operation. In some cases, it may be necessary for the patient to remain awake during the procedure so that he can follow instructions of the surgeon in moving certain muscle groups. At the same time, the patient must have an anesthetic that eliminates pain. Obviously, the anesthetist must prepare a different combination of drugs for a child, an elderly person, a pregnant woman in labor, or a man with a heart disease.

Other Members of the Surgical Team

As noted earlier, there are occasions when several surgeons are working more or less simultaneously on an accident victim with injuries to multiple organ systems. In such cases of emergency surgery, a general surgeon may supervise and coordinate the work of the other surgeons. The nursing staff in the operating room also may be headed by a Chief Operating Room Nurse, whose responsibility is to supervise and coordinate the activities of the scrub nurses who assist the surgeon in the actual operation, and the supply and circulating nurses who aid the rest of the surgical team by making available as needed the various towels, drapes, sponges, sutures, instruments, and other equipment.

One or more of the nurses wear gowns and gloves that have been sterilized so they can work directly with the surgeon and hand him equipment or supplies that he requests. Such a nurse is called a *scrub nurse* because she scrubs her hands and arms for ten minutes before the operation—just as the surgeon does. Other nurses in the operating room, who do not wear sterilized gowns and gloves, are not permitted to handle equipment directly but may be permitted to pick up sterilized materials with an instrument that has been sterilized. One or more orderlies, who are responsbile for lifting the patient and keeping the operating room in tidy condition, complete a typical surgical team.

Operating Room Equipment

When the operating room is in use by the surgical team, an impressive array of equipment is mobilized. The center of activity, of course, is the operating table, a massive metal device equipped with numerous levers and gears to permit the surface of the table to be raised, lowered, tilted to various angles, or to raise or lower the head, feet, or other parts of the

patient's body. The table is equipped with straps to hold the patient firmly in place during the surgical procedure.

Above the operating table is a very large and powerful lamp with lenses designed to focus a bright, shadowless light on the area in which the surgical team is working. Additional lights also are available to provide illumination at various sides or angles not adequately lighted by the overhead lamp.

Near the head of the operating table is a cart containing tanks of gases used as general anesthetics, plus oxygen tanks and equipment for administering anesthetics and monitoring the life processes of the patient.

Also in the operating room are a variety of other wheeled carts, small tables, and stands containing myriad instruments, and suction machines to clear mucus from the patient's throat and blood and other fluids from the incision area. Several stands in the area hold basins that, during an operation, can be filled with sterile solutions for rinsing hands, cleaning instruments, or moistening towels and sponges used by the surgeon and his assistants. One tall metal stand near the operating table is designed to hold bottles of intravenous fluids or containers of blood for transfusions. Another special stand is used to collect sponges used in the operation. One cart contains jars or bottles of alcohol and other solutions, soap, and gauze pads, all of which are available for careful cleansing and sterilizing of the skin around the area of the incision just before the surgeon begins the actual operation.

A large clock on the wall of the operating room is intended for timing various functions and procedures involved in an operation, such as the number of minutes that have elapsed since sterilization of certain instruments was started. For many patients

the clock is the last thing they see in the operating room before they begin the deep sleep of anesthesia; patients who remain conscious under a local anesthetic like to keep one eye on the clock face so they can tell how much time the operation requires.

Anesthetics and How They Are Used

Anesthesia is a word derived from ancient Greek, meaning "without perception," or a loss of sensation. During a major or minor operation, as in having a tooth extracted by a dentist, it is helpful to both the patient and the physician if there is a lack of sensation during the procedure. But eliminating pain isn't the only consideration in the choice of anesthetic and other drugs used in conjunction with it. The age of the patient, chronic ailments, the site of the operation, and the emotional status of the patient are among factors considered. If a patient has undergone surgery previously and had an adverse effect from a particular kind of anesthesia, this information would have an important influence on the choice of an alternative type of anesthetic.

For many types of surgery, the kind of anesthetic chosen may be the result of an agreement among the surgeon, the patient, and the anesthetist. Some patients, given a choice, would prefer to remain conscious during an appendectomy or hernia repair; others would rather not. The surgeon frequently recommends the use of a general anesthetic because the procedure may require more time than the patient can be comfortable with in an operating room situation. Therefore, patients should realize that when a surgeon recommends a general anesthetic for an operation in which a local or spinal anesthetic might be adequate, it is for their own welfare.

General Anesthetics

General anesthetics are those that produce "sleep," or unconsciousness, along with *analgesia,* or absence of pain. They also cause a kind of amnesia in that the patient remembers nothing that occurs during the period in which the anesthetic is effective. At the same time, general anesthetics produce a certain loss of muscle tone and reflex action. A general anesthetic, however, should not interfere significantly with such normal bodily functions as respiration and circulation, nor should it produce permanent damage to body tissues.

How They Work

General anesthetics cause the patient to fall into a kind of sleep state by depressing the central nervous system, an effect that is reversible and lasts only until the drug has been eliminated by the body tissues. The general anesthetic reaches the central nervous system rather quickly because it is introduced directly or indirectly into the bloodstream. The use of a gas to produce anesthesia is an indirect method of producing unconsciousness.

A gas-type anesthetic, such as nitrous oxide or cyclopropane, can be delivered under compression from tanks or cylinders, or it may be stored in the operating room as a liquid that is converted to a vapor, like ether or halothane. The compressed-gas anesthetics are administered with the help of an anesthetic machine. The liquid forms of gases may be dripped through a mask over the patient's face; or the liquid may be vaporized and directed to the patient by anesthetic equipment. Whether the source of the anesthetic is compressed gas or a volatile liquid, the purpose is the same: to get the anesthetic into the patient's lungs.

There the gas enters the bloodstream through the walls of the blood vessels of the tiny sacs that make up the lungs.

Kinds of General Anesthetics

Nearly a dozen different kinds of gases are available as general anesthetics. Each has certain advantages and disadvantages and interacts differently with other drugs used by the patient. The effects of each on chronic diseases of the patient must be weighed. Some gases induce anesthesia more rapidly than others; some are tolerated better by patients. These are among the many factors that can determine which gas or mixture of gases might be selected by the anesthetist for a particular surgical procedure.

Intravenous Anesthetics

Not all general anesthetics come in the form of compressed gases or volatile liquids. Several commonly used general anesthetics are administered intravenously, by injection into the bloodstream. The group includes barbiturates, such as thiopental, and narcotics, such as morphine. Ketamine is a general anesthetic drug that can be injected into the muscles as well as into the bloodstream. The intravenous anesthetics may be used instead of the gaseous general anesthetics or in combination with them. Thiopental is often administered to a patient first, to bring on sleep quickly, after which an inhaled general anesthetic is applied. Like the gaseous general anesthetics, each of the injected general anesthetics has its own peculiarities and may have different effects on different individuals. The rate of recovery from thiopental anesthesia varies according to the ability of a patient's body tissue to eliminate the drug; nar-

cotics can affect the patient's respiration; ketamine may produce hallucinations in some patients.

Regional Anesthetics

Regional anesthetics include *local anesthetics* and *spinal anesthetics.* They are more likely to be used than general anesthetics when the patient is ambulatory and the surgery involves removal of moles or cysts, plastic surgery, certain eye, ear, nose, and throat procedures, and certain operations such as hernia repair that generally are uncomplicated. Regional anesthetics also may be recommended by the surgeon for operations to correct disorders in the arms or legs.

The surgical procedure may require that the patient remain conscious so he can follow instructions of the surgeon in manipulating muscles or bones to test the function of a body part being repaired. In such cases, a regional anesthetic would be preferred; a regional also would be advised for a patient with severe heart or lung disease that might be complicated by the effects of a general anesthetic. A restless child, on the other hand, might be given a general anesthetic for a relatively minor operation, because the youngster would not be likely to remain motionless for the duration of the operation.

Topical Anesthetics

Regional anesthetics generally are administered by infiltration of a drug into the tissues involved or into the nerve trunks leading into the area of incision. A simple kind of regional anesthesia is the topical application of a substance to a sensitive membrane of a body organ. For example, the eye drops applied by an ophthalmologist may anesthetize a patient's eyes to make it easier for him to examine them. Topical anesthetics are not very effective when applied to the skin, which forms a tough barrier against most invasive substances, but they can effectively anesthetize the inner surfaces of the mouth, nose, throat, and other inner body surfaces. The anesthetic might be administered by sprays, gargles, or by direct application. Topical anesthetics commonly are used to prepare the throat and upper lung passages for examination with medical instruments.

Local Anesthetics

Local anesthetics, which are similar to those used by the dentist, are usually injected via a hypodermic needle into the tissues surrounding the area to be operated on. The injection of an anesthetic into the tissue area sometimes is referred to as a *field block*. A variation of this technique is the *nerve* or *plexus block,* in which a hypodermic needle is used to inject the drug into the region of one or more key nerve trunks leading to the site of the incision. Local anesthetics are not recommended by most surgeons if there is an inflammation or infection of the tissues around the surgery site. The drugs used for local anesthetics can lower the patient's resistance to the infection while at the same time the inflammation may reduce the effectiveness of the drug as a pain-killer.

Intravenous Administration

Sometimes a regional anesthetic is administered intravenously by injecting it into a vein that runs through the site of the surgery. The drug is confined to the area, such as an arm or leg, by applying a tourniquet about the limb. Because of the possible dangers in suddenly releasing a potent anesthetic drug into the general bloodstream after the operation is ended, the tourniquet is intermit-

tently tightened and released to slow the flow to a mere trickle. A sudden release also would quickly end the pain-killing effect in the area of the incision.

Spinal Anesthetics

Spinal anesthesia is similar to a nerve or plexus block method of eliminating pain sensation in a region of the body, except that the nerves receive the drug at the point where they leave the spinal cord. The drugs may be the same as those used as local anesthetics. They are injected either by hypodermic needle or by catheter into tissues surrounding the spinal cord. Although there are several variations of spinal anesthesia—each involving the precise layer of tissue or space around the spinal cord which is the immediate target area of the injection—for all practical purposes the objective is the same. They are all intended to produce a lack of sensation in the spinal nerves along with a loss of motor function so there will be no movement of the body area to be operated on during surgery.

The spinal anesthetic may affect not only the targeted nerve system but neighboring spinal nerves as well, generally all the spinal nerves below the point of drug injection. For its purposes, spinal anesthesia can be a highly effective alternative to a general anesthetic. However, side effects are not uncommon. Severe headache is one of the most frequent complaints of patients. Temporary adverse effects can occur after use of other regional anesthetics as well and may be owing in part to individual allergic reactions to the drug used.

Care after Surgery

The last thing you may remember as a patient, before receiving a general anesthetic, is being wheeled into the

operating room and lifted by hospital orderlies onto the operating table. You may not see the surgeon, who could be scrubbing for the operation or reviewing the information compiled on your case. The anesthetist and a few nurses may be in the operating room. You are feeling relaxed and drowsy because of the preanesthetic medications. A tube may be attached to your arm to drip an intravenous solution into a vein. The anesthetist may administer a dose of a drug such as sodium pentothal, a not unpleasant medication that brings on a deep sleep within a matter of seconds.

The Recovery Room

You will probably remember nothing after that point until you gradually become aware of the strange sounds and sights of a recovery room. The recovery room may contain a number of patients who have undergone surgery at about the same time, especially in a large hospital. Each is reclining in bed equipped with high railings to prevent a groggy, confused patient just recovering from a general anesthetic from falling onto the floor.

Nurses move briskly about the room, checking the conditions of the various patients. As each patient gains some awareness of the situation, a nurse puts an oxygen mask over his face and explains the purpose: to help restore the tiny air sacs of the lungs to their normal condition. During administration of the anesthetic, the air sacs can become dry and partially collapsed. The humidified oxygen mixture helps restore moisture to the inner surfaces of the lungs; by breathing deeply of the oxygen, the patient expands the air sacs to their normal capacity. Before the use of oxygen masks in the recovery room and deep-breathing techniques for patients recovering from the effects of an anesthetic gas, there was a much greater danger of pneumonia developing as a postoperative complication.

Nurses assigned to the recovery room are given a report on each patient arriving from the operating room and instructions about such matters as the position of the patient in the bed. One patient may have to lie flat on his back, another on his side, a third in a sitting position, and still another with the head lower than the feet. If the patient has received a general anesthetic, the nurses may be instructed to turn him from one side to the other at regular intervals until he is able to turn himself.

The patient's blood pressure, pulse, and respiration are checked at regular intervals by the recovery room nurses, who also watch for any signs of bleeding or drainage from the area of incision. The surgeon is notified immediately of any signs of complications. Because the recovery room usually is located next to the operating room, the surgeon can quickly identify complications and attend the problem without delay. Most surgical patients will remain in the recovery room for a few hours at the most, and when they appear to be able to manage somewhat on their own they are returned to their beds in the regular nursing area of the hospital.

The Intensive Care Unit

Critically ill patients or those with heart, lung, kidney, or other serious disorders usually are assigned to an intensive care unit where each bed may be isolated from the others in a glass booth designed to provide privacy and quiet during the recovery period. Patients can still be clearly observed from the central nursing station.

Patients in an intensive care unit are given continuous care by nurses.

Electronic equipment is used to monitor pulse, blood pressure, heartbeat, and, when needed, brain function and body temperature. Other devices are available for making bedside measurements of bodily function and to obtain laboratory data such as blood chemistry without moving the patient from his bed.

Pain

Most surgical patients will be concerned about how much pain they will feel after leaving the operating room. It is not unusual to expect greater pain than is actually experienced; the incision may cause no more discomfort than the problem that required surgical therapy. Obviously, a minor operation will result in less painful discomfort than a major operation. Generally, the pain or discomfort associated with a surgical incision may last for one or two days, then subside over a period of perhaps three or four days. After that an occasional twinge may be felt in the area of the incision when shifting the body puts extra stress on the muscles or other tissues involved in the operation. During the hospital stay, medications will be available to help relieve any serious pain resulting from the operation.

Signs of Recovery or Complication

While the patient may be concerned about pain following surgery, the physicians and nurses are more likely to direct their attention toward other signs and symptoms that will help them to gauge the rate of recovery, such as the patient's body temperature, skin coloring, urine output, and his ability to cough. The health professionals are well aware that surgery, and drugs or anesthetics administered in conjunction with surgery, can be disruptive to normal bodily ac-

tivities. A major operation is more likely to cause changes in the patient's physiology than a minor operation.

Vital Signs

Nurses can be expected to make regular checks of temperature, pulse, and respiration because these common measures of the body functions (sometimes called *vital signs*) can provide early-warning signals of possible post operative complications. A patient may have a temperature of 100° F. even after a major operation, but because of increased metabolic activity of the body following surgery, a slightly elevated thermometer reading is considered normal. The pulse and respiration also may be slightly above the patient's rate before surgery, but the mild change again is caused by the normal stress reaction of the body. However, a temperature rising above 100° F. and/or a significantly faster pulse or respiration rate suggests that a complication may have developed.

If a nurse seems interested in the patient's ability to cough, it is because the cough reflex helps the patient get rid of mucus accumulation in his lungs, especially after the use of a general anesthetic. If coughing is difficult, a plastic tube may be inserted into the patient's throat to help clear the breathing passages. Normal breathing can also be restored by steam inhalation, aerosol sprays of water or special medications, or positive pressure breathing equipment that forces air into the lungs. Failure to expand the air passages of the lungs leads to serious respiratory complications.

Urine output is also checked. This is just one more way of watching the rate of recovery of a patient and alerting the staff to any signs of complications. If for some reason the patient is unable to pass urine, a *catheter,* or plastic tube, is inserted into the bladder to drain it. The volume of urine drained is collected and measured.

The Incision Area

Some blood may accumulate under the skin in the area of the incision or in nearby tissues, causing a discoloration of the skin. But this effect is seldom a serious matter, and the discoloration gradually vanishes. In some cases of excess blood accumulation, the surgeon may simply remove one or two sutures and drain away the blood. Any continued bleeding about the incision would, of course, be a complication.

A more common complication is infection of the incision area by bacteria that enter the wound. An infection may develop any time from one day to one week after an operation. However, most postoperative infections of incision wounds are easily controlled by antibiotics, drainage, or natural defenses against disease. The surgeon or other physicians will make regular inspections of the incision during the first few days after surgery to make sure it is healing properly.

Postoperative Nourishment

A light meal may be offered the patient a few hours after surgery. The patient may or may not feel like eating, especially if he still feels a bit nauseated from the effects of a general anesthetic. At this stage fluid intake is probably more important, especially if the patient has not been allowed to have even a sip of water since the previous evening. If the surgery was not performed on the stomach or intestinal tract, a small amount of water or tea may be permitted within a few hours after the operation. It is unlikely in any case that the patient will feel a great desire for fluid, because intravenous solutions

may have been dripping slowly into a vein since he entered the operating room. Intravenous solutions can satisfy hunger as well as thirst because they may contain proteins, carbohydrates, and essential vitamins and minerals dissolved in a finely formulated broth. Perhaps unnoticed by the patient, the amount of fluid intake will be routinely measured by members of the hospital staff.

Ambulation

Ambulation—getting the patient out of bed and moving about—is an important part of postoperative care. Experience has shown that recovery from surgery is more effective if the patient spends increasing amounts of time each day in simple physical activity. The degree of ambulation depends upon the magnitude of the surgery and the general physical health of the patient. But in a typical case of hernia surgery or an appendectomy, the patient may be asked, on the first or second day after the operation, to sit on the edge of his bed and dangle his legs for a while. On the second or third day, he may be allowed to walk about the room, and may in fact prefer to walk to the bathroom rather than use a bedpan or urinal. On the following day, he may walk up and down the halls with the help of a nurse or other hospital staff member.

Each patient is encouraged to handle the ambulation phase of recovery at his own pace, and there are few hard and fast rules. Of two persons entering the operating room on the same day for the same kind of elective surgery, one may feel like walking to the bathroom a few hours after surgery while the second may prefer to remain in bed and use a bedpan a week after surgery. The surgeon and attending physicians may encourage and in some cases even insist upon early ambulation, however, because it reduces the rate of complications.

Back at Home

Dressings used to cover the incision are changed regularly, as the incision is inspected once each day, more frequently if warranted. If the patient is anxious to be discharged from the hospital as early as possible, the surgeon may give him instructions for changing his own dressings. The surgeon will also outline a plan for recovery procedures to be followed after he leaves the hospital. The plan will include a schedule of visits to the surgeon's office for removal of stitches that may remain and a final inspection of the incision. The surgeon will also offer his advice on how the patient should plan a return to normal activities, including a return to his job and resumption of sports or recreational programs.

Special Diets

Proper foods are as important as proper medicines in helping a patient recover from surgery. Despite the common complaints about hospital meals, the nutrients that are provided in certain special diets for surgical patients are as carefully prescribed and prepared as are some medications that are served in pill or capsule form.

Surgical nutrition has become increasingly important in recent years because of an awareness by physicians that an operation, minor or major, is not unlike an organic disease that creates physiological stresses and a nutritional imbalance in the patient's body. To help compensate for alterations in the patient's physiology as it recovers from the effects of surgery, special diets may be ordered.

Bland Soft Diet

A bland soft diet frequently is ordered for patients who are unable to handle a regular diet but whose condition is not serious enough to require a liquid diet. The foods are selected because they are low in cellulose and connective tissue; they are bland, smooth, and easily digested. The choice of food, nevertheless, represents as great a variety as one might be served in a restaurant or at home, except for an absence of spices and other substances that would be stimulating to the gastrointestinal tract. Included in the surgical soft diet might be lean meat, fish, poultry, eggs, milk, mild cheese, cooked tender or pureed fruits and vegetables, refined cereals and breads with butter or margarine, plus gelatin desserts, puddings, custards, and ice cream.

Liquid Diet

Liquid diets for surgical patients may be prepared with or without milk. They are usually ordered for patients with impaired function of the gastrointestinal tract. A liquid diet without milk may include a cereal gruel made with water, clear bouillon or broth, gelatin, strained fruit juce, and coffee or tea. Liquid diets with milk are similar but may also include creamed soups, sherbets, ice cream, cereal gruel made with milk instead of water, cocoa and beverages of milk or cream. Beverage options permitted are tomato juice and some carbonated beverages such as ginger ale.

Diets Following Particular Kinds of Surgery

Peptic Ulcers

A special diet for peptic ulcer patients may include a half-and-half mixture of milk and cream, plus mashed potatoes, eggs, toast and butter, pureed vegetables, cottage cheese, rice, plain puddings and gelatin desserts. But meat soups, tea, coffee, raw vegetables, and fried foods are prohibited.

Rectal Surgery

Following rectal surgery, and other procedures in which it is necessary to prevent bowel movements for a period of several days, a low residue diet is ordered. A low residue diet (or *minimal residue diet,* as it is also called) might offer eggs, poached or boiled, rice, soda crackers, cereals made with water, butter, bouillon or clear broths, carbonated beverages, tea, coffee, and certain meats, including oysters, sweetbreads, and tender bits of beef or veal. An alternative low residue diet is the bland soft diet with all milk-containing items eliminated.

Gallbladder Surgery

Gallbladder surgical patients may expect a modified fat diet that eliminates as much as possible fats and gas-producing food items. It includes foods that provide protein and carbohydrate sources of energy to replace fats and includes primarily fish, poultry, lean cuts of beef, cottage cheese, cereal products and bread, and certain fruits and vegetables. However, foods prohibited are mainly pork products and fatty cuts of other meats, cream, chocolate, melons, apples, fried foods of any kind, onions, cabbage, turnips, cucumbers, radishes, green peppers, and dried beans and peas.

Restricted Salt Intake

Chronic heart failure patients and those with liver ailments or edema are placed on a low-sodium diet before and after surgery. The low-sodium diet is fairly simple in that it is prepared mainly with foods from which sodium or salt either is naturally absent or has been removed. Many salt-free or low-sodium foods are available commercially from manufacturers that also supply special dietetic foods for persons suffering from diabetes.

Fractures or Burns

Special consideration is given the diets of patients who are recovering from accidents that result in fractures or burns. Because of complex body responses to such injuries, there may be an abnormal loss of nitrogen from the tissues and a breakdown of muscle tissue, which is a rich source of nitrogen, an important component of protein. As a result, adequate amounts of protein need to be provided to surgical patients with burn injuries and broken bones.

Potassium Loss

Normal body stores of potassium also may be diminished during and immediately after surgery, but potassium can be replaced in the tissues by including in the meals adequate amounts of meats, fish, poultry, bananas, raisins, figs, dates, and prunes, as well as dried peaches and dried apricots. Prune, tomato, orange, and pineapple juices also are a rich source of potassium for postoperative patients.

Replacement of Water Losses

While water is not always thought of as a food, it is an important part of the gastronomic intake of the surgical patient; adequate amounts of water need to be provided the person recovering from an operation. The postoperative patient usually requires larger than normal amounts of water even though he may not feel inclined to help himself to as much fluid intake as he would at home or on the job. In addition to normal water losses through perspiration, urine, and breathing, there may be additional water losses through vomiting. Water replacement may be provided through sufficient amounts of fruit juices and other beverages offered during meals and between meals.

Apprehensions about Surgery

Most people feel anxious when faced with the need for surgery. This is to be expected. After all, a certain amount of anxiety normally accompanies any prolonged or incapacitating illness or infirmity. When surgery is the recommended therapy, it's natural for the patient to feel some anxiety about the surgery even if he's optimistic about a favorable result.

Factors That Reduce the Risk of Modern Surgery

Much of the risk of surgery these days is eliminated through the careful preoperative screening examinations reviewed earlier. A patient with a chronic disease who might have been a surgical risk a generation ago may have one or more options not available in past years, such as regional anesthetics that allow surgeons alternatives to general anesthetics that would be less than satisfactory. Antibiotics and other backup medications are available to control possible complications after surgery. Recovery room techniques and intensive care units with electronic monitoring of vital life systems provide added insurance of safe recovery. And, of course, surgeons today have the added experience of many millions of successful operations involving a range of procedures such as kidney and heart transplants, open heart surgery, and replacement of important organ parts with plastic substitutes. These and other procedures, including the implanting of electronic heart pacemakers, were beyond the dreams of surgeons of past years.

Surgery for the Older Patient

With the rapid increase in the proportion of older people in the population, the surgical patient is more likely to be an older person with problems associated with aging. An older man who underwent surgery to remove his prostate gland before World War II had a life expectancy of a few years after the operation. Today, such procedures in older men are considered routine cases with little or no effect on longevity. It is not unusual nowadays to find men and women in their 70s and 80s who have undergone five or six major operations since reaching the traditional retirement age and without any significant restrictions on their physical activities.

Part of the reason for the greatly improved outlook for surgery on older patients may be that older persons today are simply in better health because of the improved medical care available. Thus they are better surgical risks than their parents would have been at the same age. Advanced preoperative and postoperative care has also improved the outlook for the older patient. He may be admitted to the hospital a few days earlier than the younger patient for more intensive examinations, and he may remain a few days longer for postoperative care. Convalescence for the older patient may take longer, and in some instances the recovery may not be as complete as that of a younger person. But in general, modern surgical techniques are likely to offer a safe and effective therapy for people of advanced age with complaints that can be corrected by an operation.

In addition to the physical benefits, surgery may improve the mental capacity, personality, and sensitivity of older persons who had been depressed about a disorder before surgery. The patient who complained that he is no longer the person he used to be physically may have assumed that his medical problem was simply a result of growing old and overlooked the possibility that the complaint was due to a disease that might respond to treatment.

Surgery for the Child

A child, on the other hand, may have his own reasons to be apprehensive about the trip to a hospital for surgery. Most children seem to worry that the operation will hurt or that other procedures, such as taking a blood sample for testing, will be painful.

Telling the Truth

Many surgeons recommend that the child be told as realistically as possible, in terms he can understand, what can be expected. The youngster should not be given a sugar-coated story about the operation which might give the impression that he is embarking upon a happy adventure. At the same time, the child should not be frightened by suggestions that he may be given drugs to make him unconscious while he is strapped to a table so that strangely masked and gowned strangers can cut him open with sharp knives.

Children are more likely to appreciate surgery if they are told that a friendly person will help them go to sleep; that the operation will hurt a little but the pain will go away after a while; and that the operation will make them feel better or help correct a problem so they can be more active like other children. A small child should always understand that he may have to remain overnight at the hospital without his parents, but that he will have other adults to take care of him and there probably will be other children at the hospital to keep him company.

Common Surgical Procedures

In this section some of the more

common surgical procedures are described. The operations discussed are organized by the system or region of the body with which they are concerned. The following areas are covered in this order:

- Male Reproductive System (for surgical procedures involving the female reproductive system, see Ch. 25, *Women's Health*);

- Urinary Tract;

- Abdominal Region;

- Oral Cavity and Throat;

- Ear Surgery;

- Eye Surgery;

- Chest Region;

- Vascular Surgery;

- Orthopedic Surgery; and

- Neurosurgery.

Many of the conditions treated in this chapter from a surgical point of view are also treated elsewhere, in the chapter devoted to diseases of the appropriate body system or organ; the reader is invited to turn to those chapters for additional information. For example, although heart surgery is discussed in this chapter, heart disease is treated in greater detail in Ch. 10, *Heart Disease.*

Male Reproductive System

Surgical procedures of the prostate, testis, scrotum, and penis are considered in this section. Undescended testicles and vasectomy are also among the subjects discussed.

Prostate Surgery

The prostate gland is a small cone-shaped object that surrounds the male urethra, the tube that carries urine from the urinary bladder to the penis.

It is normally about one-half inch long and weighs less than an ounce. Ejaculatory ducts empty through the prostate into the urethra, and other ducts drain glandular secretions of the prostate into the urethra. Because of the intimate association of the prostate gland and the urinary tract, a disorder in one system can easily affect the other. A urinary infection can spread to the prostate and an abnormality of the prostate can interfere with the normal excretion of urine.

Enlargement of the Prostate

A relatively common problem is the tendency of the prostate to grow larger in middle-aged men. The gradual enlargement continues from the 40s on, but the symptoms usually go unnoticed until the man is in his 60s. At that point in life, the prostate may have become so enlarged that it presses on the urethra and obstructs the flow of urine from the neighboring bladder. The older man may experience various difficulties in emptying his bladder. He may have to urinate more frequently, and suddenly find himself getting out of bed at night to go to the bathroom. He may not be able to develop a urine stream of the size and force he had in earlier years. He may have trouble getting the stream of urine started and it may end in a dribble.

In addition to the somewhat embarrassing inconveniences caused by prostate enlargement, the urinary bladder may not drain properly and can eventually lose its own muscle tone needed for emptying. Residual urine in the bladder can become a source of infection, and backflow into the ureters can gradually affect those tissues and the kidneys. It has been estimated that 20 percent of all older men may need treatment of some kind, including surgery, for correcting this problem of the prostate gland.

Factors Indicating the Need for Surgery

Factors that may decide in favor of surgical removal of the prostate include residual urine in the patient's bladder; blood in the urine, with evidence that the blood comes from the prostate; the severity of the inconveniences associated with irregular urination; and complications such as the presence or threat of failure of the wall of the urinary bladder, the formation of stones, and symptoms and signs of infection.

Surgical Methods

There are several methods of performing a *prostatectomy* (excision of all or part of the prostate) for relief of the symptoms of an enlarged prostate, a condition that may appear on the patient's medical records as *benign prostate hyperplasia.* All of the methods are relatively safe and in none of the techniques is the entire prostate removed. One method, called *transurethral resection,* requires insertion of an instrument into the urethra through the penis. The instrument, a *resectoscope,* uses a high-frequency electric current to cut away the tissue inside the gland. This technique avoids open surgery and requires a postoperative hospital stay of only a few days.

Open Surgery

The other techniques involve *open surgery,* that is, surgery in which an incision is made in the pelvic or rectal area to make the prostate gland accessible so that its inner tissues can be removed. The differences in the various open surgery techniques depend upon such factors as where the incision should be made and the risks associated with the approaches. The incision is made either in the *perineum,* the region between the rectum

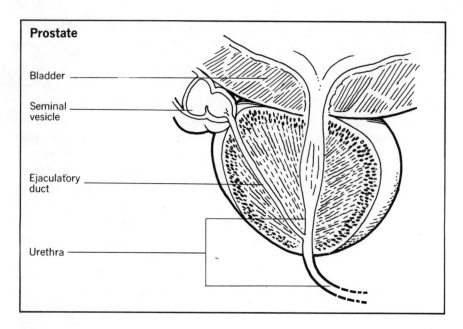

Prostate

Bladder

Seminal vesicle

Ejaculatory duct

Urethra

and the testicles, or through the abdomen. Only a small percentage of patients experience complications or regrowth of the prostate tissues to produce a second enlargement problem. Impotence is usually not an aftereffect of the surgery, and libido is normal.

Infections of the Prostate

Infections of the prostate gland can involve obstruction of the urethra, but the problem usually can be resolved by the use of medications and techniques other than surgery. An abscess, however, may require an incision to drain the prostate. Surgery also may be recommended for the treatment of stones, or calculi, that develop in the prostate and cause obstruction or contribute to infections.

Cancer of the Prostate

Cancer of the prostate also may occur in older men, causing obstruction or the urinary flow or contributing to infection of the urinary tract. If examination including biopsy studies confirms the presence of cancer, the surgeon may recommend radical prostatectomy. In this procedure an incision is made either through the lower abdomen or through the perineum to remove the entire prostate gland and surrounding tissues, such as the seminal vesicles. Hormonal therapy, chemotherapy, and radiation treatments also may be administered.

Tumors of the Testis

Tumors of the testis occur most frequently in men between the ages of 18 and 35. Such a tumor appears as a firm and enlarged testis and usually without pain unless bleeding is involved as a symptom. Testicular tumors generally are malignant and spread rapidly to other parts of the body, including the lungs. The onset of the disorder can be so insidious that the patient may seek medical advice for a more obvious secondary problem, such as the apparent development of mammary glands on his chest, the result of disruption of his normal male hormonal balance.

Special laboratory tests and other examination techniques usually are required to determine which of several possible kinds of testicular tumors may be involved and the extent of the metastasis of the cancer cells to other body areas. If cancer of a testicle is confirmed, it is removed by an incision through the groin area, and neighboring lymph nodes also will be taken out. The surgical procedure usually is supplemented with chemotherapy and radiation. The prognosis, or chances for recovery, following surgical removal of a testicular tumor depends upon the particular kind of cancer involved and how far the disease had progressed before medical treatment was begun.

Tumors of the Scrotum and Penis

Tumors of the scrotum and penis are relatively uncommon but do occur. Cancer of the scrotum is usually associated with exposure to cancer-causing chemicals. Boys who worked as chimney sweeps a century ago tended to develop cancer of the scrotum from body contact with soot in coal-burning fireplaces. Cancer of the penis occurs usually in men who have not been circumcised. In either type of cancer, the treatment usually requires removal of the affected tissues. This can mean castration in the case of scrotal cancer or amputation of a part or all of the penis, depending upon the extent of the cancerous growth. Surgery that requires removal of a part of the reproductive system can have a devastating psychological effect on a man, but the alternative is likely to be early death from the spread of cancer.

Undescended Testicles

About 10 percent of cases of tumors of the testis occur in men with an undescended testicle. Because the chances of a tumor developing in an undescended testicle are as much as 50 times greater than the incidence for the normal male population, the existence of an undescended testicle can warrant corrective surgery.

Ordinarily, the testicles descend

from their fetal location in the abdomen into the scrotum about two months before birth. But in one case in 200 male births, a child is found with a failure of one or, less commonly, both testicles to descend properly into the scrotum. In addition to the risk of cancer, undescended testicles are associated with lack of fertility and other problems, such as hernias.

Cryptorchidism

In male babies and young boys, an undescended testicle sometimes can be encouraged to enter the scrotum by manipulation or administration of hormones. Many surgeons recommend that the developmental problem of undescended testicles, or *cryptorchidism,* be corrected before a child enters school, although the surgical procedure for correcting the situation can be postponed until adolescence or adulthood. The operation for correcting an undescended testicle is called *orchidopexy* and involves an incision in the groin to release the testicle and its attached cord from fibrous tissue holding it in the abdomen. The testicle may be brought directly down into the scrotum, where it may be anchored temporarily with a suture, or it may be brought down in stages in a series of operations to permit the growth and extension of blood supply to the testis. The original location of the undescended testicle determines which procedure is used.

Vasectomy

Vasectomy is a birth control technique that is intended to make a man permanently sterile. It does not involve the removal of any of the male reproductive system and does not result in a loss of potency or libido. A vasectomy is a relatively simple operation that can be performed in a physician's office in less than 30 minutes and requires only a local anesthetic. The operation is similar to but much less complicated than the procedure in which a woman may be sterilized by cutting or tying her Fallopian tubes. A vasectomy requires no hospitalization, and the man is able to return to work or other normal activities after a day or two.

How the Procedure Is Done

The vasectomy procedure requires a small incision, about one-half inch in length, on either side of the scrotum. The surgeon removes through the incision a short length of the *vas deferens,* the tube that carries spermatozoa from the testicles, and ties a piece of surgical thread at two points about an inch apart. Then a small piece of the vas deferens between the tied-off points is snipped out of the tube. The procedure is done on each side. With the ducts of the vas deferens cut and tied, sperm from the testicles can no longer move through their normal paths to the prostate, where they would become mixed with semen from the prostate and seminal vesicles and be ejaculated during sexual intercourse.

Sterility Is Usually Permanent

A vasectomy does not immediately render a man sterile. Sperm already stored in the seminal "pipeline" can still be active for a period of a month to six weeks, and a woman who has intercourse with a vasectomized man during that period can become pregnant. On the other hand, a man who undergoes a vasectomy should not expect that the severed ducts can be connected again should he want to become a father in the future. Sperm banks have been offered as a possible alternative for the man who might want to store some of his spermatozoa for future use, but there is little

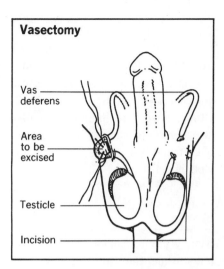

Vasectomy

Vas deferens

Area to be excised

Testicle

Incision

evidence that the sperm will remain fertile in a sperm bank for more than a year or 18 months. In rare cases, men who have undergone vasectomies have unintentionally become fertile again because of *canalization,* or creation of a new channel connecting the severed ends of the vas deferens; in one case the canalization occurred 8 years after the vasectomy was performed.

The vasectomy is regarded as an extremely safe operation, and complications are infrequent. Some swelling and discomfort are reported by a small percentage of men undergoing the operation. Steroid hormone drugs are sometimes administered to control these aftereffects.

Urinary Tract

Surgical procedures involving urinary stones and tumors of the bladder, ureter, urethra, and kidney are considered in this section. Also discussed are kidney cysts and conditions affecting the adrenal glands which might require surgery.

Urinary Stones

Most stones that occur in the urinary tract are formed in the kidneys, but kidney stones can travel to other areas, such as the ureters, and cause problems there. Various types of stones can develop in the kidneys from several different causes. A common cause is a metabolic disorder involving calcium, proteins, or uric acid. Other causes are infections or obstructions of the urinary tract, the use of certain drugs, such as diuretics, or vitamin deficiency.

Symptoms

Kidney stones seldom cause problems while they are forming, but movement of the stones irritates the urinary tract and can cause severe pain; the irritation of the tissues may cause bleeding that will ultimately show up in the urine. Other symptoms may indicate obstruction of the flow of urine, and infection. In some cases obstruction of a ureter can lead to failure of the kidney. X-ray techniques can usually verify the cause of the patient's symptoms and locate the urinary stone. Most stones cast a shadow on X-ray film, and by injecting special dyes into the urinary system, the degree of obstruction by a stone can be determined.

Ureter Stones

Most stones released by the kidney are small enough to pass through a ureter to the bladder and be excreted while urinating. But if a stone is large enough it can become lodged in a ureter, causing excruciating pain that may be felt both in the back and in the abdomen along the path of the ureter. Ureter stones often can be removed by manipulation, using catheter tubes that are inserted through the bladder. If the stuck stone cannot be manipulated from the ureter, an operation in a hospital is required. However, the surgical procedure is relatively simple and direct. An incision is made over the site of the stuck stone, and the ureter is exposed and opened just far

enough to permit removal of the stone. The operation is safe and requires perhaps a week in the hospital.

Kidney Stones

If the urinary stone is lodged in the kidney, the surgical procedure also is a relatively safe one although more complicated and requiring a longer hospital stay. The surgeon must work through skin and muscle layers to reach the kidney, then cut into the kidney if necessary to remove the stone. If the obstruction has been serious enough to impair normal kidney function or if infection has damaged the kidney tissue, the surgeon may elect to remove the affected kidney. Fortunately, the human body can get along fairly well with one good functioning kidney, so a *nephrectomy,* as the procedure is called, may not be as drastic a maneuver as the patient might imagine. If, on the other hand, the affected kidney has not been seriously damaged, the stone or stones can be removed with instruments or by the surgeon's fingers and the incision in the kidney sewed up so that it can resume its normal functions.

More modern techniques for removing kidney stones include two that hold promise of eliminating nearly all surgical methods. One involves the use of the lithotriptor, a machine that shatters the stones with an electrical shock wave. The wave is focused on the stones with the aid of a reflector and two sophisticated X-ray machines that "aim" the target beam. No surgery is required, and the patient is usually back at work within a week. A second means of attacking kidney stones is a drug, *potassium citrate,* which keeps the stones from forming. The drug actually corrects the metabolic disorders that cause the formation of kidney stones.

Vesical Stones

Occasionally, urinary stones are found in the neck of the bladder or in the bladder itself. They are called *vesical stones* and, depending upon their size and other factors, may be removed by several techniques, including use of a cystoscope inserted through the urethra. In some cases the stone can be broken into smaller pieces for removal. If it appears unlikely that the stone can be removed directly or by crushing it, the surgeon can make an incision directly to the bladder in a manner similar to the approach used in removing a stone from the ureter.

Bladder Tumors

About three-fourths of the tumors of the bladder occur in men past the age of 45. Although the specific cause of bladder tumors is unknown, physicians suspect that a cancer-producing chemical is involved. Several studies have found an association between the disease and cigarette smoking or occupations that require contact with organic chemicals used in making dyes. Tumors that appear in the female bladder are less likely to be cancerous than those that occur in the male bladder.

Symptoms and Diagnosis

The first symptom of bladder tumor is blood in the urine. The tumor itself may cause no pain, but an early complication could be an infection producing inflammation and discomfort in the region of the bladder. If the tumor blocks the normal flow of urine, the patient may feel pain or discomfort in the area of the kidneys; this condition is most likely to happen if the tumor is located at the opening of a ureter leading from a kidney to the bladder. An early examination of the bladder may fail to locate a small tumor, although X rays might show the growth as a bit of shadow on the film, and obstruction of a ureter could be seen. Nonetheless, examination of the interior of the bladder by a cystoscope is necessary to confirm the presence of the tumor. A biopsy can be made by removing a few tissue cells from the area in a manner quite like the procedure for making a Pap-smear test for possible cancer of the cervix in a female patient.

Treatment

Most early and simple cases of bladder tumor can be corrected by a procedure called *saucerization* by an instrument that removes the abnormal tissue, leaving a shallow wound that normally will grow over with healthy tissue cells. But a tumor that invades deeply into the wall of the bladder requires more radical therapy, such as surgery to cut away the part of the bladder that is affected by the growth. Radiation also may be employed to control the spread of tumor cells, particularly if laboratory tests indicate that the type of tumor cells involved are sensitive to radiation.

Surgical Procedure

If it is necessary to cut away a part of the bladder, the surgeon simply shapes a new but smaller organ from the remaining tissues. If a total *cystectomy* is required to save the life of the patient, the entire bladder is removed, along with the prostate if the patient is a man. When the bladder is removed, a new path for the flow of urine is devised by the surgeons, usually to divert the urine into the lower end of the intestinal tract.

Tumors of the Ureter or Urethra

Tumors of the ureter, above the blad-der, or of the urethra, below the bladder, may begin with symptoms resembling those of a bladder tumor, although X rays might show the growth as a bit of shadow on the normal flow of urine. Treatment also usually requires removal of the affected tissues with reconstructive surgery as needed to provide for a normal flow of urine from the kidneys.

Kidney Tumors

Wilms' Tumor

Tumors of the kidney generally occur either in children before the age of eight or in adults over the age of 25. The type of tumor that affects children usually is the Wilms' tumor, one of the most common kinds of cancer that can afflict a youngster. The tumor grows rapidly and may be painful even though there may be no obvious signs of urinary tract disorder in the child's urine. The tumor frequently becomes so large that it appears as an abdominal swelling. A Wilms' tumor usually occurs only on one side of the body, but in a small percentage of the cases the disorder can develop in both right and left kidneys. Kidney function may continue normally during growth of the tumor, but cancerous cells from the tumor may be carried by the bloodstream to other parts of the body, by metastasis, causing the problem to spread to the lungs and other vital organs.

Treatment usually requires surgical removal of the affected kidney and radiation therapy; the tumor cells responsible for the growth are sensitive to radiation. The younger the child and the earlier treatment is started, the better are the child's chances for recovery from a Wilms' tumor.

Adult Kidney Tumor

The adult type of kidney tumor, which is more likely to affect men than women, may also appear as an enlarged abdominal mass. But, unlike the Wilms' tumor, the adult kidney tumor presents as an early symptom blood in the urine. Bleeding from the kidney may be painless. X-ray studies may show an enlarged and sometimes distorted kidney. The patient may have symptoms indicating metastasis of the tumor cells to the lungs, bones, or other body systems. Adult kidney tumors are almost always malignant.

Treatment usually requires nephrectomy, or surgical removal of the diseased kidney. Radiation therapy may be provided in addition to the surgery, although the kind of tumor cells involved in the adult type of kidney tumor usually are resistant to radiation. Chemotherapy also may be offered. The chances for complete recovery from a kidney tumor depend upon several factors, such as the location of the tumor in the kidney and the extent of metastasis of the cancerous cells to other organ systems.

Kidney Cysts

A cyst is a small pouch enclosed by a membrane; technically, the urinary bladder and gall bladder are cysts. But the cysts of medical disorders are small pouches or sacs filled with a fluid or viscous substance; they may appear on the skin, in the lungs, or in other body systems, such as the kidneys.

Symptoms

Kidney cysts produce symptoms that resemble the symptoms of cancer of the kidney; in a few cases kidney cysts are associated with tumors that cause bleeding into the cysts. In addition to the troublesome symptoms of flank pain and blood in the urine, untreated cysts can grow until they damage normal kidney tissue and impair the function of the organ's functions. Simple or solitary kidney cysts usually do not occur before the age of 40.

Diagnosis

X-ray techniques are made to determine the exact nature of kidney cyst symptoms, but in some cases exploratory surgery is recommended to differentiate a cyst from a tumor. The cyst is excised, frequently by cutting away the exposed wall of the growth. The chances of the cyst reforming are very slight.

Polycystic Kidney Disease

A different kind of kidney cyst disease, consisting of many small cysts, may be found in younger persons, including small children. The symptoms again may be flank pain and blood in the urine; examination may show some enlargement of the kidney. This form of the disease, sometimes called *polycystic kidney disease,* can be complicated by uremia and hypertension as the patient grows older. Treatment usually is medical unless the cysts interfere with urine flow by obstructing the upper end of the ureter. If the outlook for recovery through conservative treatment is poor, the surgeon may consider a kidney transplant operation.

Adrenal Glands

The adrenal glands are small hormone-producing organs that are located just above the kidneys. Although the combined weight of the two glands may be only one-fourth of an ounce, the adrenals affect a number of important body functions, including carbohydrate and protein metabolism and fluid balance. Surgery of the adrenal glands may be needed for

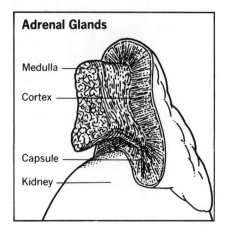

Adrenal Glands

Medulla

Cortex

Capsule

Kidney

the correction of various bodily disorders associated with oversecretion of the adrenal hormones; it may also be indicated to help control of cancer of the breast in women and cancer of the prostate in men.

Tumors of the Adrenal Glands

Tumors of the adrenal glands produce a disorder known as *primary hyperaldosteronism,* which is marked by symptoms of muscle weakness, hypertension, abnormally large outputs of urine, and excessive thirst. Another kind of tumor invasion of the adrenal glands can produce symptoms of hypertension with headaches, visual blurring, and severe sweating. Still another adrenal-related disorder, called *Cushing's syndrome,* tends to affect women under the age of 40. The symptoms may range from hypertension and obesity to acne, easy bruising, and *amenorrhea* (cessation of menstruation). Adrenal tumors may also alter secondary sex characteristics of men and women; they may result in body hair and baldness in women and increased sex drive in men.

Despite the tiny size of the adrenal glands, they are complex organs, and the varied disorders caused by tumors of the glands may depend upon the precise kind of tumor cells involved and the precise area of the glands affected by the tumor, as well

as the interactions of the adrenal hormones with hormones from other glands, such as the pituitary, or master gland of the body, located at the base of the brain.

Preoperative Tests

Before adrenal surgery for correction of a disorder is begun, the surgeon may ask for detailed laboratory tests and other diagnostic information. A radioactive scan to help locate and identify the kind of tumor more precisely may be ordered. Women patients who have been using oral contraceptives usually have to discontinue use of "the pill" for two months or more, because the medication can interfere with laboratory studies of hormones in the bloodstream.

Long-Range Effects

Physicians handling the case also must evaluate the long-range effects of an adrenal gland operation because normal metabolism is likely to be disrupted by removal of the glands, if that should be necessary. Hormone medications usually are needed in such cases to replace the hormones normally secreted. An *adrenalectomy* (removal of an adrenal gland) sometimes is explained as the substitution of a controllable disease for a life-threatening disease that cannot be controlled by medical therapy. If only one of the adrenal glands must be removed, however, the patient may be able to recover and resume a normal life without the need for hormone medications.

Surgical Procedure

The surgical approach to the adrenal glands is similar to that used in kidney operations. The incision may be made through the abdomen or through the flank. The surgery may be primarily exploratory, or the surgeon may excise a part of a gland, an entire gland, or both glands, depending upon the extent of the disease, or upon other factors, such as the need to control cancers in other parts of the body.

Abdominal Region

This section discusses the following procedures or conditions: appendicitis, peptic ulcers, hiatus hernia, adhesions, cancer of the stomach and of the intestines, gallbladder surgery, inguinal hernia, and hemorrhoids.

Appendicitis

Inflammation of the appendix is one of the most common causes of abdominal surgery today, particularly among children. But appendicitis was not recognized as a disease until 1886, leading some doctors to believe that this digestive tract infection may be related to a change in eating habits that occurred within the past century. The vermiform appendix, the site of the inflammation, is a short, wormlike (or *vermiform*) appendage at the junction of the small and large intestines. Its function in humans is unknown; plant-eating animals have an appendix, but carnivorous animals, like cats, do not. Humans live quite well without an appendix, so it seems reasonable to have a diseased appendix removed.

Symptoms

The appendix can cause trouble if it becomes obstructed by a foreign body, a tumor, an infection, or other cause of inflammation. Pain is a common symptom; there may be two kinds of pain at the same time: one, localized on the lower right side of the abdomen, near the site of the appendix; the other, more generalized and colicky, of the kind sometimes associated with gas in the intestine. Some patients experience diarrhea or a constant urge to defecate, an effect attributed to irritation of the bowel by the abnormal activity of the appendix. Frequently there is loss of appetite, nausea and vomiting, and a fever.

The symptoms of appendicitis may begin suddenly, but frequently take from 6 to 18 hours to develop into a pattern typical of the disease, so most cases permit ample time for a doctor to examine the patient and make a diagnosis before the problem becomes critical. During the period that any symptoms suggest a possibility of appendicitis, the patient should avoid the use of any laxatives.

Ruptured Appendix

A potentially serious complication of untreated appendicitis is rupture of the appendix, which can produce a slightly different set of symptoms because of the onset of *peritonitis,* a dangerous inflammation of tissues outside the intestinal tract. The contents of the ruptured appendix leak into the body cavity, spreading the bacterial infection and irritating the lining (peritoneum) of the abdominal cavity. Diarrhea and a fever of more than 101° F. are frequently associated with a perforated or ruptured appendix. The colicky pain may disappear suddenly, because the internal pressure ends with perforation of the wall of the appendix, but it is quickly replaced by the pain of peritonitis. The severe pain of peritonitis usually is made worse by any body movement, including the abdominal muscle movement required for coughing or sneezing.

Appendicitis with perforation is much more common in older persons, perhaps because the early symptoms of colicky pain that younger people notice are not felt by older people, so the disease is not detected until it has reached an advanced stage. Appendicitis also requires special attention in pregnant women, because the enlarged uterus crowds and repositions segments of the intestinal tract and the potential threat grows more serious during the last trimester of pregnancy.

Surgical Procedure

Laboratory tests usually are checked before surgery proceeds if there is no evidence of perforation. The usual symptoms of appendicitis can be produced by a number of other ailments, and the symptoms may diminish with bed rest, time, and medications. However, appendicitis must be considered in any case of acute abdominal complaints, and many surgeons and physicians follow the rule of "When in doubt, operate." Surgery for appendicitis is fairly simple and safe if the appendix has not perforated. An incision is made in the lower right side of the abdomen, the connection between the end of the large intestine and appendix tied off with surgical thread, and the appendix cut away from the stump. The actual operation, if uncomplicated by peritonitis or other factors, may require only a few minutes. A hospital stay of a few days is usually required during which the diet is readjusted from nothing by mouth at first, to a liquid diet, then a soft diet, etc. Normal work activities usually can be resumed within two or three weeks following surgery. Complications other than those related to peritonitis are rare. In untreated cases involving peritonitis, however, the risk is very high.

Peptic Ulcers

The cause of peptic ulcers is still unknown, although the disease affects about 10 percent of the population at some time in life. Men are four times as likely as women to develop ulcers; the incidence is highest in young and middle-aged men. Peptic ulcers may occur in the stomach, where they are called *gastric ulcers,* or in the duodenum, where they are called *duodenal ulcers.* Ninety percent of the ulcer cases that reach the physician's office for treatment are in the duodenum, a short length of the small intestine just beyond the stomach. Autopsy studies indicate that gastric ulcers may be as common as duodenal ulcers, but are frequently not detected during the life of the individual.

Causes

The development of ulcers is associated with the possible action of gastric acid on the lining of the stomach and duodenum in people who may have inherited a sensitivity to the substances. Ulcers are also related to the use of certain drugs and exposure to severe burns, injury, emotional stress, and disease.

Symptoms

A common symptom is a gnawing pain in the area of the stomach from 30 minutes to several hours after eating; the pain is relieved by food or antacid medications. The pain sometimes is likened to heartburn and may be described as radiating from the abdomen to the back. Some patients report the discomfort is more like a feeling of hunger or cramps; they may be awakened from sleep by the feeling that is relieved by a midnight snack of milk or other foods. Attacks of ulcers may be seasonal, occurring in certain patients only in the spring and autumn. In severe cases there may be bleeding without any sensation of abdominal pain; bleeding occurs from erosion of the lining of the stomach or duo-

denum and penetration of blood vessels in those membranes.

Complications other than bleeding can include perforation of the wall of the stomach or duodenum by continued erosion, or inflammatory swelling and scarring by an ulcer at a narrow part of the digestive tract, causing an obstruction. A duodenal ulcer can erode into the head of the pancreas, which secretes its digestive juices into the small intestine in that area. The pain may then become more or less continuous regardless of efforts to palliate it with food or antacids.

Symptoms vary only slightly between duodenal and gastric ulcers. Gastric ulcer pain usually begins earlier after a meal, attacks generally last longer, and symptoms, including vomiting and loss of appetite, may be more severe than in duodenal ulcer. But because of the similarities, physicians usually rely on laboratory tests and X-ray studies to determine the precise location in the digestive tract of the peptic ulcer.

Duodenal Ulcers

Duodenal ulcers nearly always occur within an inch of the pyloric valve separating the stomach from the small intestine. The pain or discomfort follows a cycle. The patient may experience no pain until after breakfast. The pain is relieved by the noon meal but returns in the afternoon and occurs again in the evening. Milk or other bland food or medications relieve the pain that may appear at various times in the cycle. The symptoms of duodenal ulcers also go through periods of remission and recurrence over months or years. Most duodenal ulcers are treated with diet, drugs, and measures that encourage rest and relaxation.

Surgical Procedures

Surgery for either duodenal or gastric

ulcer is designed to reduce gastric acid secretion rather than simply to excise the ulcer from the normal digestive tract tissue. One surgical approach, called *subtotal gastrectomy,* involves cutting away a portion of the stomach in the area where it joins the duodenum. There are several variations of this technique, including one in which the remaining portion of the stomach is attached to the jejunum, a segment of the small intestine. The ulcerated portion of the duodenum may be removed during the reconstructive surgery of the digestive tract, or it may be left in the duodenal segment that is closed during the gastrectomy procedure. An interesting effect is that a duodenal ulcer usually heals, when left in place, after the gastric juices are routed into the intestine through the jejunum. The reconstructed stomach and stomach-to-intestine connection cause no serious problems in eating after the patient has recovered.

A second surgical approach, called a *vagotomy,* involves cutting a part of the vagus nerve trunk that controls the secretion of stomach acid. There are several variations of vagotomy, each technique affecting a different portion of the vagus nerve distribution to the stomach.

Gastric Ulcers

Stomach or gastric ulcers tend to develop in older persons more often than duodenal ulcers, and the problem seems to be less importantly related to the overproduction of gastric acid. The real hazard of stomach ulcers is that a significant percentage are found to be a kind of cancer and do not respond to the usual therapies for controlling peptic ulcer symptoms. If it is determined that a stomach ulcer is a malignant growth, a partial gastrectomy is performed in the same manner as an operation of the type for duodenal ulcers. The vagotomy approach is not used for treatment of a stomach ulcer unless the ulcer is excised at the same time.

Hiatus Hernia

The term *hiatus hernia* actually describes a diaphragmatic hernia or weakness in the diaphragm, the horizontal muscular wall separating the organs of the chest from the organs of the abdomen. A *hernia* is an abnormal protrusion of an organ or tissue through an opening. A *hiatus,* or opening, occurs naturally to permit the esophagus to carry food from the mouth to the stomach. Blood vessels and nerves also pass through the diaphragm. The diaphragm is an important group of muscles for contracting and expanding the lungs, forcing air in and out of the lung tissues.

Hiatus hernias are rare in children, but as people grow older, there may be a weakening of the diaphragm muscles and associated tissues. Aided by a tendency toward obesity and the use of girdles and other tight garments, a portion of the stomach may be pushed through the opening designed by nature for use of the esophagus. Aside from the discomfort of having a part of the stomach in the chest, there are potential dangers of incarceration of the stomach, with obstruction, strangulation, and hemorrhage with erosion of the stomach lining. In severe complications, the entire stomach along with intestines and other abdominal organs may be forced through the hiatus hernia into the chest area.

The most common kind of hiatus hernia is sometimes called *sliding hiatus hernia* from the tendency of the stomach to slide in and out of the thorax, or chest cavity, when the patient changes body positions or as a result of the pressure of a big meal in the gastrointestinal tract. Sometimes

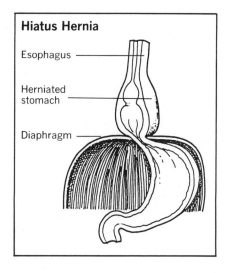

Hiatus Hernia

Esophagus

Herniated stomach

Diaphragm

the herniated stomach does not move at all but remains fixed, with a significant portion of the stomach above the diaphragm. Hiatus hernia causes heartburn symptoms, including regurgitation of digested food and gastric acid from the stomach, when one is lying down or straining or stooping. The effect also may be noticeable in a woman during pregnancy.

Nonsurgical Treatment

Many cases of hiatal hernia can be treated without surgery through a change of eating habits and the use of antacid medications. The patient may be advised to eat small amounts more frequently during the day with dietary emphasis on high-protein, low-fat foods. Some physicians recommend that patients use liquid antacid medications rather than antacid tablets or lozenges.

Surgical Treatment

When surgery is recommended to correct hiatus hernia, the repair may be performed either through the abdominal wall or through the chest. About three-fourths of the procedures are handled through abdominal incisions, because surgeons often find other abdominal problems that need to be corrected at the same time,

such as peptic ulcers or gall bladder disease. The opening through the diaphragm is firmly closed with sutures to prevent upward movement of the stomach. The stomach and lower end of the esophagus may be anchored in place in the abdomen. The chances of recurrence are about one in ten, although some patients may continue to have a few of the symptoms of the disorder for a while after the hernia repair.

Adhesions

Adhesions may develop between various abdominal organs and the peritoneum, the membrane lining the abdominal cavity. The bowel may acquire adhesions that result in obstruction of the intestinal tract. Adhesions may form between the liver and the peritoneum or between the liver and the diaphragm. The symptoms may be pain or cramps in the area where tissues are literally stuck together; in more serious cases that involve bowel obstruction, symptoms may include constipation, vomiting, and distension of the abdomen. Adhesions do not show on X-ray film and can be difficult to diagnose unless the patient's medical history suggests a cause for the bands or filaments of tissues responsible for the adhesions.

Causes

The causes may be peritonitis, injury, infection, internal bleeding, or foreign objects. Adhesions occur after an operation, perhaps because of a bit of blood resulting from surgery or as a result of a speck of talc from the surgeon's glove or a fiber from a surgical drape which produces a foreign-body reaction, much like an allergic reaction, when it comes in contact with abdominal tissues. Disease organisms may enter the female abdominal cavity through the Fallopian tubes to produce adhesions, especially in the case of gonorrhea, which can escape early detection in women because of the lack of obvious symptoms.

Complications

Adhesions can cause complications, such as changing the position of the intestinal tract through twisting or otherwise distorting its path so that bowel movements are obstructed. If the involved portion of the intestine becomes so seriously damaged that it no longer functions properly, the surgeon may have to remove that section. Generally, when the surgeon is correcting the problem of adhesions, a relatively simple procedure of cutting away the tissue bands or filaments holding organs in abnormal ways, he inspects the organs to determine if they appear to be in good working order. That part of the operation may add 15 or 20 minutes to the time spent on an operating table, but it helps insure that the patient will not have to be returned soon for further surgery.

Cancer of the Stomach

There are several possible types of stomach tumors, but one kind, called *adenocarcinoma,* is one of the greatest killers of men over the age of 45. Although the incidence of stomach cancer in the United States has declined considerably since the end of World War II, the death rate from this problem in the United States alone is about 15,000 per year. In central and eastern Europe the incidence of stomach cancer is about four times, and in Japan seven times, that of the United States. Almost two-thirds of the stomach cancers develop near the pylorus, the opening from the stomach into the small intestine; only five percent involve the entire stomach area.

Symptoms

Symptoms include a feeling of heaviness rather than pain following a meal. The patient in many cases mysteriously loses his appetite for meat and begins to lose weight. There may be vague symptoms of an upset stomach, with some vomiting, especially if the tumor begins to obstruct the pylorus such that stomach contents cannot be emptied into the intestine. The vomitus usually is the color of coffee grounds, suggesting a loss of blood from the stomach lining because of the tumor, and the patient's stools also may be dark in coloration because of internal bleeding. The physician frequently can confirm his suspicions about the cause of the symptoms by laboratory analysis of a specimen of cells from the stomach, by X-ray studies of the stomach, or by an examination with a gastroscope that permits a direct view of the interior of the stomach. In some cases the physician will be able to feel an abnormal mass in the stomach by palpating the stomach area of the abdomen with his hands.

Treatment

Treatment is by cutting away the tumor and surrounding tissues that may be involved, including parts of neighboring organs. The lymph nodes in the region of the stomach are also removed. The remaining part of the stomach is used to build a new digestive organ, as in a case of partial gastrectomy for correcting a peptic ulcer problem. However, before beginning reconstructive surgery, the physician usually orders biopsy tests of the remaining tissues to make sure the new stomach will not be made of tissues in which tumor cells have spread. If the edges of the remaining stomach wall are found to contain tumor cells, the surgeon simply extends the area

to be removed. As in subtotal gastrectomy for peptic ulcers, the remaining portion of the stomach may be connected directly to the upper portion of the small intestine, at the duodenum or the jejunum.

Meals are provided in the form of intravenous feedings for the first few days following surgery. Sips of water may be permitted on the second or third day after the operation with the amounts gradually increased to one or two ounces of water per hour as the new digestive system adjusts to fluid intake. Then soft or bland foods can gradually be taken orally in a half-dozen small feedings each day. It may take three or four months for the new stomach to distend and adjust to normal eating habits of the patient.

Postoperative Effects

Some patients may experience a variety of symptoms ranging from nausea to cramps and diarrhea while recovering from stomach surgery. The symptoms form what is known as the *dumping syndrome,* which occurs within a half hour after a meal, presumably by rapid distension of the upper portion of the small intestine as fluid rushes, or is dumped, into that part of the digestive tract from the new stomach. The effects can be controlled by a change of diet to eliminate starches and sugars, by delaying the intake of fluids until after the meal, by medications, and by training the patient to lie in a recumbent or semi-recumbent position to lessen discomfort following a meal. The symptoms occur in only a small proportion of stomach surgery patients, and they usually diminish gradually during the period of recovery.

Cancer of the Intestines

Small Intestine

Tumors of the small intestine are not

common, but they also are not rare. It has been estimated that less than five percent of all tumors of the gastrointestinal tract occur in the small intestine. Of tumors that do develop in this portion of the gastrointestinal tract, about 90 percent are benign, or noncancerous, growths. The symptoms of small intestine tumors may include bleeding, obstruction, and perforation of the intestinal wall. However, most tumors of the small intestine produce no symptoms at all. When tumors are found in the small intestine they usually are found at the same time in other parts of the body, and usually in a patient over 40 years of age, although the more malignant growths can occur in younger persons. Treatment of a cancer of the small bowel is by removing the affected section and administration of radiation therapy for certain kinds of cancerous tumors.

Large Intestine

Tumors of the large intestine, unlike those of the small bowel, account for a large proportion of cancers of the human body and for most of the malignant growths of the entire gastrointestinal tract. More than 40,000 deaths each year in the United States are a result of cancers of the colon and rectum portions of the large bowel. And about three-fourths of all large-intestine tumors develop near the rectal portion of the bowel, where, ironically, they should be easily available for detection during physical examination.

Tumors of the large intestine can be found in persons of any age, but they occur most frequently in patients who are of middle age or older, reaching a peak of incidence around the age of 65. Men are more likely to develop cancer of the rectum, but women are more frequently affected by cancer of the colon. While cancer of the large intestine tends to occur among members of the same families at a rate that is two or three times the normal incidence, it is believed that family environment factors, such as life style and diet, are the causative influences, rather than hereditary factors. People who develop cancer of the large intestine usually eat foods that are low in cellulose and high in animal fats and refined carbohydrates.

Bowel cancers appear to grow in size at a very slow rate, doubling about once every 20 months, so a number of years may elapse between the start of a bowel tumor and the appearance of signs or symptoms of cancer.

Symptoms

The location of the growth can influence the types of symptoms experienced. Cancer in the right colon may be found as an abnormal mass during a physical examination by a physician after complaints of fatigue and weakness and signs of anemia. The tumor can develop to a rather large size without producing signs of blood in the stools. Cancer in the left colon, by contrast, may be found after complaints of alternate periods of constipation and frequent urge to defecate, pain in the abdomen, and stools marked by dark and bright red blood. When the cancer is in the rectum, the patient may find blood mixed with the bowel movements but experience no pain in the early stages. Other symptoms of cancer of the large intestine may mimic those of appendicitis, hemorrhoids, peptic ulcer, or gall bladder disease.

As noted above, most cancers of the large bowel are close enough to the end of the intestinal tract to be observed directly by palpation or the use of fiberoptic instruments, such as a sigmoidoscope or colonoscope, which can be inserted into the rectum or colon. Biopsy samples can be removed for study and X-ray pictures taken after administration of a barium enema, which coats the bowel membrane in such a way that abnormal surfaces are clearly visible.

Surgical Procedures

Surgical procedures for treatment of cancer of the large intestine vary somewhat according to the location of the growth, but the objective is the same: to remove the affected portion and reconstruct the bowel so that normal digestive functions can resume. Radiation therapy and chemotherapy may be used in the treatment of certain advanced cases. When surgical treatment is begun soon after the first symptoms are diagnosed, the chances of curing cancer of the large bowel are very good.

If there are complications, such as obstruction of the portion of the large intestine, the surgery may be conducted in a series of stages over a period of several weeks. The several stages involve a colostomy procedure in which an opening is made in the wall of the abdomen to permit a portion of the intestinal tract to be brought to the surface of the body. After the complicating problem is treated and resection of the cancerous segment is completed, the colostomy is closed by sewing the open end of the bowel to the remaining portion and closing the opening in the abdomen.

Preoperative Steps

Some special preoperative measures are ordered for patients awaiting surgery for treatment of bowel cancer. They consist primarily of several days of liquid diets, laxatives, and enemas to make the interior of the intestinal tract as clean as possible. Other measures will be directed toward correction of anemia and compensation for possible loss of blood resulting from the cancer's invasion of bowel tissues.

Gallbladder Surgery

Gallbladder disease is one of the most common medical disorders in the United States. It has been estimated that more than 15 million Americans are affected by the disease and about 6,000 deaths a year are associated with it. The incidence increases at middle age; 1 of every 5 women over the age of 50 and 1 of every 20 men can expect to be treated for gallbladder symptoms. Approximately 1,000 people in the United States enter operating rooms each day for removal of gallstones, a primary cause of the symptoms of the disorder.

Gallstones

Gallstones generally are formed from crystals of cholesterol that gradually increase in size in the gallbladder; some, however, are formed from other substances, such as bile salts and breakdown products of red blood cells. Because they are very small in size, the stones may produce no symptoms at first. But as they grow in size they become more threatening and eventually can block the normal flow of bile from one of the bile ducts emptying into the intestine. Bile contains substances needed by the body to digest fats in the diet.

Symptoms

A common symptom of *chronic cholecystitis,* or gallstone disease, is a pain that appears suddenly in the upper abdomen and subsides slowly over a period of several minutes to several hours. The pain may occur after a meal or with no apparent relationship to meals. There can be tenderness in the upper right side of the body, with pain extending to the shoulder. The pain also can appear on the left side or near the center of the upper abdomen, producing misleading

symptoms suggesting a heart attack. Nausea, heartburn, gas, indigestion, and intolerance to fatty foods are among other possible symptoms. The gallbladder attacks may occur frequently or there may be remissions (periods without symptoms) lasting for several months or years.

A careful and extensive physical examination, including X-ray studies of the gallbladder area, may be needed to confirm the presence of gallstones. Until recently, the most commonly used test was the oral cholecystogram (OCG), in which the patient swallowed an iodine-based "dye," or contrast agent. X rays taken about 12 hours after administration of the dye might or might not provide useful "pictures" of the gallstones. As a result, ultrasound has largely replaced X rays as a primary test for suspected gallstones.

Acute Cholecystitis

About three-fourths of the cases of acute cholecystitis are patients who have had previous attacks of gallstone disease. In the acute phase there is persistent pain and abdominal tenderness, along with nausea and vomiting in many cases and a mild fever. Complications may include perforation, or rupture, of the gallbladder, leading to peritonitis, or development of adhesions to neighboring organs such as the stomach or intestine.

Treatment

Surgical treatment of chronic or acute cholecystitis is basically an elective procedure that can be scheduled at a time convenient to the patient. But acute cases with complications may require emergency operations. The patient can usually be maintained, after surgery, on intravenous fluids and pain-killing medications.

A number of alternatives to surgery have been developed. A gastroenterologist may use an endoscope on older patients or those in poor health. The endoscope, a tube inserted through the chest wall, enables the physician to view the gallbladder's duct area and to widen its opening so that small gallstones can slip through the small intestine. Using a small basket on the endoscope, the physician can sometimes catch and withdraw or crush the stones.

In gallstone surgery, the abdomen is opened so that the surgeon can examine the gall bladder and the ducts leading from it for stones. The gallbladder may be freed of stones and a temporary drainage tube inserted, with an opening to the outside of the upper abdomen. But usually the surgeon removes the entire gallbladder in an operation called a *cholecystectomy.* The bile duct, which remains as a link between the liver and the small intestine, gradually replaces the gallbladder in function. Most patients require no more than ten days to two weeks of hospitalization, and can resume normal work activities in a month to six weeks.

Other nonsurgical treatments include chemical preparations. Chenodeoxycholic acid, or chenodiol, has been given orally to dissolve smaller, floating cholesterol stones. But the drug has little effect against pigment stones or stones with a high calcium content, and can cause diarrhea as a side effect. Researchers have worked experimentally with ursodeoxycholic acid and other drugs that have been found to dissolve gallstones in both animals and humans.

Among the most advanced techniques is *choledocholithotripsy,* a nonsurgical method using shock waves to destroy gallstones. Already in use as a method of shattering kidney stones, lithotripsy requires only a local anesthetic and the recovery period lasts only a few days. The physician uses a hollow tool—the lithotriptor—that is inserted through the patient's chest until it approaches the stones. With a foot switch, the physician then triggers a jolt of high-voltage, low-current electricity that shatters the stones.

In another advance, drugs have been utilized to dissolve gallstones. A drug called *methyl tertbutyl ether* (MTHE) has been found to break down gallstones as large as golf balls. Still partly experimental, the compound could replace most surgical operations for gallstones.

Inguinal Hernia

An inguinal hernia (hernia of the groin) can develop in either men or women at almost any age from infancy to late adult years. But the incidence of inguinal hernia is much more common in males. An inguinal hernia is one in which the intestinal tract protrudes through the opening of one of the inguinal rings on either side of the groin. In males, the inguinal rings are temporary openings through which the testicles descend into the scrotum before birth; in females, the openings permit the passage of a ligament supporting the ovary.

Causes

Normally, the inguinal rings are closed after the birth of the child. However, they may fail to close completely or the muscles and connective tissues may become stretched or weakened in later years to permit a portion of the abdominal contents, usually part of the intestine, to protrude. A number of factors can contribute to the development of a hernia, including physical strain from exercise or lifting, straining over a bowel movement, coughing spells, pregnancy, pressure of abdominal organs, or obesity.

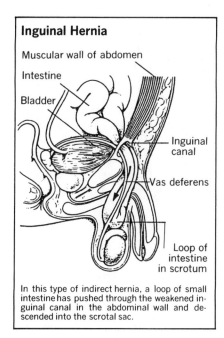

Inguinal Hernia

Muscular wall of abdomen

Intestine

Bladder

Inguinal canal

Vas deferens

Loop of intestine in scrotum

In this type of indirect hernia, a loop of small intestine has pushed through the weakened inguinal canal in the abdominal wall and descended into the scrotal sac.

Reducible and Irreducible Hernias

The hernia may be *reducible,* that is, the bulge in the abdominal wall may disappear when the body position is changed, as in lying down, only to reappear upon standing. An *irreducible* hernia does not allow the hernia sac contents to return to the abdominal cavity; an irreducible hernia also may be called *incarcerated,* a term aptly describing the hernia as being trapped. A serious complication is strangulation of the hernia contents, which usually involves obstruction of normal blood flow and resulting damage or destruction of the incarcerated intestines. A strangulated hernia may be life-threatening because of the possibility of gangrene in body tissues damaged by incarceration.

Surgical Procedure

Some hernias are called *direct,* some *indirect,* for purposes of medical records. These terms indicate to the surgeon specific layers of muscle and connective tissue that have been breached and are of no real significance to the patient, because the sur-

gical repair procedures are essentially the same for either type. In the absence of complications, the operation is fairly simple and usually can be performed with either a general or a local anesthetic. An incision is made in the lower abdomen in the area of the hernia, the protruding organ is returned to its normal position, and the weakened or ruptured layers of muscle and connective tissue are repaired and reinforced to provide a strong internal wall that will hold the abdominal contents in place. In some cases the surgeon will use available tissues from the patient's own body in building a new wall against future hernias. The surgeon also may use a variety of materials, including silk, catgut, stainless steel, tantalum mesh gauze, or mesh screens made of plastics, in building a new barrier.

Recovery

The hospital stay for hernia repair is relatively brief, usually from three days to a week; some healthy children undergo surgery early in the morning and return home in the evening of the same day. The patient usually is instructed to avoid exercise or exertion for a couple of weeks and can return to work in a month to six weeks, depending upon the work load expected. Hernias tend to recur in only a small percentage of cases among adults and very rarely in children.

Femoral Hernia

About five percent of all hernias of the groin area are femoral hernias, with the hernia bulge appearing along the thigh. Femoral hernias occur about four times as frequently among women and usually appear in middle age. While a femoral hernia is not necessarily limited to obese patients, it is more likely to be associated with being overweight, and the movement

Femoral Hernia

Inguinal ligament

Femoral vessels

Bowel hernia

Bladder hernia

of a bowel segment or the urinary bladder into the hernia frequently is preceded by a fat pad—a mass of fatty tissue. Femoral hernias are more prone to incarceration and strangulation than inguinal hernias. The surgical treatment of femoral hernias is similar to that used in the repair of inguinal hernias, although the incision may be made through the thigh in a few cases.

Hemorrhoids

Hemorrhoid, a term derived from Greek words meaning "blood flowing," refers to a system of arteries and veins that serve the rectal area. The medical problem known as *hemorrhoids,* or *piles,* is a tortuous enlargement of the hemorrhoidal veins, a problem similar to the varicose veins of the legs. Causes of the varicosities of the hemorrhoidal veins include the human peculiarity of standing and walking in an erect posture—animals that walk on all fours do not get hemorrhoids.

Women during pregnancies are particularly subject to hemorrhoidal problems because of the pressure on the veins of the lower body area. Other causes are constipation and straining at stool; diseases of the digestive tract resulting in anal infec-

tion; and cirrhosis of the liver, which obstructs blood flow and puts increased pressure on the hemorrhoidal veins.

Symptoms

Symptoms usually include bleeding, which may stain the patient's clothing; irritation and discomfort, including itching, in the anal region; and occasionally pain with inflammation. Because rectal bleeding also can be a sign of a number of other diseases, the physician usually makes a thorough examination to rule out other possible causes, such as cancer or ulcerative colitis.

Treatment

If the hemorrhoids do not warrant surgery, medical treatments may be

Hemorrhoids

Internal

External

prescribed. *Prolapsed hemorrhoids* (veins that protrude from the anus) can be reduced by gentle pressure. Bed rest, warm baths, and medications are also a part of medical treatments. A type of injection chemotherapy sometimes is used to control bleeding and eliminate the varicosed veins.

Surgery can be used to excise all the affected tissues, and the disorder also can be treated by cryosurgery in which the hemorrhoids are destroyed by a probe containing supercold liquid nitrogen or carbon dioxide. The patient usually is able to recover and return to work within one or two weeks after surgical removal of the hemorrhoidal tissues.

Oral Cavity and Throat

This section discusses oral cancers, tonsils and adenoids, and surgery of the thyroid. For a discussion of cosmetic surgery of the face area, see "Plastic and Cosmetic Surgery" later in this chapter.

Oral Cancers

There are many potential problems of the mouth, or oral cavity, besides an occasional toothache. Surgical treatment frequently is needed to correct a disorder or to prevent a life-threatening situation from developing. Cancers of the lips, tongue, hard and soft palate, and other areas of the mouth, for example, affect about 25,000 people in the United States each year. Elsewhere in the world, the incidence varies considerably according to sex and location; the rate in Hong Kong for men is three times the figure for women, and the incidence of oral cancer for women in Hong Kong is nearly 10 times as high as that of women in Japan. Environmental factors such as tobacco and contact with chemical and physical agents have been suggested as causes, although one form of oral cancer, known as *Burkitt's lymphoma,* is believed to be transmitted by a mosquito-borne virus.

Cancer of the Lip

Oral cancers tend to occur after the age of 45. Some types of oral cancer, particularly when the lips are affected, are found most frequently in persons exposed to a great deal of sunlight. Farmers, sailors, and other outdoor workers develop such tumors around the age of 60, with the lesion appearing on the lower lip. Like other cancers, cancer of the lip may begin as a tiny growth, but, if untreated, can spread through neighboring tissues and eventually destroy part of the chin. Treatment may include both radiation therapy and surgical excision of the growth; if surgery is performed when the tumor is small, the scar is likewise small. Obviously, the larger the tumor is allowed to grow, the more difficult the treatment.

Cancer of the Cheek

Similarly, cancers that develop on the inner surface of the cheek usually can be excised and the wound closed with simple surgery if treatment is started early. If the cancer is allowed to grow before treatment, the surgery becomes more complicated with removal of tissues extending to the outer skin layers and repair of the wound with skin grafts. Radiation therapy also may be used to augment the surgical repair.

Cancer of the Mouth

Cancer of the floor of the mouth may be second only to lip cancer in rate of occurrence of oral cavity tumors; together they may account for half of the oral cavity cancers in the United States. A tumor of the floor of the mouth may involve the under surface of the tongue, the lower jawbone, and other tissues of the area. A small lesion detected early can be controlled in most cases by excision of the growth and radiation therapy.

Cancer of the Tongue

The tongue may be the site of cancerous growths beginning in the 30s of the patient's life, particularly if the individual is a heavy user of tobacco and alcohol and has been neglectful of proper oral hygiene, such as brushing the teeth regularly. If the growth is at the tip of the tongue rather than underneath or along the sides, the operation is easier and there is less chance that the normal function of the tongue will be impaired by removing the growth and surrounding tissue cells. Radiation therapy for cancer of the tongue sometimes involves the implantation of needles containing radium into the tongue. The procedure is done while the patient is under a general anesthetic. Tumors at the base of the tongue, as well as some growths on the floor of the mouth, sometimes are approached through an incision in the neck.

Other Surgery

Apart from cancers, surgery of the oral cavity may be needed to treat genetic defects, such as cleft lip and cleft palate, damage to tissues from injuries, and noncancerous tumors of the soft tissues, such as cysts.

Tonsils and Adenoids

Tonsils and adenoids are glands of lymphoid tissue lying along the walls near the top of the throat. The tonsils are located on the sides of the pharynx, or throat, near the base of the tongue. Unless an adult's tonsils are inflamed, they may not be easily visible to a physician or other person looking into the throat, but when inflamed and swollen they can be seen without difficulty. The adenoids are located higher in the pharynx and cannot be seen by looking into the back of the mouth without special instruments, because the palate, or roof of the mouth, blocks the view.

Tonsillitis

The function of the tonsils and adenoids apparently is that of trapping infectious organisms that enter the body through the nose and mouth. But sometimes the glands do such a good job of collecting infections that they lose their effectiveness, becoming enlarged and inflamed, a condition known as *tonsillitis.* The patient develops fever and sore throat and the breathing passages become obstructed. The infections can spread through the nearby Eustachian tubes to the ears, causing *otitis media* (inflammation of the middle ear), resulting in deafness. Disease organisms also can spread from the tonsils and adenoids to the kidneys, joints, heart, eyes, and other body areas. Many youngsters survive occasional bouts of tonsillitis, and the infections can be treated with antibiotics and medications to relieve pain and fever symptoms. But many surgeons recommend that the tonsils and adenoids be removed if tonsillitis occurs repeatedly.

Tonsillectomy

A *tonsillectomy* (removal of the tonsils) is not a complicated operation, but it usually is performed under a general anesthetic if the patient is a child. A local anesthetic may be used for an adult. The adenoids usually are removed at the same time; they consist of the same type of lymphoid tissue in the same general area, and adenoids develop similar problems from the same kinds of infectious agents. An overnight stay in the hospital may be required or it may be possible for the patient to have the tonsils and adenoids removed in the morning and be released from the hospital in the evening of the same day, after a few hours of postoperative rest under medical observation.

Preoperative and Postoperative Care

The patient may receive antibiotic medications two or three days prior to surgery and is instructed to avoid eating foods or drinking fluids for at least 12 hours before the operation. If the patient has a cold or other viral infection, the surgery may be delayed or postponed. Some surgeons also prefer to avoid tonsillectomy operations during the hay-fever season. If there is any evidence of bleeding after the patient is released, such as spitting blood, he is returned to the hospital and the surgeon is notified; the bleeding usually can be controlled without difficulty. The patient also returns for checkups a couple of weeks after the operation and again about six months later.

Adenoidectomy

In some cases, a surgeon may recommend an *adenoidectomy* (removal of the adenoids) without a tonsillectomy. This is particularly true when the patient suffers from recurrent ear infections and hearing loss. An adenoidectomy is a relatively simple operation performed under a local anesthetic when the patient is an adult or older teenager; a general anesthetic is preferred for younger patients.

The surgeon can reach the adenoid mass through the open mouth of the patient. The tissue grows on a palate ledge near the point where the nasal passage enters the back of the mouth cavity. Using a special instrument, the surgeon cuts away the adenoid tissue within a few minutes. A medicated pack is inserted into the postnasal area to help control bleeding and the patient is moved to a recovery room. The only aftereffects in most cases are a soreness in the postnasal area for a few days and, occasionally, a temporary voice change that is marked by a nasal tone while the wound heals.

Thyroid Surgery

The thyroid gland lies along the trachea, or windpipe, at a point just below the Adam's apple. Secretions of the thyroid gland are vital for metabolic activities of the body, and the gland's functions are closely orchestrated with those of other endocrine glands of the body. When the thyroid is less active than normal, mental and physical functions are slow and the patient gains weight. When the gland is overly active, body functions operate at an abnormally fast pace, with symptoms of weight loss, irritability, heart palpitations, and bulging eyes. Occasionally, lumps develop on the thyroid, requiring medical or surgical treatment. A lump on the thyroid gland may be a nodular, or nontoxic, goiter. Or it could be a tumor. A nodular goiter poses several threats: it can make the thyroid gland become overactive, it can press on the windpipe and cause hoarseness, or it can develop into a cancer. Some growths of the thyroid gland can be treated effectively with medications, radiation, or a combination such as radioactive iodine. However, when conservative forms of therapy no longer appear to control the condition, or when it is suspected that a thyroid growth may be a malignant cancer,

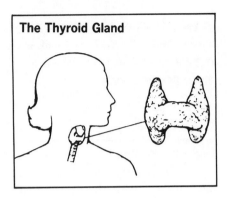

The Thyroid Gland

surgical removal of the affected area is advised promptly.

Surgical Procedure

The operation itself is fairly simple. An incision is made through the skin folds of the neck, neck muscles beneath the skin are separated, and the affected portion of the gland is cut away. The neck and throat area may be sore and painful for a few days after the operation; within a few weeks the patient can resume normal activities. A thin scar remains at the line of incision, but it is usually partly concealed by skin folds of the neck.

Ear Surgery

Surgical treatment of the ear usually is directed toward restoring the function of normal hearing which may have been lost or impaired by disease or injury. The eardrum, or tympanic membrane, can be perforated or ruptured by direct injury, by the shock waves of an explosion, or by an infection of the middle ear. Infection or injury also can disrupt hearing function by damaging the ossicles, a chain of tiny bones that transmit sound waves from the eardrum to the inner ear. Disease, aging effects, and exposure to loud noises can cause hearing loss or impairment.

Surgery of the ear usually involves working with the middle ear, the compartment between the eardrum and the inner ear, which contains the nerve endings that carry impulses to the auditory centers of the brain. The middle ear contains three ossicles, known by their common names of *hammer, anvil,* and *stirrup*—terms that suggest their functions in translating movements of air molecules into the vibrations the brain understands as sounds.

Otitis Media

One common disease of the middle ear is otitis media, which can occur by infection from a number of different kinds of organisms. Otitis media also can develop from secretions or fluids such as milk being forced into the ear through the Eustachian tube, particularly in infants who are fed while they are in a reclining position. The symptoms of otitis media are pain in the ear, fever, and loss of hearing; a small child may indicate the symptoms by crying and tugging at the ear.

Surgical Procedure

Many cases of otitis media respond to medical treatment, such as the use of antibiotics, but for patients who suffer severe pain or who have middle ears filled with pus, a surgical procedure called *myringotomy* is performed. "Myringotomy" means simply perforating the eardrum. But the operation usually is peformed in a hospital, under a local anesthetic, and with great care to avoid disturbing the ossicles or other ear structures beyond the eardrum. The middle ear is drained and the eardrum either heals spontaneously or can be subsequently repaired with a graft from the patient's own tissues.

Surgery to Correct Hearing Loss

Occasionally surgery is required to correct a conductive hearing loss in-

volving the structures of the middle ear. Such problems happen more frequently among older persons because of abnormal tissue growths that in effect "freeze" the ossicles, so that they no longer work with normal flexibility. Ossicular disorders also can occur in younger persons, including children, because of congenital defects, injury, or repeated infections, as of otitis media. The exact procedure for restoration of hearing depends upon the type of disorder. If one of the ossicles has slipped out of position or has become rigidly attached to another structure, like the tympanic membrane, the tiny bones can be repositioned or freed from the tissues that may have immobilized them. It is not unusual for the surgeon, working in a space about the size of a pea and viewing his progress through a microscope, to literally take the middle ear structures apart, rebuild the organ with bits of plastic or metal shaped like the ossicles, and reconstruct the eardrum with tissue grafts. This kind of surgery is called *microsurgery.*

Inner Ear Disturbances

Disorders of the inner ear usually are treated with medications. Surgery in that area is seldom performed unless there is a great risk to the life of the patient. Little can be done to restore hearing loss caused by nerve deafness except with hearing aids; these are designed to pick up sounds on the affected side of the head and route the sounds by electronic circuitry to an area where they can be picked up by remaining functional auditory nerves.

Eye Surgery

Among common types of eye surgery are procedures for correcting eye muscles, glaucoma, cataracts, cornea

and retina disorders. Operations on the eye muscles are intended to correct crossed eyes or similar problems in which the two eyes fail to work together.

Crossed Eyes

The condition technically known as *strabismus,* in which one eye drifts so that its position is not parallel with the other, is caused by a congenitally weak muscle. Infants often appear to have crossed eyes, but in most cases the drifting corrects itself by the time the baby is six months old. If the condition persists beyond that time, a physician should be consulted. He may recommend the use of an eye patch over the stronger eye so that the weaker one will be exercised. If this does not achieve the desired result, he may prescribe special glasses and eye exercises as the child gets older, so that there is no impairment of vision.

Corrective Surgery

If corrective surgery proves necessary after these measures, it is usually done before the child enters school. The operation is a simple one involving the muscle and not the inside of the eye itself. Each eye has six *extraocular* muscles—muscles originating outside the eyeball—to move the eye up, down, left, right, etc.; the surgeon lengthens or shortens these muscles, as may be required, to coordinate the eye movements. The operation is safe and requires only a brief hospital stay.

Amblyopia

If the lack of eye coordination is not corrected, a kind of blindness called *amblyopia* can result in one of the eyes. This condition occurs particularly in young children who depend upon the vision of one good eye; the function of the other eye is allowed to deteriorate. It has been estimated that about two million Americans have lost a part of their vision in this manner. Crossed eyes should receive professional attention early enough to prevent a permanent visual handicap.

Cataract

Cataract is a condition in which there is a loss of transparency of the lenses of the eyes. Each lens is made up of layers of cells naturally formed to focus a visual image on the retina at the rear of the eyeball. As a result of aging, or because of an injury to the eye, the lens may develop cloudy or opaque areas, or *cataracts,* that result in a blurring of vision. About five percent of the population of the United States have cataracts. Some physicians claim that anyone who lives long enough can expect to have cataracts, although age is not the only determining factor.

Surgical Correction

The condition can be corrected rather easily by several different kinds of surgical procedures. Among these, a relatively simple, advanced technique involves a microsurgery procedure called *extracapsular extraction* followed by implantation of a new lens. Using this method, the surgeon first makes a tiny incision in the cornea. Reaching through that incision, the surgeon then makes a circle of tiny cuts in the lens. The lens and its cataract are then drawn through the opening in the cornea. The back part of the lens remains in place to support the implant lens.

Extracapsular extraction has begun to replace older techniques.

These include dissolving the tissues holding the lens in place with a liquid enzyme, freezing the lens with a supercold probe, and grinding the lens tissue with a high-speed instrument. Extracapsular extraction requires only a local anesthetic injected into the facial muscles. Because the sutures are tiny, healing time can be as short as a few weeks.

Laser surgery has also been used effectively following cataract lens replacements. The neodymium yttrium-aluminum garnet (Nd:YAG) laser has helped to clear the capsular membrane that sometimes clouds the eye after such surgery.

The timing of cataract surgery presents the patient with a difficult decision. To help you make up your mind, the physician may use a potential acuity meter (PAM) to show what kind of vision you should have after a cataract is removed. The PAM projects a light beam that flashes a standard eye chart through tiny clear areas in the cataract. Because the beam hits your retina directly, you can read the chart without interference.

Lens implants normally effect greatly improved vision. But for optimum results most patients need to wear eyeglasses or contact lenses after the operation. Because implanted lenses cannot focus as your eye's natural lens does, you will probably need reading glasses. The artificial lenses may require some adjustments to compensate for visual illusions as to distances and shapes, but the blurring of progressive blindness will have been eliminated.

Sometimes after cataract operations, patients notice that the rear part of the lens left in to support the implant has begun to cloud. In such a case a surgeon may use a laser beam to punch a tiny hole in the clouded area. The hole lets light rays reach the retina unimpeded.

Cornea Transplant

The cornea of the eye is a clear window of several cells in thickness at the very front of the eye. While it is protected by the constant sweeping of the corneal surface by the eyelid and the washing of the surface by the tears, it is vulnerable to injury and infection, allergies, and metabolic disorders. The simple habit of rubbing the eyes can distort the shape of the cornea, changing the normal round shape to a cone shape. Eventually, a cornea may degenerate from wear and tear and become so clouded that the patient can no longer see clearly, if at all. It is possible, however—and has been since the 1930s—to replace a clouded cornea with an undamaged cornea from a deceased person. Corneas are contributed by donors and stored in eye banks.

Surgical Procedures

When only a portion of the cornea needs to be replaced, as is often the case, a disk encompassing the damaged cornea is carefully cut out and a piece of new cornea of precisely the same size and shape is sewn into the remaining tissue of the old cornea. The reconstructed cornea is treated with antibiotics and bandaged for several weeks. More than three-fourths of the cornea transplants are successful; the chances of success depend upon many factors, including the health of the remaining tissues of the original cornea.

Glaucoma

Glaucoma, a leading cause of blindness, is a disease caused by a failure of the fluid produced inside the eye to drain properly. The fluid, or *aqueous humor,* is produced in the anterior chamber of the eye, between the cornea and the lens. In a normal eye it drains through a duct at the base of the cornea at the same rate at which it is produced. But if the drainage system is obstructed, fluid buildup creates pressure backward through the eye. If untreated, such pressure can cause gradual blindness by crushing the nerves at the back of the eye.

Treatment

Some cases of glaucoma can be treated with medications that control the rates of fluid production and drainage. But when medications are no longer effective or when an acute attack occurs, with symptoms of severe eye pain sometimes accompanied by abdominal pain, nausea, and vomiting, surgery within a matter of hours is recommended. Several surgical procedures for the treatment of glaucoma are available; all are designed to release the fluid pressure in the eye. One common procedure involves cutting a small opening in the iris. Another technique is to insert a fine wire into the duct that normally drains the fluid and literally ream it open.

Other surgical and nonsurgical treatments for glaucoma have been developed. For example, laser surgery has proved effective for treating both open-angle and closed-angle glaucoma. In the former, the eye's internal drain system does not work properly, causing pressure to build up in the eye. In closed-angle glaucoma, fluid cannot pass properly from the front to the back of the eye, again producing dangerous pressure. The neodymium yttrium-aluminum garnet (Nd:YAG) laser is usually used in treatment to "drill" a tiny hole and destroy swollen blood vessels that block normal fluid drainage. Because marihuana has also been found to reduce pressure in the eye, manufacture of the chemical known as THC (delta-9-tetrahydrocannabinol), the key marihuana ingredient, was authorized by the Food and Drug Administration in

1985 and begun in 1986. THC has also been used to relieve the nausea accompanying cancer chemotherapy and to slow multiple sclerosis.

An estimated 10 million people in the world are afflicted by glaucoma, and the chances of developing increase with age. Women are twice as likely to develop the disease as men, and there is some evidence that the risk is hereditary. However, it also is easily preventable and controllable, since glaucoma usually develops slowly and can be detected during routine eye examinations in its early stages.

Retinal Detachment or Disease

Retinal detachment can occur from bleeding in the retinal area, an injury, a change in the shape of the eyeball, or other causes. The surgical treatment to correct the problem usually is related to the specific cause. For example, if fluid or blood has accumulated behind the retina, it is drained away. Alternatively, pressure may be directed within the eyeball to push the retina back into its proper position. For some cases, such as those associated with *diabetic retinopathy,* a kind of retinal bleeding in diabetes patients, a laser beam is used to seal the blood vessels responsible for the tiny hemorrhages in the eye.

Chest Region

This section deals with surgery of the lungs and heart. For a discussion of cosmetic surgery of the chest area, as of the breast, see "Plastic and Cosmetic Surgery" later in this chapter.

The Lungs

Before the era of modern drugs such as antibiotics, lung disorders were the leading cause of death in the United

States. Lung diseases are still common enough. With every breath taken in, the lungs are vulnerable to damage from disease organisms, chemicals, and air pollutants, many of which did not exist 50 years ago when pneumonia and tuberculosis were among the greatest threats to human life. Because the lungs are not as sensitive to pain as some other organs, a respiratory disorder may develop insidiously with few or no symptoms. When pain is felt in the chest area, the source of the pain may be the chest wall, the esophagus, or the bronchial tubes that branch from the trachea into smaller units that distribute air through the lung tissues. Other symptoms of respiratory disease may be coughing, shortness of breath, or sputum that contains blood.

Tuberculosis

Any of the above signs or symptoms could be associated with tuberculosis, which also can cause loss of appetite, weight loss, lethargy, and heavy perspiration, especially during the night. Tuberculosis is still one of the most common causes of death in the world, and new cases are found in the United States each year at a rate of 18 per 100,000 population. In addition, an estimated 35 million Americans are tuberculin-positive, indicating they have been in contact with the infectious organism but have developed an immune response to it. For an explanation of how tuberculosis is spread and of tests devised to check its spread, see "Tuberculosis" in Ch. 12, *Diseases of the Respiratory System.*

Surgical Treatment of Tuberculosis

A dozen different drugs are available for medical treatment of tuberculosis and several types may be taken in combination by a patient. Intensive treatment may require a hospital stay of several months and use of the drugs for at least 18 months. However, because of the adverse side effects of drugs, resistance of the bacterium to the drugs, and other reasons, surgery may be required. If one of the five lobes of lung tissue—the right lung has three lobes, the left lung two—has been severely damaged by tuberculosis, it may be removed by surgeons. In some instances, physicians may recommend that surgery be undertaken to allow one of the lungs to rest while it recovers from the infection. This is accomplished by crushing the phrenic nerve, under a local anesthetic, creating a partial paralysis of the diaphragm. Partial lung collapse also can be accomplished by removing parts of the ribs over the affected lung.

Lung Cancer

Cancer of the lung may appear with early symptoms of coughing, wheezing, or the appearance of blood in sputum; in about 10 percent of cases there is chest pain or shortness of breath. However, it is not unusual for the lung cancer patient to have no complaints of illness. Chest X rays during a routine physical examination may reveal the disease. In many cases, the cancer develops from metastases of cancers that have spread from other body systems. Medical therapy for lung cancer patients, including the use of radiation, is primarily for the purpose of relieving pain or other symptoms. The only effective cure is surgical excision of the affected lung tissue along with the nearby lymph nodes. Surgical treatment is most effective in young adults when the tumor has not invaded neighboring tissues, although the five-year survival rate for lung cancer is still poor.

Heart Surgery

Heart surgery procedures that are routine in many hospitals today were unheard of a generation ago. Since World War II, techniques have been devised to permit attachment of a heart-lung machine to the human body so that the patient's blood can be circulated and refreshed with oxygen while the heart itself is stopped temporarily for surgery.

Heart Valve Repair

While the blood flow is shunted away from the heart, surgeons can replace a diseased heart valve that may have become calcified with deposits that keep it from closing normally. An artificial valve made of metal and plastic may be used to replace the patient's diseased mitral valve that no longer effectively controls the flow of blood from the left atrium to the left ventricle of the heart. Artificial valves also can be installed between the right chambers of the heart. In some cases, a diseased valve leaf may be repaired with a graft of tissue from the patient's body.

Installation of artificial heart valves

has had a remarkably good record of success; some surgeons recommend the procedure over other techniques for treatment of heart valve diseases and report the operation has been well tolerated by patients over 70. While some activites may be restricted, life expectancy is increased for most patients, and they are able to have comfortable and more normal lives after such operations.

Septal Defect

Another kind of heart surgery is used to correct a septal defect. The right and left atria of the heart are separated by a septum, a wall of muscular tissue. A similar but much thicker septum separates the left and right ventricles. Occasionally, usually because of a birth defect, the septum does not close completely and blood flows from one side to the other through the opening in the heart wall. The problem is solved by putting the patient on a heart-lung machine while the heart is opened and the septum closed either by sewing the opening or by stitching into the septum a patch of plastic material.

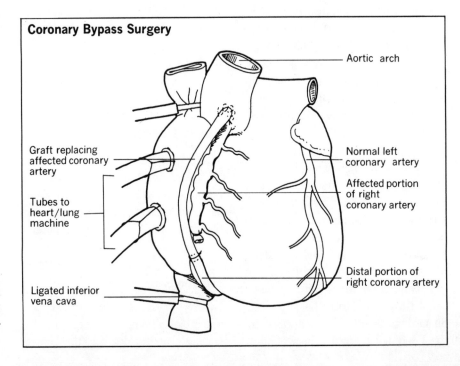

Coronary Bypass Surgery

Aortic arch

Graft replacing affected coronary artery

Tubes to heart/lung machine

Ligated inferior vena cava

Normal left coronary artery

Affected portion of right coronary artery

Distal portion of right coronary artery

Coarctation of the Aorta

An equally dramatic bit of heart surgery is used to correct a defect called *coarctation,* or narrowing, of the aorta, the main artery leading from the heart. This short, pinched section interferes with normal blood flow. If untreated, the patient may die of a ruptured aorta or heart failure. Treatment requires an operation in which the narrowed section of the aorta is cut away and the two normal-sized ends sewed together. In some cases, a piece of plastic material is sewed into the reconstructed aorta to replace the coarctated section.

Aortal-Pulmonary Artery Shunt

A comparatively simple bit of heart surgery is employed to correct a defect that occurs in some newborn children. Before birth, when the lungs are not needed because fresh blood is supplied from the placenta via the umbilical cord, the aorta is connected by a shunt to the pulmonary artery. After birth the shunt closes in most cases so the pulmonary artery can carry the blood from the heart to the lungs for oxygenation. In some children this shunt fails to close. To correct the defect and prevent heart failure, the surgeon opens the child's chest, ties off the open shunt, and cuts the ligated connection.

Vascular Surgery

This section consists of discussions of aneurysms, varicose veins, phlebitis, and intermittent claudication.

Aneurysm

When a blood vessel develops a balloonlike malformation the defect is called an *aneurysm.* A common complication of the aneurysm is that it may rupture if not treated. A ruptured

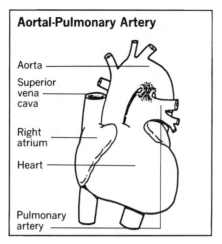

Aortal-Pulmonary Artery

Aorta
Superior vena cava
Right atrium
Heart
Pulmonary artery

aneurysm of a large blood vessel, or of a small blood vessel in a critical area such as the brain, can be fatal or severely disabling.

Surgical Procedures

If the aneurysm develops at a vital site such as the aorta, heroic surgical measures may be required to correct the problem. Before the important artery can be clamped off, the patient may have to be attached to a heart-lung machine and the body temperature lowered so as to reduce normal body functions to a minimum. After the aneurysm is removed, that section of the aorta may have to be replaced with a piece of plastic artery. Not all aneurysms require such complicated methods of repair; if the ballooning section of artery develops as a saclike appendage, it frequently can be tied off and removed while the relatively small opening between the blood vessel and the sac is sewed closed.

Surgical removal of an aneurysm is the only available treatment for the disorder. The surgery is much less complicated if the abnormal section of the blood vessel is replaced before it ruptures than after. When the patient has recovered from correction of the aneurysm, he can resume a rather active, normal life style.

Varicose Veins

Varicose veins can develop in many parts of the body. But they are most obvious and commonly a problem when they appear in the legs, especially in the *saphenous veins,* large veins that lie close to the surface of the skin.

Causes

The cause of varicose veins is a failure of tiny valves in the blood vessels to function properly, so that venous blood destined for the heart flows backward and forms pools that can make the veins distended, tortuous, and painful. Varicose veins are related to the erect posture of humans; the heart pumps blood through arteries to the extremities, but the return flow must fight the pull of gravity. Ordinarily, venous blood gets a boost up the legs by a pumping action of leg-muscle contractions. Valves in the legs are designed to let the blood move upward but are supposed to block any backward flow. People whose jobs require them to stand all day are among those likely to suffer from a breakdown of the normal functioning of the valves. Women who have had multiple pregnancies and obese individuals are also apt to develop varicose veins.

Ulceration

Varicose veins can cause ulcers in the lower leg near the ankle that bleed through the skin after an injury to the area.

Treatment

One kind of surgical treatment of the varicosed vein is *ligation,* which means "tying" or "binding". An incision is made in the leg, usually in the area of the groin. The diseased saphenous vein is severed from its connection with the larger, femoral vein and is tied off. The function of a ligated vein is taken over by other veins in the leg. An alternate kind of surgery for varicose veins, sometimes called *stripping,* requires either a series of small incisions along the path of the vein, from the groin to the ankle, or an internal stripping by use of a special, long, threadlike instrument. The diseased vein is then removed and any connections with other veins ligated.

Varicose vein surgery is used for treatment of the *superficial* veins—those that are close to the skin. The operation is simple and can be performed under a local anesthetic in many cases. When multiple varicose veins are on both legs, all of the problem veins can be stripped and ligated at the same time. A hospital stay of several days may be required, and dressings are needed on the treated legs for two or three weeks after the operation.

Phlebitis

A problem related to varicose veins is *phlebitis,* a disease that usually involves the larger, deep veins of the legs with inflammation, pain, and swelling. Phlebitis is much more serious than varicose veins because a large vein is involved and a clot usually forms, obstructing return blood flow of the limb. The danger is that the clot will break loose—that is, become an *embolus*—and travel to the lungs, where it can obstruct a vital blood vessel, with serious or even fatal results. The obstructing clot is called an *embolism.*

Causes and Treatment

Causes of phlebitis can be injury, infection, poor circulation, or simply sitting for long periods of time. Medical therapy may include wet dressings and medications, especially anticoagulant drugs to thin the blood and reduce the chances of clot formations. Supportive bandages, leg exercises, and elevation of the legs may also be recommended.

Surgical Procedure

Surgery is reserved usually for cases in which medical therapy fails to control the risk of emboli forming. The surgical procedure is directed toward treatment of the deep vein that is the source of the phlebitis symptoms. The surgeon may open the vein to remove the clot, or a device can be inserted in the vein to strain out any clots that may form in the vein and travel toward the lungs. In some cases the surgeon may block the upward flow of blood from the affected vein, allowing other veins in the leg to assume that function. However, if other veins already have been stripped or ligated in the treatment of varicose veins, it is unlikely that a surgeon would occlude or block the flow of blood in a deep leg vein.

Intermittent Claudication

Intermittent claudication is a disorder of blood circulation of the legs involving the arteries. It is primarily a disease of aging, with gradual, progressive narrowing of the lumen (interior space) of the arteries by atherosclerosis. Atherosclerosis of the arteries occurs in other parts of the body, including the arms. Intermittent claudication is marked by muscle fatigue and pain when the leg muscles are used, as in walking. The symptoms are relieved by rest. The condition can be relieved by drugs, particularly medications that help dilate the arteries, but in severe cases surgery to reconstruct the leg arteries is the solution.

Surgical Procedure

The surgeon may build a bypass artery by grafting a length of plastic tubing into the affected blood vessel and around the area blocked by atherosclerotic narrowing. Sometimes surgeons will use a piece of a vein from the patient's body to make a bypass artery; for example, a vein from the arm may be transformed into an artery for the leg. Another procedure involves simply removing the portion of the artery blocking the normal flow of blood.

Orthopedic Surgery

Orthopedics originally was the name given the subject of treating deformities in children; the original Greek term could be translated as "normal child." But the medical world now uses the word to describe treatment of the bones, muscles, joints, and associated tissues of the body's locomotion apparatus. Orthopedic surgery, therefore, might involve repair of a broken big toe, as well as treatment of a whiplash injury to the neck.

This section discusses disorders of the spine, including herniated (or "slipped") disk, fractures, and torn ligaments.

Slipped Disk

The spinal column of 33 stacked vertebrae is a common source of painful problems that require orthopedic treatment. In addition to helping support the weight of the body above the hips, the vertebrae are subjected to a variety of twists, turns, and strains during a typical day. Much of the nearly continuous shock exerted on the spinal column is absorbed by the gel-like disks between the vertebrae.

Symptoms

Eventually, one of the disks may *her-*

niate, or slip out of place, causing pressure on a spinal nerve. The result can be severe pain that radiates along the pathway of the nerve as far as the lower leg. The pain may be accompanied by muscular weakness and loss of reflexes, even perhaps by a loss of feeling in part of the leg affected by a pinched or squeezed nerve. This condition, known popularly as a *slipped disk,* has symptoms of low back pain or leg pain that are similar to those of other disorders, such as intermittent claudication, arthritis, strained muscles, and prostatitis. Also, a herniated disk can occur near the top of the spinal column with symptoms of head and neck-area pains. But more than 90 percent of herniated disk cases involve the lumbar region of the spinal column, in the lower back.

Diagnosis

Physicians usually can confirm a herniated disk problem by a technique called *myelography,* in which a dye is injected into the spinal canal and X-ray pictures taken. Another procedure, called *electromyography,* can help determine which nerve root is involved.

Treatment

Conservative measures generally are used at first to reduce the pain and other symptoms. They include bed rest on a hard mattress, medications, and sometimes the use of traction and back braces. If conservative therapy fails to correct the problem and the diagnosis has been well established by a myelogram, surgery may be advised to remove the herniated disk.

Spinal Fusion

The surgeon may recommend a procedure called *spinal fusion,* in which

Herniated Disk

Spinal cord

Spinal column (vertebra)

Herniated disk pressing against cord

Intervertebral disk

Lumbar region

Spinal Fusion

Scrapped vertebra

Pelvis

Pelvic bone chips

Sacrum

the edges of several of the vertebrae are roughened and a piece of bone from the pelvis grafted onto the roughened edges. The bone graft will fuse with the vertebrae and in effect make the several vertebrae a single bone. However, the fused vertebrae will not interfere noticeably with body movements after the fusion is completed, which takes about six months. The operation requires a hospital stay of from one to two weeks and the patient must wear a body cast for the first few weeks and then use a back brace for a period of possibly several months. The patient usually can return to work and resume some normal activities within a couple of months after the operation. Strenuous activity, however, is usually restricted after an operation on the spinal column.

Other Spinal Disorders

Spondylolisthesis

Spinal fusion surgery also may be used to correct two other kinds of spinal disorders. One disorder is known as *spondylolisthesis*, a condition in which one of the vertebrae slips out of alignment. Spondylolisthesis usually occurs at the bottom of the group of lumbar vertebrae, where that section of the spinal column rests on the sacrum.

Scoliosis

The other disorder is *scoliosis*, or abnormal curvature of the spinal column. If the case of scoliosis is mild and causes no severe symptoms, it may be treated with conservative measures such as braces and special exercises. Surgical treatment of scoliosis may involve not only spinal fusion but reinforcement of the spinal column with metal rods attached to

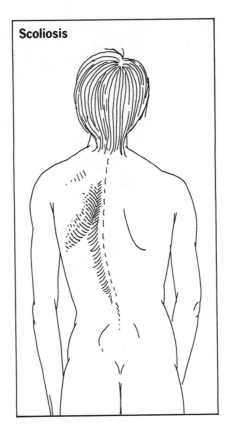

Scoliosis

the vertebrae to hold them in proper alignment.

Disorders of the cervical portion of the spinal column, in the area of the neck, may cause symptoms similar to those of a herniated disk in the lower back. But there is pain in the neck and shoulders and weakness in the arms. Surgical treatment also is similar, with removal of a herniated disk portion or fusion of cervical vertebrae when conservative therapy, with bed rest, neck braces, and medications, does not prove helpful.

Fractures

Many fractures of the spinal column also are treated by fusion operations, use of casts, braces, bed rest, or traction, in addition to therapy directed toward the specific problem. Spinal fractures frequently are compression fractures of vertebrae caused by falling in a sitting or standing position or mishaps in which a bony process of a vertebra is broken.

Spinal fractures that result in permanent damage to the spinal cord, with resulting paralysis, are relatively uncommon.

Reduction of Fractures

Fractures of the long bones of the arms and legs are treated by a method called *reduction*, the technique of aligning the broken ends of the bones properly so the healing process will not result in a deformity. Reduction also requires that the muscles and surrounding tissues be aligned and held in place by immobilizing them as the break heals.

If the break is simple enough, the limb can be immobilized by putting a plaster cast around the part of the involved limb after the fractured ends of the bone and associated tissues have been realigned. In complicated cases with a number of bone fragments resulting from the fracture and surrounding tissues in some disarray, the patient usually is given a general anesthetic while the surgeon recognizes the shattered limb like a player assembling pieces of a jigsaw puzzle. If some of the needed pieces are missing, the surgeon may fill the gaps with bone from a bone bank, although bank materials usually are not as effective in the healing process as pieces of the patient's own bones.

Use of Internal Appliances

A common technique of modern fracture surgery is the application of wires, screws, pins, metal plates, and other devices to provide internal fixation of a broken long bone during the healing process. Nails and pins may be used to fasten the fractured neck of a femur, the long bone of the upper leg, to the shaft of that bone. A steel rod may be driven through the shaft of a long bone to align the broken sections. Screws may be used to hold together bone ends of a fracture in which the break runs diagonally across the shaft. Screws also may be employed to hold a metal plate or strip of bone from the patient's own body across the break. The screws, nails, and other devices generally are well tolerated by the body and may be left in the bones indefinitely if they do not cause adverse reactions after the healing process is completed.

Traction

Traction frequently is employed to hold a limb in alignment while a fracture is healing. A clamp sometimes is placed at one end of the fractured limb and a weight attached by wires over a pulley is connected to the clamp. Depending upon the kind of fracture and type of traction prescribed, a system of several weights and pulleys may be rigged around the bed of a patient to fix the bone and related tissues in correct positions.

Torn Cartilage

Joints of the body can be vulnerable to damage from sudden twisting and turning actions, particularly when the force of the individual's body weight is added to the pressure on the joint. The effect of such forces on the knee joint can result in tearing of the half-moon-shaped cartilages that cushion friction of the upper and lower leg bones where they are joined. Sports fans are particularly aware of the vulnerability of the knee joint because of the high incidence of knee injuries to athletes, especially in football and basketball. Obese individuals are also particularly liable to develop cartilage problems in the knee.

Symptoms

When a cartilage of the knee joint is torn, the patient may feel pain and weakness in the area of the injury. Swelling usually occurs, and in more than half the cases the knee cannot be straightened, because it has become "locked" by the cartilage. There may be a remission of symptoms, but surgery frequently is required sooner or later.

Surgical Procedure

The surgeon makes an incision in the area of the kneecap and cuts away the torn cartilage. Full recovery takes several weeks after the first few post-operative days, during which the patient remains in bed with the affected leg elevated. Special exercises are required to overcome muscle weakness in the leg and to help the patient learn to use the leg with part of the cartilage cushion missing.

Neurosurgery

Neurosurgery may be employed to treat a wide assortment of disorders involving the nervous system, from the brain to nerve endings in the fingers and toes. Neurosurgery may involve treatment of epilepsy, Parkinson's disease, and psychiatric disorders, as well as herniated disks of the spinal column and aneurysms that affect the nervous system. Causes of neurosurgical problems can be injury, tumors, infectious diseases, or congenital disorders.

This section includes discussions of trigeminal neuralgia, brain tumors, and head injuries.

Trigeminal Neuralgia

Trigeminal neuralgia is one of many types of pain that sometimes can be treated by surgery. The disorder, also known as *tic douloureux* or *facial neuralgia,* tends to develop in persons between 40 and 60 years of age, causing attacks of acute pain and muscular twitching in the area of the face containing branches of the trigeminal nerve. The painful attacks occur with no apparent reason but seem to be associated with certain stimuli, such as touch or temperature changes, at points around the face and mouth. During periods of attacks, the patient may avoid eating, shaving, or any other activity that might trigger a spasm of severe pain. But the pain attacks also may cease, with or without treatment, for three or four months, only to resume for weeks or months.

Treatment

Alcohol injections and medications may offer relief of symptoms, but when symptoms continue, surgery frequently is recommended. The operation consists of an incision to reach the root of the nerve and cut the divisions that appear to be involved with the painful symptoms. However, cutting the nerve can result in loss of feeling for the entire side of the face, including the cornea of the eye, so that the patient must wear special glasses to protect the cornea. An alternative procedure that is not always effective involves exposing the nerve root and rubbing it, a technique that seems to produce a temporary loss of sensation in the nerve fibers.

Brain Tumor

Brain tumors are popularly associated with neurosurgery skills. And while brain surgery requires great skill and knowledge of brain anatomy, which in itself is quite complicated, most brain tumor operations are conducted safely and successfully. Diagnosing, locating, and identifying a brain tumor are challenges faced by the physician before surgery begins. There are a

Brain Tumors
Frequent locations of common lesions

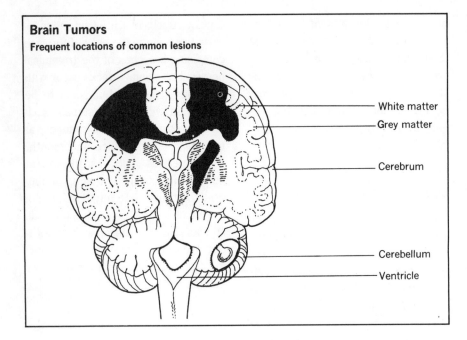

White matter
Grey matter

Cerebrum

Cerebellum
Ventricle

dozen major types of brain tumors plus some minor types. The types of tumors tend to vary according to the age of the patient; the patient's age and the type of tumor may suggest where it develops.

Symptoms

Because brain tumors can cause organic mental changes in the patient, the symptoms of changed behavior can be mistaken for neurotic or psychotic disorders, with the result that a patient may spend valuable time receiving psychiatric treatment rather than surgical treatment; autopsies of a significant number of patients who die in mental hospitals reveal the presence of brain tumors. In addition to mental changes, the person suffering from a brain tumor may complain of headaches, experience convulsions, or display signs of neurological function loss, such as abnormal vision.

Diagnosis

The specific signs and symptoms, along with X-ray studies, electroen-cephalograms, and other tests, help the physicians determine the site and extent of growth of a brain tumor. A recently developed technique called *CT scanning* (for *computed tomography*) aids the neurosurgeon by producing a series of X-ray pictures of the interior of the skull as if they were "slices" of the brain taken in thicknesses of about two-thirds of an inch. The detailed anatomical portrait of the patient's brain helps pinpoint the disorder and indicate whether it is a tumor or another kind of abnormality.

Surgical Procedure

The usual method of removing a brain tumor after it has been diagnosed and located is a procedure called a *craniotomy*. The entire head is shaved and cleaned to eliminate the possibility that a stray bit of hair might fall into the incision that is made in the scalp. After the scalp has been opened, a series of holes are drilled in a pattern outlining the working area for the surgeon; a wire saw is used to cut the skull between the drilled holes.

Removing the tumor is a delicate operation, not only because of the need to avoid damage to healthy brain tissue but because accidental severing of a blood vessel in the brain could produce a critical hemorrhage. The surgeon tries to remove the entire tumor, or as much of the tumor as appears possible without damaging vital brain tissues or blood vessels. All the various types of brain tumors are considered dangerous, whether malignant or benign, because within the rigid confines of the skull there is no opportunity for outward release of pressure. Therefore any growth may compress or destroy vital brain tissues if left untreated.

After the tumor is removed, the piece of skull removed at the start of the operation is replaced and the scalp flap is sewed in place. Radiation therapy may be administered for a month to six weeks after surgery to destroy any tumor tissue left behind or tumor cells that may have drifted into the spinal canal. Some tumors near the base of the brain may be treated effectively with radiation alone if the tumor cells are radiosensitive. Tumors of the pineal gland and the pituitary gland also may be treated with radiation.

Laser Surgery

In an alternative procedure, *laser neurosurgery,* a brain surgeon may use a laser beam to vaporize the tumor. The hair is removed from all or part of the skull; a section of the skull is removed with a power or hand saw after being marked out with tiny holes; and the surgeon then uses the laser to destroy the tumor. Typically, the surgeon may actually control two laser beams: a helium-neon type that guides the surgical work, and a carbon dioxide (CO_2) laser that does the vaporizing.

Because the "no-touch" CO_2 laser works slowly, an operation may require 10 or more hours. The laser beam can focus on and destroy one tumor cell at a time, targeting areas of tissue 1/50th the thickness of a human hair, or it can attack a number of cells in a group. The surgeon controls the electrical power that activates the beam with a foot pedal. In effect, the laser causes the tumor cells to heat up beyond the boiling point and then to explode into vapor. At the same time, the beam coagulates the tiny blood vessels that it passes through, preventing bleeding.

Head Injuries

Brain Hemorrhage

Head injuries, such as a blow to the head, can produce massive hemorrhages within the skull. As in the case of brain tumors, the expanding pool of blood within the skull gradually compresses the brain tissue and can result in death unless the problem is corrected. The damage of a brain hemorrhage can be insidious, with no immediate signs or symptoms of the problem until irreversible changes have occurred in the brain tissue. The patient may receive what may appear to be a minor head injury, for exam-

Brain Hemorrhage

Displaced brain

Cyst

Blood

ple, and not lose consciousness. Or he may be unconscious for a brief period, then recover and seem very alert. But gradually, over a period of hours or even days, neurological signs of disintegrating brain function appear.

Treatment

The treatment requires a procedure similar to that used for removing brain tumors. An opening is made in the skull to remove the blood or blood clot and relieve pressure upon the brain tissues. The chances for full recovery depend somewhat upon the extent of brain damage caused by the hemorrhage before treatment.

Skull Fracture

Surgical treatment for a skull fracture may combine techniques of various other methods for fractures and brain injuries. The scalp is shaved and cleaned carefully so the surgeon can determine the extent of the injury and its location with respect to vital tissues under the skull. With the help of X rays and signs of neurological damage, the surgeon frequently can tell how severe the fracture may be and whether there is bleeding beneath the skull.

Treatment

If the skull appears to be intact but there are signs of a brain hemorrhage, the skull is opened to remove the blood or blood clot and relieve pressure on the brain. If the skull fracture is compound and depressed, or with skull fragments in the brain tissue, efforts also must be made to elevate the depressed bone section so it does not press on vital brain areas and to remove bits of bone or other foreign materials that may have en-

tered the brain.

Surgeons frequently can rebuild a fractured skull by replacing missing bits of bone or adding appropriate synthetic materials such as a piece of metal plate. Full recovery depends upon such factors as the age of the patient and the severity of damage before treatment was started. Younger patients generally respond better to the repair procedures, but full recovery from a severe skull fracture may take as long as a year.

Aneurysm in the Brain

Aneurysms can develop in blood vessels of the brain, and like aneurysms in other parts of the body they can be corrected surgically. A ruptured aneurysm produces a brain hemorrhage. The condition is most likely to develop in people over the age of 30; in patients over 40, women are more likely than men to be victims of the disorder. The approach to repair of an intracranial aneurysm depends upon the condition of the patient and the location and size of the aneurysm, which frequently can be identified by X-ray pictures after an opaque dye has been injected into the bloodstream. The diseased blood vessel may be ligated, reinforced, or repaired, depending upon the conditions found by the surgeon after the aneurysm has been exposed and examined.

Plastic and Cosmetic Surgery

The use of surgical techniques for the correction of physical deformities is by no means a modern development. The practice goes back to ancient India, where as early as the sixth century B.C. Hindu specialists were reconstructing noses, reshaping ears, and grafting skin for reducing scar tissue.

Through the centuries, improvements in procedure and new types of operations became part of the common fund of information. During World War I, great technical advances were made when the Medical Corps of the United States Army created a special division of *plastic surgery* to treat the deformities caused by battle injuries. Today's plastic surgery is based on many of the procedures perfected then and during World War II.

In recent years, attention has been focused not only on birth and injury deformities but on lesser irregularities as well. Surgeons in the field of *cosmetic surgery* perform such procedures as nose reconstruction, face lifting, reshaping of breasts, removal of fatty tissue from upper arms and legs, and the transplanting of hair to correct baldness.

There is no longer any reason for someone to suffer from the emotional and professional problems caused by abnormalities in appearance. No child should be expected to live with the disability of a cleft lip or crossed eyes. A young woman tormented by what she considers to be a grotesque nose can have it recontoured to her liking. An older woman who finds wrinkles a social liability can have them removed. Anyone interested in undergoing any form of cosmetic surgery should stay away from so-called beauty experts, and deal only with a reputable surgeon or physician.

Some surgical specialists, called *plastic surgeons,* perform cosmetic or plastic surgery exclusively. Other surgeons and physicians, including general surgeons, dermatologists, ophthalmologists, and others, are qualified to do some kinds of plastic surgery, usually the techniques related to their particular specialties. The kind of surgery desired should first be discussed with the family doctor, who can then evaluate the problem and recommend a qualified surgeon to deal with it.

Before undergoing any kind of plastic surgery, the prospective patient should realize that it is neither inexpensive nor totally painless. Most cosmetic surgery is performed in hospitals, which means that in addition to the surgeon's fees there can be a bill for the anesthetist, use of the operating and recovery rooms, and the hospital stay itself. Also, because cosmetic surgery is often optional surgery, surgery not needed to ensure the patient's physical health, it may not be covered by a health-insurance policy.

Reshaping the Nose

Known technically as a *rhinoplasty,* the operation for the reconstruction of the nose is not only one of the oldest but also one of the most common forms of cosmetic surgery. Depending upon the demands of facial symmetry and individual taste, the nose can be shortened, straightened, narrowed, or even lengthened. If a nose deformity has caused breathing problems, the surgeon will take the correction of this into account in planning the reconstruction.

Barring accidents, most children's noses are perfectly adequate until they enter their teens, when the facial bones begin to take on the contours determined by inheritance. Teenagers are especially sensitive about their looks. If nose surgery seems advisable, therefore, it is usually undertaken when the child is between 14 and 16 years of age, though the operation is also performed on adults.

Cosmetic Breast Surgery

Breast Lifting

Breasts that sag even though they are not too large can be lifted to a more attractive contour by an operation that consolidates the tissue. The surgical procedure consists of removing strips of skin from the base of the breasts and bringing the rest of the skin together under tension so that it is tight enough to support the tissue in an upward position.

Breast Reduction

In spite of all the publicity given to breast augmentation, most cosmetic surgery involving the breasts is concerned with reducing rather than enlarging them. Breast reduction is frequently undertaken not only to improve appearance but also for purposes of health and comfort.

The operation, called a *mastoplasty,* is performed under general anesthesia and consists in cutting out fatty tissue and skin. Although the incision may be large, the resulting scars are not thicker than a hairline and are hidden in the fold below the breasts.

The most remarkable thing about this type of surgery—and the reason for its being considerably more complicated than breast enlargement—is the repositioning of the nipples so that they are properly placed relative to the newly proportioned breast contours.

Breast Enlargement

The techniques used in this operation, called a *mammoplasty,* have changed over the years. Early operations to augment the size of the breasts involved the injection of paraffin, but this was soon abandoned as unsatisfactory. Considerable experimentation with the use of various synthetics, as well as with the use of fatty tissue taken from the buttocks, didn't provide good results either.

Silicone—a form of man-made plastic material of great versatility—

was first used in this connection in the form of sponges, and later was injected in liquid form directly into the tissue. However, the federal Food and Drug Administration has ruled that the use of liquid silicone is unsafe and illegal because its presence would mask signs of malignancy. Another problem with liquid silicone is that it has a tendency to drift to other parts of the body.

In the latest techniques of breast augmentation, a silicone gel or saline solution is placed in a flexible silicone bag shaped to resemble the breast. The bags are inserted through incisions under the breast tissue, and to date appear to be the safest and most satisfactory solution to the problem of breast enlargement.

Face Lift

Face lifting, or *rhytidoplasty,* is a form of cosmetic surgery designed to eliminate as far as possible signs of aging, such as wrinkles, pouches under the chin and eyes, and sagging tissue generally. About 7,000 such operations are performed each year with satisfactory results.

In deciding on the advisability of a face lift, a reputable surgeon will take into account the person's age, emotional stability, and physical condition. The main procedure involves tightening the skin after the surplus has been removed. The resulting scars are usually hidden in the hair and behind the ears. Those directly in front of the ears are visible only under very close scrutiny. Even after a face lift, however, the same wrinkles will eventually reappear, owing to the characteristic use of the individual's facial muscles.

Eyelids

The shape and size of the eyelids can

Face Lift — Incision line behind hairline — Separating skin from the face — Tying loose subcutaneous tissue — Excess skin to be cut off

be changed by an operation called a *blepharoplasty.* In this procedure, an incision is made in the fold of the upper eyelid, and excess skin and fat are removed. The technique can be used to correct congenital deformities, such as hanging upper eyelids that do not fully open. When a comparable incision is made below the lash line on the lower lid, the surgeon can remove the fat that causes bags under the eyes.

Ears

Surgery to correct protruding or overlarge ears is called *otoplasty.* Though it can be performed on adults, it is usually performed on children before they enter school, to prevent the psychological problems that often re-

sult from teasing. In the procedure, an incision is made behind the ear, cartilage is cut, and the ear is repositioned closer to the skull. Otoplasty can also build up or replace an ear missing because of a birth defect or accident.

Scar Reduction

Unsightly scars that are the result of a birth defect or an injury can usually be reduced by plastic surgery to thin hairlines. The procedure is effective only if there has been no extensive damage to surrounding areas of underlying tissue, as sometimes occurs in severe burns. The operation involves the removal of the old scar tissue, undermining the surrounding skin, and pulling it together with very fine stitches.

Uncommon Surgical Procedures

Organic Transplants

The notion of man's ability to rebuild human bodies from the parts of other humans or from artificial organs probably is as old as the dreams that men might someday fly like birds or travel to the moon. Some of the oldest documents, thousands of years old, tell of medical efforts to transplant organs, limbs, and other tissues to save lives or enable disabled persons to pursue normal activities. In recent decades, medical scientists have discovered how to overcome some of the obstacles to organ transplanting, just as other scientists have learned to fly higher and faster than birds and travel beyond the moon.

Tissue Compatibility

A major obstacle to organ transplants has been one of *histoincompatibility* (*histo* means "tissue"): the tissues of the person receiving the transplant tend to reject the tissues of the transplanted organs. The problem is quite similar to that of allergies or the body's reaction to foreign bodies, including infectious organisms. Each individual has a set of antigens that are peculiar to that person, because of genetic variations among different persons. The histoincompatible antigens are on the surfaces of the tissue cells. But in most cases the antigens on the cells of the transplanted organ do not match those of the person receiving the transplant, so the recipient's body in effect refuses to accept the transplant.

The major exception to this rule is found in identical twins, who are born with the same sets of antigens. The organs of one twin can be transplanted to the body of the other twin with a minimum risk of rejection. Antigens on the tissue cells of brothers and sisters and of the parents will be similar, because of the biological relationship, but they will not be as compatible as those of identical twins. Even less compatible are antigens of people who are not related.

Types of Grafts

There is virtually no problem in transferring tissues from one area to another of the same patient. Skin grafts, bone grafts, and blood-vessel transplants are commonly made with a patient's own tissues, which have the same antigens, as in spinal fusions, repair of diseased leg arteries, and so on. Tissue transplants within an individual's body are called *autografts*. Transplants of tissues or organs from one human to another are called *homografts*. *Heterografts* are tissues from one species that are transplanted to another; they offer the greatest risk of histoincompatibility and are used mainly as a temporary measure, such as covering a severely burned area of a person with specially treated pieces of pigskin. The heterograft will be rejected, but it will provide some protection during the recovery period.

Much of the experience of surgeons in handling tissue transplants between humans came from early experiments in skin grafting. It was found that histoincompatibility in transplants of skin appeared to sensitize the recipient tissues in the same way that allergy sensitivity rises. Thus, when a second skin graft from the same donor is attempted, the graft is rejected more rapidly than the first graft because of the buildup of antibodies from the first rejection. The same sort of rejection reaction can occur in transplants of kidneys, hearts, and other organs unless the problem of histoincompatibility is overcome.

Immunosuppressive Chemicals

In order to make the host body more receptive to an organ transplant, *immunosuppressive* chemicals are injected into the recipient's tissues to suppress their natural tendency to reject the foreign tissue. However, the technique of suppressing the immune response of the host tissues is not without hazards. By suppressing the natural rejection phenomenon, the transplant recipient is made vulnerable to other diseases. It has been found, for example, that persons who receive the immune response suppression chemicals as part of transplant surgery develop cancers at a rate that is 15 times that of the general population. Transplant patients also can become extremely vulnerable to infections, such as pneumonia.

Antigen Matching

The breakthrough in human organ transplantation was helped by the development of a system of matching antigens related to lymphocytes—a type of white blood cell—of the donor and recipient. At least a dozen lymphocyte antigens have been identified, and it is possible to match them by a process similar to matching blood factors of patients before making a blood transfusion. If all or most of the antigens of the donor tissue and the recipient match, the chances for a successful transplanting procedure are greatly enhanced.

Antigen matching is less important in some kinds of homografts, such as replacing the cornea of the eye. The cornea is a unique kind of tissue with no blood vessels, and therefore is unlikely to be invaded by antibodies of the recipient. Pieces of human bone also may be used in homografts with a minimum risk of rejection, although surgeons usually prefer to use bone from the patient's own body in repairing fractures and in other orthopedic procedures.

Types of Transplants

Cornea Transplant

Cornea transplants helped to pioneer the art of homografts. The first successful cornea transplants were made during the 1930s. In addition to the absence of rejection problems because of incompatible antigens, cornea transplants probably succeeded in the early days of homografts because only small pieces of the tissue were used.

Kidney Transplant

Kidney transplants began in the 1950s. Antigen typing was unknown at that time, but physicians had learned of the genetic factors of blood groups and found from experience that although kidney transplants from siblings and parents could eventually be rejected, the rejection phenomenon was delayed. The first truly successful kidney transplant operation was performed in Boston in 1954 between twin brothers; doctors had tested the tissue compatibility of the twins first by making a small skin transplant to see if it would be rejected. Knowledge acquired later of immunosuppressive drugs enabled surgeons to make kidney transplants between persons who were not twins.

More than 5,000 kidney transplant operations have been performed with an 82 percent survival rate of two years or more when the donor was related to the recipient. When a cadaver kidney was transplanted, the two-year survival rate was 65 percent. It has been estimated that as many as 10,000 kidney disease patients each year could benefit from a transplanted organ, but a lack of available kidneys in satisfactory condition restricts the number of transplants. An alternative for some kidney patients awaiting an organ transplant is hemodialysis, a process that performs as an artificial kidney.

Heart Transplant

The first successful human heart transplant was performed by Dr. Christiaan Barnard in Cape Town, South Africa, in 1968. The patient survived more than 18 months and led a relatively active life until the second heart failed because of a rejection reaction. Many heart transplant operations have been performed since 1968, with varying success, sometimes leading to complete recovery and sometimes to recovery for long periods of time. Heart transplants were found to be more difficult than some other organ transplants, such as of the kidney, because the heart must be taken from the donor at virtually the moment of death and immediately placed in the body of the recipient. Because of concern about determining the moment of death, the medical profession has offered guidelines for answering this complex ethical and legal question.

Success of a heart transplant operation may depend on the health of other organ systems in the patient's body; persons in need of heart transplants usually have medical problems involving the lungs and kidneys as a result of the diseased heart. And heart transplant patients frequently seem less able to tolerate the use of immunosuppressive drugs that must be administered after surgery. The introduction of cyclosporine as an immunosuppressant changed the picture substantially, however. Medical evidence indicated that cyclosporine would lead to a five-year survival rate among heart transplant patients of 50 percent or more. Because cyclosporine speeds rehabilitation after an operation, average hospital stays for patients receiving the immunosuppressant have been reduced from 72 to 42 days.

Conducted before cyclosporine came into common use, one study of a group of transplant patients showed that fewer than 40 percent survived beyond the first year. Several lived more than two years after the operation.

Bone-Marrow Transplant

Limited success has been reported in efforts to perform bone-marrow transplants. Bone-marrow transplants are performed to supply patients with active leukocytes to fight cancer and other diseases. The successful early cases have involved transplants between sisters and brothers who had been typed for tissue compatibility.

Other Kinds of Transplants

Surgeons also have experimented with varying success with human transplants of livers, lungs, and pancreas tissue. Lung transplant efforts have been hampered by infection, rejection, and hemorrhage. Because the lungs are exposed to pathogenic organisms in the environment they are especially vulnerable to infections when the host tissues have been treated with immunosuppressive chemicals. Liver transplants are difficult to perform because of a lack of satisfactory donor organs and the complex circuitry of arteries, veins, and bile duct that must be connected to the recipient before the liver can begin to function.

Most major organ transplants are considered only in terms of a "last ditch" effort to prolong the life of a patient who is critically ill. While homografts are not always a perfect success and may lengthen a patient's life by only a few years, remarkable strides in these surgical techniques have been made over a relatively short period of time. Surgeons who specialize in organ transplants state that even greater progress could be made if a greater supply of donor organs were available.

Reattachment of Severed Members

Because an individual's tissues present no histocompatibility problem with other parts of his own body, severed fingers and other members can be rejoined to the rest of the body if vital parts are not damaged beyond repair. Children sometimes suffer amputation of a part of a finger during play or in accidents at home. For example, a finger tip can be severed when caught in a closed door of an automobile. If the severed part of the finger is saved and the patient is given immediate medical care, the finger

usually can be rejoined and sutured in place with a very good chance of survival of the graft.

Rejoining a Severed Limb

One of the most dramatic cases of a rejoined limb in American medical annals involved a 12-year-old whose right arm was severed at the shoulder when he was crushed between a train and a tunnel wall in 1962. Railroad workers called an ambulance, and the boy, his severed arm still encased in his sleeve, was rushed to a hospital. The boy was given plasma by physicians who packed the severed arm in ice and flushed out the blood vessels of the arm with anticoagulant drugs and antibiotics. During three hours of surgery, the major veins and artery of the arm were carefully stitched to the vessels at the shoulder. For the next five hours, surgeons joined the bones, located the main nerve trunks and connected them to the nerve ends in the shoulder, and repaired the muscles. The boy was released from the hospital three weeks after the accident but returned for additional operations to connect various nerve fibers. That operation was a success,

but similar attempts to rejoin severed arms of middle-aged men have failed despite heroic attempts by surgeons to restore the limbs as functioning parts of the body.

A Chinese factory worker suffered accidental amputation of his right hand when it was caught in a metal-punching machine, and was rushed to a hospital in Shanghai. Chinese medical reports of the case indicate that a procedure similar to the one used on the American boy was followed. Blood vessels were rejoined first to permit the flow of blood to tissues. This was followed by surgery to connect the tendons and main nerve trunks. The bones of the forearm, where the amputation occurred, were joined and held in place with metal plates and screws. Physicians reported that the graft was successful, and the patient, a 27-year-old man, was able to move his fingers again within three weeks after the accident.

Medical records indicate that major reattachments of severed limbs are still rare, although rejoined finger tips, ears, and other parts not involving main arteries, veins, or nerve trunks are not as uncommon.